**PERGAMON INTERNATIONAL LIBRARY**
of Science, Technology, Engineering and Social Studies
*The 1000-volume original paperback library in aid of education,*
*industrial training and the enjoyment of leisure*
Publisher: Robert Maxwell, M.C.

# JONES'S
# ANIMAL NURSING

**FOURTH EDITION**

## THE PERGAMON TEXTBOOK
## INSPECTION COPY SERVICE

An inspection copy of any book published in the Pergamon International Library will gladly be sent to academic staff
without obligation for their consideration for course adoption or recommendation. Copies may be retained for a period
of 60 days from receipt and returned if not suitable. When a particular title is adopted or recommended for adoption
for class use and the recommendation results in a sale of 12 or more copies, the inspection copy may be retained with
our compliments. The Publishers will be pleased to receive suggestions for revised editions and new titles to be
published in this important International Library.

# JONES'S
# ANIMAL NURSING

*Edited by*

## D. R. LANE

FOR THE BRITISH SMALL ANIMAL VETERINARY ASSOCIATION
WITH CONTRIBUTIONS FROM TWENTY-SIX AUTHORS

## FOURTH EDITION

**PERGAMON PRESS**

OXFORD · NEW YORK · BEIJING · FRANKFURT
SÃO PAULO · SYDNEY · TOKYO · TORONTO

| | |
|---|---|
| U.K. | Pergamon Press, Headington Hill Hall, Oxford OX3 0BW, England |
| U.S.A. | Pergamon Press, Maxwell House, Fairview Park, Elmsford, New York 10523, U.S.A. |
| PEOPLE'S REPUBLIC OF CHINA | Pergamon Press, Qianmen Hotel, Beijing, People's Republic of China |
| FEDERAL REPUBLIC OF GERMANY | Pergamon Press, Hammerweg 6, D-6242 Kronberg, Federal Republic of Germany |
| BRAZIL | Pergamon Editora, Rua Eça de Queiros, 346, CEP 04011, São Paulo, Brazil |
| AUSTRALIA | Pergamon Press Australia, P.O. Box 544, Potts Point, N.S.W. 2011, Australia |
| JAPAN | Pergamon Press, 8th Floor, Matsuoka Central Building, 1-7-1 Nishishinjuku, Shinjuku-ku, Tokyo 160, Japan |
| CANADA | Pergamon Press Canada, Suite 104, 150 Consumers Road, Willowdale, Ontario M2J 1P9, Canada |

First edition 1966
Second edition 1972
Reprinted with minor corrections 1973
Fully revised second edition 1976
Third edition 1980
Fourth edition 1985
Reprinted 1987

**Library of Congress Cataloging in Publication Data**

Main entry under title:
Jones's Animal nursing.
(Pergamon international library of science, technology, engineering, and social studies)
Includes indexes.
1. Veterinary nursing.   2. Pets—Diseases.
I. Jones, Bruce V.   II. Lane, D. R.   III. British Small Animal Veterinary Association.   IV. Title.   V. Title: Animal nursing. VI. Series.
SF774.5.J66   1984      636.089'073      84–14814

**British Library Cataloguing in Publication Data**

Jones's Animal nursing.
1. Veterinary nursing.   2. Pets—Diseases.
I. Lane, D. R.
636.089'024613      SF981

ISBN 0-08-031982-3 (Hardcover)
ISBN 0-08-031983-1 (Flexicover)

*Printed in Great Britain by A. Wheaton & Co. Ltd., Exeter*

# Preface to the Fourth Edition

"Let Distemper suspend their malignant Influence, and Powders, Pills, and Potions, their Operations"

Since this comment on medical care was printed 265 years ago, the treatment of small animal disorders has advanced very considerably. When the Register of Animal Nursing Auxiliaries was established by the Royal College of Veterinary Surgeons in 1961, the standard of nursing care for animals further improved and now has been transformed by the skill and professionalism of the RANAs. The need for a Fourth Edition of this standard textbook shows how rapidly new information on nursing procedures has become available, the first edition under the editorship of B.V. Jones was published by the BSAVA in 1966.

At the time the Third Edition was in preparation, the disease of Canine Parvovirus became endemic in this country. The value of fluid therapy in the treatment of those unfortunate dogs that were so ill with acute CPV, was unmistakable. Animal nurses were ready trained for this challenge and gave sterling value in the administration of replacement fluids. In many other ways, small animal practice could not have developed as it has done without the support of RANAs. "Parvo" also led to a greater awareness of the need for effective vaccines to protect puppies. The problems that arose with choosing the correct age for vaccination, maternal immunity and the frequency of revaccination were made easier when the trained nurses were at hand to explain and advise dog owners.

It is fitting that this fourth edition devotes more space to these new important areas of animal nursing. The chapter on Medical Nursing provides much needed facts, Fluid Therapy is dealt with by another new contributor and here, as elsewhere, the practical aspects are emphasized. Advances in other areas too have been provided for in this edition: First Aid has been written with a positive approach to life saving and new sections on nursing care and of post-operative care of fractures have been introduced. The Glossary has been further extended and may be used by the trainee to answer some of the new style of questions asked in their examinations.

This edition is of necessity larger than previously and more work was involved. Dr Bush and Dr Jones were both invaluable as an editorial sub-committee in preparing the edition, the support of the BSAVA Officers and individual members was admirable. RANAs have played an increasing role in writing and providing criticism of the text. All 26 contributors showed great willingness to improve the information provided in the new edition. It is some return for the dedicated work of so many animal nurses, that the editorial work has been a pleasure to complete. The veterinary profession as a whole, has benefited from the vocation of animal nursing.

47 Newbold Terrace                    D. R. LANE, BSc, FRCVS, ARAgS
Leamington Spa
Warwickshire
England

# Contents

# List of Authors

R.S. ANDERSON, BVMS, PhD, MRCVS
Animal Studies Centre
Freeby Lane
Waltham-on-the-Wolds
Melton Mowbray
Leicestershire LE14 4RT

K.A. APPLEBEE, FIAT
The Royal College of Surgeons of England
35–43 Lincoln's Inn Fields
London WC2A 3PN

H. BRIGGS, BVMS, MRCVS
Berkshire College of Agriculture
Hall Place
Burchetts Green
Nr Maidenhead
Berkshire SL6 6QR

B.M. BUSH, BVSc, PhD, FRCVS
Department of Clinical Studies
Royal Veterinary College
Royal College Street
London NW1 0TU

E.M. CARR, RANA
Department of Clinical Veterinary Studies
University of Cambridge
Madingley Road
Cambridge CB3 0ES

J.E. COOPER, BVSc, DTVM, FIBiol, MRCVS
The Royal College of Surgeons of England
35–43 Lincoln's Inn Fields
London WC2A 3PN

S.W. DOUGLAS, MA, MRCVS, DVR
5 Dodds Mead
Haslingfield
Cambridge CB3 7LD

D.G. EARNSHAW, MA, BSc, MRCVS
102 Shepherd Street
Chippendale
Sydney
New South Wales
Australia 2008

A.T.B. EDNEY, BA, BVetMed, MRCVS
Animal Studies Centre
Freeby Lane
Waltham-on-the-Wolds
Melton Mowbray
Leicestershire LE14 4RT

F.W.G. HILL, PhD, BVetMed, MRCVS
Faculty of Veterinary Science
University of Zimbabwe
PO Box 167 Mount Pleasant
Harare
Zimbabwe

S. HISCOCK, BVetMed, MRCVS
9 Ashridge Close
Chandlers Ford
Hants SO5 1SA

R.S. JONES, MVSc, DrMedVet, FRCVS, DVA
University Department of Anaesthesia
4th Floor
Royal Liverpool Hospital
Prescot Street
PO Box 147
Liverpool L69 3BX

A.R. KEELEY, RANA, FIAT
The Animal Department
St Mary's Hospital Medical School
Paddington
London W2 1PG

I.O. KNAPP, RANA
Templecarrig House
Greystones
Co Wicklow
Ireland

A. LEYLAND, BVSc, MRCVS
2 Comberton Place
Kidderminster
Hereford & Worcs DY10 1UA

S.E. LONG, BVMS, PhD, MRCVS
Department of Animal Husbandry
University of Bristol
Langford House
Langford
Bristol BS18 7DU

D.P. McHUGH, RANA
Department of Clinical Veterinary Studies
University of Cambridge
Madingley Road
Cambridge CB3 0ES

A.R.W. PORTER, MA
Barrister-at-Law
Registrar of the Royal College of Veterinary Surgeons
32 Belgrave Square
London SW1X 8QP

N.J. PRICE, RANA
181 Cheltenham Road
Evesham
Hereford & Worcs WR11 6LF

N.J.H. SHARP, BVetMed, MRCVS, MVM
The Veterinary Hospital
University of Liverpool
Crown Street
Liverpool L7 7EX

R.N. SMITH, PhD, DSc, FRCVS
Department of Anatomy
School of Veterinary Science
University of Bristol
Park Row
Bristol BS1 5LS

G. SUMNER-SMITH, BVSc, FRCVS
University of Guelph
Veterinary Teaching Hospital
Ontario Veterinary College
Ontario N1G 2W1
Canada

L.C. VAUGHAN, DSc, FRCVS, DVR
Department of Clinical Studies
The Royal Veterinary College
University of London
Hawkshead House
Hawkshead Lane
North Mymms
Hatfield
Herts AL9 7TA

S.B. WATKINS, MA, VetMB, MRCVS, DVA
Department of Clinical Veterinary Medicine
Madingley Road
Cambridge CB3 0ES

G.T. WILKINSON, MVSc, MRCVS
Department of Veterinary Medicine
University of Queensland
St Lucia
Brisbane 4067
Australia

J.S. WILKINSON, BSc., PhD, MRCVS
Department of Veterinary Paraclinical Studies
University of Melbourne
Veterinary Clinical Centre
Princes Highway
Werribee
Victoria 3030
Australia

# CHAPTER 1

# Anatomy and Physiology—I

R. N. SMITH

### Introduction

Dogs and cats are mammals, that is, animals that have backbones and warm blood and whose females feed their newborn young on milk produced in mammary glands (hence the class name mammals). They also always have hair.

Most, but not all, mammals are placental; in other words, they have an arrangement called a *placenta* which develops in the pregnant female and from which the unborn animal gets its nourishment. Dogs and cats are placental mammals; so also, for example, are humans, bats, cattle and mice. However, these are all classified into divisions, called orders, of mammals. Humans are primates (have hands and feet); bats, having wings, belong to the chiroptera; cattle are ungulates (their feet have hooves); mice are examples of the rodentia, gnawing animals. Dogs and cats, like bears and lions, are in the order carnivora, the flesh-eaters.

Not all the animals that are brought to the surgery are mammals; for instance, birds are often presented and so sometimes are tortoises. Nevertheless, these have backbones and so, like the mammals, they belong to a section of animals called vertebrates. Some animals of great importance to the veterinary surgeon do not even have backbones. These are the inver-

tebrates, and examples of these that are rather too common are external parasites such as fleas and internal parasites such as roundworms and flatworms.

The first two chapters of this book on nursing are concerned with how animals are constructed (their anatomy) and how they work (their physiology). This form and function are closely interrelated and interdependent and it is helpful to think of them together and not as separate disciplines.

Most sciences have their own language: this enables precise communication between colleagues. Sometimes a word in general everyday use is given a very exact meaning in some branch of science. At one time only Latin names were acceptable in biological nomenclature and some of these are still in current use in the original Latin form. It would be a great convenience if only one name were used for each structure. Unfortunately, over the centuries that some of these sciences have been studied, a variety of names has grown up and it is not a case of which is right or wrong, but which is the best term in common use. Opinions on this will vary and so some of the names used here may not be those used by the veterinary surgeon that you are assisting.

A series of terms is used to indicate

1

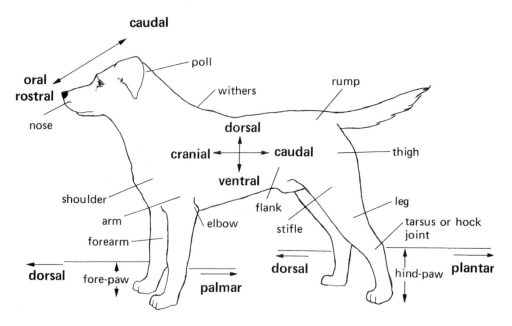

FIG. 1.1.   Some points of the dog and anatomical directions: these latter are in bold type.

directions with reference to parts of the body; some of these are common to all regions. *Superficial* and *deep* indicate relative distances from the surface of the body. *External* and *internal* refer to the relations of depth in organs and cavities. *Medial* and *lateral* give the position nearer to and farther from the mid-line of the body.

However, many terms are used only in specific regions. When the animal is standing evenly on all four limbs with the head and the tail fairly level, the surface of the head, trunk and tail nearer to the ground is *ventral:* the opposite side of the animal is *dorsal. Caudal* means that the part is nearer to the tail-end of the animal: the term is used for all the animal except the lower regions of the limbs. For this part of the forelimb the direction is *palmar* (volar is still frequently used) and for the hindlimb it is *plantar.*

The opposite to caudal is *cranial* except for the head. Here the term is *oral* (nearer the mouth) or *rostral* (towards the nose). *Anterior* and *posterior* are occasionally also used for directions in the head. For the lower parts of the limbs the *dorsal* surface is the opposite to palmar and plantar. (The conventions used for these limb regions fit best with human nomenclature and make comparison simpler.) *Distal* is another term used for the limbs and means away from the trunk; the opposite is *proximal.* These terms and some of the regions (points) of the dog are shown in Fig. 1.1.

### Tissues and Systems

All the materials of which an animal is made are arranged in **tissues**. This name is taken from the French word *tissu* which means "woven" and was used by a French scientist in the eighteenth century who noticed the resemblance of the layers and structures of the body to woven material and so classified them according to their texture or *tissu*.

Later work showed that these tissues, which together form the entire substance of the body, consist of three main components:

1. Cells. These are minute individual living entities. Nearly all cells are nucleated,—i.e. they contain a control centre (sometimes more than one) called a **nucleus**.
2. Intercellular materials. These are produced by cells and as the name suggests, they are found between the cells.
3. Fluid, either bathing the cells themselves or flowing in specially formed channels between them.

A structure in which one tissue predominates and where there is some special function is called an **organ**. A **system** is a collection of tissues, organs, parts and structures related by position or function.

### Basic tissues

A tissue can be defined as a collection of cells and their products which has a common fundamental function and in which one particular type of cell predominates.

There are four basic tissues; (1) muscular, concerned with movement; (2) nervous, enabling the animal to be aware of the environment and to make any changes it needs to adapt to it; (3) epithelial, a covering tissue; (4) connective tissue which plays a general supporting role and also weaves itself through all the other tissues, connecting and binding them together.

### *Muscular Tissue*

Muscular tissue is the one in which the property of contractility is well developed.

It has a very high proportion of muscle cells, which, since they are usually long, thin and thread-like, are often called fibres. The cells are divisible into three types: skeletal, smooth and cardiac.

**Skeletal muscle cells** are found in muscular tissue attached to the skeleton. The cells are usually cylindrical and vary from about 1 mm to 5 cm in length although they are only about one-hundredth of a millimetre in thickness. Since skeletal muscular tissue often responds to the will of the animal, the cells may be called **voluntary** muscle cells. Skeletal muscles are formed of parallel muscle cells (fibres) held together in small bundles by connective tissue. These are collected into larger groups which are also enclosed in connective tissue, and ultimately form the muscle which is surrounded by yet more connective tissue commonly called the **muscle sheath**. Where muscles are close to one another, the muscle sheaths may thicken to form **intermuscular septa**. All the connective tissue within and around the muscles continues into the connective tissue of the structure to which the muscle is attached. Sometimes the muscle appears to attach directly but usually the connective tissue leaves the muscle as a fibrous band known as a **tendon** or as a fibrous sheet called an **aponeurosis**. Muscles vary greatly in their shapes and some are named according to the shape they have in the *human* body, although this may not be the same as in other animal bodies. Some muscles are named according to their functions and yet others according to their position in the body. When looked at under a light microscope, skeletal muscle cells have regular stripes (striations) at right angles to their long axes and so this type may be called *striated muscle tissue*.

**Smooth muscle cells** are spindle-shaped and may be up to about half a millimetre in length although most are very much shorter. They are called "smooth" because they do not have the microscopic striations of skeletal muscle cells. Small amounts of connective tissue usually bind them together to form sheets or layers of *smooth muscle tissue.* However, they are sometimes found grouped together in small numbers, and in some parts of the body smooth muscle cells occur singly. Smooth muscle tissue is often associated with involuntary actions; that is, actions that are not usually controlled by the will of the animal. For this reason smooth muscle cells may be called **involuntary** muscle cells.

**Cardiac muscle cells** are confined to the heart and are involuntary in action. The cells are elongated and are the only muscle cells which frequently branch. They are held together by relatively scanty amounts of connective tissue.

*Epithelial Tissue*

Epithelial tissue covers the outside of the body and also lines the inner cavities and tubes: its main function is protection but in some areas it has other properties. The tissue is composed almost entirely of epithelial cells and these are fixed on to connective tissue by an intercellular substance.

It is necessary in some situations to allow absorption or filtration through the epithelial membrane (layer of cells). Obviously, it is better here to have a membrane only one cell in thickness and this is called a **simple** epithelium.

There may be cells in a simple epithelium that are specially designed to absorb material: these have a tremendous number of small processes (only recognizable under magnifications of about 40,000) on their free surface that increase the absorptive area. There may also be cells whose special function is to secrete (produce) a slippery protective fluid called **mucus**. Yet other epithelial cells may have very fine hair-like projections called **cilia** whose function is to move the mucus along over the epithelial tissue by their continuous waving action.

In some regions of the body the protective function is more important than absorption or filtration and a simple epithelium would prove to be too delicate. Here there will be several layers of cells and the tissue is called a **stratified** epithelium. Where even more protection is required, and especially where the surface is dry, the outermost layers of a stratified epithelium undergo changes known as **keratinization** to become **keratin**. It is a material that is very resistant to chemical change and to bacterial invasion, as well as being fairly waterproof. This tough, resilient substance protects the underlying cells from drying out and also from other forms of damage.

There are certain areas of the body where a large amount of the epithelial secretion is required, more than could be produced by cells occupying the outermost surface. The necessary epithelial cells including, of course, the secretory type, are clustered together and push down into the connective tissue to form a **gland**. Those glands which retain a connection with the free surface and whose secretion can pass up a collecting tube or duct are called **exocrine** glands. The connective tissue in which the gland is embedded may divide it into small units or **lobules**: the gland is said to be lobulated and the connective tissue divisions are called interlobular septa. Groups of lobules may be collected by stronger connective tissue to form **lobes**. Such a gland will then be lobated and have interlobar septa.

There are some glands which do not have any connection with the free epithelial surface. Since there is no duct they may be called **ductless** glands or **endo-**

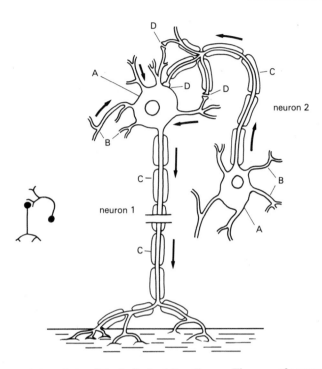

FIG. 1.2. Neurons consisting of: A, cell body: B, dendrites; C, axon. The axon of neuron 1 splits up to supply an effector organ (muscle or gland). The axon of neuron 2 forms several synapses (D) with neuron 1. Details like these can only be seen under very high magnification. Arrows indicate the direction of the impulse. The small diagram illustrates a simple convention often used for neurons.

**crine** glands. They secrete very important substances called **hormones**, which have special effects on the various body systems: since there is no duct, the secretion leaves the glands in one of the other fluids of the body.

*Nervous Tissue*

The cells of nervous tissue have the ability of responding to a stimulus by producing a wave of electrical excitation called a *nervous impulse* and of conducting the impulse rapidly over large areas of the body.

Each cell is a **neuron** and consists of a **cell body** and a number of processes (Fig. 1.2). They vary tremendously in shape and in the arrangement of the processes.

When the processes are thin and long (and in some cases they may be many centimetres long) their thread-like appearance gives rise to the name fibres as it does in so many other structures with this particular form.

All the processes carrying impulses *to* the cell body are called **dendrites** or **dendrons**. Only one process carries the nerve impulse away: this one is called the **axon**, and it may end by splitting into a number of branches. The nervous impulse which the axon is carrying away from its cell body may be destined immediately for an effector organ, in which case this is where the terminal branches end. It may, however, have to travel via another neuron to reach its destination. There is no continuity between successive neurons and the impulse has to pass over a junction or **synapse**. The arrangement is always one-way: the impulse leaves the axon and passes either to the cell body or to the dendrite of the next neuron, never in the reverse direction.

*Connective Tissue*

Connective tissue is the material that is found binding all the other tissues together, acting as a supporting medium for them and also conducting nutrition to, and waste material away from, the various cells of the body. To help perform these functions adequately, a large amount of intercellular material or **matrix** is often found in connective tissue. This is thought to be formed by some of the cells of the connective tissue and it may take one of several forms. The intercellular material may be fluid; in other cases, when it is sometimes called **ground substance**, it is gelatinous or even hard. If fibres occur in the matrix it is said to be **fibrous**; if not, then the material is considered **amorphous**. The intercellular material, its physical nature and the associated cells, to-

gether provide a variety of connective tissues depending on the proportions of each that are present. This will be decided by the function that the connective tissue has to perform: it will, however, be covered generally by the term "supporting" whether this refers to support by structure or by nutritive supplies and waste removal. The connective tissues will be described in order of increasing viscosity of their intercellular materials; that is, blood and other fluids, haemopoietic tissue, loose connective tissue, dense connective tissue, cartilage, bone.

Blood

Blood is a fluid connective tissue that circulates in all adult vertebrates in a continuous system of tubes called **blood vessels**. It comprises about 7% of the body weight and has a supporting role for other tissues by conveying nutritive material and removing waste products. It consists of a fluid matrix called **plasma** which makes up between 55% and 70% of the blood, and in this are found special blood cells called **corpuscles** and cell fragments

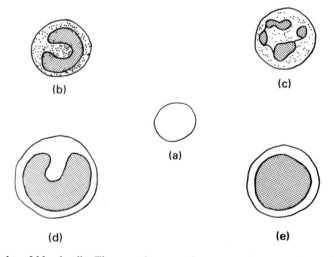

Fig. 1.3.   Examples of blood cells. They are drawn to the same scale: (a) erythrocyte; (b) eosinophil or basophil; (c) polymorphonuclear leucocyte (neutrophil); (d) monocyte; (e) lymphocyte.

known as **blood platelets**. The corpuscles are divided into "red blood corpuscles" (RBCs) called **erythrocytes** and "white blood corpuscles" (WBCs) called **leucocytes** (Fig. 1.3).

*Erythrocytes* circulating in normal dogs and cats have no nucleus. They are responsible for the colour of blood and in every cubic millimetre ($mm^3$) there are about 7 million. Like all the cells in the dog and cat they can only be seen under very strong magnification, and in size they are about seven–thousandths of a millimetre in diameter (7 micron or $7\mu$).*

The erythrocytes are concerned with the transport of gases. All the tissues of the body require a substantial supply of oxygen and they have to be relieved of the carbon dioxide which they produce. **Haemoglobin** is found in the erythrocytes and is the cause of their colour: this substance is also responsible for the carriage of oxygen. Iron is a very important component of haemoglobin and a reduction of the iron in erythrocytes affects their ability to function properly. An iron-deficient animal will usually have smaller erythrocytes than normal, and this can result in one of the forms of the pathological condition called **anaemia** (blood shortage).

There is a continual destruction of erythrocytes which has been estimated at about 100 million every minute in an average-sized dog. This takes place in the liver, bone marrow and perhaps also the spleen. When the cells are destroyed the iron of the haemoglobin is retrieved to be used for more erythrocytes. The remainder of the part responsible for the colour of the red blood cell is converted into bile pigment which is carried in the plasma to the liver where it is excreted.

Although this is a tremendous rate of destruction, the number of circulating

erythrocytes is kept fairly constant since new ones are poured into the blood stream at about the same rate. The production of red blood cells is called **erythropoiesis** and after birth this takes place in the bone marrow. (Before birth, the liver and spleen are also involved.) During its formation the erythrocyte goes through a stage when, like all other cells, it has a nucleus. But before the red blood cells enter the circulation the nuclear material has disappeared. However, if there is a shortage of normal erythrocytes (another form of anaemia), immature cells are released and these may still contain some nuclear material. This can be demonstrated by special histological staining techniques as a net-like arrangement within the cell which is then called a reticulocyte (a reticulum is a net). The life span of erythrocytes in normal healthy dogs is thought to be **about 120 days**.

The *leucocytes* are nucleated and support the body in general by taking an active part in body defence mechanisms. In dogs and cats, the number of leucocytes can vary from about 6,000 to about 18,000 per cubic millimetre of blood. The cells are colourless and are divisible into two major groups. Those that have very small granules within the cell body are called **granular** leucocytes or **granulocytes**: the others are **non-granular** or **agranular** leucocytes.

The granulocytes can be divided into **neutrophils**, **eosinophils** and **basophils** according to the way the granules stain when they are prepared for microscopic examination (i.e. histology). In neutrophils they are coloured by neutral dyes, in eosinophils by acid dyes and in basophils by alkaline dyes. Special stains are used for the examination of blood and these contain a mixture of dyes which stain the various granules differently during the one process.

The granulocytes also have the nucleus

*This Greek letter, mu, pronounced mew, is the scientific symbol for a micron.

divided into lobes or segments connected by filaments: such an arrangement is said to be polymorphonuclear. It is most marked in the neutrophils and this is the cell type usually meant by the term "polymorphonuclear" leucocyte (sometimes abbreviated to "polymorphs" or even "polys"). The eosinophils and basophils also have lobed nuclei but not usually to the extent of the neutrophils (Fig. 1.3).

The non-granular or agranular leucocytes are classified as **lymphocytes** and **monocytes**. These have large nuclei which in the case of monocytes are often kidney-bean-shaped. (They are sometimes called mononuclear leucocytes.) One of the prime functions of the leucocytes seems to be **phagocytosis**, that is, the ingestion (taking in), and consequent removal of pieces of broken-down cells and tissues. This they do mainly outside the blood vessels which they leave by active movements on their own accord: they use the blood stream as a route to travel round the body. The lymphocytes, which are usually the second most common leucocyte in circulating blood (the neutrophil is the first) are believed to be primarily concerned with immunity. This is the ability

of the animal to defend itself against infections and against the introduction of material which it has not produced itself.

An estimate of the number of blood cells is a useful guide in diagnosing some diseases. This is found by counting the cells under a microscope in a diluted measured quantity of blood. These estimates are called **blood cell counts** and may be of red or of white cells. A differential white cell count gives an estimate of the various types of leucocytes. Details of these techniques are given in a later section on diagnostic aids.

In addition to erythrocytes and leucocytes there are also small rounded non-nucleated bodies called platelets (or sometimes thrombocytes) circulating in the blood. Their main function seems to be to prevent haemorrhage and they play a very important role in the coagulation of blood.

The fluid which suspends all these cells is the plasma. This is colourless, perhaps slightly yellow in large quantities, and has a very complex composition. Just over 90% of it is water but it contains some important compounds including **plasma proteins**. One of their functions is to control the amount of water in the circu-

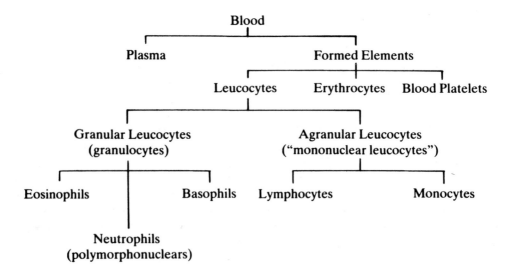

lating blood by preventing it passing out of blood vessels and into the surrounding tissues. **Osmosis** is the term used for this passage of water through partitions such as the walls of blood vessels (and of cells) and **osmotic pressure** is the force which controls which way the flow will go. The osmotic pressure depends on several features including the compounds in the fluids on each side of the partition.

In physiology the osmotic pressure is usually compared to that of blood plasma. If a solution has the same osmotic pressure as plasma it is said to be **isotonic**. There will be no forced movement between isotonic solutions. If the osmotic pressure is higher than that of plasma it is **hypertonic**: the proportion of water in the solution would need to be increased to balance the pressure, perhaps by movement from the plasma. A **hypotonic** solution has an osmotic pressure lower than that of plasma. Three very important plasma proteins are *albumin, globulin* and *fibrinogen*. All are produced in the liver and since albumin is present in the greatest quantity it is the major contributor to maintaining osmotic pressure. The globulins have a role in the immunity reactions of the body and in the transport of hormones. Fibrinogen is an essential substance for the clotting of blood.

Plasma does contain very many other substances since blood is involved in the transport of all nutrients to the cells and all the waste products from the cells. Knowledge of the levels of the various chemicals in the blood can give most useful help in diagnosing some pathological conditions and the various tests that are used will be described in Chapter 7 on diagnostic aids.

If the blood stops moving or if it breaks out of blood vessels which have been breached in any way it coagulates into a jelly-like mass, a phenomenon that is known as **clotting**. Blood platelets play an important role in the mechanism of the clotting, especially if a vessel wall becomes damaged. They immediately stick to the ruptured edge and also to each other. Platelets will also stick to foreign bodies in the circulation and to any clot that is in the process of formation. They disintegrate and liberate an enzyme that plays an active role in the production of fibrin from the fibrinogen, which is a normal constituent of circulating plasma. The fibrin forms into threads which become a network trapping the blood cells; in this way a clot forms. The fluid that remains after clot formation is **serum**.

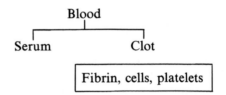

Comparison of the tables of blood constituents and blood coagulation will show that plasma consists of serum and the substances that go to form fibrin (i.e. fibrinogen). The table of blood constituents could be produced as:

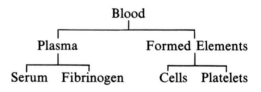

When blood is taken from an animal it has to be combined with an **anticoagulant** if it is to be kept in a fluid form; otherwise the blood settles out into the clot and the serum. Even in a sample of blood that has had an anticoagulant added the cells will gradually drift to the bottom of the container. The rate at which the red cells settle is called the **erythrocyte sedimentation rate** (ESR), and this figure is sometimes required in blood analysis. If the sample of unclotted blood is whirled round in a centrifuge the cells will be forced to the bottom of the centrifuge tube and form three layers. The thickest layer is of red cells and the percentage of the sample formed by these erythrocytes is called the **packed cell volume** (PCV). A thin pale layer above this is formed by the blood platelets and on the top is the "buffy coat" formed by the leucocytes. This method of blood separation is sometimes called **haematocrit**. The ESR and PCV techniques are explained in Chapter 7 on diagnostic aids (p. 459).

## Tissue Fluid and Lymph

The gases carried by the erythrocytes have to be transported to and from the other cells of the body and yet it is unusual for the red blood corpuscles to leave the blood vessels. The gaseous exchange is achieved through the medium of **tissue fluid**. Other nutritive material and waste products also use tissue fluid as a transfer medium and the mechanism of exchange takes place through blood vessels which have walls of extreme thinness. These vessels are known as **capillaries** and their walls consist of a single layer of epithelial cells.

The capillary wall acts as a semipermeable membrane; that is, it is permeable to some, but not all, of the constituents of the blood. The part of the blood that can diffuse into and out of the lumen (cavity) of the capillary is tissue fluid, the transfer medium for many of the cells' nutrients and waste products.

Outside the blood vessels, the tissue fluid bathes the cells of surrounding tissues. Much of the fluid that diffuses out of the capillary blood vessels will diffuse in again. However, not all of it takes this direct route back. Some of it diffuses through the thin walls of another system of capillary vessels which permeate the tissues to form another complex network. Once the tissue fluid has passed into the lumen of this alternative set of capillaries it is called **lymph**. These *lymph capillaries* join up to form larger *lymph vessels* and they eventually discharge their lymph into the system of blood vessels.

## Haemopoietic Tissue

The cells that circulate through the body wear out in a relatively short time. They must be continually replaced by new ones and the old cells must be continually removed. These two functions, replacement and removal, are both performed in one type of connective tissue. This is called haemopoietic tissue. There are two sorts of haemopoietic tissue, the main difference being the types of blood cells produced. The haemopoietic tissue producing erythrocytes and granular leucocytes is the **myeloid** tissue of bone marrow: that producing the agranular leucocytes is called **lymphoid (lymphatic)** tissue.

## Loose Connective Tissue

In this form of supporting tissue the intercellular material consists of a semifluid gelatinous material contained in a loose meshwork of fibres. Whitish in colour, the sticky mass surrounds and supports elements of other tissues. It acts as a packing material and when it is cut and exposed to the air it often has a bubbly appearance. It is sometimes called **areolar** tissue.

The fibres of the intercellular material may be collagenous, elastic or reticular. The **collagenous** fibres are often arranged in bundles which run in all directions. Although of a soft nature they are very resistant to tensile stress, that is, to being pulled. They consist of collagen. The **elastic** fibres are not as common as the collagenous ones. They tend to run singly, to branch freely and to join up to make networks. If they are present in any great number they give a yellowish tint to the tissue. **Reticular** fibres are very delicate and are common where connective tissue borders on to another tissue. One of the characteristics of loose connective tissue is that it can stretch in any direction. Fibres therefore are neither very numerous nor are they woven closely together.

The jelly-like but slightly fibrous matrix is infiltrated by several types of cellular elements such as **fibroblasts** which are usually associated with the collagenous fibres and are thought to play an important part in their formation, and **fat cells** which are characterized by the presence of a large drop of fat. When these occur in large numbers the nature of the connective tissue is so altered that it may be called fat or **adipose** tissue.

One of the functions of loose connective tissue is to attach the skin to underlying structures. In this way, the skin can be freely movable (it also allows the skin to be fairly readily removed from underlying tissues). In this position, the connective tissue may also be called **hypodermis**; it is sometimes called **subcutaneous** tissue. Both words mean "beneath the skin" and it is into this tissue that a "subcutaneous" injection is given using a "hypodermic" syringe. It is also called **superficial fascia** and it may be found arranged in definite layers.

### Dense Connective Tissue

In this form, the proportion of fibres is very much greater than in other forms of connective tissue: it is found where great tensile strength is an advantage. Some-

times the fibres are interwoven and give the appearance of a dense mass: this is called **irregular dense** connective tissue. If the fibres are nearly parallel and tend to run in bundles or sheets they are said to form **regular dense** connective tissue.

The tissue between the epithelial layer of the skin and the superficial fascia that has just been described is irregular dense connective tissue. It is called the **dermis** and is fixed firmly on its outer surface to the epithelial **epidermis** (Fig. 1.28). On its inner surface it continues into the loose connective tissue of the superficial fascia (hypodermis or subcutaneous tissue). The skeletal muscles, especially in the limbs, are often ensheathed in a tough sheet of irregular dense connective tissue. This is called the **deep fascia**. It dips down between the muscles and is continuous with the connective tissue of the intermuscular septa and the connective tissue between the muscle fibres. The deep fascia attaches in places to the skeleton; in some areas it is continuous with muscles. Irregular dense connective tissue is also found around many of the organs of the body where it is said to form a **capsule**. Sometimes the fibres in a particular part become more regularly arranged than in the remainder of the capsule. Such localized areas, which are often thicker than the surrounding connective tissue and may therefore be raised above it, are called **ligaments**.

Regular dense connective tissue is usually associated with muscles. The connective tissue fibres are nearly parallel and leave the muscle as a fibrous band known as a **tendon** or as a fibrous sheet called an **aponeurosis**.

### Cartilage

Cartilage is a connective tissue which whilst being rigid can also be flexible and resilient. It is able to bear a certain amount of weight and it possesses quite considerable tensile strength.

There are relatively few cells. The intercellular material consists of a mass of fibres embedded in gelatinous material. In some cartilage the fibres are of collagen and are not easily seen: this is called **hyaline cartilage** and the fibres are randomly arranged to form a mat. In **fibrocartilage** there is an increase in the number of collagenous fibres and they are organized in a parallel form. Fibrocartilage is found where it is essential that the tissue has great tensile strength. There are some areas of cartilage with a very high proportion of elastic fibres: this is called **elastic cartilage**, and, whilst still retaining the rigidity characteristic of all cartilage, this form of connective tissue is more resilient.

Perhaps the most unusual feature of cartilage is that, given a slight amount of lubrication, surfaces coated with this tissue can move and slide on one another with very little friction or wear. With the exception of such surfaces, i.e. those that move on one another, the periphery of a piece of cartilage has a less "cartilaginous" appearance than a more central zone. The collagenous fibres appear more obvious and they form a fibrous layer, the **perichondrium**. This will merge imperceptibly into cartilage.

### Bone

In this form of connective tissue the matrix contains collagenous fibres and a cementing substance with a substantial proportion of chemicals such as calcium phosphate. The cells occur in microscopic cavities in this ground substance.

Mature bone is arranged in thin layers (or **lamellae**) with the collagenous fibres running in different directions in adjacent lamellae. This increases the resistance of the bone tissue to mechanical forces.

The shape and arrangement of the lamellae allow a separation into spongy (cancellous) and compact bone tissue. **Spongy** bone consists of bars and plates called **trabeculae** and these form a three-dimensional network. Each trabecula consists of a few lamellae generally arranged parallel to one another or in concentric layers. In **compact** bone most of the lamellae are arranged in cylindrical systems (**osteones** or *Haversian systems*) around narrow axial canals. The canal is called an *Haversian canal* and contains minute blood vessels and fine nerve fibres in loose connective tissue.

Bone formation is termed **ossification** or **osteogenesis**; semi-fluid ground substance already at the site of ossification condenses and undergoes a chemical change: this masks any fibres that are also present. The resulting substance is **osteoid** tissue; it becomes calcified almost immediately, and undergoes a subtle chemical change to become bone. There is a constant remodelling of bone tissue.

In the developing young animal, bone formation in some regions of the body is preceded by cartilage. When it is time for bone to be produced the cartilage becomes calcified and acts as a scaffolding. Bone is laid down on this scaffolding and the calcified cartilage is then gradually removed. *Calcified cartilage is not bone.* Bone tissue formed on a calcified cartilage scaffolding is commonly called **endochondral** bone and the process is said to be endochondral ossification. It is essential to realize that this bone tissue is formed in the same way as any other bone tissue: it is only the environment that is different. Where bone tissue is formed without the aid of a cartilage scaffold, it is said to be **intramembranous** bone and to have formed by intramembranous ossification.

## Systems

The body systems are all interdependent and the fundamental purpose for which they are designed is the survival of the animal and the species. Life depends entirely on chemical reactions and many of these are so precise that they can take place in conditions that vary within only the narrowest limits. The temperature, acidity, etc., of the internal environment needs to be kept constant no matter what is happening outside the body. This is achieved by an all-pervading fluid arrangement.

The **vascular system** of heart and vessels (tubes) keeps the blood and lymph circulating through the entire animal. Tissue fluid bathes all the structures of the body and substances such as nutrients and waste products can pass between the fluid inside and outside the cells and also through the vessel walls between the tissue fluid and the blood and lymph. The vascular system ensures a constant mixing of all the fluids of the body with a resulting levelling of extreme conditions that might occur locally.

Nutrients are brought from outside the animal into the **digestive system,** a tube open at both ends. The chemical and physical extraction they undergo is **digestion**, a process helped by substances secreted (the act of producing useful material) by the cells of this system. Digestion breaks down the complex chemicals of the food into very small packages that can pass through the **intestinal wall** (part of the lining of the digestive system) and into the vascular system. This process is **absorption** and the fluid then passes the packages along to other cells where they are needed. The unwanted part of the food continues on through the digestive system and is eventually passed to the outside of the animal as **faeces** (droppings) during the act of **defaecation.**

While it is travelling along the digestive system other unwanted substances are added which have passed through the wall into the lumen (cavity) of the tube. Removal of waste products from the cells and from the body is called **excretion**.

The small packages of nutrient substances that have been absorbed into the blood and lymph may be used by the cells without any further alteration. Sometimes special products need to be manufactured and this can only be done by cells in certain regions such as the liver. **Metabolism** is the term used to describe all the chemical reactions that go on in the body and this special manufacture is called *intermediary metabolism.*

An essential chemical in the vast majority of reactions in the animal body is the gas oxygen, and this is obtained from the air by the **respiratory system**. The air is pulled into the lungs inside the body and the oxygen passes into the blood through the extensive but very thin membrane of the lungs which terminates the respiratory system in the thorax (chest). The dissolved oxygen is carried by the ubiquitous fluid system to the cells to play its role in chemical reactions which usually end in the production of another gas, carbon dioxide. This is passed back into the blood stream and taken into the lungs where it flows back across the very thin membrane and is excreted to the outside air by the respiratory system.

There are other waste products besides carbon dioxide which result from cell metabolism and which are excreted into the blood stream. However, these are not gaseous and many are removed from the blood through the numerous small tubes within the paired kidneys. These excretory products help to form the **urine** and from the kidneys this fluid passes to the urinary bladder to be voided at intervals to the outside during the act of **urination**. This excretory arrangement forms the **urinary** system and is very closely linked with the organs used in producing the young.

The male animal produces **sperms**, small cells carrying fundamental and chemical information from this parent. A tubular part (the **penis**) of the urinary system is used to deposit them inside the female. The potential mother produces **ova**, cells containing the contribution of the female parent to the basic chemical store of the young. Eventually the sperms meet and penetrate the ova and the resulting **fertilized** cells develop within the female. All the parts of the male and female concerned with this function of producing young constitute the **reproductive system**. Its closeness to the urinary system in the male has been outlined and there is a similar relation in the female. To get the sperms naturally into the correct place, the penis of the male has to be positioned partly in the passage of the female that is also used for voiding urine. But the male reproductive cells then pass into an adjacent tubular structure (the **uterus**) to fertilize the female germ cells and this is where the young develop. The reproductive part may also be called the **genital system** and the two closely linked arrangements are often referred to as the **urogenital system**.

But how do the male and female animals get together and how do they get around to the food they must take in? For this there is the **locomotor system**. A complex arrangement of contractile ropes (muscles) and fairly rigid rods (bones of the skeleton) is used to move the animal from place to place and, in addition, this **musculoskeletal** apparatus acts as a fairly efficient protective casing for the delicate structures forming all the other systems.

The **integumentary system** embraces all these parts of the body, keeping them together, to a certain extent insulating them from the outside and helping to keep the internal environment constant. The most extensive part of the integument is the skin and in addition to the multiple functions just outlined, it also plays an important role in excretion.

Information about the outside environment, about the position of the animal, about the relation of one part to another, about the internal environment, is all collected together by the **nervous system**. This information gathering part is the **sensory** component and its integration and evaluation takes place in the **brain** and **spinal cord**. From here instructions are sent throughout the body to deal with each situation as it arises. This part is the **motor** component and the pathways used may run side by side with those of the sensory component. The tissues forming these pathways are the **nerves** of the body and like the vessels of the vascular system, they are all-pervading.

## Chemistry and Structure of the Cell

All the tissues of the body are made of chemicals and only of chemicals. These can all be purified and, if necessary, bottled and put on display. The preceding section on tissues and systems should have afforded a glimpse into the complete integration of the body, a condition requiring a fantastic interplay of delicate chemical reactions that together constitute life. However, cells are not just small compartments filled with a haphazard collection of dilute solutions of chemicals. They have their own individual structure and an appreciation of this is necessary as well as an insight into some of the chemical processes that takes place there.

### Chemistry of the cell

Chemical substances found only in living material were originally classified as

**organic** compounds, as opposed to those found elsewhere which were grouped as **inorganic**, since it was thought that they were quite different and imbued with some wonderful extra "vital spirit". However, the chemists eventually showed that organic compounds could be isolated and synthesized in the same ways that were used for other compounds. Nevertheless, they did have one curious common factor: these organic compounds all contained the chemical element carbon and to a certain extent organic chemistry can be considered the same as carbon chemistry. It is a branch of science that exists in its own right and so it is quite customary to continue discussing the chemistry of living material in organic and inorganic terms. Water is the commonest compound in the body and is itself an inorganic substance. Other inorganic compounds found in animals are often referred to as minerals (a very special use of the word) and since the remaining materials would all be destroyed by heat leaving only inorganic substances they are also said to make up the ash content of the body.

### Inorganic Content of the Body

The body consists of 60–80% water and the other inorganic substances include calcium, phosphorus, magnesium, sodium, potassium, chlorine, iron and copper. Some others such as iodine and manganese exist in such small amounts that they are called trace elements. None of these exist as the purified element: one no more finds pure chlorine than one does a piece of metallic copper. The chemicals are found in a special combining form called an *ion*; calcium ions, magnesium ions, chloride ions, phosphate ions, etc.

Any substance that will split up into ions when it is dissolved in water can be referred to as an **electrolyte**.

Hydrogen is a very important element that one tends to think of as a gas. But as a hydrogen ion in solution it does not exist in gaseous form. Some substances in solution can give up the hydrogen ions when they take part in chemical reactions. These are called **acids**, and in fact an acid can be defined as a substance that can give up hydrogen ions. Those that can accept hydrogen ions in a chemical reaction are alkaline and are described as **bases**. The usual way of describing the acidity (or alkalinity or basicity) of a solution is to refer to a measure of its hydrogen ion content; this is called its pH (written in this form and pronounced pee-aitch) and is marked on a scale between 0 and 14. If a solution is very acid it has a low pH, very basic (alkaline) a high pH, and neutral a pH of 7. The average pH of body fluids is 7.4, i.e. slightly basic.

*Water.* No living cell can exist without water and intracellular water (inside the cell) represents about 50% of body weight (Fig. 1.4). Extracellular water (outside the cell) is found in tissue fluid (16% body weight) and blood plasma (4%). A very small amount is found in joint and body cavities, cerebrospinal fluid and lymph. There is a constant interchange of water between these fluid compartments but there is quite a difference in the concentration of water in different tissues. It makes up about three-quarters of muscles and about one-quarter of bone; there is very little water in fat tissue.

Since water is a very good solvent it can act as a transport medium for a multitude of chemicals. It also plays a vital role in temperature regulation for not only can it be moved around to dissipate heat but also its evaporation from body surfaces including the mouth and the respiratory tract can have an extremely useful cooling effect. There is a high content of water in the lubricants of the joints and of the surface of the eye.

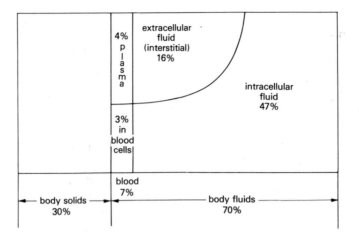

FIG. 1.4.   Diagrammatic representation of the distribution of body fluid. All figures are very approximate and represent percentages of body weight.

It is not convenient for an animal to store water in bulk and, since there is a continual loss through the urinary and digestive systems as well as through the lungs and skin, there must be continual replacement. Water enters the body as a liquid, in the food, and it is also formed there as a result of chemical reactions. An excessive intake is usually balanced by an increased urine output. When water is short and the amount of urine is low, the excretion through the lungs and the skin may exceed urine output. Illness can cause a serious loss of fluid especially when it is accompanied by vomiting and diarrhoea. Severe bleeding (haemorrhage) can also lower the fluid level of the body. (Fig. 1.5.).

But sometimes the body has an excess of fluid in the tissue spaces. This pathological condition is called **oedema** and is often associated with heart disease and kidney disease.

*Calcium, phosphorus, magnesium.* The greater part of the mineral content of the body consists of these elements and most of it is found in the bones and teeth. The calcium level is higher than that of the phosphorus and it seems that the

more of one that is present the less there is of the other. A correct balance between them seems essential for the well-being of the animal. They are necessary for satisfactory nerve function and contractibility of muscle, a deficiency leading to muscular spasms and eventually paralysis and unconsciousness. An inadequacy can also result in bone conditions such as rickets. Calcium ions also play an important role in the blood-clotting mechanism. These chemicals are of exceptional importance in the pregnant animal that is having to supply them to the developing young and also in the mother supplying milk (which contains these elements) for suckling. In both cases the parent can suffer severe illnesses through even a temporary deficiency.

*Sodium, potassium, chlorine.* Potassium is found mainly within the cell, but sodium and chlorine ions (usually in the form of sodium chloride) are major constituents of extracellular fluid. These chemicals appear to be very important in regulating fluid balance, especially in maintaining that between the inside and the outside of individual cells. They are

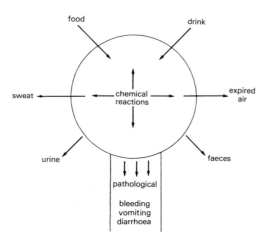

Fig. 1.5.   Water movement.

also essential for nerve conduction and muscle contraction.

*Iron and copper.* These are probably distributed in all tissues but the best known site of iron is in the blood where about two-thirds of it occurs. It is part of haemoglobin, the pigment found in red blood cells, where it is essential for the transport of oxygen. Copper seems to be needed for the proper use of iron in haemoglobin formation. When the red blood cells break down, the iron is salvaged and passes to the liver, spleen and bone marrow. From here the haemopoietic tissues reissue it as newly constituted haemoglobin.

*Organic Content of the Body*

The organic compounds can be grouped into two classes: simple and complex substances. Those that are absorbed into the cell are relatively simple ones, amino acids, fatty acids and sugars; but they are derived from more complex food substances, proteins, lipids, and carbohydrates respectively. Not only are they derived from these but they are then used by the cell as building bricks to produce other complex substances, the proteins of muscle, skin and hair, the lipids which make up the layers of subcutaneous fat, the carbohydrates that are stored in liver and muscle.

These are, of course, complicated chemical reactions and ones that can only take place in carefully controlled conditions. This has been mentioned earlier and some of the methods for achieving this equilibrium have been discussed. Not only must the conditions be ideal, but nearly every chemical reaction in the body needs the presence of one of a group of substances called **enzymes**. These are protein compounds that assist and accelerate organic chemical reactions. They are very specific substances and will usually only be of use in one particular reaction. Since each cell performs many different reactions there must be a great number of enzymes, probably at least 200, in any one cell. It is these substances that play a decisive role in the conditions under which the reaction will take place since enzymes are very easily inactivated.

*Amino acids and proteins.* Each amino acid always contains nitrogen, carbon, hydrogen and oxygen and some contain sulphur and iodine. When two join together they form a **peptide**. Many amino acids joined together form a **polypeptide** and when there are several hundred they form a protein. This joining together of simple organic substances to make the complex ones is called **polymerization**.

Proteins can be grouped into two classes: structural proteins (such as the keratin found in epithelium and collagen in connective tissue) are tough substances, resistant to acids, alkalis and quite high temperatures; functional proteins such as enzymes and hormones are associated with cellular chemical reactions.

*Fatty acids and lipids.* Fatty acids are made up of carbon, hydrogen and oxygen and result from the breakdown of lipids, one example of which is fat. Fatty acids are the main forms in which fat is transported in the blood from one part of the body to another. They are involved in many of the cellular chemical reactions as well as being used as building bricks in the formation of lipids such as phospholipids and steroids, as well as fats. Phospholipids are involved in the structure of cell membranes, including those found inside the cell as well as the enveloping one. They also act as insulators around the nerves. Probably the major steroid in the body is cholesterol, and in addition to playing a role in membrane function it is linked chemically with some of the acids used in digestion and with some hormones (and incidentally also with some important drugs and poisons). Fats are used as food stores: when excess food is available it may be converted to fats and be laid down subcutaneously and in other fat depots. Here they may also act as insulators against heat loss and when they surround delicate organs they will also act as protection.

*Sugars and carbohydrates.* Sugars also consist of carbon, hydrogen and oxygen but the oxygen forms a higher proportion than in fatty acids. Glucose is an example of the sugars (here the term is being used in a chemical sense) and forms an important source of energy for the animal. When hundreds of the simple forms of sugars like glucose are linked together they form carbohydrates (also known as polysaccharides). The simple ones dissolve easily in water, but not the more complex ones such as glycogen (sometimes called animal starch). This is the form in which animals store carbohydrates and it is found mainly in the liver and muscles. Sugars are also used in the formation of two complex substances of tremendous significance in cell chemistry and inheritance: ribonucleic acid (abbreviated as RNA) and desoxyribonucleic acid (DNA).

*Chemical Reactions of the Body*

In the description of the systems many actions were described that involve a lot of work. Fluids are being forced around the body, muscles are contracting, materials are brought from one group of cells to another, organized and joined together into complex organic substances. These survive for only a short while, longer than a few days is an exception even for apparently stable tissues like bone and cartilage. From these few examples of work, it can be appreciated that a lot of energy must be available.

Energy cannot be created or destroyed: it can be moved around and can also change its form, for instance heat energy can be converted to electrical energy and, as with an electric fire, electrical energy into heat energy. Energy can be locked up in a compound during synthesis and is then termed *potential energy*: this will be released when the compound is broken down. Some chemical reactions need energy whereas others release it.

When carbon (coal) is made to burn, a

little heat energy has to be supplied at first. As soon as it is really burning it is undergoing a chemical reaction whereby it is combining with oxygen, and this releases a tremendous amount of energy as heat. The resulting compound is carbon dioxide and the reaction can be written as follows:

$$\text{carbon} + \text{oxygen} \xrightarrow{\text{results in}}$$
$$\text{carbon dioxide} + \text{energy}.$$

Energy in this type of reaction is measured in units called **calories** and if 1000 calories of energy were released it could be written as

carbon + oxygen→carbon dioxide
+ 1000 calories of energy.
(Energy is also measured in **joules**: 1 calorie = 4.2 joules).

If we wanted to turn the carbon dioxide back into carbon and oxygen, 1000 calories (4200 joules) of energy would have to be supplied (assuming the same amounts of chemicals were being used):

carbon dioxide + 1000 calories (4200 joules) of energy→carbon + oxygen.

The same sort of procedures occur in the cell: one group of reactions release energy and this is then either stored in another compound to be called upon later or it is used immediately in another cellular chemical reaction. This may result, for instance, in a nerve impulse or a muscle twitch or the synthesis of a complex substance. Generally speaking, chemical reactions in the body which result in complex substances being broken down into simpler components usually release energy: these are called **catabolic** reactions. Building-up reactions require energy and are **anabolic** reactions. The results of all the anabolic and catabolic reactions taking place at the same time will be the total metabolism of the animal.

The body constantly loses energy to the outside environment: the rate at which the resting animal produces heat is its *basal metabolism* or *basal metabolic rate*. When an animal is fed there is an increase in the production of heat and in cold weather this may warm the body. The contraction of muscles produces heat energy as a result of the chemical reactions involved. If in so doing mechanical work results, such as moving part of the body, then this will absorb some of the energy, and the remainder appears as heat. This can be an important method of heat production: animals exposed to cold undergo rapid muscular contractions, more commonly called shivering, to achieve these results.

It is wasteful to use these chemical reactions to keep an animal warm when other methods are less expensive. An alternative is to reduce heat loss from the body and this is achieved by the insulation effect of hair and of subcutaneous fat. Clipping and starvation will reverse these particular mechanisms, and it must be remembered that new-born animals do not have the full advantage of these protective devices. To enable these to conserve their energy it may be necessary to supply the young with warmth as well as ensuring a satisfactory diet that will release energy for internal chemical reactions.

However, although heat production by muscular contractions may be a useful technique for the animal in a cool environment it may be an embarrassment at other times, when the exercise is prolonged or the outside temperature is high. At such times there must be an efficient system that allows heat to be removed, otherwise the body temperature would rise continuously and an increase in muscular activity could lead to death. About three-quarters of the heat lost by the body can be removed as dry heat from the surface if the outside temperature is lower than that of the animal. If this cannot operate then it must be lost by evaporation of water from the integument (perspiring, sweating) and from the surfaces of the mouth (panting) and respiratory system. Evaporation is a very efficient method of heat removal and even at ordinary temperatures a quarter of all the heat lost from the resting animal goes this way.

When heat loss is balanced by heat production the temperature should remain constant and this is necessary for so many of the chemical reactions of the body. The temperature of an animal varies in different parts of the body and the veterinary surgeon usually checks it at the rectum.

For the dog and cat, the average reading here is about 38.6°C (101.5°F), but there is quite a variation between animals and the conditions under which the animal is examined can also affect the reading.

There are delicate mechanisms predominantly under nervous control that regulate heat production and loss, acting somewhat like a thermostat, so that the normal temperature is maintained. When an animal suffers from a fever, the "thermostat system" appears to be disturbed, so that it operates at a higher temperature. That is, although heat is being produced by all possible means such as increasing energy releasing reactions like shivering (in this case called a chill) and the temperature rises, the heat loss mechanisms are not brought into play. At a certain point in the illness the "thermostat" is corrected, the heat-losing mechanism is switched on but the temperature is high. Evaporation processes come into play as is shown by profuse sweating. This is the "crisis" of the fever and the body temperature should then begin to return to normal and the illness recede. If the chemical reactions of the animal diminish, as happens just prior to death,

the body temperature then falls below normal.

Since energy is always leaving the animal and some is locked up in various ways, a constant supply is essential. Plants are able to use the energy from the sun to unite carbon dioxide and water to form sugars and carbohydrates. Animals are unable to do this, and so they obtain their energy indirectly from the sun by eating the plants as food: indeed, some animals go farther and achieve an energy balance by eating animals that have eaten plants. The foodstuff is broken down into simpler substances with the aid of enzymes during digestion and the resulting mixture of amino acids, fatty acids, fats and sugars is dissolved through the intestinal wall and eventually reaches the blood stream from where it can reach the individual cells. Here the chemicals combine with oxygen, a reaction which is energy-yielding. The principal source of energy is the oxidation (combination with oxygen) of glucose which results in the formation of carbon dioxide and water as well, and this metabolism can occur in all the cells of the body. (The oxygen–carbon dioxide link has already been mentioned in the reference to the respiratory system.) If the glucose oxidation occurred in one reaction there would be so much energy released locally that the cell would probably not be able to withstand the heat. Instead it goes through about thirty steps, using a large number of different enzymes, each yielding a small amount of energy: the total given up will still be the same as that resulting from the one large reaction. The released energy may be used immediately but in many cases it is stored in a special substance which can be broken down later and perhaps in another place to yield its energy content.

If there is more glucose available than is needed immediately as an energy source, the liver and muscle cells convert the excess to the carbohydrate glycogen by polymerizing 200–300 glucose units, and this is stored locally. These cells can also break the glycogen down to its component glucose units again when necessary and use these for energy production. When the glycogen reserve is full, the liver cells use the surplus glucose to make fat and this is deposited in various sites throughout the body.

When the glucose is in short supply and the glycogen has also been depleted, fats and fatty acids will need to be called upon as a source of energy and when these are low even the amino acids will be broken down. All this occurs mainly in the liver which can convert these compounds into glucose; this can then be dispatched to provide energy for less versatile cells.

During starvation or illness when carbohydrates are low, fat is transferred from the various depots to the liver ready for its processing and causes the condition of "fatty liver". When a large amount of fat is being metabolized, some of the breakdown products, called **ketones** or ketone bodies, accumulate in the liver and the blood stream and are slowly excreted in the urine. Since they are poisonous, this condition of "ketosis" is very serious.

When all else fails and the cells still need energy, amino acids have to be broken down. This also produces a problem since these compounds contain nitrogen. There is always a limited amount of amino acid breakdown occurring and the nitrogen is excreted by being incorporated by the liver cells in the harmless compound **urea** which passes via the blood stream through the kidneys and out of the body in the urine. The amount of nitrogen absorbed from the food through the wall of the digestive system equals that passed out in the urine so that the body maintains a *nitrogen balance*. When starvation dictates that amino acids shall be used,

there is no nitrogen entering the body but it is being excreted in increasing amounts due to their breakdown. The amount finally increases rapidly, followed by death.

In addition to this breakdown of complex compounds, cells must have the capacity to synthesize them. The formation of glycogen by liver and the muscle cells has already been mentioned and this is how most of the carbohydrate reserve of animals exists. Lipids can be synthesized by all cells, some for their own particular use, others for export to separate tissues. Some lipids are produced in specific areas: for instance, liver cells are of major importance in cholesterol formation although other tissues can perform the process.

All cells synthesize protein, some continuously, others for only a part of their life cycle. It is an important function of cells, since even after the maximum size has been achieved, the proteins are still being broken down and then reformed. This is where ribonucleic acid (RNA) and desoxyribonucleic acid (DNA) play such a significant role (p. 18, 23, 24).

There are about twenty different amino acids, and proteins consist of hundreds of these linked together in an individual sequence for each protein. Any change in the order produces a different material and so synthesis can be a complex undertaking. One form of RNA, soluble RNA, is responsible for the gathering together of the individual amino acids and passing them to the other form, insoluble "ribosomal" RNA. It is here that they are arranged in correct sequence, joined together (polymerized) and released as protein. Each type of soluble RNA will be responsible for only one amino acid and each ribosomal RNA will only produce one type of protein. The formation of the RNA itself is automatically controlled by DNA.

### Structure of the cell

Most animal cells are very small, from one-hundredth to one-tenth of a milli-metre (10–100μ) in diameter. It is the number of cells that mainly decides the size of the animal: small animals have fewer cells not necessarily smaller ones. Although some of the structures in the cells can be seen by using light micro-scopes, it is only by using the electron microscopes with magnifications of up to many hundreds of thousands that detail connected with the work of the cell can be appreciated.

If the cells are free they are usually spherical or oval, but when they are packed into tissues their shape becomes distorted due to pressure of other cells or because of their own growth and multipli-cation. When the cells are studied through microscopes it is usually necessary to kill and dye them with various stains to see the small structures: it is difficult to reconcile their dead appearance with their dynamic activity in life. The material of which cells are made is called **protoplasm** and even by using light microscopes it can be seen that nearly all cells consist of two main com-partments enclosed within a **cell mem-**brane (Fig. 1.6). One compartment, the **nucleus**, consists of **nucleoplasm** and is embedded in the remainder of the cell which forms the other compartment and is called the **cytoplasm**.

### *Cytoplasm*

The electron microscope has shown that this living jelly is not a substance in the ordinary sense but a highly structured organization. Within the cytoplasm orga-nized units of living material called **orga-nelles** have important specific functions; these are probably always present and include mitochondria, the Golgi appara-tus, sometimes called the Golgi body, endoplasmic reticulum, ribosomes, lyso-somes and centrioles. **Inclusions** are accu-mulations of cell products often of a temporary nature such as protein, car-bohydrates, lipids, pigment, crystals, and secretory droplets.

The cytoplasm is fluid or semi-fluid and physically and chemically it is in a state of flux. Its constitution will vary with age and metabolic state and cells will have different and characteristic variants.

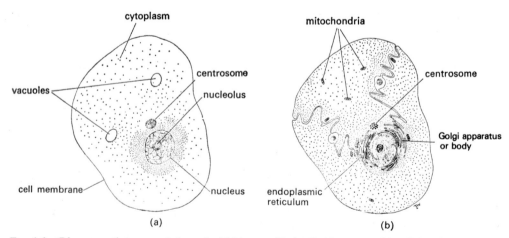

FIG. 1.6.  Diagrammatic representation of a highly magnified cell: (a) as seen with a light microscope; (b) when viewed by an electron microscope.

*Cell membrane*. This is a thin limiting membrane for the whole cell and it acts as a barrier between the cytoplasm and the surrounding materials. It has a variable and selective permeability, allowing only certain substances into and out of the cell. In some cells numerous finger-like processes may project: they increase the surface area and are called **microvilli**.

*Cytoplasmic organelles*. **Mitochondria**: the number of these small organelles varies with the state of the cell from a few hundred to a few thousand. They contain a very large number of enzymes responsible for releasing a vast amount of energy as well as for various synthetic pathways. They are sometimes called **mobile power plants**.

**Golgi apparatus or body**: this complex may be seen under the light microscope and is named after the man who first described it using that technique. Higher magnifications show that it consists of parallel flattened small bags. It seems certain that it plays a role in secretion in glandular cells, but it is found in nearly all cells and its function in non-glandular cells is uncertain.

**Endoplasmic reticulum**: this is a network of membranous tubular cavities filled by fluid. In some areas the surface of the reticulum is smooth but in others it is covered by small particles called **ribosomes** composed mainly of RNA, and these areas are described as rough-coated. The ribosomes attached to the membranes are thought to be concerned with the formation of protein that is secreted from the cell. The function of the smooth-coated reticulum is not known although lipid metabolism has been suggested.

**Ribosomes**: in addition to those attached to the reticulum there are numerous ribosomes found free in the cytoplasm. It is thought that the RNA in these is responsible for synthesizing protein to be used within that cell.

**Lysosomes**: these are membranous compartments containing enzymes that help break down the complex organic compounds. Some cells can absorb into their cytoplasm matter that is not wanted, that is perhaps even injurious to the body: this is *foreign* matter and can be taken in, for example, during phagocytosis. Once absorbed, this matter becomes surrounded by lysosomes that discharge their enzymes so that it is broken down for removal. Another use occurs when the cell is damaged: the lysosomes then release their enzymes to clear up the resulting cell debris.

**Centrioles**: small bodies found near the nucleus that play an important role in the reproduction of the cell. Their surrounding cytoplasm is usually condensed and may be called the **centrosome** or **centrosphere**.

*Cytoplasmic inclusions*. Dark brown to black granules are found in cells called **melanocytes**: the granules are **melanin** and these cells occur in pigmented areas of the body. A golden-brown pigment called **haemosiderin** may be found in cells connected with haemoglobin breakdown. Other pigments, carbohydrates, lipids and proteins can also be found as cell inclusions.

*Other cytoplasmic contents*. Many of the inorganic substances of the body are found in the cytoplasm in addition to a vast range of enzymes. Water is the commonest compound and in this the dissolved chemicals can react as necessary, either in the fluid or on the surface of the membranous organelles.

## Nucleus

Nearly all cells have one nucleus and some have more than one. Metabolism is restricted and growth is impossible in cells without a nucleus. When present it is the control centre of the cell and contains large quantities of DNA. This governs the activities of the cytoplasm as well as being the material controlling heredity from parents to the young. The DNA compounds are the **genes** and are found combined with structural proteins to form **chromatin**. The DNA controls the formation of the RNA and this spreads throughout the cell controlling the formation of the many proteins produced in a cell. There is also a discrete collection of RNA within the nucleus forming a **nucleolus** (there may be more than one). The nucleus is separated from the cytoplasm by a distinct nuclear membrane, but this is thought to be perforated by several small openings.

*Reproduction of the Cell*

There seems to be a certain size to which cells grow and this may be determined by the amount of DNA in the nucleus. In many cases the cell then doubles all its contents and divides evenly. The resulting two cells continue independently and themselves increase in size. This method of reproducing is called **mitosis** (p. 205). Growth and reproduction may be continuous in some tissues: the cells lining the surface of the intestine are one example. Other cells, such as those found in some muscle tissue, only reproduce occasionally during the life of the animal and yet others which are highly specialized such as neurons may never reproduce. Mitosis is a phase in the life of a cell and the time between the mitotic events is called the **interphase**. Although all the dynamic processes are fully active during this period, the cell is sometimes (mistakenly) said to be "resting".

The cells that result from mitotic division will be identical to each other. There is another method of cell division called

meiosis (p. 205, Fig. 3.28), when the resulting cells have only half the number of chromosomes of the parent cell, and this is the method used by the sex cells. Chromosomes are thread-like structures of condensed chromatin (the combination of genes with structural proteins). Meiosis is necessary so that when the sperm (with half the normal species number of chromosomes) fuses with an ovum (also with a half) the resulting fertilized egg (called a **zygote**) will then have the normal species number. Meiosis is only performed by the sex cells.

## The Skeletal System

The hard structures that support and protect the soft tissues form the **skeleton**. They can be taken to be organs in which bone tissue and/or cartilage tissue are predominant. For convenience, one often uses the term skeletal system to include also the joints, that is the tissues which connect such organs.

## Bones

A bone is an organ and includes several tissues (Fig. 1.7). The bone tissue itself is usually arranged in the compact form on the outer surface and this varies tremendously in thickness, depending on the part of the bone and its function. The layer of compact bone is often referred to as the **cortex**; inside this there is usually some spongy (cancellous) bone and there may also be a space called the **medullary cavity**.

This space and also those between the trabeculae of the spongy bone are filled with connective tissue known as **marrow**. In some bones this is very fatty and is called **yellow marrow**. In others, and also sometimes in the same bones that one finds yellow (fatty) marrow, there is a **red**

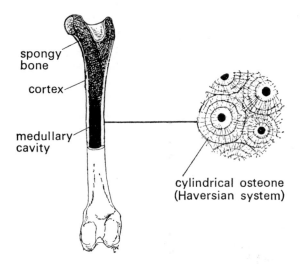

spongy
bone

cortex

medullary
cavity

cylindrical osteone
(Haversian system)

FIG. 1.7. A long bone, partly sectioned. The enlargement in the circle represents the microscopic appearance of compact bone.

**marrow**. This is myeloid (haemopoietic) tissue, the connective tissue responsible for producing erythrocytes and granular leucocytes. In the very young animal all the marrow in all the bones is the red (myeloid) variety. Gradually fat cells replace the myeloid tissue and yellow marrow becomes substituted in many of the spaces.

Blood vessels will be intimately connected with the marrow, especially when it is the red variety and if they use one definite place to pass through the compact bone this is called the **nutrient foramen**. Do not be misled into thinking that this is the point of entry of the only vessel that is responsible for the nutrition of the bone; it receives supplies from many other vessels over its surface. Fine nerves will also be found associated with the inside of the bone.

The outer surface of the bone is covered by a layer of dense connective issue, the **periosteum**. The deeper part of the periosteum in intimate contact with the surface of the bone can help in bone-tissue formation. The outermost part of the periosteum is more fibrous than the deeper layer and has a protective function. Fibres of the periosteum continue into the bone tissue itself and may make it extremely difficult to separate the periosteum.

There are a few regions where periosteum does not cover the bone. If one bone is in contact with another, and especially if there is movement between the bones, the contiguous areas are usually covered instead by a layer of cartilage. Sometimes, however, and especially if there is little or no movement, the uniting medium is dense connective tissue. Various structures attach to bones and nearly always the actual uniting medium is dense connective tissue. Its fibres are continuous with those of the periosteum and they may also run into the bone tissue itself.

Bones are sometimes classified according to their shape. This is not an all-embracing classification and also it is difficult to be certain to which class some bones belong.

*Long bones.* These bones are found in the limbs and are rather like cylinders.

The humerus in the forelimb and the femur in the hindlimb are two examples. The ends or **extremities** are often expanded and are usually filled with spongy bone. The part of the bone between the extremities is the **shaft**, and this encloses a medullary cavity.

*Short bones.* These are many-sided and have similar dimensions in length, breadth and height. Short bones consist of the outer compact bone enclosing spongy bone, and do not have medullary cavities. Bones of the carpus (wrist) are in this category.

*Flat bones.* Flat bones consist of two layers of compact bone, usually very close together and separated by a small amount of spongy bone. Some of the bones of the head are flat bones and in these the spongy bone is also called the **diploë**.

*Irregular bones.* This term is used for the vertebrae. These do not fit any of the above classes. They are found in the midline of the body and like short bones, they consist of outer compact bone enclosing spongy bone. Their shape, as the name suggests, is irregular.

### Development of Bones

There is only one way in which bone tissue forms but there are two ways in which a bone as an organ may develop (p. 12). Direct formation within the connective tissue is intramembranous ossification; on to and gradually replacing a cartilage predecessor (which goes through a calcified stage) is endochondral ossification. Many of the bones of the skull develop by intramembranous ossification, whereas the bones of the limbs develop by endochondral ossification.

Some bones have one centre where ossification begins and the bone tissue is gradually added over the surface of the centre until the final shape is attained. In others there may be two or more centres and the bone tissue around each gradually merges and obliterates the original connecting material, whether it is dense connective tissue or cartilage. Often where centres of ossification are separated, the intervening tissue continues to reproduce itself. The distance between the original centres increases but the intervening tissue is being constantly replaced by bone tissue. This is an important method whereby bones grow, usually in length. The rate of bone deposition is ultimately faster than the rate of reproduction of the intervening tissue which gradually decreases in thickness. Eventually the entire intervening tissue may be replaced by bone which is then continuous between the adjacent original centres: they are then said to have **fused**.

This method of growth is especially important in long bones and also in some of the irregular bones (Fig. 1.8). The cartilaginous shaft of the very young bone is first replaced by bone tissue (Fig. 1.8 b,c). A centre of ossification then forms in one extremity, sometimes in both extremities, of the cartilaginous remainder of the bone (Fig. 1.8 d,e). Such a centre of ossification is called an **epiphysis**. The part between the epiphyses, that is, the shaft of a growing bone, is called the **diaphysis**. Between the diaphysis and each epiphysis there will be a plate of cartilage called the **growth plate** (you may hear it referred to as the epiphyseal cartilage or plate). The intervening tissue mentioned above will be cartilage in this case. As long as the cartilage cells in the growth plate continue to multiply, the bone will grow in length. When they cease, bone will gradually replace the cartilaginous growth plate and fusion will occur. (Fig. 1.8 f,g). This takes place in different bones and even in different parts of the same bone at different times; in other words, growth does not cease at the same time in all parts of the

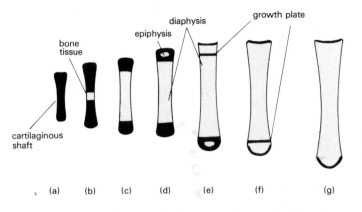

Fig. 1.8.  Development and growth of a long bone. (See text for full explanation.)

skeleton. There is quite a variation between different species; there is an appreciable difference between animals of the same species and even between littermates. After fusion is complete there appears to be a condensation of bone tissue at the site of the growth plate; this is called the **epiphysial line**.

## Cartilages

Many parts of the skeleton develop first as cartilage and this tissue is then replaced by bone. However, some parts remain as cartilage throughout the life of the animal. Sometimes, as the animal ages, the cartilage may become calcified: calcified cartilage is not bone.

## Joints

When two or more pieces of bone or cartilage are connected this is a joint. **Arthrosis** is another word for joint. We often refer to an arthrosis as an **articulation** and things relating to an arthrosis as **articular**. For instance, those surfaces of a bone that can actually appose in the articulation are the *articular surfaces*. We have, then, three words that can be used

for the connection of bones and/or cartilages; joint, arthrosis, articulation.

Joints have been classified in many different ways but the system which is receiving international recognition is that dependent on the tissue connecting the bones or the cartilages of the joint. The classes are then **fibrous, cartilaginous** and **synovial** joints.

*Fibrous joints.* The connecting medium is dense connective tissue. Many of the bones of the head are connected to each other in this way and here such joints are called **sutures**. Usually there is very little movement between the bones and/or cartilages of these joints, and they are sometimes known as *synarthroses*.

*Cartilaginous joints.* The connecting medium is cartilage and such a joint between corresponding bones on opposite sides of the body is a **symphysis**. This is the type of joint between the right and left sides of the pelvic floor.

Those cartilaginous joints that show little or no movement are sometimes also called synarthroses. If there is a reasonable amount of movement the joint may be called an *amphiarthrosis*. The bodies of most of the vertebrae are linked by amphiarthroses.

In both fibrous and cartilaginous joints, bone may eventually replace the dense

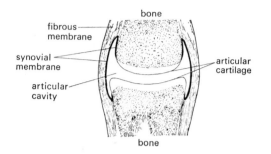

FIG. 1.9.  Section of a synovial joint between two bones. Normally there is no space between the articular cartilages.

connective tissue and the cartilage and unite the whole mass into a continuum of bone. Such an arrangement is a *synostosis.*

*Synovial joints* (Fig. 1.9). When these joints are cut, a small amount of fluid leaks out: this is called **synovia** or synovial fluid. The shoulder joint is one example of this class of articulation.

The articular surfaces in the synovial joint are always cartilage: even if the joint is basically between two bones, the contacting surfaces are covered by a layer of cartilage. The articular cartilages are never covered by perichondrium and they are only separated by the thin layer of synovia. The peripheries of the articular cartilages are connected by a dense connective tissue membrane, which, since it is responsible for the production of synovia, is called the **synovial membrane**. The membrane does not usually hold the surfaces tightly together but often pouches outward from the **articular cavity**. (Although the term cavity is used, there is actually no empty space in the joint. Only if the joint is damaged is it possible to separate the surfaces.) The synovial membrane may also merge with the periosteum of the bone supporting the articular cartilages. Dense connective tissue forms another layer outside the synovial membrane; as it is usually very fibrous it is called the **fibrous membrane**. The two

membranes are closely interconnected and together form the **articular** (or **joint**) **capsule**. Fibrous thickenings strengthen parts of the joint capsule: these are **ligaments** and usually run between the bones of the joint. The articular capsule attaches to the periosteum of the bones, or the perichondrium of the cartilages: so also will the ligaments and they will gain additional attachment by inserting into the bones or cartilages themselves.

Synovial joints are usually able to move more freely than fibrous or cartilaginous joints. They are sometimes called *diarthrodial joints.* In some situations in the skeleton the main joint is divided by an **articular disc** (or **articular meniscus**) of cartilage. The stifle joint has a pair of menisci side by side.

The articular disc (or meniscus) may be connected all round its periphery to the joint capsule and one has then, in effect, two articular cavities within the one main joint. In some the connection to the joint capsule is not complete and the articular cavities are in free communication.

*Movements in Joints*

The changes in position between the bones of a joint can be complex. The movements are generally approximately

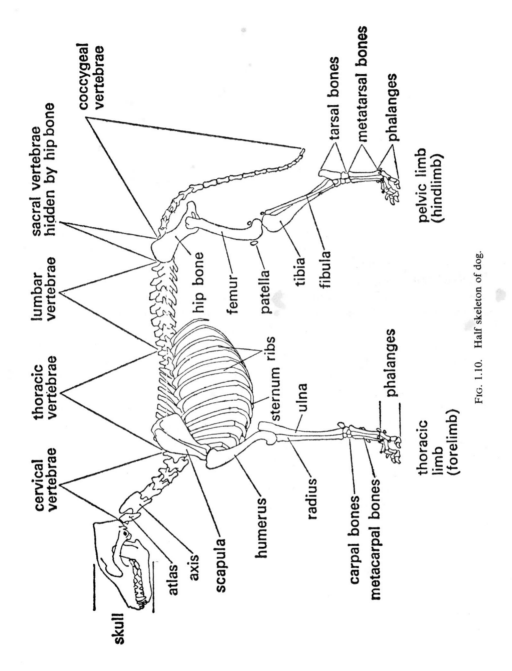

cervical vertebrae

thoracic vertebrae

lumbar vertebrae

sacral vertebrae hidden by hip bone

coccygeal vertebrae

tarsal bones

metatarsal bones

phalanges

pelvic limb (hindlimb)

hip bone

femur

patella

tibia

fibula

sternum ribs

ulna

phalanges

thoracic limb (forelimb)

carpal bones

metacarpal bones

radius

humerus

scapula

axis

atlas

skull

FIG. 1.10.   Half skeleton of dog.

classified into four types but any change in position is usually the result of a combination of these. When one articular surface slides over another this is a **gliding** movement. Altering the angle between two pieces of a joint is an **angular** movement: decreasing the angle is **flexion**, increasing the angle until the components are in a straight line is **extension**. **Rotation** takes place when one bone rotates round its longitudinal axis. In **circumduction**, one end of the bone is involved in the articulation, the other describes a circle or a segment of one.

**General arrangement of the bones and joints** (Fig. 1.10).

The skeleton may be divided into two major parts, axial and appendicular.

**Axial skeleton**: as the name suggests this part of the skeleton forms a straight line from end to end of the body. It includes the bones of the head (the skull), the bones of the vertebral column (the vertebrae) and the other bones of the thorax (the ribs and sternum).

**Appendicular skeleton**: this is the part of the skeleton in the limbs—those parts of the body that are attached or appended to the trunk.

**The axial skeleton**

*Skull* (Figs. 1.11–13)

Some dogs have long thin heads; they are classified as dolicocephalic and the Borzoi are good examples. Others, such as Bulldogs, have very short broad heads: these are brachycephalic. Dogs with heads of average length are mesaticephalic. Whatever the shape of the head, the skull will contain the same bones although their individual shapes will be different.

Part of the skull resembles a box with two joined tubes attached to one end. The box is the cranium, the tubes the nasal chambers. The mandibles (the bones of the lower jaw) and the hyoid apparatus are suspended from the cranium.

*Cranium.* The floor of the box can be considered to consist of two bones one behind the other in the midline of the head: the **occipital** and the **sphenoidal** bones. The latter is nearer to the nose.

The base of the occipital bone forms the floor of one end of the box. The actual end of the box consists mainly of a large hole

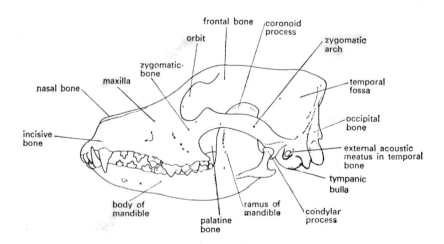

Fig. 1.11.   Average dog skull.

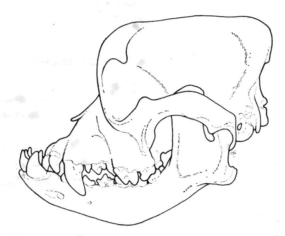

FIG. 1.12. Skull of brachycephalic (short-nosed) breed, such as Bulldog. It has the same bones as the average dog skull (FIG. 1.11) but they are shaped differently.

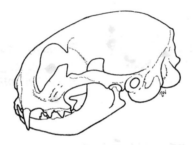

FIG. 1.13. Cat skull. The bones are the same as in the dog skull (FIG. 1.11) but they have different shapes.

(the **foramen magnum**) and the occipital bone forms the frame all round this hole.

An apparently solid pyramid of bone, forming part of the **temporal** bone, is wedged into the space between the side parts of the occipital bone and the caudal part of the sides of the sphenoid. The organs of balance and of hearing it contains need the protection of the thick bony tissue. On its outer surface is the external acoustic meatus, the opening to which the (external) ear is attached. The most ventral part of the temporal bone forms the **tympanic cavity**. This is a small bony chamber that connects with the middle ear and also with the external acoustic meatus. It has a very thin bony wall called the **tympanic bulla**.

Each side of the sphenoid is continued nearer the nose by a **frontal** bone and these form not only the walls in this region, but also part of the roof of the cranium. Each frontal bone is hollowed out and the space it contains is called the **frontal sinus**. This connects with the nasal chamber and is described in the section on the respiratory system.

The box is now nearly complete; at one end the occipital bone frames the foramen magnum. At the opposite end there is a flat plate of bone with two areas where there is a large number of holes. This bone gives the appearance of a sieve and it is called the **ethmoid** bone.

The space inside the box or cranium is the **cranial cavity** and in life it houses the brain. This part of the central nervous system will have nerve fibres flowing to and from it and will need a good blood supply and drainage. There are many holes, or foramina, in the boundaries of the cranial cavity for their passage. The brain is continuous with the other part of the central nervous system, the spinal cord, through the foramen magnum.

*Nasal chambers.* These have been described as two joined tubes and their common wall is the **nasal septum**. Much of this structure remains cartilaginous throughout life. It attaches to the midline of the ethmoid and its ventral border is strengthened by a grooved bar of bone. The floor and lateral wall of each tube are formed by three L-shaped bones; the **incisive** bone (sometimes called the premaxilla), the **maxilla** and the **palatine** bone. These bones are in line, with the palatine bone being nearest the cranium. The roof of each nasal chamber consists of the **nasal** bone.

The roots of the upper teeth are embedded in the incisive and the maxillary bones. The maxillary bone is also hollowed out and the space it contains is called the **maxillary sinus**. This connects with the nasal chamber and is described further under Respiratory System in Chapter 2 (p. 58).

All the bones of the nasal chambers are flat bones and are interconnected by sutures. The chambers are open-ended and slightly curved; they are far from being empty spaces. Attached to the ethmoid bone and to the lateral walls and roof of each nasal chamber there is a number of thin scrolls of delicate bone: these are the **conchae** and **turbinates**.

Two other small bones lie on either side of the skull, near the nasal chambers and the cranium, but forming an integral part of neither. The **lacrimal** bone is between the frontal bone, the palatine bone and the maxilla. The **zygomatic** bone (sometimes called malar or jugal bone) is bounded by the lacrimal bone and the maxilla and has a projection which joins with a similar spike from the temporal bone to form the *zygomatic arch*. In the dog and cat there is a ligament connecting this arch and the frontal bone. The connection divides the space into two parts: the region nearer the nose is the **orbit**, and the other part is the **temporal fossa**. The orbit houses the eye and its related structures, usually embedded in fat. Strong jaw muscles attach at one end to the walls of the temporal fossa and at the other end to the process of the mandible which projects into this region.

*Mandibles.* The bone of the lower jaw consists of right and left mandibles. They are joined only at the "chin". The articulating surfaces between them are rough and the projections and depressions of one side fit snugly into those of the other. They are bound together by fibrocartilage into a symphysis. Each mandible has a horizontal part, the **body**, and a vertical part, the **ramus**. Teeth are fixed in the body. The ramus has two strong processes: one, the **coronoid** process is normally in the temporal fossa and forms a point of attachment for the very strong muscle which helps to close the jaw; the other, the **condylar** process is caudal to the coronoid process and forms a synovial joint with the articular surface of the temporal bone. This temporomandibular joint is one that has a complete meniscus dividing the cavity into two parts; it forms the pivot for jaw movement. (Some people consider that the entire lower jaw is one bone, the mandible, consisting of right and left halves. There are reasons for both points of view.)

*Hyoid apparatus.* There are several parts of this, which collectively are also called the **hyoid** bone. It resembles a trapeze and each of its limbs is attached by a cartilaginous joint to the temporal bone. The tongue and the larynx are suspended by attachments to the bar of the trapeze.

### *Vertebral Column*

This is the collection of bones, the **vertebrae**, in the midline of the body, stretching from the skull to the end of the tail. The bones are classified as irregular and are divided into regions according to the part of the body in which they are found. **Cervical** in the neck, **thoracic** in the chest, **lumbar** in the loins, **sacral** in the croup, **coccygeal** (or **caudal**) in the tail. The bones in each region have characteristics similar to one another but different from those of other regions. Nevertheless, a basic plan can be recognized for all vertebrae.

### Basic Vertebra

The **body** of the vertebra (Fig. 1.14) is somewhat cylindrical; its ventral surface sometimes bears a single midline **ventral crest**. The dorsal surface is flattened and forms the floor of the **vertebral foramen**. The **arch** of the vertebra arises from either side of the body and completes the vertebral foramen. The vertebral foramina of a series of connected vertebrae together form the **vertebral canal** which houses the spinal cord and many blood vessels in their surrounding fat. Small **notches** in the cranial and caudal borders of the arch meet in the adjacent vertebrae to form the **intervertebral foramina**, through which nerves and blood vessels pass. The **spinous process** rises dorsally from the middle of the arch; it varies in shape and direction in the different vertebrae. There are a pair of **articular processes** on the cranial edge and a pair on the caudal edge of the arch. The articular processes of adjacent vertebrae forms synovial joints. The **transverse processes** are paired pieces of bone that project laterally from the junction of the body and the arch. The interior of a vertebra consists of closely arranged trabeculae of spongy bone interspersed by red marrow.

There is a pair of **intervertebral synovial joints** between the articular processes of

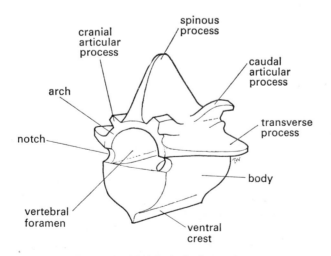

cranial
articular
process

spinous
process

caudal
articular
process

arch

transverse
process

notch

body

vertebral
foramen

ventral
crest

FIG. 1.14.　Model of a basic vertebra.

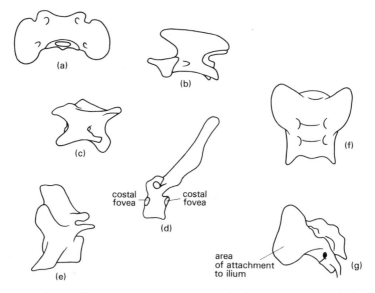

Fig. 1.15.  Vertebrae from different regions: (a) dorsal view of atlas; (b) axis; (c) cervical; (d) thoracic; (e) lumbar; (f) ventral view of sacrum; (g) left lateral view of sacrum. b-e are left lateral views.

adjacent vertebrae and an **interverte-bral disc** between the bodies. The discs are firmly attached to the vertebrae and consist of a very fibrous periphery, the **annulus fibrosus** and a softer more amorphous central part, the **nucleus pulposus**. There are also short ligaments running between two or three adjacent vertebrae and longer ligaments running between two or three regions of verte-brae.

Regional Differences

*Cervical vertebrae.* There are seven in all domestic mammals and the first two are very modified.

The first cervical vertebra is called the **atlas** (Fig. 1.15a) and it seems to consist only of a pair of large flattened transverse processes (sometimes called the *wings*) joined dorsally and ventrally to enclose a large vertebral foramen. The vertebra forms a pair of large synovial joints with articular surfaces of the occipital bone of the skull, supporting the head and allow-ing it to nod up and down. (This support-ing function is the reason for its name; Atlas was a mythical giant who supported the world on his shoulders.) The second cervical vertebra is the **axis** (Fig. 1.15b); it has a long body with a cranially projecting process, the **dens**. There are only synovial joints between the first and second cervi-cal vertebrae and these are so arranged that the head and the first cervical verte-bra pivot around the dens of the second cervical vertebra.

*Thoracic vertebrae.* There are usually thirteen or fourteen thoracic vertebrae in the dog and cat. They are characterized by tall spinous processes and also articular depressions or fovea on each side of the cranial and caudal surfaces of the body. Since the function of the depressions of adjacent vertebrae is to clasp and to make a synovial joint with the head of a rib they are called **costal foveae**. (Each one is a fovea. "Costal" is an adjective used in phrases referring to a rib.) In addition, the transverse process also makes a synovial joint with the rib, this time with its tuberculum.

*Lumbar vertebrae.* There are six or seven lumbar vertebrae and these have large flat laterally projecting transverse processes.

*Sacral vertebrae.* The dog and cat usually have three. The bodies and the arches fuse together to form one mass which is often called the **sacrum**. This is a wedge-shaped bone with lateral parts that form a firm **sacro-iliac** joint (usually cartilaginous) with the ilium of the pelvic girdle.

*Coccygeal (caudal) vertebrae.* The number of these will vary tremendously depending on the length of the tail. They decrease in size and become quite regular so that the terminal few are like small rods of bone. A dog which has had its tail amputated is said to be *docked.* Rarely is this necessary for the well being of the animal: it is more commonly done to subserve owners' ideas of fashion. (Coccy-geal vertebrae are sometimes called caudal vertebrae.)

*Ribs.* These elongated bones form the walls of the bony thorax (Fig. 1.16). There is one pair of ribs for each thoracic vertebra. One end of each rib articulates with the vertebral column and so one can talk of the vertebral extremity. This has a **head** which for most ribs forms a synovial joint with the costal foveae of adjacent vertebrae. The head is on the end of a **neck** and adjacent to this is the **tuberculum** which forms a synovial joint with the transverse process of the thoracic vertebra. The other extremity of the rib articulates with the sternum. This sternal extremity is cartilaginous and although strictly the whole organ from the vertebral column to the sternum is a rib it is common to consider the bony part to be the rib and talk of the remainder as the **costal cartilage**.

Not all the ribs articulate directly with

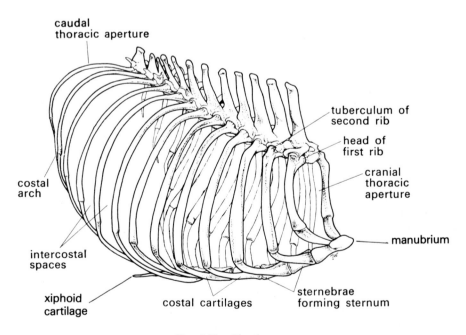

caudal thoracic aperture

tuberculum of second rib

head of first rib

cranial thoracic aperture

costal arch

manubrium

intercostal spaces

xiphoid cartilage

costal cartilages

sternebrae forming sternum

FIG. 1.16.   The thorax.

the sternum; those that do are called **true** (sternal) ribs; the others, more caudal, are **false** or asternal. The costal cartilages of the false ribs overlap and are attached to each other and so indirectly to the sternum. The line of the last rib and these overlapping cartilages forms the **costal arch**. There is no medullary cavity in a rib. The interior is filled with spongy bone packed with red marrow.

*Sternum.* The sternum completes the thorax ventrally. It is an axial structure, composed of a line of bones or **sternebrae**, which mostly articulate with each other by a series of cartilaginous joints. Internally they resemble vertebrae. The first sternebra is larger than the others and is known as the **manubrium**. The last one is flattened and is called the **xiphoid process** (or xiphisternum): it is made longer by a thin **xiphoid cartilage** which projects even further caudally. The costal cartilages form synovial joints with the sternum.

Thoracic Cavity

The thorax (Fig. 1.16) consists of the thoracic vertebrae dorsally, the sternum ventrally and the ribs and costal cartilages laterally. The gaps between the adjacent ribs are **intercostal spaces**. The **cranial thoracic aperture** (the inlet) is formed by the first thoracic vertebra, the first pair of ribs and the sternum. The **caudal thoracic aperture** (the outlet) is formed by the last thoracic vertebra, the costal arch (including the last pair of ribs) and the sternum. As the cranial thoracic aperture is much smaller than the caudal thoracic aperture the **thoracic cavity** is irregularly conical in shape with the dorsal wall much longer than the ventral.

**The appendicular skeleton**

*The Thoracic Limb*

There is no bony connection between the thoracic limb and the trunk. The attachment is solely by muscles. These run between the scapula and humerus of the limb, and the head, neck and thorax of the trunk. During movement the scapula moves slightly over the wall of the thorax and pivots round an area rather than any specific point.

*Scapula.* This is a flat bone which is closely applied to the thorax. Its outer (lateral) surface is divided into two areas by a well-marked spine (Fig. 1.17). The end which forms the synovial joint (the shoulder joint) with the humerus is expanded into the **glenoid cavity**.

*Clavicle.* The cat has only a thin sliver of bone and the clavicle is also vestigial in the dog. In both species it lies buried in a muscle running between the forelimb and the head and neck, over the point of the shoulder.

*Humerus.* This is the bone of the upper arm. The proximal extremity of this long bone has a convex articular **head** which is part of the shoulder joint. This synovial joint has no well-marked ligaments. It is normally kept in place by the surrounding muscles and although it allows movements in all directions, they are chiefly flexion and extension. The *point of the shoulder* is formed by a process of bone, the **major tubercle**, which lies craniolateral to the articular head. The distal extremity is transversely cylindrical forming the **condyle** of the humerus: this forms part of the synovial **elbow joint**.

*Radius.* This and the ulna are the two forearm bones. The radius is a long bone that articulates proximally with the humerus in the elbow joint (Fig. 1.18) and distally with the carpus. It is the medial of the two forearm bones.

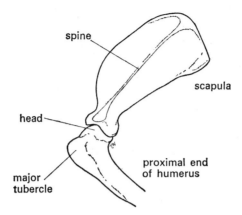

FIG. 1.17. Shoulder joint.

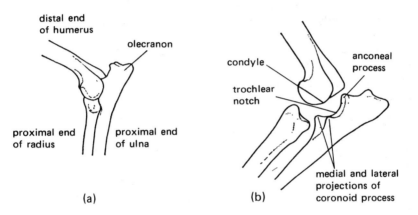

FIG. 1.18. Elbow joint: (a) bones in natural position; (b) bones separated.

*Ulna.* The proximal end is the **olecranon**, which forms the *point of the elbow* and on its cranial edge the bone has a semicircular **trochlear notch** (Fig. 1.18b). Into this fits the condyle of the humerus to help with the radius in forming the elbow joint. The proximal end of the notch is the **anconeal process**. The distal end is the **coronoid process**; this is forked producing a lateral and a medial projection. The ulna of the dog and cat is closely applied to the radius, but it is able to rotate around this bone, being attached to it by muscle tissue. The elbow joint is formed by the condyle of the humerus fitting into the

trochlea notch of the ulna and being supported by the proximal end of the radius. There are very strong ligaments on the lateral and medial sides of the joint and these, together with the shapes of the bones, restrict movement to flexion and extension.

*Carpus.* This corresponds to the wrist of the human and this term may also be used for the carpus of the dog and cat. There are several short carpal bones arranged in two rows. All the joints between them are synovial and so also are those between the upper row and the bones of the forearm, and between the lower row and the metacarpus. Most of the movement of this series of complex joints takes place between the upper row of the carpal bones and the forearm bones; some takes place between the proximal and distal rows. Mostly it is flexion and extension, but a small amount of lateral movement is possible. Some rotation can also take place and enables the animal to turn the paw so that it can lick the undersurface. This movement of the distal part of the limb is *supination.* Movement in the opposite direction is *pronation.*

*Metacarpus.* In the typical mammal there are five metacarpal bones which are numbered one to five, the most medial being the first. The dog and cat are near to the typical but even here the first metacarpal bone is very reduced.

The proximal end of each metacarpal bone is flattened and forms the synovial joint with the lower row of carpal bones. There is however very little movement at this joint. The distal end of each metacarpal bone is transversely cylindrical with a sagittal ridge on the articular surface. The synovial joint between this bone and the proximal phalanx of the digit has strong lateral ligaments. Only flexion and exten-

sion are possible. Each main metacarpal has a pair of very small sesamoid bones at the distal end of the palmar surface. They are included in the articulation between the metacarpal and phalangeal bone.

*Digits.* For every complete metacarpal bone there is a complete set of three phalangeal bones, a proximal, a middle and a distal (see Fig. 1.32). These correspond to the bones in the human fingers. The proximal phalanx has a concave proximal extremity and a convex distal extremity. The middle phalanx resembles the proximal except that it is a shorter bone. The distal phalanx conforms roughly to the shape of the claw which covers it in life.

The development of the phalanx for the reduced first metacarpal bone is variable. However, the dog and cat usually have a *dewclaw* related to the first digit.

The joints between proximal and middle, and middle and distal phalanges are synovial and are called the toe joints. All have strong lateral ligaments and are only able to flex and extend.

The fore-paw is the equivalent of the human hand and includes the carpus, metacarpus and digits.

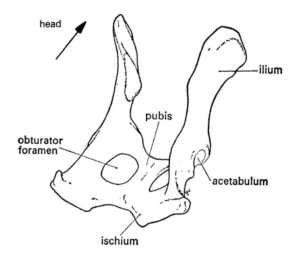

FIG. 1.19.  The hip bones of a dog viewed from behind and slightly to the right of the animal.

*The Pelvic Limb*

The bony pelvis is composed of the pair of hip (coxal) bones joined at the midline symphysis, the sacrum and the first few coccygeal bones.

*Hip bone.* Each consists of the **ilium**, the **ischium** and the **pubis** (Fig. 1.19). These are all flat bones and they meet together in an articular cavity, the **acetabulum**, into which fits the head of the femur to form the **hip joint**. The centre of the acetabulum has no articular cartilage and is called the **acetabular fossa** (Fig. 1.20b).

Most of the ilium is vertical and it forms a mainly cartilaginous joint, the sacro-iliac articulation, with the lateral parts of the sacrum. The floor of the pelvis is formed on each side by the pubis cranially and the ischium caudally. The floor is incomplete and has a large hole on each side of the midline; this is the **obturator foramen**. The ischium also forms a part of the low side-walls of the pelvis caudal to the acetabulum. The ilium, pubis and ischium fuse together quite early in life and the right and left sides meet at the midline to form a symphysis. Later in life this gradually ossifies and the hip bones fuse together. There is a ligament of dense connective tissue between the sacrum and the ischium (**sacro-tuberal ligament**).

The ventral part of the body of the sacrum, the medial surface of the iliac bones, and the dorsal aspect of the pubic bones form a ring which is the **cranial pelvic aperture** (pelvic inlet). The **caudal pelvic aperture** (pelvic outlet) is formed dorsally by the ventral part of the caudal end of the sacrum, laterally by the sacro-tuberal ligaments and ventrally by the dorsal aspect of the ischial bones.

*Femur.* This is the bone of the thigh. It is a long bone with a rounded **head** proximally, which fits into the acetabulum to form the **hip joint** (Fig. 1.20). Like all synovial joints this has a joint capsule: it runs between the rim of the acetabulum and the neck of the bone joining the head to the rest of the femur. There is also a ligament of the head of the femur (sometimes called the *teres* or the *round* ligament) which runs from a firm attachment on the rounded articular head of the femur to the non-articular acetabular fossa. The muscles surrounding the hip joint are mainly responsible for holding the femoral head firmly in the acetabulum in the normal animal. Although it would appear that this arrangement allows a wide range of movement, the hip joint usually only flexes and extends. There are roughened processes for muscular attach-

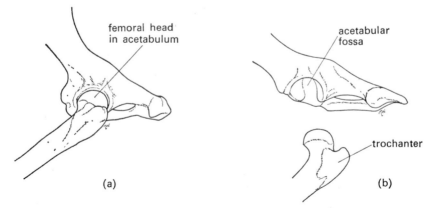

FIG. 1.20. The hip joint: (a) bones in natural position; (b) bones separated.

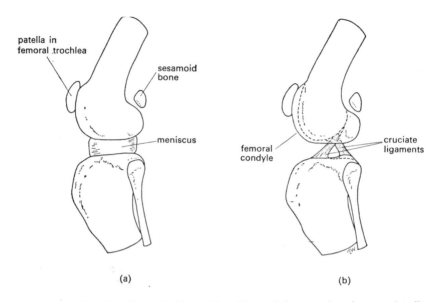

patella in
femoral trochlea

sesamoid
bone

meniscus

femoral
condyle

cruciate
ligaments

(a)

(b)

Fig. 1.21.   Stifle joint: (a) with menisci in position; (b) menisci removed to show cruciate ligaments.

ment near the head which are called **trochanters**. At the distal end, a pair of articular **condyles** take part in the formation of the **stifle** (knee) joint (Fig. 1.21). Just proximal to the condyles and merging with them the **trochlea** of the femur forms a gutter for the **patella** (knee-cap). This is a **sesamoid** bone; that is, a bone formed in a muscle or its tendon to assist its passage over another piece of bone. There are also sesamoid bones in the muscles on the side of the femur opposite to the patella. However, these are very much smaller.

*Tibia and fibula.* It is convenient to deal with these two leg bones together. The tibia is the main bone and is medial to the fibula. In the dog and cat the fibula is a complete bone but is much finer than the tibia.

The proximal end of the tibia is flattened and helps form the stifle joint with the femur. There is a pair of fibrocartilaginous **menisci** between the femoral condyles and the articular surface of the tibia. There is also a pair of strong **cruciate** ligaments which help to stabilize

this synovial joint. One is attached cranially between the femoral condyles and caudally on to the head of the tibia: the other is attached opposite to this and so they cross (hence the name, which means crossing).

The distal end of the tibia forms a synovial joint with one of the tarsal bones. To conform to this the tibia has a pair of rather deep articular grooves, separated by a ridge.

*Tarsus.* There are several tarsal bones. They all form parts of synovial joints but the one in which there is most movement is that between the **talus** (astragalus) and the tibia. This tarsal bone has a **trochlea** which conforms very well indeed to the distal end of the tibia. The **calcaneus** (os calcis) is closely associated with the talus; it has a distinct process for muscle attachment which forms the *point of the hock.* The talus and the calcaneus can be considered to form the proximal row of tarsal bones. The distal row resembles those in the corresponding position in the carpus, forming a fairly level row to

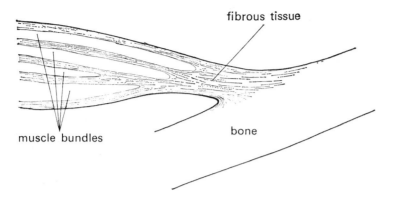

fibrous tissue

muscle bundles

bone

FIG. 1.22. The attachment of a muscle to a bone. Notice that it is the fibrous tissue which forms the attachment and that this runs into the bone.

articulate with the proximal end of the metatarsal bones and being quite firmly attached to them. One tarsal bone is found between the proximal and the distal rows: this is the **central** tarsal bone. It is also known as the scaphoid bone and seems prone to fracture in the racing greyhound.

The whole region of the distal end of the tibia, the tarsus and the proximal end of the metatarsus is called the **hock joint**: but since nearly all the movement (predominantly flexion and extension) takes place between the tibia and the talus this part of the joint is sometimes said to be the "true hock joint".

*Metatarsus and digits.* The bones of the remainder of the hind limb are sufficiently similar to those of the corresponding region of the thoracic limb that separate descriptions are unnecessary. The hindpaw is the equivalent of the human foot and consists of the tarsus, metatarsus and digits.

## Skeletal Muscles

The structure of a skeletal muscle has been outlined with the connective tissue binding the cells into bundles and the bundles into muscles enclosed in a muscle sheath (p. 3). This interweaving connective tissue continues the line of the muscle fibres as a rope-like tendon or a sheet-like aponeurosis. It is this fibrous connective tissue that forms the attachment of a skeletal muscle to another structure; the muscle cells themselves do not come into direct contact with the organs (Fig. 1.22). However, there may sometimes be little fibrous tissue and then one talks of a "fleshy", as opposed to a "tendinous", attachment. The point of attachment which moves least when the muscle contracts is often termed the **origin**: the opposite end is the **insertion**. This is not entirely satisfactory and in the limbs, for instance, the more proximal end is usually called the origin. For muscles between the trunk and the limbs the more medial attachment is often termed the origin. With some muscles the term **belly** is used for the swollen part; the tapered origin is then the **head**.

One tends to think of skeletal muscles as only causing movements at a joint. However, in addition to this important function, they may have many other uses, as the following examples will show. Complete limbs are moved; softer structures, such as the eyeball and the outer part of the ear, are reorientated; the skin is twitched; apertures, such as that between the eyelids, may be closed by circular **sphincter** muscles; the entire mass of abdominal organs is supported by the muscular body wall.

It is as well to realize, also, that a muscle may be called upon to perform more than one function. Perhaps this is best illustrated by the fact that, although so far the emphasis has been on movement, one of the most important duties of a muscle is to keep a structure still. For instance, a limb is kept rigid, and so an animal is supported, by muscles on opposite sides of the limb-joints exerting forces which balance each other. No movement as such, but a necessary use of skeletal muscles.

**Muscle contraction**

Contraction is controlled by motor nerve impulses passing from the central nervous system through hundreds of nerve fibres that enter the muscle belly. After entry, each nerve fibre splits up and innervates very small bundles of muscle fibres distributed throughout the muscle. If the muscle is used for delicate movements the number of muscle fibres supplied by each nerve fibre may be very small, perhaps only about ten: for gross movement many more muscle fibres, 200 or more, may be innervated by each fibre. All the muscle fibres innervated by a single nerve fibre form a **motor unit**.

When a muscle fibre contracts it does so to its maximum: it cannot contract partly. At the same time all the muscle fibres in that unit will contract, but since they are spread throughout the muscle, innervation of only one unit will result in an overall weak contraction. Stimulation of all the motor units in the muscle will result in maximum contraction. Grading of the contraction is achieved by varying the number of motor units innervated at any one time.

If the ends of a muscle are brought closer together when it is stimulated the contraction is said to be **isotonic** and this is common during movement. Sometimes a muscle is tensed but not shortened: this often happens while standing and the contraction is **isometric**.

Muscles are usually in a slight state of tension: this is called **muscle tone** and is accomplished by a few nerve impulses continually leaving the central nervous system. Any additional stimulus will provoke a more rapid reaction. The rate of nerve impulses, and hence the muscle tone, is increased during fear and anxiety. The animal becomes apprehensive ("jumpy" or "nervy") and may react violently to any additional stimulus. The rate of tonic impulses is reduced during sleep and muscles become more relaxed.

The more a muscle is used, the more it increases in size and strength: when the nerve supply is destroyed, however, the muscle fibres degenerate and the muscle withers and atrophies.

The complex chemical reactions of muscle contraction demand a ready source of energy and also a plentiful supply of free calcium ions. The reactions are quite inefficient and only about a quarter of the energy goes into mechanical work; the remaining three-quarters appear as heat, an occurrence that can be very embarrassing to the animal during prolonged or intense muscle activity.

*Muscles of the Head*

These can be intrinsic (muscles within the head region altering the position of parts of the head) or extrinsic (muscles altering the entire head in relation to the rest of the body).

The lower jaw pivots at the temporomandibular joint. There are very strong intrinsic muscles for closing the jaws; the

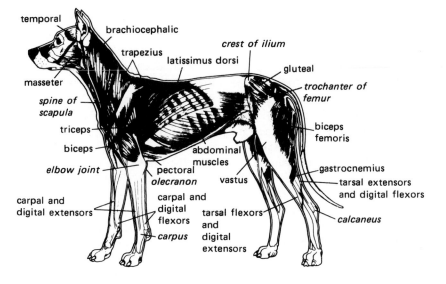

FIG. 1.23. Superficial muscles of the dog. Names in italics refer to bony features.

one in the temporal fossa (the temporal muscle) has been mentioned in the description of the skull and there are others between the upper jaw and the bodies of the mandibles such as the masseter muscle (Fig. 1.23). It is important that the jaws can be closed strongly and held tightly shut: they can be opened by relaxation of the "jaw-closing" muscles, but there are some relatively weak ones that can help by contraction.

There are several intrinsic muscles that adjust the lips, nostrils, eyelids, and ears: these are sometimes grouped as "muscles of expression". Special eye muscles within the orbit control the eyeball and muscles between the mandibles merge into the tongue.

Extrinsic muscles attach to the occipital bone and to the vertebral column dorsal to the transverse processes. These will tend to tilt the head dorsally, with the point of fulcrum being the synovial joint between the occipital bone and the atlas. Muscles running ventral to the transverse processes and to the sternum will depress the head. There are also laterally placed muscles.

All extrinsic muscles of the head harmonize to provide it with a wide range of movement.

## Muscles of the Trunk

These can be grouped into three: vertebral (spinal) muscles, the diaphragm, abdominal muscles.

*Vertebral muscles.* These attach to the vertebrae, ribs and ilium. Sometimes the end attachments are only one or two vertebrae apart, sometimes many vertebrae separate them. There is a lot of intermingling between the bundles that form this group, making it difficult to isolate specific muscles. However, those that run between adjacent ribs form an important part of the thoracic wall and are called **intercostal muscles**.

Vertebral muscles lying dorsal to the transverse processes are called **epaxial**, those lying ventral are **hypaxial**. The cervical vertebral column can be said to be ventrally concave, the thoraco-lumbar region dorsally concave. The epaxial muscles will increase the ventral concavity of the cervical region and decrease the dorsal concavity of the thoraco-lumbar region. By combination of actions the trunk can also be curved laterally to the left or right. The muscles attaching to the thorax may be used during respiration.

*Diaphragm.* This is a very important skeletal muscle and is found near the mid-point of the trunk. Its attachment to the ventral surfaces of the bodies of the lumbar vertebrae is by a pair of thickened muscle bundles called **crura** (singular **crus**). These run cranially and at the last thoracic vertebra spread out as a sheet stretching over the entire caudal thoracic aperture (thoracic outlet). It attaches all round its periphery to the ribs; dorsally, just cranial to the costal arch and ventrally, to the caudal end of the sternum. In this way the thoracic cavity is separated off from the remainder of the trunk. The cavity thus formed caudal to the dia-phragm is the *abdominal cavity*. The diaphragm does not run the shortest distance between these attachments: in the midline it bulges cranially, to take the shape of a dome. It does have a few foramina for the passage of structures between the thoracic and the abdominal cavities. In life the central parts of the diaphragm are continually moving to vary the size of the thoracic cavity and so play a major role in respiratory movements.

*Abdominal muscles.* There are several muscles concerned in forming the abdo-minal wall on each side of the body. They have to be strong and well arranged to support the contents of this cavity. The muscle fibres extend for about half the length of the muscle which is continued by a strong fibrous aponeurosis; this meets its fellow of the opposite side ventrally in the midline stretching cranially from the ster-num and caudally reaching to the pubis.

The left and right aponeuroses of most of the abdominal muscles meet at the midline and here the fibrous tissue is fused to form a strong seam which extends from the sternum to the pelvis and is called the **linea alba** (white line). The attachment to the pubis is called the **prepubic tendon**. The aponeuroses do intermingle to a certain extent other than at the midline.

The supportive action of these abdomi-nal muscles has been mentioned. In addi-tion they have the important function in the dog and cat of increasing the dorsal concavity of the thoraco-lumbar part of the vertebral column by drawing the sternum and the pubis closer together: this is part of their method of locomotion.

### Muscles of the Limbs (Fig. 1.23)

These can also be divided into extrinsic and intrinsic muscles. The extrinsic ones run between the trunk and the limbs, the intrinsic ones between the bones of the appendicular skeleton of each limb.

*Extrinsic limb muscles.* In the descrip-tion of the skeletal system it was men-tioned that the forelimb pivoted in the region of the scapula. The hindlimb pivots at the hip joint. If the lower part of the limb is drawn cranially it is said to be **protracted** (Fig. 1.24) and the protractor muscles attach on the trunk cranial to the limb and on the limb ventral to the pivot. Alternatively they can be attached on the limb dorsal to the pivot and on the trunk caudal to the limb. **Retraction** is the action of drawing the lower part of the limb caudally and the attachments of retractor muscles will be opposite to the protractors. Retraction and protraction are very important actions in locomotion (movement from place to place) and muscles acting about the pivot points of the entire limbs are very strong. Fortu-nately they are rarely damaged and conse-quently receive rather less attention than some of the intrinsic limb muscles.

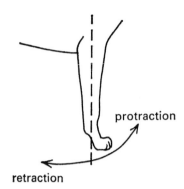

F<small>IG</small>. 1.24.   Protraction and retraction of a forelimb.

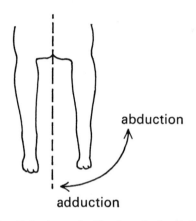

F<small>IG</small>. 1.25.   Abduction and adduction of a forelimb.

If the entire lower limb is brought nearer to the midline it is said to be **adducted** (Fig. 1.25). Adductor muscles are attached to the trunk and to the limb ventral to the pivot point. **Abductor** muscles have the opposite effect and have their attachments dorsal to the pivots.

There is a considerable overlap of action of these extrinsic muscles. Several can both protract and adduct, for instance, and contraction of separate parts of one muscle may cause both protraction and retraction at different times.

*Intrinsic limb muscles.* These cause the flexion and extension of the limb joints described in the skeletal system. Some of the muscles affect one joint only, being attached to the two components of that joint, whereas others, whose attachments are further apart, may have an effect on each joint over which they pass.

It is more important to know the action of the muscles than their names and the convention that is applied to intrinsic muscles is shown in the accompanying diagram (Fig. 1.26). When the bones are brought together as shown, the joints are considered to flex. The opposite action is extension. In describing the action of the muscle it should refer to the effect at each joint it controls. It is possible for the same muscle to flex one joint and extend another: a good example is the muscle attached to the proximal end of the tibia

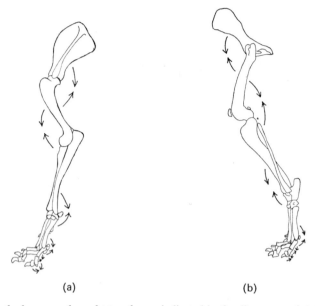

FIG. 1.26.    When the bones are brought together as indicated in the diagram, each joint is said to flex: (a) forelimb; (b) hindlimb.

and to the distal phalanges. On contraction this could flex the hock but it can extend the toe joints. It is not essential that these two actions should occur. Opposing muscles can ensure that one joint is kept still while the other is moved.

Because of their attachments, the protractor and retractor muscles of the forelimb can extend and flex the shoulder joint and similarly those of the hindlimb can effect the hip joint.

*Muscle of the Skin*

The skin over various parts of the bodies of domestic mammals can be made to move or twitch. This is achieved by contractions of the **cutaneous muscle**, a thin layer that is widely distributed in the superficial fascia. It is only attached to the skeleton in a few places and the connective tissue between the muscle cells is continuous with that of the dermis and hypodermis.

**Special arrangements**

A whole variety of muscles has now been described, some with short fibrous attachments, others with vast aponeuroses. Sometimes the muscle takes origin from two or more sites: likewise there may be more than one insertion, the end of the tendon being split. Some of the limb muscles have very long tendons, the muscle belly being near the proximal end of the limb and the insertion being at the distal end.

Long tendons running beside bones are sometimes covered with fascia which is attached to the bone. Such an arrangement of dense fibrous tissue is a **retinaculum** (sometimes called an annular or vaginal ligament).

Several muscles, especially those with long tendons, have special modifications where they pass over skeletal prominences, whether this is in the normal position of the bones or as a result of movement at a joint. The bony prominence usually has a

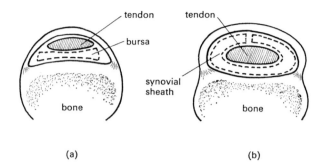

FIG. 1.27. (a) A bursa between bone and a tendon; (b) a synovial sheath wrapping round a tendon.

cartilage covering and the tendon may thicken and itself contain cartilage. In some muscles a small bone may develop at the point of contact, especially where there is a slight change of direction. Such a structure is a **sesamoid** bone and it may form in the fleshy part of the muscle or in the tendon. The part of the sesamoid that faces the prominence is covered with cartilage (in keeping with the arrangement that moving parts of a bone are covered with cartilage) and the opposing surfaces form part of the synovial joint. All the sesamoid bones are closely related to joints between larger limb bones. The joint cavity between the sesamoid bone and the bony prominence is in free communication with the joint cavity of the major limb bones. The synovial membrane is continuous around the periphery of the articular surfaces of the main bones and of the sesamoid bones.

In some joints the synovial membrane also pouches out to lie between tendons and the extremities of bones. These extensions of the cavity are called **bursal elongations**.

Similar to these, and often, but not always, separate from a joint cavity, structures called **bursae** lie between tendons and the bone (Fig. 1.27a). The lining of the bursa secretes the small amount of synovial fluid and the effect is that of a fluid-containing cushion minimizing pressure and friction. These functions may be useful in situations other than between tendons and bones; for instance, bursae are also found between the skin and bony prominences at sites where pressure and friction occur. The loose connective tissue in these regions becomes more open in texture and eventually a sac is formed, with the local cells capable of producing the small amount of synovial fluid that is required to form the cushion. Sometimes abnormal or excessive pressure and friction cause the formation of a bursa in an unusual place: this is called an *adventitial bursa*.

If one imagines the bursa to wrap all around the tendon, the structure so produced is a **synovial sheath** (Fig. 1.27b), and several of these occur at the carpal and tarsal joints.

Joints, bursae and tendon sheaths all have a lining synovial membrane. This consists mainly of intercellular substances such as collagen with cells in among the fibres. The synovial membrane, although it is lining a cavity, is not therefore an epithelial membrane, which is a continuous sheet of cells fitting tightly together.

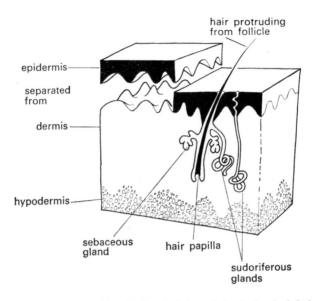

FIG. 1.28.    A section of skin showing epidermis, dermis, hair and glands. On the left the epidermis is shown as if it could be accurately separated from the rest of the skin.

### The Integument

The integument is the covering of the body. In addition to protecting the animal mechanically, it is a sensory structure, conveying information on pain, touch and pressure as well as about the temperature of the environment. It forms a barrier against the inward penetration of many chemical agents (including water) and also reduces their escape outwards. Since epithelium is the tissue that forms a covering layer, the outermost part of the integument consists of epithelial cells. There are several layers of these constituting the **epidermis**; over most of the body this is quite elastic and forms part of the **skin** (Fig. 1.28). The surface cells of the epidermis of the skin die and become dry and hard. As these superficial cells have a very high content of the protein *keratin*, they are said to be *keratinized* or *cornified*. There are some regions of the body where extra protection is needed and here there is a vast increase in the amount of keratin. In this way claws are formed to protect the ends of digits (horns, used as weapons, are produced in the same way). These may be described as *modified epidermal structures*; the fundamental difference between these and skin is the increase in proportion and amount of keratinization.

The epidermis, whether it is relatively lightly keratinized as in the skin, or heavily keratinized as in a claw, is avascular (has no blood supply). It is firmly attached to the underlying **dermis** (Fig. 1.28) which consists of irregular dense connective tissue carrying blood vessels and nerve fibres. The **hypodermis** is deep to the dermis; it may also be called the **subcutis** and is actually the superficial fascia formed of loose connective tissue.

The epidermis and dermis together constitute the skin. In addition to the functions already mentioned, the skin, often helped by an underlying layer of fat, plays an important role in temperature control by acting as a blanket to conserve heat.

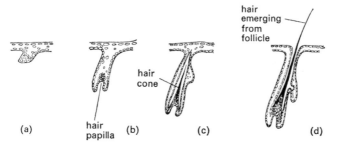

FIG. 1.29.  Formation of a hair.

## Epidermis

The epidermis of the skin consists of two main layers. The deeper layer is very closely attached to the dermis. By the active reproduction of its cells, more layers are formed which are gradually pushed towards the surface. The more superficial cells contain an increasing proportion of keratin and constitute the *cornified layer.*

The surface adjacent to the dermis is pitted and furrowed, with dermis fitting into all the holes and undulations that this forms. In addition to this irregular surface some epidermal structures such as hairs and glands project much further into the dermis.

## Hairs

Hairs are epidermal structures formed by the epidermis thickening and extending down into the dermis (Fig. 1.29a). The deeper end flows over a knob of dermis which is then called the **hair papilla** (Fig. 1.29b). The epithelial cells immediately over the papilla produce a central **hair cone** which eventually forms the hair (Fig. 1.29c). The cells around the point of the cone disintegrate and make a canal which the growing hair uses to reach the surface of the skin. The canal opens on to the surface and can then be called the **hair follicle** (Fig. 1.29d). The cells of the deeper layer of the epidermis continue to produce the hair shaft while the hair grows. When this ceases that particular hair dies in its follicle. At any time after this it may fall from the skin, that is, it may be *shed.* The deep epidermal cells may by then be producing another hair as a replacement.

Small numbers of hairs group together to share common openings on the surface of the hairy skin of dogs. One hair in the bundle is larger and stiffer than the others and is called a **cover** or **guard** hair: the smaller, softer hairs in the bundle are **under** hairs. The number of hairs in the bundle varies with the type of hair coat.

Hairs are most common on the dorsal and lateral sides of the dog and cat but there are few inside the flanks, on the abdomen, or under the tail. There are no hairs around the nostrils nor on the foot pads but long sensory hairs (**vibrissae**) are found for instance on the sides of the nose and above the eyelids.

The hair coat is thicker in winter than in summer which is when some of it is normally shed: however, in house pets there is a tendency for shedding to occur throughout the year. It does not grow very quickly in the summer, but when the cool weather begins the rate increases. During

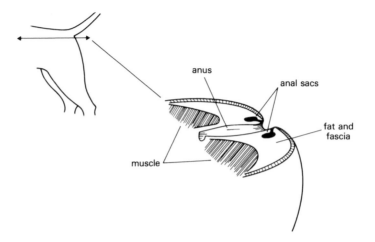

FIG. 1.30.   Section of pelvic region of a dog to show position of the anal sacs.

active growth, about a millimetre of hair shaft is produced each week by the hair follicle. The hair coat gives good protection against cuts and abrasions and the layer of air trapped by the hair assists the insulating properties of the skin to control heat loss from the body.

Cutaneous Glands

Some of the epithelial cells of the wall of the hair follicle proliferate and form glandular masses which surround the follicle and open into it (Fig. 1.28). These masses are **sebaceous** glands and their secretion, called **sebum**, keeps the skin and hair pliable and is also a protection against both drying and moisture. **Sudoriferous** or **sweat** glands may also open into the hair follicle, developing from the epithelium between the sebaceous glands and the surface of the integument. Glands may fail to function adequately during illness and malnutrition: the hair coat then becomes dull and dry. Sebum and sweat also contain some of the excretory waste of the body. The glands of some regions produce odoriferous substances which

may be influential in reproductive behaviour. In some animals sweat production plays an important role in temperature control but not to any significant degree in the dog and cat.

There is an opening on either side of the anus, where the terminal end of the digestive tube joins the skin, which leads into an **anal sac** (also called **para-anal sinus**) (Fig. 1.30). These paired cavities vary from about the size of a pea in cats and small dogs up to as large as a walnut in bigger animals. The secretory glands lining these pockets of integument produce an unpleasant smelling sticky liquid which is stored in the sacs and intermittently evacuated. The openings may occasionally become blocked and the animal will show symptoms of irritation and annoyance.

*Mammary glands* (Fig. 1.31). These are another group of modified cutaneous glands and their function is to produce milk. There are usually eight to twelve arranged as pairs on either side of the midline, extending from about the fourth rib to the region of the pubis. They are most obvious in the female, especially towards the end of pregnancy and during

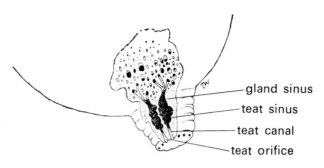

FIG. 1.31.   Section of a mammary gland.

and after suckling. Rudimentary structures are present in the male.

Each gland is provided with a conical teat (nipple) bearing several openings, ranging in number between about eight and sixteen. The secretory epithelium of the gland is embedded in a mass of connective tissue which varies in its nature with the age and condition of the animal. The secretions collect in dilatations called **gland sinuses**; these are drained by **teat sinuses** occupying most of the teat. Nearer the apex of the teat, the sinuses narrow to become **teat canals** that open as the **teat orifices**.

The production of milk is **lactation** and this is usually associated with the nursing of the young progeny. During pregnancy the glandular material increases in amount and size and the first milk associated with each pregnancy is called **colostrum**. This contains many substances that are vital to the new-born: after a few days the proportion of proteins, lactose (milk sugar), minerals and small fat globules changes and then stays fairly constant for the rest of the lactation.

### Dermis

This may be called *corium* and is a dense feltwork of connective tissue fibres with blood vessels and nerves freely scattered in its substance. The dermis is continuous throughout the body, whether it is deep to the skin or to modified epidermal structures. Hair follicles and glands form downgrowths into its substance and the dermis forms ridges, bumps and papillae into the under-surface of the epidermis. There are many smooth muscle cells in the dermis, especially related to the hair follicles: these can alter the slope of the hair relative to the skin surface.

### Hypodermis

This is very variable in amount, being virtually absent in some situations. It may merge imperceptibly into the dermis. It is the superficial fascia and consists of loose connective (areolar) tissue often arranged in sheets. Fat infiltrates between these to form the subcutaneous layer that can be such a useful insulating blanket, protection and energy store, but which when present in excess not only inconveniences the animal but also the surgeon who has to incise through these layers at an operation site.

### Modified Integument of the Foot

The foot consists of four toes, each of which has a **claw** and a (digital) **footpad**; there is in addition a metacarpal and a metatarsal pad. (The **paw**, as opposed to

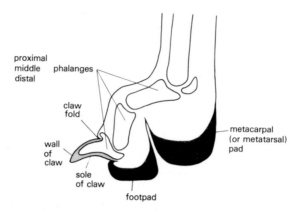

proximal
middle    phalanges
distal

claw
fold

metacarpal
(or metatarsal)
pad

wall
of
claw

sole
of claw

footpad

FIG. 1.32.    Section of a toe of a dog.

the foot, includes, in the forelimb, the carpus, metacarpus, phalanges and the associated sesamoid bones. The paw of the hindlimb is composed of corresponding hindlimb bones.) The metacarpal (or metatarsal) and phalanges medial to these four toes are not well developed and are known as **dew-claws**. They may be completely absent: this is commonly so in the hindlimbs, especially in cats. Dew-claws do not reach the ground and may cause more trouble than claws that do. They are removed from some dogs within a few days of birth.

*Footpads*

The keratinized, hairless epidermis of a footpad is thick and pigmented. In the dog it is arranged in conical papillae which may become worn down on hard surfaces. Those of the cat have smoother surfaces with ridges producing a branching connected pattern. Sweat glands open on to their surface.

The subcutaneous tissue helps to form **digital cushions** deep to the footpads: they consist of fibrous adipose tissue. Sweat glands are found in this layer.

The digital pads are oval and support

the distal interphalangeal joints (Fig. 1.32). The metacarpal and metatarsal pads of the dog are somewhat "heart-shaped"; the apex is distal and the two lobes are unequal in area. Those of the cat are more rounded. The joints between the proximal phalanges and the metacarpus (or metatarsus) rest on them when the paw supports weight.

There is also a carpal pad situated palmar and distal to the carpal bones.

*Claws*

The claw of the carnivore (Fig. 1.32) is the horny covering of the distal phalanx. The beak-like shape is quite characteristic; there are two **walls** that are continuous dorsally but on the ground surface the free edges embrace a soft flaky horn which forms the **sole** of the claw. The free edges of the walls may meet, thereby covering part of the sole; sometimes the part of the sole nearest the apex of the claw is visible.

The proximal end of the claw, which may also be called its base, root, or **coronary border**, fits into a groove. There it is continuous with the epidermis of hair-free skin which, as it leaves the groove to continue as the hairy skin, constitutes the

**claw fold**. The ground surface of the claw is separated from its corresponding digital pad by a furrow.

The claw of the cat is narrower than that of the dog; it is very pointed and often the edges are quite sharp. Cats tend to keep their claws pulled back into a pocket of skin. This is achieved by the strong elastic ligaments which stretch between the middle and distal phalanges. The claws can be very rapidly unsheathed and brought into use by muscle action overcoming the tension of the elastic ligaments.

The claw of the dog and cat is produced mainly from cells in the groove housing the coronary border; as it is produced the horny covering curves over the dermis that is tightly attached to the distal phalanx.

The dermis between the bone of the distal phalanx and the horn of the claw is very vascular and great care should be taken when trimming claws to ensure that only the epidermis is cut. The extent of the dermis can be seen by shining a light through the claw, providing it is not pigmented.

The claw grows at a rapid rate, and if it is not worn off or trimmed it will sometimes continue growing in a circular fashion until the point penetrates the ground surface of the foot. Especial notice should be taken of dew-claws which are unable to be worn down in the same way as the main claws (p. 178).

# CHAPTER 2

# Anatomy and Physiology—II

R. N. SMITH

## The Cavities of the Body and the Visceral Systems

### Body cavities

The **viscera** (singular, viscus) are those organs found in body cavities, i.e. the thoracic cavity, the abdominal cavity and the pelvic cavity (Fig. 2.1).

The **thoracic cavity** is within the chest and is bounded by the cranial thoracic aperture (first thoracic vertebra, first pair of ribs and the cranial end of the sternum), the diaphragm, the bodies of the thoracic vertebrae, the ribs (including costal cartilages) and the sternum.

The **abdominal cavity** is within the "belly" of the animal. It has as its cranial boundary the diaphragm and as its caudal limit the cranial pelvic aperture: the dorsal boundary is formed by the lumbar vertebrae and the diaphragm, and the muscles of the abdominal wall form the dorsolateral, lateral and ventral limits.

The **pelvic cavity** has the cranial pelvic aperture (pelvic inlet) and the caudal pelvic aperture (pelvic outlet) at either end as limits, the sacrum and first few coccygeal vertebrae dorsally, and the pubis and the ischium of the left and right sides as the floor. The lateral boundaries are muscles; in the dog, but not in the cat, these are stiffened by a narrow sacrotuberal ligament between the sacrum and the ischium.

Tissue is attached to the inner surfaces of these body cavities to form two sacs in the thoracic cavity and one sac in the abdominal and pelvic cavities. This tissue consists of a continuous layer of epithelial cells on the inner surface of the sacs and a thin supporting layer of connective tissue on the outer surface. The epithelial cells produce a very small amount of watery serous fluid; the epithelium and the layer of connective tissue are therefore said to form a **serous membrane** or serosa and the sacs surround *serous cavities*. The serous membrane lining the thorax is **pleura** and this surrounds two pleural cavities. The serous membrane in the abdomen and most of the pelvis is the **peritoneum** and this surrounds peritoneal cavity (Fig. 2.1).

There is a left and a right pleural sac and the space between them is the **mediastinum**. Most of the organs, such as the heart, and other structures of the thoracic cavity are in the mediastinum. However, the largest viscera, the **lungs**, and one or two closely related tissues including their vascular and nerve arrangements, push laterally out of the mediastinum, taking pleura with them and reducing considerably the size of the pleural cavities. The pleura which actually covers the lungs is called **pulmonary pleura** (visceral pleura), the remaining pleura is **parietal pleura**. This is subdivided into that forming the limits of the mediastinum, **mediastinal**

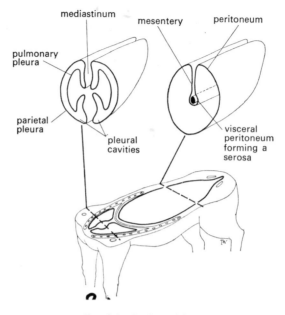

FIG. 2.1.   Body cavities

**pleura**, that covering the diaphragm, **diaphragmatic pleura**, and that lining the ribs, etc., **costal pleura**. The pleural cavity is so reduced that it is virtually non-existent and the pulmonary pleura is separated from the parietal pleura by only a thin film of *pleural fluid* produced by the pleura itself. This acts as a lubricant between the serous membranes, which will therefore be moist, shiny and slippery.

The peritoneal cavity fills the abdominal cavity and the more cranial part of the pelvic cavity. In describing the pleural cavity it was seen that the growth of the viscera laterally from the mediastinum reduced the cavity to a potential space. In the case of the peritoneal cavity a similar phenomenon can be imagined (it does not actually occur like this) but the "growth" would be downward from the *dorsal* surface of the abdominal cavity. There are many parts of several viscera involved in this "growth" and they are all coated with peritoneum which will be **visceral perito-**

**neum**. The part closely applied to the viscus is often described as a part of that viscus; then it is called its **serosa**. The **parietal peritoneum** lines the limits of the abdominal cavity and the more cranial part of the pelvic cavity. The part of the peritoneum between the viscus and the parietal peritoneum has a variety of names depending on the viscus, e.g. **mesentery, omentum, ligament**. This part, which is very thin, consisting of a little connective tissue between the two layers of serous membrane, will carry the vessels and other structures to and from the viscus. The peritoneum-coated viscera and their attachments fill the peritoneal cavity, leaving room only for the small amount of the serous *peritoneal fluid* to act as a lubricant between the serous membranes. All the surfaces are normally moist, shiny and slippery.

It should be emphasized in completing these comments on the pleural and peritoneal cavities that only fluid is to be found within the cavities themselves and that this acts as a lubricant between the serous membranes which are constantly apposed to each other.

**Visceral systems**

There are three visceral systems: **respiratory, digestive** and **urogenital**. Not every organ of these three systems is within one of the three body cavities, but since the major part of these systems is truly visceral they are included in this group. Conversely, because an organ is in a body cavity (and hence it is a viscus) it is not necessarily part of a visceral system.

The system consists primarily of tubes contained within the body which eventually open to the outside. In the case of the digestive system the tube opens to the outside at both ends. In the respiratory and urogenital systems only one end of each system opens to the outside. These tubes have a continuous lining of epithelium which is usually very thin. One of the methods of protecting this membrane is by lubrication with mucus (p. 4), produced either by glands or by individual cells. The epithelium of the tubes of the visceral system is therefore called **mucous membrane** or **mucosa**. (Note that the noun is spelt **mucus** and the adjective **mucous**.)

**Respiratory System**

Respiration is the gaseous exchange between a living structure and its environment. Oxygen is necessary for the chemical reactions essential to animal life and carbon dioxide is an end-product. In discussing blood, it was mentioned that this tissue is capable of carrying these gases (p. 7). The transfer of oxygen from blood to all the cells of the body and of carbon dioxide from these cells to the blood is called *tissue (or internal) respira-*

*tion.* The transfer of the gases between the external environment and the blood is called *external respiration* and in mammals this takes place in the lungs. The structure of these organs and of the passageways from the outside to the site of external respiration will be considered in this description of the respiratory system. It will include the nasal cavities, the pharynx, the larynx, the trachea, the bronchi and the lungs (Fig. 2.2). Occasionally the mouth is used as an additional air-way during mouth breathing and panting. The thorax, pleural cavities, diaphragm and other muscles, such as those of the abdominal wall, which can affect the size of the thoracic cavity are also essential parts of the respiratory system.

Some regions of the respiratory system are used for other functions in addition to the passage of gases: for instance, parts of the nasal cavities play a role in the sensation of smell, the larynx helps in the production of sound and part of the lining of the respiratory system is effective in heat and water loss. In the section on the visceral systems the respiratory system was described as a tube within the body that had an opening to the outside at one end only. This tube has a continuous lining called a mucous membrane, the epithelial cells of which vary with the region.

*Nasal Cavities* (Fig. 2.3)

The nasal chambers, and the turbinates they contain, are lined with **nasal mucous membrane** to form the **nasal cavities**. The continuation with the epithelium of the skin takes place at the **nostrils**. The animal is able to increase and decrease the size of these apertures. The openings are strengthened by cartilage and are surrounded by a zone of hairless skin to form the nose.

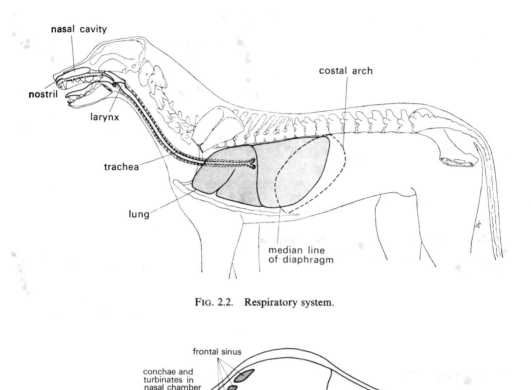

FIG. 2.2.   Respiratory system.

FIG. 2.3.   Median section of a dog's head to show part of respiratory tract.

The scrolls of bone in the nasal chambers are covered by a vascular mucous membrane, that is, one rich in blood vessels, many of which are wide-bored and have thin walls. Near the cranial cavity, i.e. in the depths or *fundus* of the nasal cavity, the epithelium over the turbinates has a special arrangement to register the sensation of smell and convey the information to the brain. This part of the mucous membrane is the **olfactory region**: the remainder is the **respiratory region** and most of the mucous membrane bears minute hair-like projections called **cilia** which are constantly in wave-like motion. The mucous membrane moistens, warms and cleans the incoming air. Any small particles are trapped in the mucus which is continuously produced by the membrane. This secretion, together with any trapped material, is wafted by the cilia into the throat and then swallowed.

The mucous membrane forms a lateral pouch called a **maxillary sinus** in the spongy interior of the maxillary bone. The epithelium of the cavity differs from that in the nasal chamber.

More of these outpouchings of the nasal mucous membrane take place between the turbinates. Here the bone that is invaded is the frontal bone and so **frontal sinuses** are formed.

All these sinuses retain their connections with the nasal cavities and all are lined by a continuation of the nasal mucous membrane. The outpouchings are collectively known as the **paranasal sinuses**.

The nasal cavities are continued into the single midline **pharynx** through paired openings.

### *Pharynx* (Fig. 2.3)

This chamber is common to the respiratory and the digestive systems. Both systems have entrances to it but these are separated by a musculo-membranous partition, the **soft palate**, into a dorsal **nasal part** and a ventral **oral part**. At times of respiratory distress, the mouth is used for an additional opening, and the oral part of the pharynx then becomes an air-way.

In the dorsal region of the nasal part of the pharynx, there are paired openings into the **auditory** (Eustachian) **tubes**. The tube of each side connects the middle-ear cavity with the pharynx and its lining is continuous with that of the pharynx.

The opening into the larynx is in the floor of the pharynx and just caudal and slightly more dorsal is the opening into the **oesophagus**, the continuation of the digestive system.

The wall of the pharynx is muscular and its lining is continuous with that of all the tubes which enter and leave it.

### *Larynx* (Fig. 2.3)

The **larynx** is a complex valvular mechanism of interconnected cartilages, muscles, fibrous tissue and mucous membrane, whose function is to stop the entry of material other than gases into the more distal part of the respiratory system; if any food touches the pharynx the larynx immediately closes. The larynx also controls the flow of these gases, as well as producing sounds. It lies in the midline between the rami of the mandibles.

There are fundamentally three single, and one pair of cartilages. The single midline **epiglottis** is the most rostral cartilage and it points towards the soft palate. Caudal to the epiglottis is a pair of **vocal ligaments**. Since each vocal ligament is attached dorsally to cartilages which are slightly separated and yet ventrally they attach to a midline structure their arrangement will represent the two limbs of a V, one limb on either side of the midline.

The continuous action of the two cartilages swings these two limbs alternately nearer to and further from the midline. The mucous membrane lining the cavity of the larynx covers the vocal ligaments and the combined ligament and mucous membrane forms the **vocal fold**. The space bounded by the folds and the mucous-membrane-covered cartilages to which they are attached is the **glottis**. Movement of the cartilages controls the size of the glottis and therefore regulates the flow of gases. Forced passage of gases through the glottis causes the vocal folds to vibrate and so produce a sound. This is modulated by the size of the glottis and the tension of the folds and further modified by the resonance effects of the remainder of the head region.

In anaesthetizing an animal with a gas it is often convenient to lead the anaesthetic vapour straight from the machine into the trachea, using an **endotracheal tube**. It is also a very useful technique even with anaesthesia by other methods as this ensures that the animal can continue to breathe without anything being able to block the "upper airway" (i.e. that part of the respiratory system in the head and neck). When the animal has been lightly anaesthetized the mouth is held open, the tongue is pulled forward and the lubricated endotracheal tube is pushed carefully into the mouth. The end of the tube is used to lift the soft palate so that the epiglottis can be seen pointing forwards. The tube is then turned so that its tip will depress the cartilage and expose the entrance of the larynx more clearly. The tube is slowly advanced so that it passes into and through the glottis.

*Trachea*

The **trachea** is a permanently open tube attached to the laryngeal cartilages. It lies on the ventral aspect of the neck and passes through the cranial thoracic aperture into the mediastinum of the cranial half of the thorax. Here it ends by splitting at the **bifurcation** into **right and left bronchi** (Fig. 2.5).

The tube is kept open by a series of incomplete **tracheal cartilages**, which vary in shape but resemble a C. The open part of the cartilage is dorsal; this means that the part nearer the skin is always the solid part of the cartilage. They are connected into a tube by fibrous tissue with which smooth muscle cells are associated. The ciliated mucous membrane is continuous with that of the larynx and the bronchi and is attached to the inner surface of the cartilages.

*Bronchi and Terminal Air Passages* (Fig. 2.4).

The bronchi that leave the trachea branch continually in such a manner that the very apt descriptive name of the bronchial tree is given to the arrangement (see Fig. 2.5). The successive branches decrease in size and the smaller tubes are called **bronchioles**. Although the larger tubes have a cartilage arrangement resembling that of the trachea this becomes reduced to a series of small overlapping plates and eventually the cartilage tissue ends. These tubes, which are lined by a continuation of the ciliated mucous membrane, are of a very small diameter. Ultimately the stage of the smallest bronchioles is reached. These are called **respiratory bronchioles** and each branches into several **alveolar ducts**. Each duct ends as **alveolar sacs** which consist of a large number of **pulmonary alveoli**. The epithelium of the walls of these respiratory bronchioles and their ramifications is extremely thin and has no cilia; it is sometimes called the **pulmonary membrane**. This is the level at which gaseous exchange takes place and so these structures are covered by equally thin-walled capillaries accompanied by just a trace of connective tissue. Oxygen continually leaves the air in the alveoli, diffuses across the pulmonary membrane and passes into the blood. It is replaced in the alveoli by carbon dioxide which has left the blood by a similar mechanism. As the blood vessels are followed away from this alveolar level they get larger and have thicker walls. The amount of connective and other tissue also increases. Blood leaving the lungs in an oxygenated state circulates to capillaries permeating the body and there the oxygen passes into tissue fluid and into the cells where it rapidly used for oxidation. Most of the oxygen has been carried in combination with haemoglobin although a small

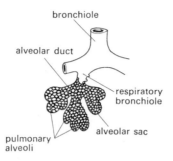

bronchiole

alveolar duct

respiratory
bronchiole

alveolar sac

pulmonary
alveoli

FIG. 2.4.   Terminal air passages.

amount is dissolved in the plasma. At normal times the haemoglobin only gives up about a quarter of its oxygen to the tissues; however, at times of distress it can probably release about three times as much as this.

The collection of air passages, blood vessels and surrounding connective tissue forms the lung tissue. Only the proximal parts of the bronchi are outside the lung tissue, that is, are extra-pulmonic. All the lung tissue is enclosed in pulmonary pleura to form the **lungs**.

### Lungs

The right and left lungs fill nearly all the thoracic cavity not taken up by the heart. They are not very similar to one another in shape and the right one is larger than the left. The bronchi and the blood vessels, nerves, etc., associated with a lung, enter it at its **root**. The lung tissue in dogs and cats is completely divided by fissures into a group of **lobes** (Fig. 2.5). A cranial (apical), middle (cardiac) and caudal (diaphragmatic) lobe can be seen in both lungs. The right lung has, in addition, an accessory (intermediate) lobe which lies between the two lungs.

### Breathing

This is accomplished by alternately enlarging and contracting the thorax. The diaphragm and some of the trunk muscles enlarge the thorax by their contractions. During quiet respiration the thorax may reduce in size by virtue of the elasticity of the tissues and the relaxation of muscles. Contraction of abdominal muscles can force the contents of that cavity against the diaphragm and so help reduce the size of the thorax. The lungs slide freely in the pleural cavity and follow the excursions of the thorax. As the lungs enlarge during inspiration air is pulled into the alveoli; as they reduce in expiration air is forced out. The muscles of respiration are not used to their maximum during quiet breathing, but have an enormous reserve that can be called upon in respiratory distress.

During quiet respiration the dog breathes 10–30 times per minute, the cat 20–30. This is called the **respiratory rate**.

When the lungs are distended nerve impulses are sent to a respiratory centre in the brain; this transmits information which inhibits the inspiratory muscles. A similar mechanism is used at expiration and so a rhythmic control is established. There are other nerve patterns used in a similar manner so that this vital function does not rely on only one. The rate and depth of respirations are affected by many factors, including carbon dioxide and oxygen levels in the blood.

The motor-nerve impulses leave the spinal cord in nerves at appropriate levels

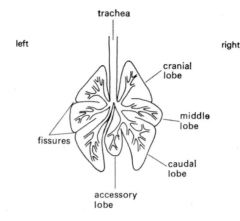

FIG. 2.5.    Diagram to show bronchial tree within the lobes of the lungs.

to reach the respiratory muscles. Some leave the cervical part of the cord and together form a **phrenic nerve** on each side which runs through the mediastinum to reach the diaphragm.

The air that passes into and out of the lungs with each respiration is the **tidal air** and the amount is the **tidal volume**. Even at the end of the most forceful expiration there is some air left in the lung; the amount is the **residual volume**. That which is left after normal expiration is the **functional residual capacity** and this is the air that allows gaseous diffusion between breaths. A lot of the air drawn in at each inspiration is exhaled again before it reaches the alveoli; this amount is called the **dead space** and is the same as the volume of the respiratory passages from nostrils to alveoli.

In the pathological condition **pneumonia** the alveoli fill with fluid and their walls become inflamed and "waterlogged" by excess fluid. This will obviously severely restrict gaseous exchange. Another pathological state can occur if the thorax is punctured or opened in any way. Air can then enter the pleural cavity and the lungs will collapse away from the wall; this is **pneumothorax**. It may be caused

intentionally during thoracic operations, and at the end the anaesthetist will ensure that the lungs are restored to their normal size, and the air expelled from the pleural cavity.

## Digestive System

The normal animal requires material to incorporate into its own body to help replace worn-out tissues. The breakdown of these substances can also provide the energy required to carry on life processes. The material is *food* and the function of breaking it down and altering it to make it available for absorption into the body is *digestion* and is carried out by the **digestive system**. *Absorption* is the transference of foodstuffs from the digestive system into the blood and lymph; these carry it eventually to tissues for storage or immediate use.

In the natural state dogs and cats obtain most of their food from animal, as opposed to plant, sources; that is, they are carnivorous. As pets this is certainly not so. The food must supply water, proteins, carbohydrates, lipids and inorganic compounds. It must also provide a group of chemicals called **vitamins**. These are essential in minute traces in the food since the animal is probably incapable of manufacturing them itself. It appears that many of the vitamins form parts of enzyme systems. Diseases can occur in their absence, but the average well-balanced diet probably contains an adequate supply. Vitamins will be discussed more fully in the section on feeding in Chapter 3. Some foods need no digestion, but in most cases quite elaborate changes have to take place before the complex and sometimes insoluble substances can be absorbed.

In the description of the organic content of the body (p. 17) the compounds were divided into simple and complex substances. Much of the food that is eaten consists of complex carbohydrates, proteins and fats. But only relatively simple compounds can be absorbed from the digestive system and so in the process of digestion the carbohydrates are broken down into simple sugars (mostly glucose), the proteins into polypeptides, peptides and then amino acids and the fats into fatty acids. This is only possible in the presence of enzymes found in the juices secreted into various parts of the digestive tract. Furthermore, their actions can only take place when all the conditions, especially the acidity, are correct.

The digestive system is basically a tube which is open at both ends and has entering into it ducts from glands producing secretions that help in the digestive process. The food is taken in at the mouth and here secretions from salivary glands are added; the breaking-down of this mixture is helped by the teeth and tongue. The result is carried through the pharynx to the oesophagus, a musculo-membranous tube that passes along the neck and then through the mediastinum within the thorax. The oesophagus enters the abdominal cavity through the diaphragm and there it enlarges to form the stomach, a storage organ where some digestion occurs. From here material is propelled along the small intestine, in which three consecutive parts, duodenum, jejunum and ileum, are recognized. The remainder of the tube is the large intestine and consists of the caecum, the colon, the rectum and the anal canal. It has been mentioned that salivary glands add their secretion (saliva) to the contents of the mouth. The pancreas and the liver, two other glands of the digestive system, add their secretions to the contents of the small intestine. Since these glands (salivary, pancreas, liver) are remote from the tube itself, they may be considered as *extrinsic*. Glands in the wall of the digestive tube are *intrinsic*, and these, together with individual cells, also pour their secretions into the lumen of the tube. Mucus is produced along the entire length of the digestive system to act as a lubricant and to protect the inner lining. The epithelium of the mucous membrane of the tube is continuous with that of the skin at the lips and at the anus (the opening to the outside of the anal canal). The part of the digestive tube caudal to the pharynx (i.e. from the oesophagus to the anus) may be spoken of as the **alimentary canal**.

## Mouth

The **mouth** is supported by the bones of the upper and lower jaws which move mainly in a vertical plane. The bones of the upper jaw form the floor of the nasal chambers and also act as the roof of the **mouth cavity**. They are covered by mucosa to form the **hard plate** (Fig. 2.6). The caudal end of the hard palate is continued by the musculo-membranous **soft palate**.

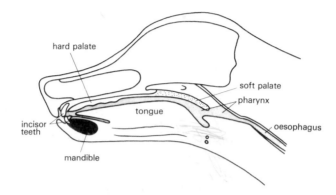

FIG. 2.6.   Median section of a dog's head to show parts of the digestive system.

This reaches as far as the larynx and in some of the short-headed breeds of dogs (e.g. Bulldogs) it may interfere with normal respiration. The skeleton of the lower jaw consists of the paired mandibles, joined in the midline. **Teeth** are found in the body of each mandible and in the opposing part of the bones of the upper jaw. The line of the teeth in each jaw is called a **dental arch**.

The sides of the jaws are connected by muscles covered on the outside by skin and on the inside by mucous membrane. These form the **cheeks**. The **lips** are also formed by muscle covered by outside skin and inside mucous membrane and it is along the edge of the lips that the epithelium of the skin becomes continuous with that of the mucous membrane. The upper lip has a furrow or **philtrum** dividing the right and left halves.

The entire inside of the mouth cavity is lined by mucous membrane. From the inside of the lips and cheeks it is reflected on to the bones of the upper and lower jaws where it is pierced by the teeth and attaches to the periosteum of the tooth-bearing bones. The reflections of the mucous membrane are the **gums** and in the upper jaw it continues onto and attaches tightly to the bones of the hard palate. The mucous membrane of the lower jaw is continuous from the gums over the free surfaces of the tongue.

Carnivores do not masticate food (i.e. mechanically reduce it in the mouth) very well. It is pushed on rapidly by the tongue and cheeks into the next part of the system.

*Teeth*

These hard structures, embedded in the jaws, are used for grinding, tearing and crushing. The sockets in which they fit are called **alveoli**.

The centre of the tooth is the **pulp**, a soft mass of nerves, blood vessels, etc., held together in connective tissue, and this is contained in the **tooth cavity** formed by the immediately surrounding **dentine** (Fig. 2.7). This resembles bone but is much harder. The part of the tooth buried in the jaw is the **root**; some teeth may have two or even three roots. Here the dentine is covered by **cement**, a tissue that resembles bone but is softer than dentine. The part of the tooth projecting out of the jaw is the **crown**. It consists of the dentine covered by a cap of **enamel**; this is an extremely hard tissue.

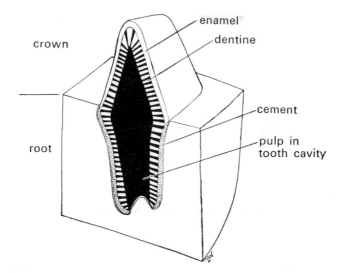

FIG. 2.7. Diagrammatic section of a tooth in an alveolus.

The surface which comes in contact with a tooth of the opposite jaw is its **masticatory surface** (grinding surface, or table).

According to their positions, four types of teeth are recognized. **Incisor** teeth are found at the opening of the mouth, and are used for tearing and cutting food. Caudal to these there is a **canine** tooth on each side in the upper and lower jaws. Continuing along the dental arch, the next teeth are the **pre-molars**. These and the yet more caudal **molars** may together be known as the *cheek teeth*, whose main function is grinding food.

The dog and cat have two consecutive sets of many of these teeth. The first set are called **deciduous** or milk teeth. Although not showing at birth (i.e. not erupted) they are usually all functional by 1 to 2 months. In this dentition the puppy has on each side three incisors, one canine and three pre-molars in the upper jaw and the same arrangement in the lower jaw (Fig. 2.8). This information can be written as a dental formula as follows:

$I^3/_3C^1/_1PM^3/_3$ (total, both sides upper and lower jaws, 28).

The dental formula for the deciduous dentition of the kitten is:

$I^3/_3C^1/_1PM^3/_2$ (total 26).

The deciduous teeth drop out and are replaced by permanent ones. Molar teeth appear in this dentition and in the dog there is an additional pre-molar. This replacement starts at approximately four months in the dog and the cat.

The dental formula for the permanent dentition of the dog is:

$I^3/_3C^1/_1PM^4/_4M^2/_3$ (total 42)(Fig. 2.9).

These teeth are larger than deciduous ones. The incisors are slender with single roots. In young dogs the crowns have a central rounded projection flanked by two smaller ones. Depending on the age of the dog and the wear the teeth receive during chewing, these projections may be ground down to various levels. The canine teeth are the longest, with a curved single root

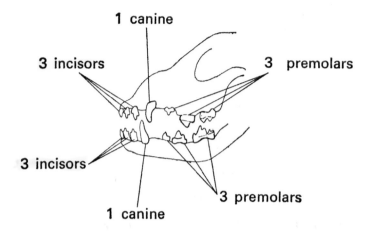

FIG. 2.8.    Skull of a puppy to show deciduous teeth.

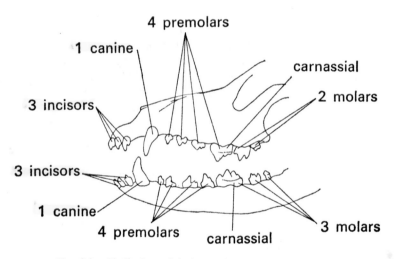

FIG. 2.9.    Skull of an adult dog to show permanent dentition.

almost twice as long as the cone-shaped crown. There are four pre-molar teeth in the upper and in the lower jaw. The first one is quite simple and has only one root. The masticatory surface of the other cheek teeth have two to four rounded cones called **tubercles** or **cusps**. The fourth pre-molar in the upper jaw is massive. It is called the **carnassial** tooth of the upper jaw and is especially important in cutting tough material. This tooth is very firmly fixed and, like the molars of the upper jaw, has three diverging roots. None of the lower jaw pre-molars or molars has more than two roots. The first molar is the carnassial of the lower jaw; it is about twice as large as the second and third put together. A dog will turn its head to one side in tackling hard food so that the carnassial teeth are brought into use.

The formula for the permanent dentition of the cat is:

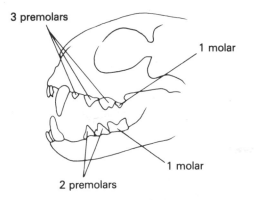

3 premolars

1 molar

1 molar

2 premolars

FIG. 2.10. Skull of an adult cat to show permanent dentition.

$I^3/_3C^1/_1PM^3/_2M^1/_1$ (total 30)(Fig.2.10).

The incisors and canines resemble those of the dog, but are, of course, much smaller. In the upper jaw the pre-molars increase in size caudally; the third is the largest tooth in the mouth and is the only one with three roots. In the lower jaw the molar is the largest tooth. These cheek teeth resemble those of the dog in having a tuberculate (i.e. rounded cusps) arrangement of their masticatory surfaces. The significance of the number of roots lies in the difficulty they cause in tooth extraction.

*Tongue*

The tongue lies on the floor of the mouth and is mainly a mass of striated muscle fibres, some of which are attached to the hyoid apparatus and the mandibles. The caudal part, the **root** of the tongue, is continuous with the larynx, and if it is necessary to pass an instrument through the glottis, pulling the tongue brings the epiglottis and other laryngeal structures nearer to the lips (Fig. 2.6). The oral end of the tongue is unattached and able to move over an extensive area, sometimes making quite delicate movements. It is made into a ladle-shape when the dog and cat lap up fluids. Most of the mucous membrane is arranged in a multitude of small projections called **lingual papillae**; some have **taste buds** containing special nerve endings associated with them. The papillae help the tongue to control the food during its treatment in the mouth and the rough surface they provide is also useful for grooming. The mucous membrane is well supplied with nerve fibres which convey general information as well as data about the taste of the material in the mouth. A large vein is very prominent on either side of the underneath surface of the tongue. This is the *lingual vein* and it is especially useful for intravenous injections in the anaesthetized animal.

*Salivary Glands*

There are several paired glandular areas which produce saliva. The largest are the zygomatic, sublingual, mandibular and parotid glands and these have several ducts opening into the mouth (Fig. 2.11).

The zygomatic gland lies within the orbit and very close to the eyeball, under the protection of the zygomatic arch. The sublingual glands lie medial to the mandible immediately under the mucosa con-

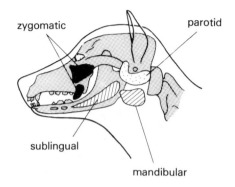

FIG. 2.11.    Position of salivary glands. The zygomatic is often in two parts. The sublingual is medial to the mandible.

necting the tongue to the lower jaw. Neither the zygomatic nor the sublingual glands can normally be palpated, but the positions of the mandibular and parotid glands can be more easily defined. The mandibular gland is rather oval in shape and can be felt immediately caudal to the angle of the jaw. There are two or three much smaller rounded structures between the gland and the jaw. These are mandibular lymph nodes. Although the parotid salivary gland is not easily felt it can be taken as filling the space between the mandibular salivary gland and the base of the ear (parotid means near to the ear). There is a small parotid lymph node which can be felt between the parotid salivary gland and the mandible.

The sight of food and also other signs associated with its preparation start salivary secretion. It is increased when food is in the mouth. Saliva is about 99% water and this moisture makes food easier to masticate and swallow. Since it does not stay long in the mouth, the food does not undergo any significant chemical change there.

Saliva does also have a role in heat regulation. It provides water which readily evaporates especially during panting and this helps dissipate heat.

### Pharynx

This chamber is common to the digestive and respiratory systems (Fig. 2.6). The pharyngeal wall is muscular and its mucous membrane lining is continuous with that of all the tubes which enter and leave. There are many diffuse lymphoid areas in the mucous membrane of the pharynx, forming an almost complete ring round the entrances. These areas are called **tonsils**; the palatine tonsils, however are distinct bulges of lymphoid tissue, one on each side of the pharynx, usually hidden in a small recess. When enlarged and inflamed as in *tonsilitis*, they are more obvious and can be very painful.

Food is pushed by the tongue to the back of the mouth and into oral part of the pharynx; from here the pharyngeal muscles propel it to the oesophagus. This is *swallowing* or *deglutition* and while food is in the pharynx the glottis is closed to stop food entering the respiratory system.

### Oesophagus

The oesophagus is a simple tube leading from the pharynx and in its passage along the neck it is closely related to the dorsal surface of the trachea and slightly on its

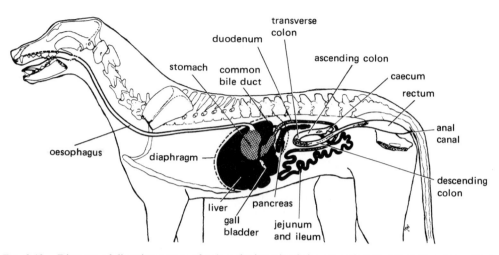

FIG. 2.12.    Diagram of digestive system of a dog: the intestine is longer and more coiled than shown here.

left side (Fig. 2.12). In the mediastinum it is still related to the trachea as far as the bifurcation and it then continues caudally to pass into the abdominal cavity through a special foramen in the diaphragm. The mucous membrane lining the tube is surrounded by a loose submucous coat: this allows the mucosa to be arranged in many longitudinal folds that become smoothed out when the oesophagus undergoes distension.

Outside the submucosa there is a muscular coat consisting of layers of striated muscle fibres. The connective tissue that surrounds the oesophagus is usually called its **adventitial coat** and this will blend with local fascia.

Food is passed along the oesophagus by **peristalsis**; this is a circular constriction of the tube by its muscle coats which moves towards the distal end of the digestive system.

## Stomach

The junction of the oesophagus and stomach is the **cardia**. The exit from the stomach into the small intestine is at the **pyloric opening** or **pylorus**. The simple tube shape is distorted by a much greater lengthening of one side (Fig. 2.12). It can adapt itself to the quantity of food and between meals it may be almost empty. Gastric digestion occurs here, and it also acts as a reservoir for the food. Nevertheless, it is not essential to life and animals that have had it removed may live apparently normally.

The glands of the mucous membrane of the stomach produce gastric juice in which are found mucus, hydrochloric acid and several enzymes used in splitting proteins and lipids.

The mucus forms a continuous layer over the surface epithelium of the stomach to protect it against the action of acid and the protein-splitting enzymes. It does also prevent mechanical damage to the lining of the digestive tract. One of the major enzymes in the gastric juice is pepsin, and a very high level of acidity is necessary for this to break down the complex proteins into much simpler substances. Some of the carbohydrates in the food are dealt with in the stomach by enzymes such as amylase which is contributed by the saliva. However, the acidity prevents complete carbohydrate breakdown. There is also some of the enzyme lipase present to begin the digestion of fats.

Food has not normally been simplified sufficiently for absorption to occur in the stomach. The fluid or semi-fluid mixture leaving the stomach is called **chyme** (pronounced *kime*). The submucous coat consists of loose connective tissue and allows movement of the mucous membrane. The muscular coat has at least two layers of smooth muscle fibres. At the cardiac and pyloric openings, the smooth muscle layers tend to be arranged as sphincters; the pyloric sphincter is quite strong. The stomach wall is moved by its muscle layers to mix the food with the gastric juice and to pass it on to the small intestine. The movements are rhythmic segmentations which chop the food at different places by isolated constrictions and also peristalsis similar to that described for the oesophagus.

Peristaltic waves also occur in an empty stomach. These are hunger contractions and seem to be linked with a low level of glucose in the blood. (Thirst, however, appears to be more closely connected with a dehydration of the mucous membrane of the mouth and throat.) In antiperistalsis, the waves of contraction pass toward the head. This occurs in vomiting, the act of ejecting stomach contents through the oesophagus and mouth. The pylorus closes, the cardia opens and the abdominal muscles contract to press the stomach against the diaphragm and force its evacuation. Some drugs called **emetics** can cause this automatic act, which may be necessary to remove swallowed poisons rapidly.

## Small Intestine

This is a long and relatively narrow tube and is the chief site of absorption.

The peritoneal covering which forms the serosa is attached to the dorsal abdominal wall, the connection being called **mesentery**. Blood and lymph vessels and also nerves use the mesentery to reach and leave the intestine. For most of the intestine the mesentery is quite long and allows it to form numerous coils (Fig. 2.12). The first part of the small intestine, however, is close to the roof of the abdominal cavity; it has only a short mesentery and so is fixed in position. This is the **duodenum** and the general arrangement is somewhat U-shaped. The **pancreas** lies between the limbs of the U and the secreted pancreatic juice passes along its **ducts** (usually two, but occasionally only one) which open into the lumen of the adjacent duodenum. The **common bile duct** from the liver also opens into the duodenum, a very short distance from the pylorus and closely related to the pancreatic duct openings. Immediately following the duodenum, the rest of the small intestine is attached by relatively long mesentery. These parts are the **jejunum** and **ileum**.

The mucous membrane of the small intestine is arranged in numerous fine projections called **villi** (singular, *villus*) which greatly increase the surface area available for absorption (Fig. 2.13). This is also a profusion of glands whose secretion is called *intestinal juice*. Areas of lymphoid tissue are freely distributed in the intestinal mucous membrane. The submucous coat is surrounded by two layers of smooth muscle, one encircling the tube, the other running longitudinally. The ileum, the terminal part of the small intestine, joins the large intestine. Pancreatic juice, intestinal juice and bile all combine with the chyme in the small intestine. The wall of this part of the digestive system undergoes peristalsis and rhythmic segmentation movements to ensure that the food is moved from place to place, that it is brought close to the

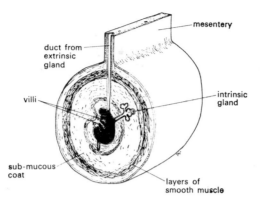

FIG. 2.13.  Hypothetical transverse section of intestine showing possible structures.

absorptive surfaces and that it undergoes a thorough mixing.

Pancreatic juice is a clear fluid with a very high concentration of bicarbonate ions; it contains a number of digestive enzymes. The bicarbonate ions produce an alkalinity which partly neutralizes the acidity of the chyme from the stomach. The pancreatic enzymes require a much more alkaline environment to be able to do their work. Amylase is one of these and is used to continue the breakdown of the carbohydrates. Trypsin acts on the proteins and also on the breakdown products from the pepsin treatment in the stomach. Lipase is another of the pancreatic enzymes and this continues the fat digestion.

Bile is essential for the proper breakdown of fats: if it is absent fat digestion is markedly reduced and fat can appear unchanged in the faeces. The important components in the bile for fat digestion are the bile salts. These reduce the surface tension between the fats and water and allow them to be broken down into an emulsion of very small globules. (Bile salts act in exactly the same way as detergents.) The fat-splitting enzymes (the lipases) are then able to act much more effectively. The other major constituent of bile, the pigments, are waste products of blood pigment breakdown and are being excreted via the digestive system. They are the main cause of the colour of faeces.

Intestinal juice from the glands of the mucous membrane has a high bicarbonate content; it contains also a wide variety of enzymes that help complete the breakdown of food.

Absorption by the small intestine is facilitated by the villi. These projections have a large lymph capillary, called a **lacteal**, in their centre and this drains into lymph vessels in the wall of the intestine (Fig. 2.14). From here the lymph passes into mesenteric lymph vessels to mesenteric lymph nodes and then into a collecting chamber called the **cisterna chyli** in the roof of the abdominal cavity.

Chyle (pronounced *kile*) is the name often given to lymph from the wall of the intestines. Lymph leaves the cisterna chyli in the **thoracic duct**, a vessel that runs through the thorax to open into large veins near the cranial thoracic aperture.

There is a plexus of blood capillaries around each lacteal and these together with other vessels of the intestine unite to form the venules and veins which join to become the **portal vein**. This enters the liver where the blood is discharged to circulate round the liver cells.

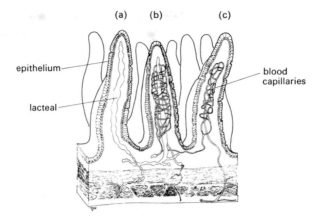

FIG. 2.14.   Arrangement of intestinal villi (highly magnified): (a) shows central lacteal; (b) lacteal and blood-vascular system; (c) blood-vascular system only.

The surface of each villus is covered by the epithelial lining of the intestine. The villi are continually waving about, shortening and lengthening, either singly or in groups. Inorganic compounds and the simplified products of protein and carbohydrate digestion are absorbed through the intestinal surface and are mainly carried to the liver by the blood in the portal system. The fatty acids resulting from lipid breakdown and also very finely divided fat globules are absorbed into the lacteals of the villi. This causes the lymph in the mesenteric vessels (chyle) to appear milky-white. It passes eventually into the venous system.

### Large Intestine

Most of the large intestine has a greater diameter than the small intestine. The arrangement of this region of the digestive tube is **caecum, ascending colon, transverse colon, descending colon, rectum, anal canal** (Fig. 2.12). There are no villi in the large intestine. Its main function is to absorb water from what is left of the foodstuffs and the secretions that have been added earlier in the system. There is practically no absorption of organic compounds. Mucus is secreted by the glands of the mucous membrane and bacteria flourish in this part of the gut. They split up some of the protein which is still present and the resulting products are responsible for the odour of faeces. The contents are passed on by intestinal movements caused by the muscle layers surrounding the submucosa.

The caecum is a short blind-ending sac. The ileum joins the large intestine at the junction of the caecum and ascending colon. The latter is on the right side of the abdominal cavity closely applied to its roof. The transverse colon crosses the more cranial part of the abdominal cavity and the descending colon is on the left side.

The rectum is that part of the large intestine between the cranial aperture of the pelvis and the anal canal. The piece of rectum immediately continuous with the descending colon is covered by peritoneum. More caudally the limit of the peritoneal cavity is reached and so the last piece of the rectum is covered by fascia and also by extrinsic muscles attaching this part of the gut to the vertebrae near the root of the tail.

The terminal piece of the large intestine, the anal canal, is a very short length of the digestive tube that is usually closed by the action of the sphincter muscles. One sphincter results from a thickening of the circular smooth muscle fibres. Around this, extrinsic striated muscles also form a sphincter, attached in part to the local skeleton. The continuation of the epithelium of the mucous membrane and that of the skin occurs at the anus, the terminal external orifice of the digestive system.

The anal sacs (para-anal sinuses) which occur at this junction are described with the cutaneous glands of the integument (Fig. 1.30).

The act of passing faeces to the outside is *defaecation.* As the rectum fills, sensory nerve impulses pass to the spinal cord from which motor impulses are sent to relax the internal smooth muscle sphincter. However, the external sphincter is under voluntary control and is opened only when the animal decides the time and place are appropriate.

## Assimilation of the Results of Digestion

The activities of the digestive system in breaking down the foodstuffs into simple units that can be absorbed has been described. Much of the very large volume of the digestive secretions must also be reabsorbed and almost all the absorption will take place in the small intestine. It is essential for the well-being of the animal that this activity is not impaired by poisons or by pathogenic microbes. After the absorption of the breakdown products they need to be transported to the tissues where they are to be assimilated.

### Carbohydrates

By far the largest proportion of carbohydrate absorption is in the form of glucose and this passes through the intesti-

nal epithelium and into the blood in the capillaries of the intestine. The blood enters the portal venous system which empties into the liver, and here the glucose may undergo some processing before further distribution. In fact the liver acts as a glucose bank, taking out the excess glucose in the blood that occurs immediately after a meal and converting it into **glycogen**—a form in which it can be stored. When the blood glucose level falls the stored glycogen can be converted back to glucose and passed out into the blood.

All the cells of the body rely on circulating glucose for the production of energy, and, in fact, dietary carbohydrates provide well over half the energy needs of the body. The breakdown of glucose by the cells results in carbon dioxide, water and the release of energy. The energy is essential for all the functions of the body. But first the glucose must get into the cells where the enzymes can release the energy. This requires the presence of the hormone **insulin** which is produced in the pancreas and released directly into the blood stream. (It is not part of the pancreatic juice; it is produced by islands of special cells in the pancreatic tissue. This is how the hormone gets its name, *insula* being the Latin word for island.) Insulin helps the passage of glucose through the cell membrane and the rate of carbohydrate metabolism is regulated according to the rate of insulin production by the pancreas. When it is plentiful the concentration of glucose in the blood and in extracellular fluids diminishes. When the insulin is deficient the glucose is dammed back in the blood instead of entering the cells.

Diabetes mellitus is the disease resulting from the failure of the pancreas to produce insulin, and in this condition the blood glucose level rises three to four times the normal level. Although the kidneys do not normally allow glucose to pass out into the urine, they are unable to operate their usual control at the high level circulating in diabetes. Not only will the glucose appear in the urine but this has an effect also on the water balance of the tissues. Another result of diabetes mellitus is therefore a great increase in the excretion of water.

### Proteins

Each of these consists of several amino acids of which there are about twenty altogether. The animal is able to manufacture some of these itself given the right building bricks, but those that it cannot must provided in the food. These are known as essential amino acids and further details of these will be given in Chapter 3f on nutrition and feeding. The proteins in the food are broken down by enzymes of the digestive tract into their component amino acids (p. 186). These are absorbed through the wall of the small intestine and pass into the blood stream of the villi. Cells needing amino acids for repair, for growth and for synthesizing other proteins abstract what they want from the circulating blood. Proteins are in a constant process of being broken down and being re-built so the turnover of amino acid is continuous. Any surplus amino acids are broken down in the liver and eventually converted into urea. This passes into the blood stream and is excreted through the kidneys into the urine (see also p. 83).

### Fats

The digestion of fats is made easier by their emulsification by the bile salts and the lipases of the digestive system can then break them into simpler compounds which will pass through the intestinal wall. Here they enter the lacteals of the villi and are absorbed into the lymphatic system which carries them eventually to the blood circulation. (Some of the breakdown products do go via the portal venous system direct to the liver.) The fat may be converted directly to release energy or it may be stored by the cells. There are often preferred sites for storage and these are called **fat depots**. When these stores need to be called on the fat is transported to the liver where it is converted into fatty acids and glycerol. The fatty acids can be used directly for energy production by further splitting. The glycerol is converted into glycogen, the storage form of glucose.

### Pancreas

This organ consists of a mixture of exocrine and endocrine tissue found in the loop of the duodenum near the roof of the abdominal cavity (Fig. 2.12). Most of the gland is exocrine and this is responsible for providing pancreatic juice which passes into the duodenum via one or more, usually two, ducts. The contents and the action of the juice are described in the section on the small intestine which is the part of the alimentary tract where the juice helps in digestion. Since it contains large quantities of enzymes which act on virtually all the constituents of food, pancreatic juice plays a very important role in digestion. In its absence, due to disease of the pancreas, food passes through incompletely processed. The faeces, which will smell particularly rancid, will contain exceptional amounts of fat and muscle fibres from undigested meat.

Embedded in the exocrine tissue are small islands of endocrine tissue which produce the hormones insulin and glucagon (p. 525). The secretions of this tissue are passed directly into the blood stream. Insulin is essential for the passage of glucose into cells, where its breakdown can release energy. Absence of insulin produces the condition of diabetes mellitus; this is described in the section on the assimilation of carbohydrates (p. 189).

Glucagon causes the breakdown of glycogen (the storage form of glucose) in the liver cells into glucose. Glucagon production results directly from a low level of glucose in the blood. As it flows through the pancreas, the glucose-low blood has the direct effect of stimulating the production of glucagon; this is itself released into the blood. The glucagon-containing blood circulating through the liver causes its cells to release glucose and restore blood glucose levels.

## Liver

The liver is a large, rather flattened gland which fits into the concavity of the abdominal side of the diaphragm (Fig. 2.12). It is divided into several lobes, which are separated peripherally. It has been described as the largest chemical factory in the body and its numerous functions can be summarized as:

(1) Production of bile.
(2) Special roles in metabolism of carbohydrates, proteins, fats.
(3) Storage.
(4) Synthesis.
(5) Detoxification.

### Production of Bile

Bile is a greenish-yellow fluid produced continuously by liver cells. It contains bile salts, bile pigments, and very small amounts of cholesterol and electrolytes such as chlorides and bicarbonates. It is alkaline and, like pancreatic juice, it helps neutralize the very acid chyme which enters the duodenum from the stomach. From its sites of formation in liver cells

bile is collected into small tubes, the bile ducts, of increasing order of size that join with one another until one main **common hepatic duct** is formed (hepatic is an adjective used in phrases referring to the liver). This joins the **cystic duct** of the **gall bladder**. The **common bile duct** results from this union and enters the duodenum a short distance from the pylorus.

Bile is produced all the while and when it does not pass directly to the digestive tract it is stored in the gall bladder. Here it becomes concentrated, ten to twentyfold in the dog, by the extraction of water by the wall of the gall bladder. Presence of food in the stomach and duodenum stimulates the release of stored bile.

Bile salts are formed mainly from cholesterol. They are necessary for the absorption of fats and of vitamins that are fat soluble. They act by lowering the surface tension around the fat globules so that they can be formed into a fine emulsion. This occurs in the small intestine, and further along the alimentary tract most of the bile salts themselves are absorbed and return to the liver for re-use.

The bile pigments are predominantly bilirubin. This results from the breakdown of haemoglobin wherever the red blood cells are destroyed. It travels in the blood stream to the liver where it is removed from the plasma and excreted in the bile. Bile pigments have no digestive function but they do colour the faeces. A small amount is normally present in blood.

An excessive accumulation of bilirubin causes a yellowing of the tissues called **jaundice** or **icterus**. This may occur in three ways:

(i) There may be an over-destruction of red blood cells so that the liver is unable to convert the breakdown products into bile pigments. This is haemolytic jaundice.

(ii) The liver may be damaged or diseased and thus unable to turn the bilirubin into bile pigments.

(iii) The bile is unable to flow away from the liver cells due to some physical blockage; this is obstructive jaundice.

The level of bilirubin in the blood plasma rises and it becomes deposited in the tissues, especially in fat.

### Special Roles in Metabolism

Carbohydrate, protein and fat metabolism occurs in nearly all the cells of the body but the liver cells have specific roles over and above the general ones.

*Carbohydrates.* The end products of carbohydrate digestion pass by the portal vein to the liver before entering the remaining circulation. The liver cells extract the excess carbohydrate that occurs after a meal and converts it to glycogen (a process called glycogenesis). This is the storage form of glucose, and the liver has the highest glycogen content of all the tissues. When the glucose level in the blood drops the glycogen is converted to glucose. The liver is also able to produce glycogen from amino acids and fatty acids.

*Proteins.* The portal blood flow also takes the digested protein products direct to the liver. The amino acids may then be passed on to other cells for their synthetic processes or they may be used by liver cells themselves to produce proteins; nearly all the plasma proteins (p. 8) including fibrinogen, essential for blood clotting, are produced in the liver. Amino acids are also used by the liver to release energy. This results in the production of ammonia which is toxic (poisonous) to the body; the liver cells have to convert this to urea which can then be excreted through the kidneys.

*Fats.* The liver is very important in fat metabolism. It converts fat into substances, for instance cholesterol and phospholipids, which are used elsewhere in the body. The two examples given are major components of cell membranes and structures inside cells. If the animal is starved the liver will use fats to release energy, but this will only happen if no glucose is available. The fat is transferred from fat depots to the liver where it may accumulate sufficiently to cause the condition "fatty liver". When large amounts of fats are being metabolized, the ketones or "ketone bodies" that result from fat breakdown may accumulate in the blood stream and be excreted slowly in the urine. Since ketones can be toxic, a serious accumulation (ketosis) is a dangerous state for the animal.

When the carbohydrate stores of an animal reach a certain level, the excess is converted into fat by the liver. Fatty acids are used by many cells to provide energy, but nearly half of these are split by the liver into simpler substances which can be used more easily.

### Storage

The liver is a store for glycogen, fat, certain of the vitamins and for iron (essential for erythrocytes). It does also act as a blood reserve since decreasing the flow through the portal vein releases a large volume to go to other parts.

### Synthesis

The role of the liver in synthesis of various components has been included in the comments on metabolism.

## *Detoxification*

Many materials foreign to the body and also several of the metabolites (substances resulting from metabolism) above certain levels can poison the animal. They are said to be toxic and detoxification is the process of rendering them relatively harmless and in a form suitable for excretion. Since much of the material absorbed from the intestines goes directly to the liver, harmful substances can be detoxified almost as soon as they are absorbed. There may, of course, be too much or it may be too potent for the liver to be able to cope. The detoxification into urea of the results of protein breakdown has already been mentioned.

## Urogenital System

The urogenital system consists of the **urinary system** and the **genital system**. The urinary system is responsible for removing waste products and excess water as **urine**. The genital system includes the organs, called **gonads**, which produce the cells used in procreation. Those of the male are the **testes** and produce **sperms** whereas the gonads of the female are **ovaries** and produce **ova**. The system also includes the means whereby the male and female products (sperms and ova) can unite and in the female provides an environment in which the resultant organisms (embryos) can develop properly.

For part of their course, the urinary and genital systems have common use of certain structures. In the male the products of the genital system are poured into the terminal part of the urinary system and the urethra is used as a common tube to the outside. The products of the urinary system of the female use the terminal part of the genital system and here the vestibule and vulva are the shared parts of the urogenital apparatus.

The urinary system will be described first. In the case of the male this includes the complete tract that conveys the urine to the outside of the body; the description of the female urinary system will finish where it joins the reproductive tract. The male genitalia will then be described as far as its junction with the urinary system. The description of the female genitalia includes all the parts of the tract.

## Urinary system

The urinary system is responsible for removing several waste products and also chemicals, including water, that are present in the body in excessive amounts. This is done by clearing them from the blood plasma but conserving those that are present in normal or subnormal quantities. The materials are brought in the blood stream to the left and right **kidneys** and in these organs they are passed into thousands of small blind-ending **renal tubules**. There are in the region of half a million in each kidney of a dog. ("Renal" is an adjective used in phrases referring to the kidney. Renal tubules are often called *nephrons* although this is not strictly accurate. The root of the word nephron is also used in terms referring to the kidney: for instance, nephritis is an inflammation of the kidney.) The tubules unite and eventually one tube, the **ureter**, leaves each kidney to transport urine (the material to be excreted) to the single **bladder** (see Fig. 2.17). From here the fluid is voided at intervals to the outside through the **urethra**.

In addition to its role in producing urine the kidney also has an endocrine function in that it is one of the sites where erythropoietin (also called erythropoietic stimulating factor or haemopoietin) is formed. This passes in the blood to the

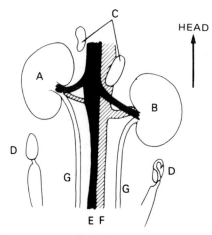

HEAD

FIG. 2.15   Kidneys in position in abdominal cavity of a bitch viewed from ventrally: A, right kidney; B, left kidney; C, adrenal glands; D, ovaries and tips of uterine horns; E, caudal vena cava; F, aorta; G, ureters.

bone marrow where it stimulates red blood cell production.

*Kidney* (Fig. 2.15)

One kidney is found on each side of the midline ventral to the lumbar vertebrae. They lie in the abdominal cavity where they are related to the large blood vessels, the aorta and the caudal vena cava. The kidneys are between the parietal peritoneum and the roof of the abdominal cavity. The organ itself is invested in a strong **fibrous capsule** of dense connective tissue which can be stripped easily from the healthy structure.

The blind end of each renal tubule is the **glomerular capsule** and this is invaginated by a knot of capillaries known as a **glomerulus** (Fig. 2.16). The remainder of the tubule follows a very long and tortuous course during which it is surrounded by a complex arrangement of capillaries. The whole system is an intricate mechanism for the control of body fluids by the physiological process of **renal filtration**.

The renal tubules finally empty into

**collecting ducts** and these amalgamate to form eventually a few large **papillary ducts** which open into a collecting area called the **pelvis**. (This is not related to the skeletal pelvis, both names are derived from the Latin word for a basin.)

The pelvis, the renal blood and lymph vessels, and the nerves may be surrounded by fat and are situated in the cavity of the kidney called its **sinus**. This opens on the medial edge of the kidney at the **hilus**. The renal blood vessels and nerves pass through the hilus and here also the renal pelvis narrows rapidly to be continued to the bladder by the ureter.

**Renal filtration**

Material is filtered from the blood through the wall of the glomerular capillaries and through the capsule lining. The pressure of the blood in the capillaries is higher than that inside the lumen of the capsule: the difference between them is called the **filtration pressure** and this causes the continual passage of filtrate. Anything which affects the filtration pressure will alter the filtration rate. Control of

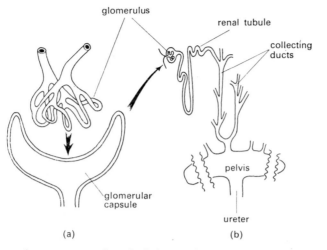

FIG. 2.16. Diagrams of arrangements of renal tubules: (a) glomerular capsule (very highly magnified) with glomerulus removed; (b) remainder of the tubule and connection with renal pelvis.

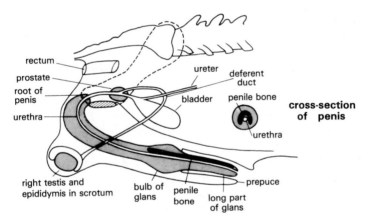

FIG. 2.17. Lateral view of part of the urogenital system of the dog in section. The small diagram is a section through the penis.

local blood pressure will be very critical; if this falls, e.g. due to loss of blood as with a haemorrhage, less filtrate will pass. The volume of blood and extracellular fluid will not suffer further reduction via the kidneys until blood pressure is restored to normal level. When arterial pressure is low, the kidneys will produce an enzyme called **renin** which converts one of the plasma proteins to **angiotensin**. This causes constriction of blood vessels and so increases arterial pressure. It is thought

the angiotensin also stimulates the cortex of the adrenal gland (part of the endocrine system) to produce the hormone **aldosterone**. This affects the kidneys so that they reduce the output of salt and water; this in turn maintains the volume of water and interstitial fluid in the body. It is sometimes necessary in treating a sick animal to increase the rate and the amount of filtrate. One way of doing this is to dilate the capillaries of the glomerulus. This will effectively increase the filtration pressure and the amount of fluid that will pass. Therapeutic substances that increase the amount of filtrate are called *diuretics.*

The capillaries and the glomerular capsule will not normally allow blood cells or very much plasma protein (p. 8) to filter through. Glomerular fluid is often called an "ultrafiltrate of plasma" and in fact it is almost identical to plasma except that it has only a very small amount of protein.

As the filtrate passes along the remainder of the renal tubule most of it is reabsorbed through the tubule wall into surrounding tissue fluid and so into the network of adjacent capillaries. Most of the water, glucose, amino acids, proteins and electrolyte are conserved in this way. Undesirable substances and excess amounts of even useful materials are left in the tubule fluid. There has been a "selective reabsorption". There is a definite control on the amount of each that is reabsorbed from the filtrate; some substances are completely readmitted whereas very little is taken back of an unwanted compound, such as urea. The reabsorption will depend on the rate that the fluid passes along the tubules; the faster this is the less efficient the reabsorption. This depends very much on the filtration rate and hence the filtration pressure. The absorption of water by the tubules is also regulated by the presence of the **antidiuretic hormone** (also called vasopressin or ADH). This is produced by the posterior part of the pituitary gland of the brain and circulates in the blood stream. In its presence the tubules are able to reabsorb water but when it is not available little absorption takes place. The very dilute fluid passing the glomerular filter stays that way right through the tubules and a very copious quantity of dilute urine is excreted. This condition (associated with malfunction of the production site in the pituitary) is called diabetes insipidus (diabetes refers to the production of large quantities of urine; insipidus, meaning tasteless, differentiates it from mellitus, sweet, resulting from the glucose excreted in insulin deficiency) (p. 75).

As well as absorbing needed material, the walls of the tubules do empty some excretions directly into the fluid. As little as 1% of glomerular filtrate may end up as urine.

In removing waste products and preserving the right balance of materials in the blood the kidneys have a key role in maintaining **homeostatis**, that is, the conditions in which cells can function at their best. The effect of the kidneys on blood volume and extracellular fluid has been mentioned: when these fall the kidneys will reduce the quantity of fluid leaving the body. By its selective reabsorption of some electrolytes and its excretion of others it firmly regulates the levels of ions in the extracellular fluids. The role of some of these will be described later (p. 311–15). Included in the regulation of ions will be that of hydrogen and so the pH (p. 15) of all body fluids will depend on the kidneys. Since these electrolytes affect the osmotic pressures of the body fluids, even these will be determined by the efficiency of the kidneys.

*Ureters*

This pair of tubes conveys the urine from the kidneys to the bladder by peristalsis. They are each suspended in a peritoneal fold and consist of a lining mucous membrane surrounded by a coat of smooth muscle which in turn is covered by an adventitial coat. The ureters enter the neck of the urinary bladder at an angle that ensures that they travel for some distance in its wall (Fig. 2.17). In this way a very effective valve is formed to prevent the return of urine from the bladder into the ureters.

*Bladder* (Fig. 2.17)

The bladder is shaped something like a pear, with the more caudal narrower end being the **neck** and the other end the **apex** (or **vertex**). Between these ends is the **body**. The size, shape and position of the organ varies with the quantity of its contents, but ventrally it is usually in contact with the abdominal floor.

The mucosa is attached to the muscular coat by a very elastic submucous layer and forms many folds when the organ is empty. The muscle coat consists of fibres running in all directions, but around the neck the circular fibres form sphincters. Not all of the bladder is covered by peritoneum since the most caudal part (i.e. near the neck) is beyond the level of the peritoneal cavity. The neck of the bladder is continuous with the urethra.

When the bladder is sufficiently full, sensory nerve impulses pass to the nervous system. Motor impulses to the bladder wall cause it to contract and the innermost smooth muscle sphincter to relax. There is, however, an outer voluntary muscle sphincter that only relaxes when the animal finds it convenient to *micturate*. The act of passing urine is *micturition*.

## Urethra of the Female

This is a very short tube which leaves the neck of the bladder and opens into the floor of the vestibule of the female genital tract.

It is sometimes necessary to pass a catheter (a tube) into the bladder (p. 323). If the lips of the vulva are held apart by an instrument such as a speculum and a light directed into the exposed interior of the urogenital tract, the opening of the urethra will be seen as a small cleft a short distance inside and on the floor. The catheter (which will need to be quite narrow) is passed through the cleft. Pass-

ing a catheter requires patience, practice, and especially a detailed knowledge of the anatomy of the region. For the queen cat, pulling the lips of the vulva downwards towards the hocks forms a small channel in the floor of the vestibule which helps guide the catheter to the relatively large urethral opening. The initial direction of the catheter will be towards the sacrum, but when the urethra has been entered, the catheter will then need to be slid cranially.

## Urethra of the Male

The urethra of the male starts at the neck of the bladder and runs caudally on the floor of the pelvis. As it leaves this at the ischial arch it continues as the tubular part of the penis. The urethra can be considered for descriptive purposes to have a pelvic and a penile part.

At the start of the urethra, that is near its junction with the bladder, the pelvic part in the dog has a small projection into the dorsal side of its lumen. Near this are the duct openings associated with its genital system; these are the deferent ducts and those of the prostate gland. In fact, at this point the urethra is passing through the prostate gland. From the entry of these ducts the urethra will carry both urine and seminal secretions. The arrangement is slightly different in the cat in that there is a length of urethra (called the pre-prostatic urethra) between the neck of the bladder and the prostate gland. Near the caudal end of the pelvis the urethra of the cat receives ducts from the bulbourethral glands which lie on either side (Fig. 2.18). The dog does not have these particular accessory genital glands.

The urethra is lined by mucous membrane and this is surrounded by a layer of cavernous erectile tissue. This consists of connective tissue divisions and trabeculae which condense peripherally to form a limiting layer. The spaces ("caverns") between the trabeculae are lined with endothelium and usually filled with blood. When the passages by which the blood leaves are markedly narrowed, the local pressures rises and the tissues becomes engorged. The turgid organs may then stiffen and for this reason the descriptive term of erectile tissue is used for those situations where such vascular engorgement is possible.

As the urethra surrounded by its erectile tissue and muscle coats leaves the pelvis it is joined by more erectile tissue, and the whole mass forms the **penis**. The urethra runs the entire length and opens at the end of this organ.

*Penis*

The penis is attached to the ischium of each side by fibrous tissue forming a crus. These crura (plural of crus) contain erectile tissue and come together uniting in the midline forming the **root** of the penis. Here they are joined by the urethra with its erectile coat. Together they (the ure-thra, its coat and the continuations of the two crura) constitute the penis. The parts following the root is the **body** of the penis. The terminal free end is the **glans** of the penis and in the male cat (the tom-cat) its surface is covered by tiny curved papillae which are hard and sharp (see Fig. 2.18). The penis of the tom points caudally and the urethra with its surrounding layers lies on the dorsal aspect. Ventral to this the erectile tissue of the remainder of the penis becomes partly replaced in the glans by bone (cartilage in the young cat) which stiffens the organ even when it is not engorged. The lumen of the penile part is smaller than that of the remainder of the urethra.

The penis of the dog curves cranioventrally at its root turning to point between the thighs. The root and body are firmly attached to the ventral body wall and only the glans is free. The urethra becomes ventral to the continuations of the crura because the penis is directed cranially. As the glans continues from the body of the penis the first quarter is markedly swollen forming the **bulb** of the glans. This is formed by the erectile tissue of the urethra and when the penis is erected it forms a hard collar round the base of the glans.

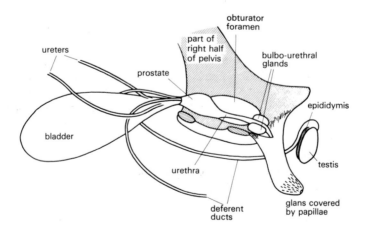

FIG. 2.18.    Genital system of tom (male) cat. (The left testis and part of the left half of the pelvis have been removed.)

The remaining three-fourths of the glans is called the **long part**: it forms the tip of the penis and has its own erectile system.

In the male dog there are no papillae on the glans but there is a well-developed **penile bone** (or **os penis**) which lies dorsal and on each side of the urethra which is thus in a bony tunnel and unable to expand very much (Fig. 2.17). Although the dog and cat are the only domestic mammals in which this penile bone is found, it occurs in a large number of other mammals.

The function of the cavernous erectile tissue is to stiffen the penis for insertion during copulation; it has no special use during urination.

The entire relaxed organ lies within a sheath of skin called the **prepuce**. The epithelium of the skin is continuous with that of the inside of the prepuce. From here it is reflected on to the end of the penis and becomes continuous with the epithelium of the mucous membrane of the urethra where that tube opens to the outside.

Passing a cathether in the dog and tom cat needs extreme care. The length of the urethra is much greater than in the females and great care must be taken not to damage the inside of the tube. The penis of the cat is extruded by gently pressing with the fingers towards the base of the organ. The penis is kept pointing straight caudally and the catheter is inserted towards the sacrum until the caudal brim of the pelvis is passed. The catheter is then slid cranially. To catheterize the dog the prepuce should be retracted by pushing with the fingers against the caudal edge of the bulb of the glans; the penis can be kept out by maintaining this pressure. The catheter is inserted into the urethral orifice. It must be remembered that the penile urethra runs through the tunnel of the penile bone and that it then curves dorsally to pass over the caudal brim of the pelvis. A flexible catheter and patient carefulness are essential.

## Urine

The ultrafiltrate of plasma forming the glomerular fluid has many of its constituents reabsorbed by the tubules. Waste products are excreted into the fluid by other regions of the tubules and the resulting solution is urine. It will reflect in some ways the state of the blood (and hence of the whole animal) and also of specific regions such as the kidneys, ureters, bladder, etc., through which it has to pass. By physical and chemical analyses it is possible to assist diagnoses as to sites of pathology: at least into pre-renal (before blood passes through the glomerulus), renal and post-renal (ureters, bladder, urethra) areas.

Species, feeding, exercise, medicaments and even environment will affect the condition of the urine, and so there is a wide range that may still be normal. The dog is recorded as voiding 20–100 ml per kg body weight per day: comparable figures for the cat are 10–12 ml. The colour is usually yellowish and the specific gravity will depend on the relative properties of the dissolved material: large frequent quantities of urine (polyuria) usually have a low specific gravity. The "normal" range for dog urine is 1.016–1.060 and for cat 1.020–1.040.

When fresh, the urine is acidic (pH 5–7) if the animal is on a normal carnivorous diet with an acceptable level of protein. There should, however, be little protein in the urine itself. The normal glomerular filter does not allow much to pass from the plasma, but if the permeability is increased due to irritation, etc., protein will appear in the urine. Protein may also be present due to other renal disease and also to inflammation of the urinary bladder (cystitis). Damage to the liver and blockage of the normal passage of bile to the small intestine usually increases the amount of bile pigment and bile salts in the blood. As it flows through the kidneys, the plasma will allow these to pass into the urine. If the glucose level of blood reaches abnormal levels, as in diabetes mellitus, the excess will leave the body in the urine. Ketones (ketone bodies) (p. 478) in the urine are associated with a deficient carbohydrate intake or faulty carbohydrate metabolism leading to imperfect oxidation of fats. Blood pigment or even blood cells may also be present in abnormal urine. An analysis of urine may be a very useful aid in diagnosis and the various tests are outlined in Chapter 6 on diagnostic aids. Damage to the kidneys will also result in the increase of certain breakdown products appearing in the blood. Examination of plasma for creatinine and blood urea nitrogen (BUN) can greatly assist diagnosis in these cases.

Various deposits may also be found if urine is allowed to settle out. These may be cells from various parts of the urinary tract (and also from the genital system, especially in the male), crystals due to abnormal chemical constituents or small cylinders which are casts of the inside of renal tubules. These form during some disease processes in the kidneys and may contain precipitated protein, fat, epithelial and blood cells. Small (sometimes quite large) beads of chemicals may form in the urinary tract most commonly in the bladder. These may be called calculi, stones or uroliths. In cats the material is like sand and is then said to be *sabulous*. These structures are quite solid with layers of mucoprotein and minerals, but the causes of urolithiasis (urine stone formation) are not fully understood. However, the dangers are very apparent since the stones may get into the urethra and block the flow of urine, a condition that may lead to acute distress. Blockage usually occurs at the narrowest part of the urethra—at the base of the penis or sometimes where the urethra passes through the prostate gland (p. 86).

### Genital system of the male
(Figs. 2.17, 2.18, 2.19)

This system is responsible for producing cells that will fertilize the ova of the female and also a suitable fluid medium for their transport and maintenance. It is another visceral system that consists of several tubes joining together to have eventually only one opening to the outside. The many blind-ending tubes are **seminiferous tubules** and into their cavities are shed the sperms which are the fertilizing cells (Fig. 2.19). These tubules are all in the paired **testes** and they collect together to form eventually the **deferent duct (ductus deferens)**. This pair of tubes open into the urethra near the neck of the bladder and the sperms use the urethra to reach the outside of the body of the male. Accessory glands add their secretions so that the sperms are part of the fluid mixture called **semen**. This is ejaculated during sexual union via the temporarily stiffened penis which has been inserted into the female genital system.

The testes are surgically removed if the animal is not to be allowed to breed. It is then said to have been **neutered** or **castrated** as opposed to the unoperated animal which is called an **entire**. The erectile tissues of the penis do not develop fully if the animal has been castrated when young.

Secondary sex characters (characteristics) are also affected by early castration. These are features which differ between the sexes. There are few obvious ones in the dog: musculature and skeleton are usually heavier in the male. The tom cat

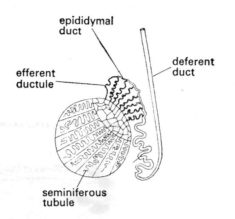

FIG. 2.19. Section of testis: there are very many more seminiferous tubules than are shown here.

does have definite male characteristics, shape, smell, voice, that can differentiate it from the female.

### Testes

The walls of the seminiferous tubules consist of two types of cells—those from which sperms are produced (spermatogenic cells) and supportive cells which produce fluid that is thought to be nutritive to the sperms. These are also known as Sertoli cells, and in the dog—in addition to providing for the sperms—these supportive cells produce oestrogenic hormones (see p. 523). There are also cells between the seminiferous tubules: these are interstitial cells (of Leydig) and they produce the hormone testosterone (see p. 126).

The spermatogenic cells divide and from these spermatids are formed. These become transformed into sperms by undergoing a series of modifications including the formation of a tail. At this stage they detach from the sperm-producing wall of the seminiferous tubule and are released into its lumen.

The tubules form a network of channels through which the sperms pass. They can then leave the testis by several **efferent ductules** which unite to form one **epididymal duct (ductus epididymis)** outside the testis.

Spermatogenesis (production of sperm) involves a special method of division of nuclear material called **meiosis**. This was mentioned in the section on reproduction of the cell (p. 24). In mitosis, the usual method of division, each chromosome splits into half and a half of each chromosome goes to each of the two resulting cells. This means that all the cells undergoing mitotic division always have the same number of chromosomes (the species number). But in meiosis there is no splitting of individual chromosomes. Instead the total number of chromosomes is divided equally between the two resulting cells, each ending up with half the species number.

The same meiotic division happens in the production of ova so that each ovum also has only half the species number of chromosomes. When the sperm joins the ovum at fertilization, each parent will have provided half the chromosome number (and incidentally the characteristics (genes) the chromosomes carry) and the species number will be restored. Normal mitotic division of the resulting zygote will then be established.

### Epididymis

The sperms are stored and mature in the epididymal duct which slowly transports them away from the testis. This is very long but by close coiling it forms **lobules** which are attached to the long border of the testis, and it is then usually referred to as the **epididymis** (Fig. 2.19). The epididymal duct is continued by the deferent duct **(ductus deferens)**.

### Deferent Duct

Each one of this pair of tubes connects the epididymis to the urethra. At its termination the wall thickens and becomes very glandular; the secretion of the glands is poured directly into the lumen of the duct. The opening of each tube into the urethra occurs near the junction of the urethra and the bladder.

### Accessory Genital Glands

These structures add their secretions to the semen, producing, in fact, most of its volume. The only accessory genital gland in the dog is the **prostate** (Fig. 2.17). The cat has, in addition, a pair of **bulbo-urethral** glands (Fig. 2.18). The prostate of the dog surrounds the urethra near the neck of the bladder; in the cat the gland is further caudal with a portion of urethra between the bladder and the prostate. The gland has several openings into the urethra and the deferent ducts pass through its substance to open near by. The prostate normally lies on the floor of the pelvis and may, when pathological, enlarge to almost fill the pelvic cavity. A gland in such a state can severely interfere with defaecation by pressure on the rectum.

In the cat the bulbo-urethral glands flank the urethra caudal to the prostate, lying just cranial to the ischial arch. They also have ducts which pass the secretions into the urethra.

### Scrotum

The testes of the adult domestic mammals are contained in a diverticulum of the abdominal cavity called the **scrotum**, which in the cat is ventral to the anus near the ischiatic symphysis. The scrotum of the dog lies between the thighs. Smooth muscle tissue and collagenous and elastic fibres form a **septum** between the right and left halves of the scrotum and each of the pouches which are thus formed contains a testis.

Each testis is surrounded by a diverticulum of peritoneum which is called the vaginal tunic or coat (**tunica vaginalis**) as it leaves the main abdominal cavity. The deferent duct, the nerves, the blood vessels and the lymphatic vessels which are connected with the testis are also covered by the vaginal coat. These structures which pass to and from the testis, and the layer of tunica vaginalis which covers them, constitute the **spermatic cord**.

Each cord runs between the abdominal cavity and the pouch of the scrotum in a passage called the **inguinal canal**. The abdominal opening of the canal is called the **deep inguinal ring**; the other end is a slit in an abdominal muscle and is called the **superficial inguinal ring**.

The diverticulum of peritoneum remains opens throughout life, and omentum or intestine may occasionally slip down it into the scrotum. This condition is called a **scrotal hernia**. A similar condition called an **inguinal hernia** occurs if the abdominal contents protrude through the inguinal canal outside, but along with, the tunica vaginalis.

### Genital system of the female
(Figs. 2.20, 2.21)

The organs of this system produce the female sex cells (ova) and provide situations in which these can be fertilized and develop during *pregnancy*. This is the period, also known as *gestation*, between the fertilization of the ova and *parturition* (the act of birth). The genital system is also arranged to receive the penis during copulation.

The time of year at which sexual union normally takes place is the *breeding season* and during this time there is at least one period of sexual activity on the part of the female known as *oestrus* or *heat*. The release of ova (*ovulation*) is closely related to oestrus and the rhythmical changes undergone by the female genital system at this time constitute the *oestrous cycle*. It is unusual for signs of oestrus to appear during pregnancy.

The ova are produced by paired **ovaries** and pass into the open ends of **uterine tubes** (one of which is associated with each ovary) (Fig. 2.20). These continue into the **uterus**. If the ovum is fertilized by a sperm it becomes an **embryo** and as this enlarges it is called a **fetus** (foetus). The development takes place in the lumen of the uterus which undergoes marked changes during pregnancy. The uterus of a pregnant animal is said to be *gravid*. When the animal is pregnant for the first time it is *primigravid*; during later pregnancies the animal is *multigravid*. When several young are developing in the one uterus as in the dog and cat, the animal is *multiparous*; if only one is developing the animal is *uniparous*.

The caudal end of the uterus is modified to form the **cervix**, through which the cavity of the female genital system continues into the **vagina**. Caudal to this the **vestibule** continues into the **vulva** consisting of a pair of lips through which the female genital system opens to the outside.

The surgical removal of ovaries to prevent breeding is **ovariectomy**. If the uterus is also removed, the operation is **ovariohysterectomy**, more commonly called **spaying**.

### *Ovary* (Fig. 2.22)

Each ovary consists of a framework of connective tissue which condenses peripherally. A layer of epithelial cells attached to its outer surface is continuous with the epithelium of the peritoneum. As it leaves the ovary to attach to the wall of the abdominal cavity the peritoneum is called

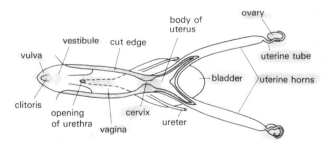

FIG. 2.20.   Dorsal view of female genitalia. The dorsal wall of the tract has been opened from the horns caudally.

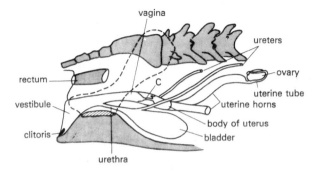

F<small>IG.</small> 2.21.   Lateral view of female genitalia. The right uterine horn and ovary are removed. The tract is sectioned from the horns caudally. C, cervix.

the **mesovarium**. This helps form a pouch (**ovarian bursa**) which in the bitch completely encloses the ovary, hiding it from view even when the rest of the tract is exposed.

In the very young animal, cells in the ovary group together to form **follicles** and eventually **follicular fluid** is formed within the cluster. Some of the inner cells of the follicles give rise to the ova (eggs). Their formation resembles that of sperms in that meiosis occurs and each ovum will have only half the species number of chromosomes.

The follicles move slowly towards the surface of the ovary while these events are beginning. At some physiologically opportune moment the outer surface of the follicles rupture, expelling the follicular fluid and the mature ova. This phenomenon is ovulation and in the dog and cat several ova are released at the same time. Adult ovaries will usually show follicles at all stages of development and at varying depths from the surface.

Some bleeding into the ruptured follicle occurs after ovulation. The blood clot that forms is gradually resorbed and replaced by cells which grow in with their products from the wall of the ruptured follicle. This structure is called a **corpus luteum**. Each ruptured follicle is succeeded by a corpus luteum which then undergoes a slow diminution in size. However, if the ova liberated by the ruptured follicles are fertilized and so the animal becomes pregnant, the regression of the corpora lutea (plural of corpus luteum) is delayed.

Adult ovaries, then, may show not only follicles at all stages of development and at varying depths from the surface, but also corpora lutea at different levels of maturity and degeneration.

Follicular fluid and corpora lutea are both responsible for hormone production (p. 127). Those associated with follicular fluid help produce the outward signs of sexual desire (heat, p. 648) and prepare the genitalia for coitus. The hormones released by the corpora lutea help first in preparing the animal for pregnancy and then later in maintaining the condition. Towards the end of pregnancy the corpora lutea hormones affect structures that will be involved in parturition.

*Uterine Tube* (Fig. 2.20)

The ova are expelled from the ovary into the peritoneal cavity. However, the open end of a uterine tube (also called a Fallopian tube) is very close to the ovary and the ova are passed along this and into the uterus. The ovarian end of the tube flares out and may be split into irregular

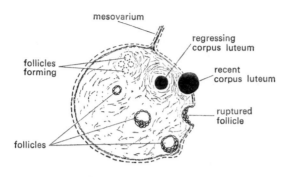

Fɪɢ. 2.22.    Diagram of ovary.

processes called **fimbriae**. The uterine end of the tube opens into the uterus.

It is in the uterine tubes that the sperms usually fertilize the ova. A large number of sperms surround the small number of ova and eventually a single sperm penetrates into each egg. This seems to affect the surface of the ovum so that no more sperms can then enter. The nuclear material contained in the sperm begins to separate out and so does that of the female. The chromosomes from the male (half the species number) join with the chromosomes from the female (also half the species number) (see p. 207). The species number has been restored and mitotic division starts the ever-increasing production of cells that will constitute the new animal.

*Uterus* (Figs. 2.20, 2.21)

The entire uterus is somewhat Y-shaped with a pair of **uterine horns** joining to form a single **uterine body**. Each horn is about five times the length of the uterine body. The uterus undergoes tremendous changes in shape and position during pregnancy and afterwards it never completely returns to its non-gravid morphology. It lies usually in the abdominal cavity but in the young animal some of it may be in the pelvis.

In structure it resembles other parts of a visceral system. The mucous membrane forming the inner layer is called the **endometrium** and the muscle layer the **myometrium**.

Probably the most important function of the uterus is to retain the embryos within the body of the mother and these are distributed in the two horns. As the fertilized ova develop they each produce a group of structures called **extra-embryonic**, and later **fetal, membranes**. In addition to providing a container for fluid in which the embryo develops, the membranes form an intimate attachment to the endometrium whilst remaining in complete continuity with the embryo. The membranes have an extensive blood supply and in this way the local blood streams of the mother and of the embryos are brought very close together (*but do not intermingle*) and an exchange of nutrient and waste material can take place between the mother and the offspring. This arrangement of embryonic and maternal tissue constitutes a **placenta**, having a **fetal** and a **uterine** part.

In the dog and cat each placenta forms a broad ring encircling the fetal membranes. The blood vessels and other attachments to the fetus come together to form the **umbilical cord** which enters its abdominal region; apart from this connection the developing animal floats freely in the fluids within the membranes. At parturition the fetal membranes are usually expelled shortly after the young; hence the origin of one of their names, the *afterbirth*.

The cavity of the body of the uterus connects with that of the vagina through the narrow **cervical canal** of the cervix. The thick walls of this region act as a sphincter which relaxes only during oestrus to allow the passage of sperms and during parturition to allow the expulsion of the young. During pregnancy the cervical canal is closed by muscular contraction and by a plug of mucus. The peritoneal suspension of the uterus and ovary is part of the **broad ligament**.

*Vagina*

The vagina extends from the cervix to the **external urethral orifice**, the opening of the urethra into the floor of the female genital system. The vagina is a highly dilatable part of the tract and lies entirely in the pelvis. Only the cranial part has a peritoneal covering forming its serosa. The caudal part is surrounded by connective tissue called **pelvic fascia**.

*Vestibule*

The vestibule extends from the vagina to the external opening of the female urogenital system. Since the external urethral orifice is its cranial limit the vestibule is a part that is common to the genital and the urinary systems. Muscle fibres in the wall of this part of the tract form a very strong sphincter mechanism.

*Vulva*

This vertical slit marks the external opening of the urogenital system and consists of a pair of **lips** which join dorsally and ventrally. A small knob-like structure called the **clitoris** formed partly of cavernous erectile tissue is found just inside the ventral angle of this vulvar cleft.

## Reproductive Patterns

### General

The pattern of sexual activity common to many animals is not completely followed by either the dog or the cat. However, it will be useful to outline the stages and control of this general pattern first (Fig. 23a) and then to describe the signs in the bitch and queen.

**Oestrus** is the only time that the female will accept a male (a notable exception to this is the human). The animal may then also be said to be "on heat" or "in season". The length of oestrus varies between species: although it may last for 10 days in the bitch it is less than one day for a cow. Just prior to oestrus the follicles in the ovary start increasing in size and this phase is called **pro-oestrus**. During oestrus, follicles rupture spontaneously and from each of the ruptured follicles a corpus luteum forms (p. 88). The period during which corpora lutea develop is **metoestrus**. Once corpora lutea are established the female is in a **dioestrous** phase and this continues until their hormonal activity fades considerably. The animal may then go into pro-oestrus and the cycle pro-oestrus, oestrus, metoestrus, dioestrus, pro-oestrus be repeated.

It is not uncommon for reproductive patterns like this to occur only during certain times of the year. In that case, after several of the cycles just described, the "breeding season" will come to an end and a period of **anoestrus** with no activity on the part of the reproductive organs will follow the dioestrous phase. When another breeding season comes along anoestrus will be replaced by pro-oestrus, follicles will develop and the cycle will recommence. Animals with these reproductive patterns are "seasonal breeders".

So far it has been assumed that no males have been involved with the female but it could be that the animal was successfully mated during oestrus. The corpora lutea will form and so there will be a metoestrus: but now pregnancy will replace the dioestrus. The corpora lutea will remain active longer and are then called the corpora lutea of pregnancy. They will produce hormones that will help maintain pregnancy and prepare the animal for parturition. This will eventually happen and then anoestrus (which may be very short, or even absent in some species) will follow till the next breeding time.

## Bitch (Fig. 23b)

The reproductive behaviour of the bitch differs from the general pattern in that she is "mon-oestrus", i.e. there is only one oestrous period in each breeding season. When the bitch has been "on heat" once she will not be attractive to a dog again for several months.

A bitch first comes "on heat" between 6 and 12 months of age with small breeds being earlier than large ones. Although it is often said that oestrus occurs twice a year this is not strictly true in all cases; some bitches only have one breeding time in a year, while others may have three. Oestrus can happen at all times of the year but it is certainly most common during the spring.

During the pro-oestrous phase the vulva swells up and all the tubular genital tract thickens and produces an increased amount of secretions. These will be blood-tinged and appear as a sanguineous (bloody) discharge at the vulva. Pro-oestrus usually lasts about 9 days but then will come the time when the bitch will accept the male. In fact, the smell of the vulval secretions positively attracts and invites many males. In addition, the bitch will make all efforts to escape to find a male. The first day of acceptance is day 1 of oestrus. This phase of accepting matings lasts between 1 and 2 weeks usually, although ovulation will normally occur within the first 3 days of oestrus.

Ovulation takes place whether the animal is mated or not and so the bitch is said to be a **spontaneous ovulator**. Corpora lutea form after the ovulation resulting in the period of metoestrus. If the bitch has been mated successfully pregnancy will follow; after parturition the bitch will then become anoestrus until the next breeding season.

Corpora lutea also form if the bitch is not mated or if the mating is not successful. In the description of the general pattern outlined above this period was called dioestrus. The activity of the corpora lutea of the bitch is slightly different from that of other species and some authorities prefer to call this period a second stage of metoestrus. Although the bitch is not pregnant the hormones produced by the corpora lutea may cause the animal to show some of the signs usually associated with pregnancy. So this period of dioestrus which is also known as a later stage of metoestrus may be given yet other names, pseudopregnancy, false pregnancy, pseudocyesis. (In the introduction on page 1, it was pointed out that several names exist for the same thing and that it was not possible to say that any one was necessarily the only correct term. This is one such case and all these names have been mentioned because they appear in books and articles that may be read during your studies.) Whatever name is given to this period it is followed by anoestrus and this continues until the next breeding season.

Although the term **pseudopregnancy** (false pregnancy, pseudocyesis) is used by some workers for one of the normal periods of the oestrous cycle there may be no obvious similarity to pregnancy. On the other hand, in some cases there are very marked signs such as swollen mammary glands which can leak milk, an enlarged uterus and the bitch may even indulge in bed-making. These can be accepted as normal physiological events that will subside in time as the bitch approaches anoestrus.

### Queen (Fig. 2.23c)

The majority of female cats are "seasonal breeders" and are not receptive over the winter. During the breeding season, unless pregnancy takes place, oestrus keeps recurring. Because of this, the cat is said to be poly-oestrus (and is, therefore, seasonally polyoestrus).

One major difference between the cat behaviour and the others that have been described is that the ovarian follicles only rupture and allow ova to escape if the queen is mated (or has some similar artificial stimulation). Because of this the cat is described as an **"induced ovulator"** as opposed to spontaneous ovulators such as the bitch.

The queen reaches sexual maturity between 6 and 12 months of age and during the next nearest spring or autumn will undergo a pro-oestrus lasting from 1 to 3 days. Ovarian follicles will develop. She will then go into oestrus when she will freely accept the male. Her behaviour may be so unusual that the owner considers she is ill. She may go off food, cry out and adopt apparently strange postures which

are really positions for copulation. If mating does not occur oestrus lasts for about 10 days and then the follicles reduce in size without rupturing: corpora lutea do not form. The cat will then come into oestrus in another 1–3 weeks with another wave of follicular development. This cycle will be repeated several times if no mating takes place and then anoestrus will occur for several months during which the ovary is non-active until the next breeding time.

If the queen is mated ovulation occurs and corpora lutea form. This marks the phase of metoestrus. When the mating is fertile this is followed by pregnancy. If the mating is infertile, the corpora lutea continue hormonal activity and the queen undergoes a period of pseudopregnancy (false pregnancy, pseudocyesis. This may also be referred to as dioestrus.) Like the bitch at a similar time, signs of this vary from being very marked to being negligible. A short anoestrus phase follows if it is still the breeding season. The return to oestrus for a cat that has been pregnant is usually 1–2 weeks after weaning.

### Mating

#### Dog

The male is able and willing to mate at all times of the year although there are probably periods when he is more excitable.

The female will only accept the male during oestrus. This occurs first sometime after about 6 months of age.

As has been described above, just prior to every oestrus of the bitch, the vulva becomes swollen and there is a haemorrhagic vulval discharge. Although the male may be attracted he is not allowed to serve (mate). After about a week the discharge is replaced by a clear amber-coloured secretion and the female posi-

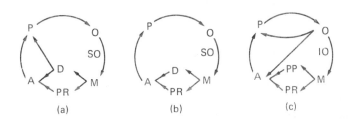

FIG. 2.23. Reproductive patterns (a) general (b) bitch (c) queen. A anoestrus, D dioestrus (in the bitch this may be called pseudopregnancy, false pregnancy, pseudocyesis or a later stage of metoestrus; see text), M metoestrus, O oestrus, P pro-oestrus, PP pseudopregnancy (false pregnancy, pseudocyesis or it may be called dioestrus), PR pregnancy, IO induced ovulation, SO spontaneous ovulation.

tively invites **coitus,** the act of sexual union. This stage also lasts for about a week; thereafter the vulva returns to normal size and mating is no longer allowed.

If conditions are favourable, the dog mounts and pushes the penis between the lips of the vulva. Thrusting movements follow and the penis becomes engorged with blood. Semen is being ejaculated into the female at this time. The bulb of the glans of the penis swells up to form a hard collar round the base of the glans. The sphincter muscles around the female vestibule contract behind the bulb and hold the male in position even after ejaculation is complete; this constitutes the **tie** that often (but not always) occurs with dogs. The male is able to dismount from the female and they even turn tail to tail without the tie being broken. This may last for up to 30 minutes or so before the engorgement subsides and allows the genitalia to separate.

A tie (or "locking") is quite natural to the dog and should not be interfered with. It may facilitate the entry of the ejaculate into the uterus and, in any case, a forced separation may damage the animals.

*Cat*

The cat also becomes sexually mature after about 6 months and during each of the breeding seasons the queen comes into oestrus about every 21 days and stays in this condition for about 1 to 4 days. Inviting postures such as raising the hindquarters and flattening the back accompanied by "calling" usually occur for a day or two before she will accept the tom. Mating can then occur several times a day for the period of oestrus. In the non-erect (flaccid) state the penis points caudally but during erection it turns cranio-ventrally. The mating posture and realignment of the penis enable the vulva to be entered. Ejaculation is immediate and the animals soon separate.

Sperms move very rapidly and may be found in the uterine tube within half a minute of being deposited near the cervix.

**Pregnancy**

Pregnancy in the dog and cat lasts about 9 weeks tending to be slightly longer in the cat (see also pp. 654). During that time the fertilized eggs develop from single cells into the complicated organisms

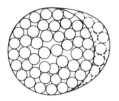

FIG. 2.24.    Ball of cells forming zygote cut in half.

that are born at parturition. The uterus in which they develop also undergoes massive changes and so do other maternal tissues. The study of the development of the unborn animal is called **embryology** and an appreciation of some of the changes is useful in understanding the care and welfare of pregnant animals and their young.

The eggs, as single cells, are released from the ovaries into the uterine tubes. There they are met by the sperms from a successful mating and the penetration of an ovum by a sperm is fertilization. It takes place 2–3 days after ovulation and has been described in the section on the uterine tube (p. 89). The fertilized egg is called a *zygote* or a *conceptus.*

Fertilization provokes the zygote into dividing into more cells which all stay clumped together. During this time the zygote is still free in the uterine tube and is gradually making its way towards the uterus, dividing as it goes, from 2 cells to 4, then 8, 16, 32, etc. (Fig. 2.24). The zygote of the dog takes 8–10 days to pass along the uterine tube before it reaches the uterus: that of the cat takes about 3 days. The uterine tube helps the conceptuses along by muscular movements and by the beating action of the delicate hair-like projections (the cilia) of the cells in its lining. The tube also produces secretions for the nutrition of the zygotes.

In cases where mating has taken place and the pregnancy is not wanted (a misalliance), the conditions inside the tube and the rate of passage of the zygote can be interfered with by an intra-muscular injection of a compound containing one of the oestrogen hormones. This usually results in the death of the zygotes and the very early termination of the pregnancy.

Even when the ball of cells resulting from the continuous division of the zygote reaches the uterus it still floats freely in the cavity until about 2–3 weeks after the original ovulation (slightly less than this in the cat).

During this time the zygotes are being arranged along the inside of the uterine horns. Some conceptuses migrate from one horn to the other but eventually they settle within the wall of the uterus at fairly regularly spaced intervals. Although the zygotes are still less than 5 mm in diameter they cause the uterus to show slight swellings. During the free-floating time the zygotes are being nourished by secretions of the uterus.

While it is still moving around in the uterus, changes are going on inside the ball of cells. A fluid-filled cavity forms, and instead of a solid mass the conceptus becomes a ball filled with fluid with one area rather thicker than the rest (Fig. 2.25). The thick area is called the *inner cell mass* and it will eventually form the body of the animal. The thinner area is called the *trophoblast* and this helps form the membranes that will eventually attach the conceptus to the inside wall of the uterus.

Two waves of cells migrate from the

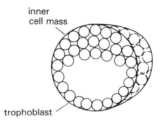

FIG. 2.25.  Cavity formation of zygote cut in half.

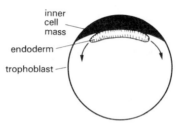

FIG. 2.26.  Endoderm formation. Layers of cells now shown as lines.

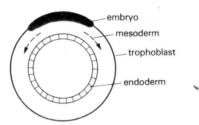

FIG. 2.27.  Mesoderm formation. Inner cell mass can now be called embryo. In all the diagrams spaces are shown between the layers. This is only for clarity.

deep surface of the inner cell mass. This itself begins to lengthen so that two ends are formed: the inner cell mass can now be called an **embryo**. The first wave of cells is called the *endoderm* and the cells spread all round the inside of the ball (Fig. 2.26). The second wave is the mesoderm and this itself splits into two layers (Figs. 2.27, 2.28).

The mesodermal layers push up and over the embryo which has now a slight curl at both ends (Fig. 2.29). (It is convenient to describe the development as if the embryo were at the top of the ball of cells, but this certainly need not be so.) The folds are meeting from all round the embryo (the diagrams are only sections of the complete structure) and in this way the embryo becomes trapped inside a complete bubble of fluid: this is the *amniotic cavity*. The outer wall of the bubble is formed by the membrane consisting of mesoderm and trophoblast and is called the **amnion**. Close contact between the mesoderm and trophoblast in other parts of the conceptus makes the membrane called the **chorion**.

In addition to forming the amniotic folds the mesoderm also begins to push into the ball of endoderm making it into a very small top part and a very large spherical bottom part (Fig. 2.29). This large part is the **yolk sac**. It does not contain any yolk but it joins with the trophoblast in supplying the embryo with its nutrition. By now the conceptus (zygote) is loosely attached by all these membranes to the endometrium and sustenance is obtained from here and from the uterine secretions. The small top part of the endoderm is very closely associated with the embryo itself and it narrows out into a tube running the length of the inside of the developing animal. It becomes the *primitive gut tube* and from this some of the other visceral organs will develop (Fig. 2.30). One structure that immediately arises as a balloon-like outpouching from the tube of endoderm is the **allantois**. It develops at the caudal end of the embryo and pushes outside the developing body of the embryo and into the layers that are surrounding it. The yolk sac, the amnion, the chorion and the allantois are called extra-embryonic membranes (that is, they are outside the embryo) (Fig. 2.30).

The allantois continues to expand and eventually it virtually encircles the embryo floating in its amniotic cavity (Fig. 2.31). The yolk sac shrivels into a very small structure. The chorion and allantois fuse together (forming the allanto-chorion) and produce small finger-like processes called **villi** that burrow into the endometrium. Blood vessels covering the surface of the allantois extend to the tips of the villi and so there will be very little tissue between the blood inside the vessels of the embryo and the blood inside the

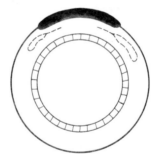

FIG. 2.28.   The mesoderm splits into two layers.

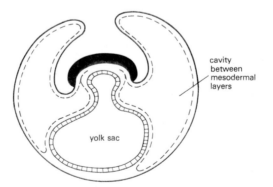

FIG. 2.29.   Mesodermal folds extending over embryo and also pinching the hollow ball of endoderm.

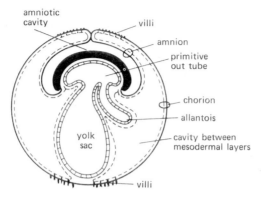

FIG. 2.30. Amniotic folds meeting over embryo and forming amniotic cavity. Yolk sac attaches by small neck to primitive gut tube. This has allantois developing from caudal end. Villi are forming around the extra-embryonic membranes.

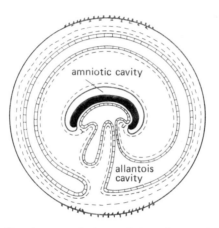

FIG. 2.31. In this section the allantois surrounds the amniotic cavity containing the embryo. Almost all the fluids are now in the allantoic and amniotic cavities (sacs). The villi are strong structures forming a band round the extra-embryonic membranes. This is the placenta.

vessels of the uterus of the mother. The villi develop as a broad band around the outside of the membranous sacs that are now surrounding the embryo and form a thick vascular arrangement with the uterus (Fig. 2.31). This is the **placenta**, an arrangement of embryonic and maternal tissues that allows the transfer of nutrient from the mother's blood to the embryo's blood. In the reverse direction the waste products of the embryo's metabolism pass out through the layers of the placenta and into the mother's blood who then excretes them with her own waste products.

The placenta of the dog and cat is called a *zonary placenta* since it is restricted to the band around the middle of the extra-embryonic membranes. (Fig. 2.32). (Different species have different sorts of placentae.) The extra-embryonic membranes on each side of the placenta are in contact with the uterine wall but they do not form the same intimate arrangement.

There is a narrow band between the

placenta and the rest of the membranes where maternal blood has escaped from the uterus and becomes trapped. This band runs along each edge of the placenta and is called the *marginal haematoma* (Fig. 2.32). It is coloured green in the bitch and brown in the cat, and at parturition it stains the discharges and vulvar region a similar colour.

The blood vessels use the neck of the allantois as a route to enter and leave the body of the embryo. Together with special supporting connective tissue these all form the **umbilical cord** which attaches the extra-embryonic membranes to the umbilical region of the embryo.

While these membranes have been developing the embryo has undergone changes. The head and tail become obvious and the limbs begin to push out from the sides of the trunk. The shape of the final animal is becoming recognizable and it is now called a **fetus** (or foetus) and so the extra-embryonic membranes are **fetal membranes**.

## The developing animal

These are approximate stages and lengths for puppies of average-sized dogs. Kittens seem to be slightly more advanced at each age (except for the time of birth) and they are not quite as long as puppies at the same time of pregnancy.

By the end of the third week of pregnancy the amnion is complete and the allantois has formed. The embryo is just under 5 mm long and the forelimbs and hindlimbs are small buds sticking out from the trunk. By the end of the fourth week the limbs have developed into small cylinders with indications of the shape of the paws (Fig. 2.33). The embryos are about 20 mm long, the eyes are pigmented and the external ear has appeared as a ridge of skin. At the end of the fifth week the ear flap is more distinct and eyelids partly cover the eyes (Fig. 2.34). The digits have become definite shapes in the paws and the external genitalia can be seen near their final positions. There are tactile

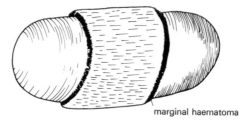

marginal haematoma

FIG. 2.32.  Zonary placenta around fetal membranes. The marginal haematoma is shown along the edge of the placenta.

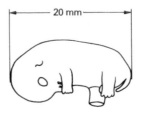

FIG. 2.33.  Embryo at end of fourth week. Eyes are pigmented, ear flap just shows, limbs are small cylinders with indications of paw shape.

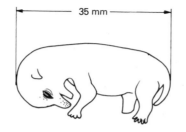

FIG. 2.34. Fetus at end of fifth week. Eyelids partly cover eyes, ear flap well developed; limbs have recognizable shapes with distinct digits; tactile hair follicles above eyes and mouth.

hair follicles on the upper lip and above the eyes. The fetuses are about 35 mm long.

By the end of the sixth week the fetuses are about 60 mm long. The scrotal and vulval tissues are prominent. The digits are widely spread and the eyelids have fused. Hair follicles are present on the body and tactile hairs have appeared. Claws have also formed. Radiographs of the mother will show signs of ossification of the fetal skeleton. The fetuses are about 100 mm long at the end of 7 weeks. Body hair is forming and the colour markings are appearing. By 8 weeks the hair covering is complete and the digital pads are present. The fetuses are about 150 mm long by the end of 8 weeks and are ready for birth by the end of 9 weeks.

### Recognition of pregnancy

This can be done in most cases by palpating the uterus and its contents through the abdominal wall. The non-pregnant uterus is between the colon dorsally and the bladder ventrally. In the average-sized bitch the cervix will be 3–5 cm cranial and ventral to the pelvic brim.

At about the end of the third week of pregnancy the uterus has a series of oval distensions just over 1 cm in length. These can be felt through the abdominal wall, separated by the very slightly enlarged parts of the uterine horns. By 4 weeks the swellings become spherical and about 1.5 cm in diameter. From 5 to 6 weeks they increase to 2.5 cm in diameter and the uterus between them is swelling up; the constrictions are becoming obliterated. The abdomen is beginning to enlarge about now and changes start in the mammary glands. The teats get larger and stick out and they become bright pink in unpigmented areas.

From this time on there is a rapid increase in the size of the fetuses and soon it will be possible to palpate the puppies themselves through the uterus and the membranes. Radiographs of the mother will show signs of ossification in the fetal skeletons. The mother's teats continue to enlarge and become softer and swollen. They may also become pigmented especially around their tips. There is usually a marked rise in the weight of the bitch from the fifth week on.

After the seventh week the uterus and its contents almost fill the abdominal cavity and there should be no difficulty in recognizing pregnancy. The mammary glands are now very obvious, forming two parallel swollen ridges from the pelvis to the thorax. They produce a watery secretion 1–2 days before parturition and milk from the time of whelping.

### Parturition

During the latter part of pregnancy the

pelvic tissues, muscles and ligaments gradually relax, but this increases greatly in the last few days before parturition. The soft tissues of the perineal region and the vulva relax and become enlarged and flabby. Clear mucus may be passed.

Just prior to parturition the mother becomes restless and her nesting behaviour becomes intensified. Birth usually takes place with the mother lying down on her side. The first stage consists of the rhythmic contraction of the uterus leading to movement of the most caudal fetus towards the cervix. Usually the allantochorion has ruptured and the fetus is propelled along in the fluid-filled amnion. The contractions are concentrated towards the end of the uterus near the cervix so that other fetuses do not become disturbed too soon. Early contractions are associated with body twitches and increased panting by the bitch.

The fluid-filled fetal membranes get pushed into the slightly opened cervix. Each uterine contraction forces them further and further through the gradually widening canal. Finally it is wide enough to allow the fetus to begin its passage. This may be head first or tail first.

During the second stage the fetus is expelled from the birth canal. Fetal membranes full of fluid appear at the vulva and gradually balloon out. They may rupture spontaneously or the mother may help. The uterine contractions intensify and are reinforced by abdominal pressure. Expulsion of the newborn (*delivery*) usually follows four or five contractions. The umbilical cord is still intact at the birth of the puppy and this will be torn by the mother. She licks the membranes off the puppy and also licks clean the discharges and all round her vulva.

The expulsion of the fetal membranes left within the uterus (the after-birth) is the third stage of parturition and this takes place intermittently. In the bitch, it is associated with the discharge of dark greenish material due to the breakdown of the marginal haematoma of the placenta. This staining is quite normal. The bitch may deliver puppies at intervals of 10–30 minutes, but there may be even longer intervals between them. The puppies will soon find the way to the mammary glands which will be letting down the milk at this time. Parturition is usually complete in 4–6 hours from the onset of labour, but there are many exceptions to this.

Parturition in the cat is similar to that in the dog except that the staining associated with the marginal haematoma is brown and not green. There may be quite long intervals between the birth of kittens on some occasions (p. 659).

## Vascular System

This is an arrangement of tubes for the circulation of fluid. Two parts can be recognized and considered separately, although they are very closely related and are connected. The *blood vascular system* conveys blood throughout the body; it is sometimes called the cardio-vascular system. ("Cardiac" is an adjective used in phrases referring to the heart.) The *lymph vascular system* carries lymph and eventually opens into the blood vascular system. These systems are also described as the circulatory systems; there are, however, other regions which can be said to constitute a circulatory system.

### Blood vascular system

In the section on connective tissue (p. 6) blood was described as circulating in a continuous system of tubes called blood vessels. The organ which plays a major role in causing circulation is a mass of muscle associated with a restricted part of this system of tubes; the structure is the

**heart**. As blood is carried away from the heart, the vessels split into branches with smaller diameters and thinner walls than the parent vessel. With every branching the total diameter of the resulting vessels increases. At the level at which there is an interchange of fluid between the inside and the outside of the vessels, they are very small in diameter and the walls consist almost entirely of a single layer of epithelial cells constituting the endothelium. At this level they are called **capillaries**. The first parts of the vessels carrying blood from the heart to the capillaries have quite thick walls of smooth muscle and elastic fibres and are called **arteries**. Between these and the capillaries they are known as **arterioles** and have thinner walls and smaller diameters than arteries.

The large arteries form a pattern that is fairly constant in animals of the same species and there are often striking similarities between animals of different species. The arterioles can contract rhythmically and control the flow of blood into the capillaries. In this way the supply to major sections of the body is regulated so that each tissue gets the amount it needs to function properly. Constriction and dilatation of the blood vessels is controlled by the rate of motor nerve impulses to the smooth (involuntary) muscle of their walls. Arteries may unite with one another to form **anastomoses** and the smaller the vessels the more frequently anastomoses occur. An **arterial plexus** is a network of arteries. Blockage of one vessel does not necessarily cut off the blood supply to a region; using the anastomotic pathways, a *collateral circulation* is set up.

Capillaries form a complex network in nearly all the organs of the body; on the whole the more active the organ the larger its supply of blood and the smaller the spaces between the capillaries forming the strings of the net. The term *capillary bed* is also used for the network. It is at this level

that nutrients and waste products leave or enter the blood. The capillary wall acts as a semi-permeable membrane, being permeable to some, but not all, of the constituents of blood. The part of blood that can diffuse into and out of the lumen of the capillary is tissue fluid and this is the transfer medium for the nutrients and waste products of the body cells.

Blood passing on from the capillaries returns to the heart through vessels called **venules**, which gradually increase in diameter. Their walls, however, are very thin, the endothelium being supported only by a small amount of collagenous connective tissue. The venules unite to form **veins** and these have a wider lumen and thinner walls than the corresponding arteries. Some veins, especially those in the limbs, have a system of **valves** which open towards the heart and prevent a backflow of blood. Each valve usually consists of a pair of flaps (*cusps*) formed by a fold of the endothelium strengthened by a small amount of connective tissue. When a limb is moved or even when a muscle contracts, the blood in the local veins is compressed. Because of the valves, it is only able to flow towards the heart. Veins, like arteries, anastomose very freely with one another; they may thus form **venous plexuses**.

Some veins are called **sinuses**: for instance, the large vessel which receives smaller veins from the tissues of the heart itself is called a sinus; so also are the veins in the cranial cavity. It is best, where possible, always to use the term **venous sinuses** for these structures, to distinguish them from other recesses of the body which may be called sinuses (e.g. paranasal sinuses). The venous side of the blood vascular system acts as a reservoir for blood, holding it in the plexuses and sinuses as well as in the large veins. If it is required rapidly, the vein walls are constricted and transfer the blood to where it is needed.

Some veins break up into a plexus of capillaries instead of continuing directly into main venous trunks. This is a *portal system* and ensures that material absorbed from one region by the first capillary network can be transferred to another region by the second (portal system) capillary network without having to circulate very far or without being widely distributed. The blood leaves the portal system in venous trunks.

*Cavernous erectile tissue* consists of connective tissue partitions separating intercommunicating spaces which can be filled with blood. The spaces are lined with endothelium and in some cases will act as capillaries, occurring between arteries and veins; in other cases the cavernous erectile tissue occurs as part of the course of a vein. Engorgement of the spaces with blood causes a stiffening and hardening of the tissue. Cavernous erectile tissue has been described in the section on the urinary system (pp. 81, 82).

In some regions of the body the arterioles and venules are in direct communication by **arterio-venous anastomoses**. Blood can thus bypass the capillary network.

*Heart*

This can be considered in effect as a localized increase in the muscle layer surrounding the endothelial lining of the blood vascular system. It is situated in the mediastinum of the thoracic cavity and there forms an invagination into a sac of tissue called the **pericardium** which is attached to the sternum and to the mediastinal pleura (Fig. 2.35).

Its position varies slightly with individuals and breeds but in general it extends from the third rib to the caudal border of the sixth. The pericardial sac has a continuous layer of epithelial cells on its inner surface; part is closely attached to the heart muscle and this region of the epithelial cells is considered as the outer layer of the heart wall and is called the **epicardium**. The inner surface of the sac produces serous *pericardial fluid* and is termed the **serous pericardium**. This is surrounded by the **fibrous layer** of the pericardium which is continuous with adjacent tissues and with the external coat of the vessels entering and leaving the heart. In life the inner surfaces of the pericardium are separated only by a thin film of pericar-

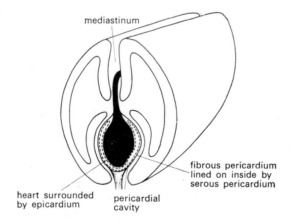

FIG. 2.35.   Heart in pericardium within mediastinum.
(Heart and vessel represented in black; see also FIG. 2.1).

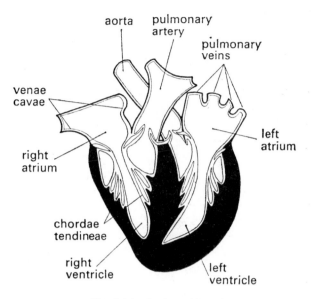

FIG. 2.36. Section of heart.

dial fluid; nevertheless, the potential space is called the **pericardial cavity**.

Normally the lungs cover most of the heart and its pericardial sac but in these regions the lungs are thin and the beating heart can be easily heard and felt through the thoracic wall.

The wall of the heart consists of three layers. The outermost is the epicardium which has just been described. The innermost is the **endocardium**, consisting of a layer of epithelial cells; this is continuous without a break with the epithelial lining (*endothelium*) of blood vessels attached to the heart, the whole presenting a very smooth surface lining the blood vascular system. The endocardium is connected by a thin layer of loose connective tissue to the muscular middle layer of the heart wall. This is the **myocardium** and consists entirely of cardiac muscle cells; these were mentioned with muscle tissue (p. 4).

The heart has right and left halves (which, however, are not strictly in the right and left halves of the body); in the adult there is no communication between the cavities in each half, which are kept

separate by a muscular division. Each half has two chambers, an **atrium** and a **ventricle** (Fig. 2.36).

The blood enters an atrium and is then forced through a corresponding **atrioventricular valve** into a ventricle. The atrioventricular valve of each side of the heart consists of a number of flaps or cusps lined on each side by endocardium enveloping a thin layer of connective tissue. The free edge of each cusp is attached to the inside of the muscular wall of the ventricles by fibrous threads (**chordae tendineae**) covered by endocardium. In this way the blood is allowed into the ventricles but the reverse flow is prevented by the cusps meeting together to form a barrier; the chordae tendineae prevent the cusps being turned inside out even under the great pressure to which they are subjected.

Blood leaves the ventricles through great vessels: from the left part of the heart through the **aorta**; from the right through the **pulmonary artery**. The reverse flow of the blood from each of these vessels is prevented by a valve at the junction with the ventricle. There are three cusps in each

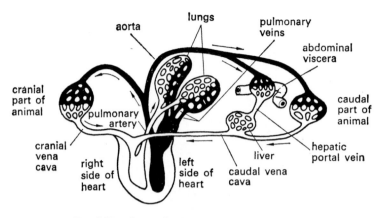

FIG. 2.37.   Generalized pattern of blood circulation.

of these valves; their connective tissue is covered on each side by epithelial cells which will be called endocardium on the heart side and endothelium on the vessel side. There are no fibrous threads attaching to the edges of the cusps of these aortic and pulmonary valves.

When the blood leaves the right ventricle in the pulmonary artery it is carried to the lungs (Fig. 2.37). Here it is oxygenated and returns via a few **pulmonary veins** to the left atrium. From this chamber it passes through the left atrioventricular valve (sometimes called the mitral valve) into the left ventricle. The oxygenated blood is then forced through the aortic valve into the aorta to spread throughout the entire body with the exception of a very few restricted areas. The oxygen will be given up to the tissues and the blood will take up the waste carbon dioxide and return to the heart via the **venae cavae**. These are large veins which drain the deoxygenated blood into the right atrium. From here it passes through the right atrioventricular valve (sometimes called the tricuspid valve) to the right ventricle and so again through the pulmonary valve.

The flow of blood from the heart via the pulmonary artery to the lungs and its return through the pulmonary veins to the left atrium is the *pulmonary circulation.* The path from the aorta and back through the venae cavae is the *systemic circulation.*

*Systemic Circulation* (Fig. 2.38, 2.39)

As soon as the aorta leaves the heart it gives off two **coronary** arteries whose sole function is to supply the heart with oxygenated blood. Much of the venous return is through cardiac veins which join to form the **coronary sinus**. This opens into the right atrium. Some small veins opens directly into the heart chambers.

The next arteries that arise from the aorta (and this is still near to the heart) are vessels which will supply the neck, the cranial end of the thorax, the head and the forelimbs. These originate very close to one another usually as two main branches which then give regional vessels. The supply to the head uses the paired **common carotid** arteries (one on each side of the neck) which, on reaching the jaw, split into several branches to the superficial and deep structures (including the brain).

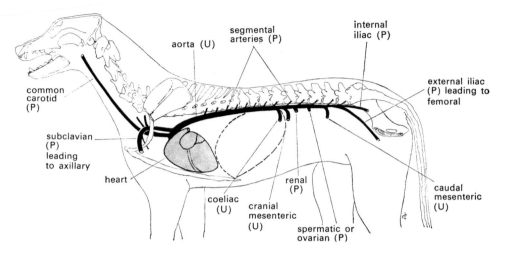

FIG. 2.38.   Arterial pattern of a dog. P, paired vessel; U, unpaired vessel.

The main returning blood leaves the head as several veins which unite just caudal to the mandibles to form the left and right **external jugular** veins. One of the head veins that is used for intravenous injections is the **lingual** vein. This lies fairly superficially on the underside of the tongue and can be used when the animal is under general anaesthesia. The jugular veins are large vessels closely related to the common carotid arteries on the ventral side of the neck. The veins are the more superficial and lie directly under the skin. If pressure is applied at the base of the neck to dam back the venous blood and prevent it continuing to the heart, these veins will become engorged, enlarged and stiffened. They are then convenient for **venipuncture** (entering with a hypodermic syringe needle), either to obtain a blood sample or to give an intravenous injection.

The vessels inside the thorax which will supply the forelimbs are the pair of **subclavian** arteries. One runs to each limb leaving around the first rib through the cranial thoracic aperture. There the name of the vessels is changed to **axillary** artery and this continues to the forelimb, dividing up into many more named arteries.

The major continuation of the axillary is the **brachial** artery and this lies against the bones as it passes on the medial side of the elbow joint. This is a pressure point; that is, a place where an artery can be pressed against a bone. In this way the arterial supply to more distal structures can be greatly reduced and this may be necessary as a first-aid measure in haemorrhage from the forelimb. The venous return from the forelimb can be divided into deep and superficial vessels.

The deep ones run very close to the arteries that supply the limb and usually have similar names; the superficial ones are subcutaneous. One of these is the reasonably large **cephalic** vein which runs proximally on the cranial aspect of the radius and presents another site for venipuncture (Fig. 2.40). Pressure can be applied on the cranial side of the elbow joint to cause venous enlargement (p. 222).

Arteries to the neck and the cranial part of the thorax radiate out to supply these

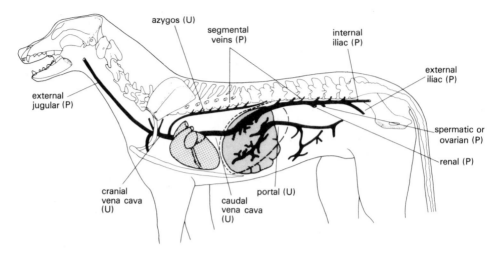

Fig. 2.39.    Venous pattern of a dog. P, paired vessel; U, unpaired vessel.

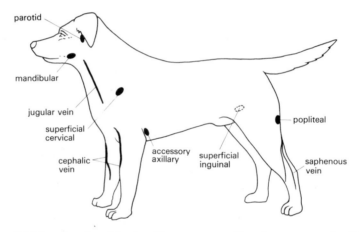

Fig. 2.40.    Superficial lymph nodes of the dog. The accessory axillary does not occur in all dogs but when present it is palpable on the side of the thorax. The superficial inguinal lies between the thigh and the abdominal wall in the inguinal region. Vessels commonly used for intravenous injections are also shown.

regions and the returning veins are found very close to them. These veins join those from the forelimbs and the head; the resulting large vessel is the single **cranial vena cava** which empties directly into the right atrium.

The aorta leaving the heart curves to reach the ventral surface of the vertebral column at about the fourth thoracic vertebra and continues in this relation as far as the lumbo-sacral junction. At approxi-mately each vertebra a pair of vessels is given off dorsally to supply the vertebral column and adjacent muscles, the spinal cord and the local region of the body wall. Within the thorax relatively small arteries run to the lungs to supply these structures with oxygenated blood. (Although this is where oxygenation takes place, the supporting connective tissues of the lung require oxygenated arterial blood for their nutrition. Blood in the pulmonary arteries comes to the lungs to receive, not to release, oxygen.)

Within the abdominal cavity, the aorta continues to give dorsal segmental vessels and it also supplies the abdominal part of the digestive tract through three ventral midline unpaired vessels, the **coeliac**, **cranial mesenteric** and **caudal mesenteric** arteries. The venous return from this system will contain a large amount of the absorbed results of digestion and the veins unite to form the large **portal** vein which enters the liver. Here it breaks up into a second set of capillaries which penetrate the hepatic tissue. The abdominal part of the aorta also gives paired **renal** arteries to the kidneys and **spermatic** or **ovarian** arteries to the gonads.

The termination of the aorta is by splitting into left and right **internal iliac** arteries supplying the pelvic contents and the left and right **external iliac** arteries which supply the wall of the pelvis and also give a **femoral** artery as the main supply to each hindlimb. (This is one recommended as a site for feeling the pulse. It can also be used as a pressure point). As in the forelimb, the hindlimb drainage is superficial and deep and there is also a convenient vessel, the **saphenous** vein, on the lateral side of the distal end of the tibia that can be used for intravenous injections (Fig. 2.40).

The hindlimb and pelvic veins unite to form the large **caudal vena cava** near the lumbo-sacral junction. It is closely associated with the aorta in the abdominal cavity. The venous return from the kidneys, gonads and all the body segments that have been supplied by the corresponding arteries opens directly into the caudal vena cava. That from the abdominal part of the digestive system forms the portal vein and only after it has passed through the hepatic capillary bed does this venous blood enter the vena cava. Whereas the aorta is adjacent to the vertebral column throughout the caudal two-thirds of the thorax, the caudal vena cava on reaching the liver turns ventrally and passes through the diaphragm near its centre point. As it travels through the edge of the liver it receives numerous **hepatic** veins draining that organ. In its thoracic course the caudal vena cava receives no more tributaries but empties into the right atrium. The venous drainage of the dorsal part of the thoracic wall and the corresponding part of the vertebral column is by a series of segmental vessels into an unpaired **azygos** vein which does not have a corresponding artery. This runs on the right side, dorsally the length of the thorax and discharges blood into the cranial vena cava.

Heart Beat

Most of the force necessary to drive the blood through the complex circuit comes from the cardiac muscle itself which has the intrinsic property of rhythmic contraction.

The muscle in the different parts of the heart contracts in a definite sequence. Initiation and control is the responsibility of a group of modified muscle cells forming the **conduction system**. The beat appears to be started by a mass of specialized fibres, the **sinuatrial node**, in the wall of the right atrium. The impulse then passes to the **atrioventricular node**, which is a collection of special muscle cells in the wall between the atria. From here they form an **atrioventricular bundle** which soon splits to give one limb running in each ventricle in opposite sides of their common (intraventricular) wall. The conducting system ends by merging into the regular cardiac muscle tissue.

The spread of the impulse through the heart sets up an electrical current in the surrounding fluids. This can be detected on the surface of the body by a special instrument called an electrocardiogram (ECG) recorder and will show whether or not the heart is functioning normally.

The central nervous system has an overriding control on these automatic cardiac contractions. In this way heart activity may be markedly increased in stressful situations such as exercise, excessive heat and disease.

The right and the left atria contract together to force the blood into the respective relaxed ventricles. The phase of contraction is *systole* and *atrial systole* has just been described. When the blood is forced out of the ventricles this is *ventricular systole*. The relaxed filling periods which follow systole are called *diastole*. The sequence of events between any particular phase and its next occurrence is a *cardiac cycle:* this constitutes a complete *heart beat*.

The number of heart beats per minute is the *heart rate* and is faster for smaller animals than for larger ones. A resting small dog may have a heart rate of 120 beats per minute whereas in a larger one it may be 80 or less. The cat varies between about 110 to 130. Young animals have a faster rate than older ones, and exercise, excitement, high environmental temperatures can all have an accelerating effect.

Two definite sounds are produced during each heart beat. The first is related to ventricular systole and is produced by the contraction of the muscle of the ventricle and the vibration of the atrioventricular valve flaps and the chordae tendineae. The second sound is related to the vibrations of the aortic and pulmonary valves after their closure, and this will coincide with the start of ventricular diastole.

## Blood Pressure

This usually means pressure in the **arteries** and is the force that makes blood flow through the vessels. It is governed by the beat of the heart, the volume of the blood, the resistance and elasticity of the blood vessels. It is measured like barometric pressure in millimetres of mercury.

The pressure is highest at systole and this is the systolic pressure; diastolic pressure is the lowest. The mean pressure is the average of the systolic and diastolic pressures over a given period of time and for the dog is about 150, for the cat about 160 mm of mercury. Blood pressure in capillaries is very low.

It is sometimes necessary to know the venous pressure; for instance, when giving fluids intravenously this will give a guide to the rate and quantity to be administered. Venous pressure will vary according to where it is measured and especially whether the site is peripheral or very near to the heart. The pressure measured during intravenous infusions is that in the great veins near the heart and sometimes in the right atrium of the heart itself. This is called the *central venous pressure* and it is measured by passing a catheter through a peripheral vein and pushing it along until its tip is in the right position. More details will be given in the section on intravenous infusions (p. 318).

## Pulse Rate

Each heart beat is reflected in the arterial blood pressure and this causes a wave of expansion and elongation of the arterial walls, which starts at the aorta and spreads over the entire arterial system. This is the **pulse** or **pulse wave** and it may be felt in many of the superficial arteries. In the dog and cat, the most convenient site is on the medial side of the thigh, were the large femoral artery is virtually subcutaneous. The **pulse rate** will be the same as the heart rate but the experienced clinician can deduce a lot of other information on the heart and circulation by palpating the arterial pulse.

Heart Failure

The body tissues often rapidly increase their oxygen requirements; for instance, muscles during exercise may need up to fifteen times as much as they use when resting. Some of this can be met by a better use of the oxygen carried in the blood, but an increase in cardiac output will probably also be needed. *Cardiac output* is the volume of blood pumped out by a ventricle per minute and depends on the heart rate and on the output of a ventricle at each beat. The heart may well have sufficient reserve to accomplish an increase. If it is unable to cope, blood will accumulate in the pulmonary system and the right atrium, and the condition is that of heart failure.

Circulatory Shock

In this very serious condition, there is a marked reduction in blood volume passing through the heart. This may be due to blood loss through haemorrhage, plasma loss from wounds and burns, increased water excretion from the urinary and digestive systems, and decreased water intake. Sometimes blood remains pooled in the venous system and does not return to the heart. Cardiac output is insufficient to supply the tissues and this results in inadequate nutrition and an accumulation of waste products. The heart itself becomes starved and unable to work and, furthermore, the deprived brain is not able to respond correctly to danger signals from sensory nerves monitoring the condition of the internal environment (p. 577).

**Lymph vascular system**

The tissue fluid bathing the cells can enter the blood stream by two routes. The direct way is through the thin walls of the capillary blood vessels. A very important alternative that is used extensively is the capillary lymph vessel network which also permeates the tissues. Once the tissue fluid has passed into this alternative set it is called **lymph** and these capillaries join up to form larger **lymph vessels**. They eventually discharge their fluid into the system of blood vessels. However, before the lymph drains into the blood it passes through *lymphoid (lymphatic) tissue* somewhere along its course. This may be massed together in a connective tissue capsule to form a lymph node or it may be scattered diffusely throughout various organs such as the intestines. The nodes act as filters to hold back bacteria, dust and other foreign matter from entering the blood. Lymph tissue also produces lymphocytes (a very important group of white blood corpuscles which also circulate in the lymph) as well as substances called **antibodies** used to neutralize the effect of bacterial infections. The lymph vascular system (also called the lymphatic system) includes the lymph vessels and the lymphoid tissue.

*Lymph Vessels*

The lymph capillaries, like blood capillaries, are endothelial vessels formed of epithelial cells. The blind-ending terminal tubes join together to form networks which combine to form lymphatic vessels of increasing size. These resemble veins in their structure and also possess numerous delicate valves with one or two cusps directing the lymph away from the tissues and towards the vein into which it is finally discharged. The flow of lymph is similar to the venous return from the extremities. Muscle action moves the fluid which can only go in one direction because of the valves. Eventually two major vessels can be recognized: the thoracic duct and the right lymphatic duct.

The **thoracic duct** is the main collecting channel and can be traced through the thorax from an expanded end called the **cisterna chyli** which lies partly in the abdominal region (p. 71). The cisterna chyli receives the lymph from the hindlimbs and the lumbar region in addition to that from the abdominal organs. Chyle from the wall of the intestines performs yet another important function of lymph, being responsible for transporting a major fraction of the absorbed fats. The products of lipid digestion enter the lacteals in the intestinal villi and pass through mesenteric lymph vessels and nodes to reach the cisterna chyli. After receiving many vessels from other areas, the thoracic duct opens into one of the great veins which join the right atrium.

The **right lymphatic duct** drains the lymph from the right forelimb and the adjacent part of the body. It opens into the venous system near the thoracic duct or even into the thoracic duct. A pair of **tracheal ducts** carry lymph from the head region and these open into the above-mentioned vessels or near them into the venous system.

*Lymph Nodes* (Fig. 2.40)

These encapsulated masses of lymphoid tissue vary tremendously in size and shape. Several vessels carry lymph to each node entering at various points through the capsule. Connective tissue divides the inside of the node into a series of compartments which are filled with lymphoid tissue. After filtering slowly through the lymphoid tissue, the lymph leaves in a small number of vessels which originate from one area, the **hilus**, of the node.

Each region of the body and each viscus has lymph vessels leaving which pass through at least one node before entering the venous system. Since they are important defences against the spread of disease, the condition of the nodes can help in deciding its nature and extent. Whilst many may only be seen at operation or post-mortem examination, some can be felt through the skin.

The **parotid** lymph node can be felt just caudal to the temporo-mandibular joint (p. 32). In a medium-sized dog it is about 1 cm long and is partly covered by the parotid salivary gland. It receives lymph from about the dorsal half of the head; this can be called the *drainage region* of the parotid lymph node.

The group of 2–5 **mandibular** lymph nodes can be palpated just caudal to the junction of the ramus and body of each side of the lower jaw. They vary in length from 1–3 cm each in a middle-sized dog and receive lymph from much of the head. The lymph from these and from the remainder of the head all passes to the large **retropharyngeal** lymph nodes (up to 5 cm in length) which lie close to the pharynx. They are too deep for palpation and it is from these that the tracheal ducts arise which carry the lymph along the neck. The **superficial cervical** lymph nodes can be felt through the skin. There are usually two on each side at the base of the neck just cranial to the scapula (they have been called the prescapular lymph nodes). In medium-sized dogs they cover a length of some 3–5 cm. Lymph from the lateral surface of the neck and from the forelimb drains through these nodes.

A superficial node involved in hindlimb drainage is the **popliteal**. It is about 2 cm long and lies subcutaneously caudal to the stifle joint. All the lymph from the hindlimb and also from the caudal mammary glands, or penis, and adjacent skin passes through **superficial inguinal** nodes. There may be two on each side, each one being about 2 cm in length. They can be palpated dorsal to the mammary glands or penis, between the thigh and the abdominal wall.

Within the thorax, **bronchial** lymph nodes associated with the major bronchi drain the lymph from the lungs and this, together with that from the remainder of the thoracic viscera and from the thorax, passes through **mediastinal** nodes to reach the thoracic duct. Lymph from abdominal viscera drains through their specific nodes, **mesenteric, hepatic, colic**, etc., before reaching the cisterna chyli from where it passes along the thoracic duct.

## Lymph Follicles

Masses of lymphoid tissue, usually associated with mucous membrane may occur as small discrete areas but they are also found grouped together as large patches called follicles.

## Tonsils

These have been mentioned in the description of the pharynx in the section on the digestive system. They help form a complete ring of lymphoid tissue around the opening of the mouth into the pharynx.

## Spleen

This organ is closely adjacent to the stomach in the abdominal cavity. It is, however, a haemopoietic organ and contains regions of lymphoid tissue. Its functions are still imperfectly understood. In addition to the blood-cell formation and destruction carried out by all haemopoietic tissue the spleen is a very efficient storage area for blood, a function that

produces considerable variations in its size.

## Thymus

This lymphoid organ is in the thoracic inlet and the cranial part of the thoracic cavity, cranial to the heart. It is very important in the production of lymphocytes and these are essential for the development of *immunity*. This is the ability of the animal to defend itself against infection and against the introduction of "foreign substances", i.e., materials that the animal has not manufactured itself.

The thymus is lobulated, greyish-pink in colour and quite large at birth. It grows rapidly for about 4 or 5 months and then gradually decreases in size, with the lymphoid tissue being replaced by fat.

## Nervous System

In the notes on nervous tissue (p. 5), the neuron (nerve fibre) is described as a cell body with processes. The processes carrying impulses to the cell body are called dendrites (dendrons) whereas the one process that carries impulses away from the cell body is called an axon. When the impulse passes from one neuron to another it does so at a synapse (Fig. 2.41). The impulse can only pass one way across the synapse. The axon termination may be composed of a very large number of filaments and these will not necessarily all synapse with one neuron; in fact, the termination of one neuron, by virtue of its large number of terminal filaments, will usually synapse with a large number of other neurons. Conversely, any neuron may receive impulses (via synapses) from many other neurons. This arrangement of terminations allows extensive interaction and integration of impulses.

The function of the nervous system is to

receive stimuli from the environment (inside and outside the body), to analyse and integrate these stimuli and then cause such response by the tissues of the body as is necessary. The stimuli are received by neuron processes which may be free endings or may be attached to more complicated structures. The receptors are known as **sensory nerve endings** and the processes which transmit the impulses are **sensory fibres**. The first part of the fibre will be a dendrite and this will end at the cell body. The impulse will then be carried by the second part of the neuron, the axon. If a response is evoked, an impulse has to be transmitted to muscle tissue or to a gland. The neuron process carrying this impulse is a **motor fibre**. The simplest functional unit of the nervous system consists of a sensory unit synapsing with a motor unit. At least one other neuron is usually involved and conveys the impulse from the sensory to the motor unit; such a neuron is an **intercalated** or **connector** neuron (Fig. 2.42).

A further classification of fibres is made which relates to the structures in which the sensory and motor nerve endings are found. Internal organs, smooth muscle, glands and mucous membrane are considered to be innervated by **visceral** motor and sensory fibres. All other structures are innervated by **somatic** motor and sensory fibres.

**Somatic sensory** fibres have receptors in, or close to, the skin which are activated by stimuli such as pain, pressure, heat and touch from the outside environment. There are also receptors in muscles, tendons and joints which are sensitive to alterations in their state, tension and position. Some sensory fibres have highly

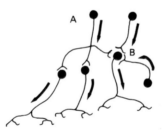

FIG. 2.41.   Diagrammatic representation of: A, one neuron synapsing with three others; B, three neurons synapsing with one. Arrows indicate direction of impulse (see FIG. 1.2.).

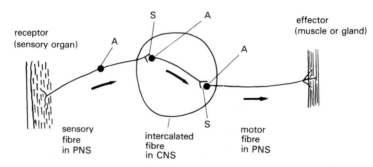

FIG. 2.42.   Diagrammatic representation of path of impulse from sensory organ transmitted via sensory fibre, intercalated neuron and motor fibre to effector organ (muscle or gland). A, cell body; S, synapse. Arrows indicate direction of impulse. PNS, peripheral nervous system. CNS, central nervous system.

specialized endings and carry impulses from organs responsible for sight, hearing and balance.

**Somatic motor** fibres: the impulses pass along these neurons to skeletal muscle cells.

**Visceral sensory** fibres; stimuli are received from blood vessels, mucous membranes and viscera. There are also special fibres that carry stimuli relating to smell and taste.

**Visceral motor** fibres: these are distributed to involuntary muscle cells and to glands.

The visceral sensory fibres, the visceral motor fibres and their connections are often said to form the **autonomic nervous system**. The term means self-governing, and refers to the fact that bodily processes (for example, blood circulation and digestion) involving the visceral sensory and visceral motor neurons, etc., are not under the control of the will. Many authorities restrict the use of the term "autonomic" to the visceral motor fibres only.

The somatic and visceral fibres, together with some connective tissue, make up the nervous system. This is a functional classification. It is often convenient to use a topographical division and so the part of the system which is situated in the midline of the body closely related to the vertebral column and the skull is called the **central nervous system** and this consists of just the brain and the spinal cord. All the other nervous tissue constitutes the **peripheral nervous system**. It is essential to understand that both somatic and visceral neurons appear in the central nervous system and that both somatic and visceral neurons are present in the peripheral nervous system. Further, that a nerve fibre can be part of the peripheral nervous system, continue into the spinal cord or brain and so become part of the central nervous system; similarly, fibres can leave the central nervous system and then continue in the peripheral nervous system.

**Central nervous system**

This topographical unit of the nervous system consists of the **brain** located in the cranial cavity and the **spinal cord** in the vertebral canal. In addition to the protection afforded by these skeletal structures, the central nervous system is enveloped in three tubes of protective membranes called **meninges**, between two of which there is a layer of liquid, the **cerebrospinal fluid** (CSF).

The outermost of the protective membranes is the **dura mater**: this is tough and fibrous and within the head it is interwoven with the periosteum on the inner surface of the bones of the cranium. In the vertebral canal the dura is quite free from the local periosteum and is surrounded by fat and blood vessels occupying the **epidural space** (Fig. 2.43). The innermost of the protective membranes is the **pia mater**; this is closely applied to the central nervous system. It is a delicate but very vascular membrane and follows all the gross irregularities of the brain and spinal cord. The meninx (singular of meninges) between the dura mater and the pia mater is called the **arachnoid** and consists of a network of delicate collagenous fibres. The **subarachnoid** space between the fibres is occupied by the cerebrospinal fluid.

*Spinal Cord* (Fig. 2.43).

This extends from the foramen magnum of the cranium as far as the caudal lumbar/cranial sacral region. The caudal end of the tube of dura mater is about mid-sacral region, but the spinal cord does not extend quite so far.

At an early stage of development, the body of the embryo is partly segmented and each segment has its own muscles, blood supply and sensory and motor nerve fibres. The sensory and motor fibres for a

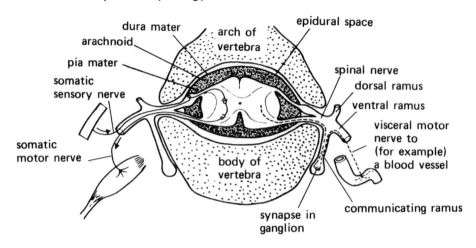

FIG. 2.43.    Section of spinal cord within vertebral canal.

segment combine to form the mixed spinal nerve for that segment. The nerve uses the intervertebral foramen between adjacent vertebral arches to enter and leave the vertebral canal. There are a pair (a left and a right) of nerves related to each vertebra. In the case of the cervical region there are eight pairs although there are only seven vertebrae; this is because the first pair emerge through the arch of the first cervical vertebra (the atlas). All the other spinal nerves emerge caudal to a vertebra. There are only a few coccygeal spinal nerves, restricted to the more cranial coccygeal intervertebral foramina. Each spinal nerve is attached to the spinal cord by a **dorsal** and a **ventral root** (Fig. 2.47).

The dorsal root has a localized swelling, the **dorsal root ganglion**, which lies close to, or in, the intervertebral foramen.

A transverse section of the cord shows the ventral part separated into halves by a **ventral median fissure** containing pia mater and blood vessels. The dorsal part is also separable into halves by the **dorsal median septum**; this connective tissue partition can usually only be seen under magnification. A very narrow bore **central canal** runs the length of the cord, in the

area between the ventral median fissure and the dorsal median septum. In life, this contains cerebrospinal fluid.

The nerve fibres that help to form the spinal cord tend to run in recognizable regions. Since many of the fibres are covered by a fatty material called *myelin,* the regions are fairly clearly defined and form the peripheral **white matter** of the cord. The more central region consists mainly of cell bodies, but there are also many nerve processes. This is **grey matter** and although usually considered to be H-shaped it will vary with the region of the cord (Fig. 2.47).

The spinal cord is formed entirely of neurons, comprising cell bodies together with their dendrites and axons and also a relatively small amount of supporting tissue.

*Brain* (Figs. 2.44, 2.45, 2.46)

The spinal cord is continued rostrally by the brain without any abrupt change. Like the cord it is formed of neurons, but the grey matter of the brain tends to be separated into discrete areas by tracts of (white) fibres that connect different

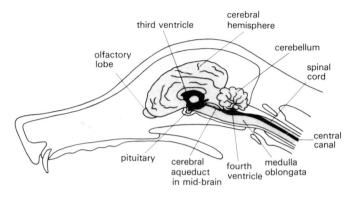

FIG. 2.44.   Median section of brain in outline of dog's head. Dotted area represents nervous tissue. Black represents ventricular system.

regions. The brain has to deal with more complex activities than the spinal cord and so certain regions are greatly enlarged by bulges of nervous tissue superimposed on the otherwise simple tube. The central canal of the spinal cord continues rostrally in the brain tissue. There it expands and has diverticuli to produce a relatively large **ventricular system** filled like the central canal of the spinal cord with cerebrospinal fluid. It is actually into the ventricular system that this fluid is produced.

The brain can be divided into a **hind-brain** continuous with the spinal cord, a **mid-brain** and a **fore-brain**.

*Hind-brain.* The part of the hind-brain continuous with the spinal cord is the **medulla oblongata** (Fig. 2.45). The central canal of the cord continues into the medulla oblongata and becomes very much wider. This enlarged part is called the fourth ventricle and is also filled with cerebrospinal fluid. The ventricle has a thin roof and is bounded on each side by large tracts of fibres entering and leaving the *cerebellum* (Fig. 2.45). This is a globular mass of nervous tissue with a surface of ridges separated by furrows; it is concerned with the maintenance of balance and equilibrium by co-ordinating muscular activity. The cerebellum lies on the

dorsal aspect of the hind-brain over the fourth ventricle and it is attached to the remainder of the hind-brain by three pairs of **peduncles**.

*Mid-brain.* The dorsal surface of this short length of the brain is covered by the overhanging fore-brain. The ventricular system containing cerebrospinal fluid is continued rostrally through the mid-brain by the **cerebral aqueduct**.

*Fore-brain.* The fore-brain consists of a mid-line portion flanked by two lateral expansions, the right and left **cerebral hemispheres** (Fig. 2.44). The midline portion and each hemisphere encompass parts of the ventricular system; the **third ventricle** is a laterally flattened fluid-filled space in the midline and diverticuli of this (called **lateral ventricles**) occupy part of each cerebral hemisphere.

The ventral surface of the midline portion consists mainly of the **optic chiasma** which is a cross-shaped arrangement of nerve fibres associated with the eye, and the **pituitary gland** (an endocrine tissue attached by a short stalk) (Fig. 2.46).

The cerebral hemispheres are large masses joined to each other by a band of nerve fibres. The surface resembles that of the cerebellum in being arranged in ridges and grooves. The most rostral parts of the

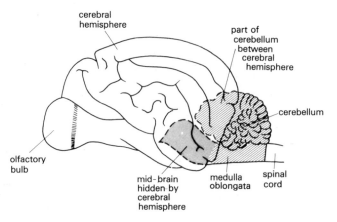

FIG. 2.45.   Left lateral view of brain. The left cerebral hemisphere covers the mid-brain and part of the cerebellum. Cerebellum and medulla oblongata form hind-brain.

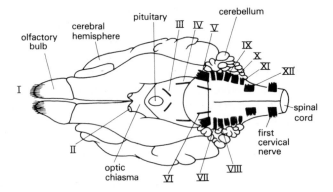

FIG. 2.46.   Ventral view of brain. Roman numerals indicate the cranial nerve number.

cerebral hemispheres, and hence of the brain, are the **olfactory bulbs**. These paired structures are closely applied to the plate of bone separating the brain from the nasal chambers and convey the stimuli concerned with the sense of smell.

The attachment to the spinal cord of motor and sensory fibres forming spinal nerves has already been described. Motor and sensory fibres are also attached to specific regions of the brain to form **cranial nerves** (Fig. 2.46). Spinal and cranial nerves constitute the peripheral nervous system.

**Peripheral nervous system**

There are four basic functional types of fibres that can make up a cranial or a spinal nerve: somatic sensory, somatic motor, visceral sensory and visceral motor.

Somatic motor fibres leave the spinal cord through the ventral root of every spinal nerve and somatic sensory fibres enter through every dorsal root. In fact, the swelling on the dorsal root (the dorsal root ganglion) is caused by the collection of cell bodies of the sensory fibres forming that root. It is likely that the dorsal roots of many of the spinal nerves also contain visceral sensory fibres. The distribution of the visceral motor fibres differs slightly from the other functional types. The ventral roots of the thoracic and lumbar spinal nerves contain visceral motor fibres. In the thoracic and lumbar regions the visceral motor fibres are called **sympathetic** fibres. The ventral roots of some of the sacral spinal nerves and the corresponding parts of some of the cranial nerves also contain visceral motor fibres; these cranio-sacral visceral motor fibres are **parasympathetic**. To summarize: sympathetic nerves are visceral motor fibres that leave the central nervous system in the ventral roots of the thoracic and lumbar spinal nerves; parasympathetic nerves are visceral motor fibres that leave the central nervous system in cranial nerves and in the ventral roots of some sacral nerves.

There are many functional differences between sympathetic and parasympathetic fibres. As a general rule it can be taken that the parasympathetic fibres are concerned with maintaining smooth muscle tone and glandular secretions sufficient for the ordinary normal state of the animal. Sympathetic stimulation is often associated with states of excitement, as suggested by the phrase "fight, flight and frolic". Physiological phenomena commonly experienced at these times, e.g. increased heart rate, more rapid respiration, are usually due to the increased activity of the sympathetic system.

*Spinal Nerves* (Fig. 2.47).

The dorsal and ventral roots fuse to form a **mixed** spinal nerve which then divides into a dorsal and a ventral **ramus**. The dorsal rami are usually smaller than the corresponding ventral rami and retain more or less their segmental pattern of innervation.

The ventral rami carry fibres that innervate the limbs and the ventral and lateral parts of the neck and trunk. In the cervicothoracic and the lumbosacral regions the ventral rami of adjacent nerves form a network or plexus where the nerve fibres related to different segments of the cord intermingle. The fibres innervating the limbs enter or leave the plexus peripherally as named, but not segmentally distinct, nerves. The cervicothoracic plexus of nerve fibres is called the brachial plexus and forms the nerves of the forelimb. It is situated between the limb and the thorax. The lumbosacral plexus contains the nerves of the hindlimb and this is found inside the pelvis.

All spinal nerves have a **visceral ramus**, or **communicating ramus** (ramus communicans), as a branch of the ventral ramus. This originates close to the continuation of the ventral ramus with the mixed spinal nerve and consists of visceral motor and visceral sensory fibres. The communicating rami have visceral motor fibres running from one to the other to form a continuous nerve on each side of the vertebral column inside the abdominal and thoracic cavities. As the visceral motor fibres in this thoracolumbar region are sympathetic the nerve linking the rami is called the *sympathetic chain* (Fig. 2.47).

*Cranial Nerves*

The nerves are numbered as they arise from the brain from the most rostral I to the most caudal XII (Fig. 2.46). Although this is a matter of convenience it does not explain the fibre types involved, nor how the nerves are distributed. The nerves do not attach to the brain with regular dorsal and ventral roots, nor do many have both motor and sensory fibres. Special sensory and special motor fibres are found in the cranial nerves. All the nerves innervate only structures in the head region with the

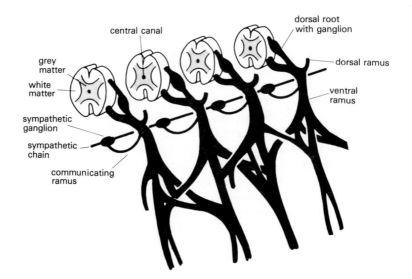

FIG. 2.47.    Formation of plexus by ventral rami of adjacent nerves. The arrangement of white and grey matter in the cord and the formation of the sympathetic chain are also shown.

exception of the **vagus** (X) nerve; this also supplies thoracic and abdominal organs.

Three nerves are concerned entirely with special senses: the **olfactory** (I) for smell, the **optic** (II) for sight and the **vestibulo-cochlear** (VIII) for hearing and equilibrium. Three nerves convey motor fibres to muscles of the eyeball: **oculomotor** (III), **trochlear** (IV) and **abducens** (VI). Another nerve with only motor fibres is the **hypoglossal** (XII), which supplies the muscles of the tongue. The remaining nerves are mixed, being formed of motor and sensory fibres. The **trigeminal** (V) carries the general sensory fibres of the head and also motor fibres to some of the muscles of mastication. The **facial** (VII) carries mainly motor fibres to the non-masticatory muscles of the head. The **glossopharyngeal** (IX), **vagus** (X) and **accessory** (XI) carry motor and sensory fibres for the mouth, the pharynx, larynx, heart, lungs and abdominal organs.

## Reflex Arcs (Fig. 2.48)

A reflex action is a fixed involuntary response which is always similar for a given stimulus. The reflex arc is the nerve pathway along which the stimuli travel; from the source of the sensory stimulus to the central nervous system, the route within the central nervous system, the motor nerve to the responding structure. Any arrangement whereby only one sensory nerve and one motor nerve (and therefore only one synapse) is involved must be a reflex arc. Where an intercalated nerve is present and this has other intercommunications, it is possible that the response would not always be the same; this would not be a reflex.

The definition stresses that the act is involuntary, but the animal may nevertheless be conscious of what is happening. If the pad is pricked, the animal will reflexly draw it away from the point, but it will become aware of the pain. The first part of this is called the **flexor reflex** and is an

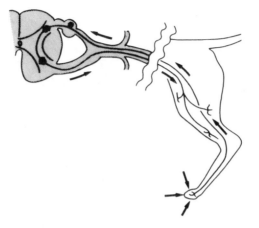

FIG. 2.48. Diagram of a reflex arc. The toe is pinched or pricked. Sensory nerve fibres convey the impulses to the spinal cord. Intercalating neurons (only one is shown) transmit impulses to the motor nerves of flexor muscles that cause withdrawal of the limb. Arrows indicate direction of impulses.

example of a normal **spinal reflex**; that is, one where the complete circuit is spinal and does not involve the brain. It can take place even if the cord is cut through, provided the damage does not occur at the segments used by the reflex. For the hindlimb flexor reflex, this would be approximately from the fourth lumbar to the third sacral segment and if the cord is damaged more cranial than this a hindlimb flexor reflex will still probably be present.

There are several other basic limb reflexes which are restricted to the spine but more complex reflexes pass through centres in the brain. Respiratory, digestive and cardiovascular reflexes are in this category, using the autonomic (visceral) nerve pathways and not reaching the level of consciousness. Nevertheless, any given stimulus still causes the same fixed response.

### Special senses

Vision, hearing, balance, smell and taste are special sensations and particular regions of the body are specifically modified to receive stimuli related to them. The stimuli are transmitted to the central nervous system by cranial nerves; to be quite accurate, in the case of vision and smell the sensory organs are extensions of the brain itself.

*Vision* (Fig. 2.49)

The **eye** is specially adapted for the reception of visual impulses. This globular mass lies in the orbit and can be moved freely in many directions. This is accomplished by a group of ocular (eye) muscles of voluntary fibres. Each muscle has one attachment to the periphery of the eyeball. The other ends of the muscles are grouped together in the depth of the orbit to attach to the skull. It is most unlikely that any one of the group operates on its own but by complex co-ordination the delicate movements of the entire eyeball within the orbit are achieved. The eye consists of three main layers which enclose two compartments, one containing a liquid called **aqueous humour**, the other a gelatinous mass known as **vitreous humour**.

The outermost layer is the tough,

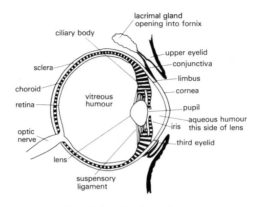

lacrimal gland
opening into fornix

ciliary body

upper eyelid
conjunctiva
sclera
limbus
choroid
cornea
vitreous
humour
retina
pupil
aqueous humour
optic
iris    this side of lens
nerve
third eyelid
lens

suspensory
ligament

Fig. 2.49.    Section of eye.

fibrous protective **sclera** which over the front of the eye becomes transparent and forms the **cornea**. The junction between the sclera and the cornea is the **limbus**. Immediately inside the sclera, the **uvea** forms a very vascular pigmented layer. It does not extend as far as the cornea but just behind the limbus it projects towards the centre of the eyeball as the **ciliary body**. This leaves a circular orifice which is occupied by the transparent biconvex **lens**: the circumference of the lens is attached to the ciliary body by the fibres of the **suspensory ligament**. The ciliary body, the suspensory ligament and the lens divide the interior of the eyeball into two regions. The aqueous humour fills the space between the cornea and this division; the vitreous humour fills the other region. The part of the uvea between the vitreous humour and the sclera is the **choroid**. In this there is a special arrangement of iridescent cells called the **tapetum**. This is a light-reflecting area which in the dog varies in colour from green through yellow to pink. In the cat it is an even brighter more colourful metallic yellowish blue or green. This is the surface that causes eyes to "shine in the dark", or to be more accurate, reflect the small amount of light that is present. Another part of the

uvea projects as a septum between the ciliary body and the cornea: this is the **iris** and it has a central orifice called the **pupil**.

The sensory endings which receive visual stimuli form the **retina**; this is the innermost of the three main layers of the eye and is found between the vitreous humour and the choroid. Light passes through the cornea and is directed by the lens on to the sensory nerve endings of the retina. Focusing is achieved by the action of the ciliary body working through the suspensory ligament to change the curvature of the lens. The amount of light entering through the lens is controlled by the smooth muscle content of the iris which is able to vary the size of the pupil. The stimuli pass from the sensory endings of the retina along fibres which emerge from the eyeball as the optic (IInd) cranial nerve.

Most of the eyeball is within the orbit of the skull. The rest of it is protected by **eyelids** which can completely cover this part. The upper and lower eyelids of hairy skin converge at the medial and lateral **canthi** (singular canthus) or angles. Deep to these a third eyelid occupies the medial canthus. The epithelium of the skin on the outer surface of the lids is continuous with that of the **conjunctiva** of the under surface and this is attached to the eyeball.

The angle formed by the reflection of the conjunctiva is the **fornix**. The third eyelid consists of a plate of cartilage projecting from the medial canthus with its free lateral edge covered on its inner and outer surfaces by conjunctiva.

It moves like a protective curtain across the eyeball if it appears that something is going to hit the eye. Sometimes it stays projecting partly across the eyeball from its attachment in the medial canthus. This is most commonly associated with illness, especially in cats.

The corneal surface of the eye must be kept constantly moist and this is achieved by **lacrimal fluid** produced by the **lacrimal gland**, situated on the dorso-lateral surface of the eyeball. The secretion passes through several small ducts into the fornix of the upper eyelid. The fluid spreads over the entire area (helped by the eyelids sweeping over the eyeball) and then collects in the medial canthus where it drains into a small tube, the **nasolacrimal duct**. The opening for the duct is in a small depression in the lacrimal bone; note that the bone gets its name because this is where lacrimal fluid is collected and not because of any direct relationship with the lacrimal gland. The nasolacrimal duct passes through the bones of the face to open into the nasal chamber. This is where lacrimal fluid normally drains to; if there is excessive production or deficient drainage it will spill over the eyelid and may then be called **tear** fluid or tears. The fluid can have an irritating scalding effect on the skin it then runs over.

*Hearing and Balance* (Fig. 2.50)

These stimuli are received by endings in the **ear**, which is clearly divisible into three parts: *external, middle* and *inner*.

The external ear starts at the **pinna**, a funnel-shaped collection of cartilages covered by skin, which can be turned in various directions so that its concavity can collect air vibrations. The funnel leads to the **external acoustic meatus**, a short tube which is firmly fixed to the temporal bone. The deepest part of the meatus is closed by the **tympanic membrane**.

The middle ear is in the temporal bone and houses three small bones or *ossicles* which form a chain stretching from the tympanic membrane to the **vestibular window** opposite. The auditory tube also opens into the middle ear cavity. The other end of this tube opens in the pharynx; in this way the pressure on both sides of the tympanic membrane will be atmospheric and therefore the same.

The inner ear is also in the temporal bone and consists of a sealed bag of fluid called the **membranous labyrinth** which

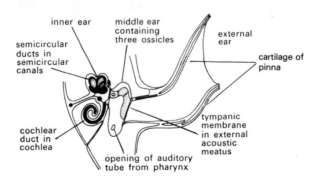

FIG. 2.50.   Section of ear.

fits into excavations called the **bony labyrinth**. This consists of three main parts. The central part is the **vestibule** and on one side of this are several openings of **semicircular canals**. Another tube that opens into the vestibule is the **cochlea**: this is coiled on itself in the form of a spiral. The bony labyrinth is filled with the fluid **perilymph** and the membranous labyrinth floats in this. However, it is not freely movable. Three tubular hoops form part of one side of the membranous labyrinth; these are **semicircular ducts** and they fit accurately into the semicircular canals of the bony labyrinth. There is also a **cochlear duct** which forms another part of the membranous labyrinth and this fits inside the cochlea of the bony labyrinth. The membranous labyrinth is filled with the fluid **endolymph**; this does not mingle with the surrounding perilymph.

The cochlear duct is concerned with hearing and the stimuli are transmitted to the brain by sensory fibres in the vestibulocochlear (VIIIth) cranial nerve. The remainder of the membranous labyrinth is affected by movement; sensory fibres carrying stimuli relating to equilibrium, posture, etc., also form part of the vestibulocochlear (VIIIth) cranial nerve.

## Smell

The **olfactory system** is concerned with smell. The sensory nerve endings are scattered in part of the mucous membrane covering the turbinates in the nasal cavity. The fibres do not form a compact nerve but run through the several holes in the ethmoid bone direct to the brain. They are considered to form the olfactory (Ist) cranial nerve.

## Taste

The sensory nerve endings are associated with special organs called **taste buds**. These are mainly scattered over the tongue but they also occur in the mucous membrane of the palate, pharynx and larynx. The fibres carrying stimuli associated with **gustatory** sensation (i.e. taste) form parts of the facial (VIIth), glossopharyngeal (IXth) and the vagus (Xth) cranial nerves.

## Endocrine System

This is a collective term for the endocrine (or ductless) glands and tissues that produce **hormones**. These secretions are spread by the blood stream to target tissues, organs and systems on which they have prolonged regulatory effects. The actions are extremely complex and very few are well understood. Some of the more important endocrine functions of the thyroid, parathyroids, adrenals, pancreas, pituitary and gonads will be outlined.

## Thyroid

The thyroid gland flanks the first few tracheal rings. It accumulates iodine and combines it into the hormone **thyroxin**. This it does under the control of a thyrotropic hormone produced by the adenohypophysis (anterior pituitary). The amount of iodine required is very small and so it is known as a trace element; nevertheless it is essential. Thyroxin has a general effect on many of the systems and especially on oxygen utilization by every cell of the body. It is necessary for normal growth, and young animals deficient in this hormone (the condition of *hypothyroidism*) suffer a form of dwarfism. Human hypothyroid dwarfs are called cretins. If the deficiency occurs after maturity, one of the main results is a lowered metabolic rate and the animal becomes fat and sluggish: this condition is called *myxoedema*. When excessive hormone is produced (*hyperthyroidism*) there is a marked increase in metabolic rate and the animal becomes nervous, irritable, overactive and often loses weight.

The thyroid gland also produces **thyrocalcitonin** (TCT, also called calcitonin), a hormone that reduces the amount of calcium in blood plasma. It seems to oppose the action of the hormone produced by the parathyroid glands and its rate of release increases greatly when the level of blood calcium rises. The effect is to reduce the rate at which bone is resorbed, so decreasing the entry of calcium from the skeleton into the plasma.

## Parathyroids

There are usually two very small parathyroid glands on each side of, and in close anatomical relationship to, the thyroid gland. The hormone produced is extremely important in maintaining a correct balance of calcium in the body. The concentration of calcium in the plasma seems to have a direct effect on the secretion of parathyroid hormone, a low circulating calcium level (*hypocalcaemia*) increasing the amount of the hormone. This increases the rate of bone resorption to transfer calcium into the blood. It decreases the excretion by the kidney by increasing its absorption in the renal tubules and it also promotes the absorption of calcium by the intestine.

Over-production of parathyroid hormone may be primary or secondary. If there is, for example, a neoplasia (tumour) of a parathyroid gland there may be a *hyperparathyroidism*. This will result in marked resorption of bone leading to weakening of the skeleton ending in fractures of the long bones and the vertebrae. Chronic renal failure due to long-standing kidney disease is often accompanied by a hypocalcaemia which results in a secondary (indirect) hyperparathyroidism. This seems to favour bone resorption from certain areas of the skeleton such as the mandibles and the maxillae. These bones become very softened and pliable giving the condition the name "rubber-jaw".

There is also a secondary hyperparathyroidism that can result from faulty nutrition such as a diet that is so low in calcium that the daily requirement is not met. It is especially seen in young cats kept on a predominantly meat diet. The secondary hyperparathyroidism that will result from the low blood calcium level again causes very marked derangements of the skeleton with the bones being very poorly mineralized and fracturing very easily. Nutritional secondary hyperparathyroidism does also occur in dogs kept on a meat diet low in calcium and has been frequently recorded in zoo and other captive animals.

## Adrenals

These paired glands lie close beside the kidneys (*ad*=near to; *renals*=kidneys). They have an inner *medullary* region and an outer *cortex* each of which produces its own hormones; there is no connection between these secretions.

*Adrenal medulla.* This produces two hormones, **epinephrine** (also called adrenalin) and **norepinephrine** (also called noradrenalin) whose actions are to prepare the body to meet emergencies. In this they are very similar to the sympathetic component of the autonomic part of the nervous system. Epinephrine seems to be mainly responsible for metabolic adjustments in emergencies, especially by raising the blood glucose level. Both the hormones increase the heart rate and raise blood pressure. They also decrease activity of and relax smooth muscle in the intestines and bladder but they do cause sphincters to contract (close).

*Adrenal cortex.* The hormones produced by this part of the adrenal gland all have a common basic biochemical structure and are called *steroids*. They can be arranged into three groups: **glucocorticoids, mineralocorticoids** and **adrenal sex hormones**. The glucocorticoids and mineralocorticoids are often called corticosteroids.

(a) Glucocorticoid secretion is regulated by adrenocorticotropic hormone (ACTH) from the pituitary. The two principal ones are **cortisol** (hydrocortisone) and **corticosterone**. Their actions are to raise the blood-sugar levels, increase glycogen storage in the liver and in this way to oppose the actions of insulin. They are also involved in the control of water and electrolyte flow between cells and the extra-cellular fluids. Glucocorticoids have an anti-inflammatory response; that is, they can suppress the body's reaction to injury such as the degree of local inflammation. This may seem a useless attribute but glucocorticoids can be of value in treatment when these reactions do not appear to be helpful, such as in arthritis, allergy and eye inflammations (conjunctivitis). These steroids are also of use, especially in humans, to control the natural rejection of transplanted tissues. It is usual to employ synthetic steroids such as prednisone and prednisolate which have similar effects but are much more potent than the glucocorticoids.

(b) Mineralocorticoids regulate electrolytes, especially sodium in the extracellular fluids. By far the most effective of the group is the hormone **aldosterone**, and it controls the resorption of sodium from the glomerular filtrate by the tubules of the kidney and so the amount of sodium that is passed out in the urine. If present in large quantities, aldosterone will reduce sodium excretion to virtually nil. The retention of sodium will be linked with a retention of chloride and of water but with an increased excretion of potassium, phosphorus and calcium. These adjustments in the electrolyte content will be associated with an increased intake of water (polydipsia) and an increase in extracellular fluids (oedema). This increase in fluid will increase blood volume, enhance the cardiac output and raise blood pressure. The possible role of the enzyme renin controlling the production of aldosterone was mentioned in the section on the kidney (p. 79).

(c) Adrenal sex steroids are known to be produced but they are not considered of great importance. They may have an important role in the spayed or castrated animal.

## Pancreas

This gland lies adjacent to the duodenum and by its exocrine production of pancreatic juice it plays an important role in intestinal digestion. Small patches of endocrine tissue form the islets of Langerhans which are responsible for producing **insulin** and **glucagon**. Insulin lowers the concentration of glucose in the blood and extracellular fluids by assisting its transfer to the interior of cells. In its absence, glucose cannot be used and so it is excreted: fats and proteins are therefore called upon to provide energy, resulting in a wasting-away of tissues. A fuller account of the action of insulin is given in the section on digestion; diabetes mellitus, the disease resulting from deficiency of insulin is also described there (p. 73).

Glucagon appears to increase the conversion of liver glycogen to glucose and so has exactly the opposite effect to insulin. It has been described in the section on the digestive system.

It would appear that the blood glucose limits are controlled to a large extent by the balance of these two hormones (although others such as epinephrine are also involved).

## Pituitary

This small gland is attached in the midline to the ventral surface of the midbrain. It is sometimes called the hypophysis and there are two major hormone-producing areas—the **adenohypophysis** (or anterior pituitary) and the **neurohypophysis** (or posterior pituitary). Between them these two produce a large number of hormones, many of which control the secretion of other endocrine organs.

*Adenohypophysis (Anterior pituitary).* Six major hormones are produced by this anterior part of the pituitary—**thyrotropic hormone, somatotropin, adrenocorticotropic hormone, prolactin** and two **gonadotropins**. (The word ending -*tropin* or -*tropic* indicates that the word beginning refers to a target organ: for example, thyrotropic hormone has a direct effect on the thyroid gland.)

*Thyrotropic hormone*: also called thyrotropin or thyroid stimulating hormone (TSH). The level of the thyroid hormone depends on the direct stimulation of the secreting cells of the gland by the thyrotropic hormone.

*Somatotropin* (STH, growth hormone). This hormone does not have a target organ but it has a general effect on several tissues. Its presence favours a build-up of muscle by making the cells more permeable to amino acids. Somatotropin also increases the retention of nitrogen which helps to produce protein. Carbohydrate metabolism is also improved. If insufficient somatotropin is produced in young

animals they will remain underdeveloped: such animals are called pituitary dwarfs. Overproduction of somatotropin in the young will produce giants if closure of epiphyses has not taken place. If the excess occurs in the adult the bones will thicken and a condition called acromegaly will result.

*Adrenocorticotropic hormone* is also known by the initials ACTH or as corticotropin. As the name suggests, the target is the cortex of the adrenal gland, which is itself responsible for producing a large number of hormones. An increase in ACTH stimulates the production of the corticosteroids.

*Prolactin.* This is the lactogenic hormone of the anterior pituitary, i.e. one which is able to stimulate mammary tissue to produce milk.

*Gonadotropins.* There are two hormones of the adenohypophysis which have gonads as the target organs. Follicle-stimulating hormone (FSH) as its name suggests, is responsible for growth of the follicles in the ovary. Luteinizing hormone (LH, interstitial cell stimulating hormone, ICSH) stimulates the maturation of the follicle and helps in its ovulation: it also stimulates oestrogen production by the ovary. Luteinizing hormone is also produced in the male, when it is known as interstitial cell stimulating hormone. It is responsible, with other hormones, for the normal development and function of the testes and it does specifically stimulate the interstitial cells of the testes to themselves produce hormones, such as testosterone, which are grouped together as androgens. These influence characteristics that are usually associated with the male animal, such as body size and shape.

Gonadotropins are used quite frequently in veterinary work and there are two other sources which are not directly associated with the pituitary. The one which resembles FSH in its activity (and so may be called FSH-like hormone) is extracted from the serum of pregnant mares. This PMSG (pregnant mare serum gonadotropin) is used to stimulate follicle growth in adult females. The luteinizing hormone-like (LH-like) hormone is found in the urine of pregnant women. It is called human chorionic gonadotropin (HCG) since it is produced by the placental chorion. It has also been known as pregnant urine hormone or PU. This product is used to cause ovulation in the female and to stimulate androgen production in the male.

*Neurohypophysis (posterior pituitary).* Strictly, the hormones are only stored in the neurohypophysis. They are secreted deeper within the brain tissue and are conducted to this site from where they are released. The two important substances are **antidiuretic hormone (ADH)**, and **oxytocin**.

The action of antidiuretic hormone, also called vasopressin, has been described in the section on the kidney (p. 80). It plays a major role in water resorption by the tubules of the kidney, increased amounts of hormone increasing the absorption. The hormone is normally released if for any reason the animal begins to get dehydrated. But if there is some malfunction of the hormone-producing area in the brain and insufficient is produced, the tubules do not take back the water from the glomerular filtrate. Copious amounts of very dilute urine will be voided (polyuria) and the animal will drink heavily (polydipsia) in an attempt to retain water balance. This is the condition of *diabetes insipidus.* It differs from diabetes mellitus resulting from insulin lack in that glucose excretion is not involved and glucose is not found in the urine.

Oxytocin is thought to be only of importance in the female. It has specific actions on the uterus, causing the muscle cells to contract. It is especially important during parturition when the uterus is expelling the fetus. Oxytocin also affects mammary gland tissue to release milk. The epithelium that produces the milk in the depth of the gland is surrounded by special types of cells (myoepithelial) and these contract to force the milk into the gland sinuses. This is called "letdown" of milk and results from the production of oxytocin which in its turn is stimulated by nerve reflexes set up from the suckling by the young.

## Male Gonad

The testis has two major functions: gametogenesis, production of sperm and steroidogenesis, production of hormones. The sperms are produced in the seminiferous tubules. One of the hormones comes from the cells (of Leydig) which pack between the tubules. These are the interstitial cells and it has been described above that they are controlled by the ICSH of the pituitary. They produce **testosterone**, a hormone responsible for the development and maintenance of the reproductive tract and the accessory sex glands and for the secondary sex characters and sex behaviour characteristic of the male.

Castration prevents the circulation of testosterone from the gonads and if performed while the animal is still sexually immature it will stay that way. None of the remaining genitalia will develop fully nor will the accessory sex glands. The animal will not show any mating activities. If castration is performed after sexual maturity, the major result of the lack of testosterone will show in an increase of depot fat due to a lowered metabolic rate. It is still possible for mating behaviour to occur as a form of "play" in these castrated animals.

Another hormone produced by the testis is secreted by the supportive cells (of Sertoli) in the seminiferous tubules. This has oestrogenic properties which will inhibit pituitary gonadotrophin production and is part of the delicate interplay of endocrine organs which helps keep a balance. However, when the balance is upset (such as in neoplasia or tumour of the Sertoli cells) there is a massive output of oestrogens which will have the effect of feminizing the dog.

### Female Gonad

The ovary also has two major functions: the production of eggs (ova) and the production of hormones. Two are produced—**oestradiol** and **progesterone**. As the follicle develops in the ovary the fluid it contains has an increasing amount of oestradiol which is being produced by the cells of the follicle wall and will pass out into the blood steam. Oestradiol is one of a group of compounds (not necessarily only produced by the ovary) called **oestro-**gens that will all have similar effects. These are to produce the outward signs of heat (sexual desire) and to prepare the genitalia for coitus. Under the influence of oestrogens the lining of the tubular part of the tract undergoes increased activity and produces large quantities of mucus. The hormone also affects the hypophysis to reduce the production of FSH but to increase that of LH. When the follicle ruptures a corpus luteum forms and the cells involved with this structure also produce a hormone. This is progesterone and this is essential for the maintenance of pregnancy. Under its influence the uterus prepares for the reception of the fertilized ovum and later in pregnancy progesterone will act on mammary tissue to prepare for lactation. It will also reduce still further the production of FSH so that oestrous cycles do not (normally) occur during pregnancy. Towards the end of pregnancy the corpus luteum produces another hormone, **relaxin**. This causes relaxation of some of the ligaments around the pelvis so that the birth canal becomes more pliable to facilitate the passage of the fetuses.

# CHAPTER 3

# Management, Hygiene and Feeding

## (a) Restraint and Handling of Dogs and Cats

G. SUMNER-SMITH

### Introduction

To love animals does not mean, unfortunately, that your love will be reciprocated, hence the necessity for restraint. But if love of animals can, as it should, comprehend a knowledge of animal psychology and behaviour patterns, the first stages in the act of restraint will have been learned. Recognition of instinctive behaviour patterns in the dog and cat when faced with stress is essential to a rational approach to handling of animal patients in hospital.

Biting or scratching through fear is the main hazard in nursing the domestic dog or cat, and to understand and alleviate that fear is one of the main duties of the RANA. Although the main emphasis of this section is on the actual manual techniques of restraint it should never be forgotten that the more knowledge the RANA acquires of instinctive behaviour and breed characteristics the less will be the necessity to resort to the cruder methods of restraint.

### Approach

The approach to a patient is of primary importance, as it should be remembered that the strange sites, noises and, more particularly, odours of a veterinary hospital may make even a normally placid patient nervous.

The RANA who is able to make friends with her charge will find it easier to restrain the animal for treatment or examination.

### The Restraint of Dogs

Approach the dog with a kind and quiet word and present the back of one closed hand for inspection; the lead and collar is taken in the other hand. Before taking charge of an animal it is essential to check that the collar is fastened on a hole that is sufficiently tight, and is not likely to slip over the dog's head should it struggle on parting from the owner. The owner should be instructed to leave the dog with the RANA, rather than the RANA take the dog from the room before the owner leaves. The dog will usually submit to being led away once the owner is out of sight. On occasions it may be considered desirable to leave the lead attached to the animal's collar when it is placed in a kennel. Should the animal later be reluctant to leave the kennel it will be far easier to reach the lead with hand or broom handle than to attempt affixing the lead whilst the animal is still in the kennel. This is particularly advisable when the patient is unco-operative, but the danger of an animal becoming entangled should always be borne in mind, and the RANA will decide in the circumstances which course is to be taken.

## Handling

When it becomes necessary to lift the dog on to the examination table the collar is grasped in the left hand, the RANA standing by the animal's left foreleg, and facing in the same direction. The right arm is passed over the back and the hand under the sternum. The hand takes the weight of the dog as it is lifted, the left hand controlling the head. The left arm should be tensed in order to respond to any sudden attempt on the part of the dog to struggle or turn on its handler. Assistance will be necessary when lifting large dogs and this may be performed by a second person standing directly behind the animal, grasping both stifles to aid the lift. Patients should never be lifted by a hand or arm under the abdomen. The small, wriggling and unco-operative dog may be picked up by first covering with a blanket that has been folded a number of times, or by the handler wearing thick pruning gloves.

## Muzzling

When handling a strange dog a muzzle should be applied if there is the slightest doubt as to the docility of the animal. A muzzle may be made of leather or wire; but in veterinary practice it is usual to apply the **tape muzzle** (Figs. 3.1 and 3.2). This muzzle may be discarded after use as

a point of hygiene and it is not necessary to stock the large range of sizes that are required when using the fixed type (Fig. 3.8). The bandage may usually be applied without a lot of fuss if the approach is gentle and reassuring. Occasionally it is necessary to have an assistant hold the forelegs if the animal attempts to remove the bandage with its claws. The bandage should be secured in position by a bow to aid a quick release. Whilst a bandage may be applied to most breeds, it will be readily appreciated that one cannot apply same to such breeds as the Pug and Pekinese, and for these animals the use of a hand towel is recommended. The towel is rolled lengthways, passed under the neck, and the two ends held firmly close to and behind the patient's head.

## Holding for examination and medication

Six methods will be described.

1. The RANA stands behind the patient who is already standing on the examination table. The collar is grasped on each side of the head, just below the ears, with the heel of the palms pressed firmly against the dog's neck to extend the head forward (Fig. 3.3).

2. The left arm is passed under the patient's neck and the palm of the hand pressed firmly on its right shoulder blade —the patient being hugged against the RANA. The right hand either forces the rear quarters to the sitting position, and holds them there; or supports the body in the standing position behind and under the quarters. The method will be determined by the position required, and it is of course possible to stand on the other side of the animal and reverse the procedure should such be required.

3. In order to restrain an animal on its side, the patient should be grasped by the

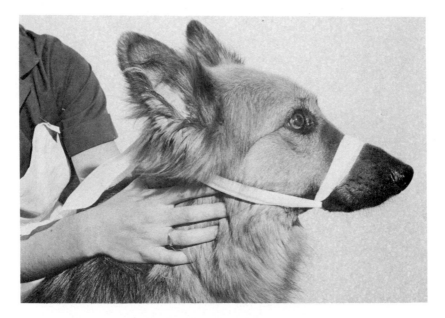

Fig. 3.1.　Tape muzzle applied to a dog.

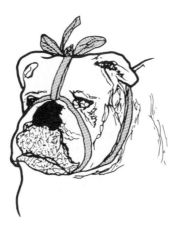

Fig. 3.2.　Tape muzzle applied to "bull-nosed" dog.

far side opposing front and hindlegs, lifted from the table, lowered slightly and then rolled on its side as the table is approached again, the operator's chest aiding in pressing the animal on to the table. Ideally, this movement should be performed by one person, enabling a second person to pass one arm over the neck and grasp the underneath foreleg and the other over the lumbar region and grasp the corresponding under hindleg (Fig. 3.4).

4. Restraining an animal on its back is accomplished by rolling from method 3, and holding each pair of fore and hindlegs in the hands. Naturally it is necessary to have the assistance of another when a large dog is being handled.

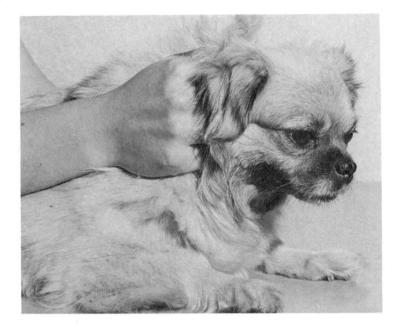

FIG. 3.3.   Holding for examination—method 1.

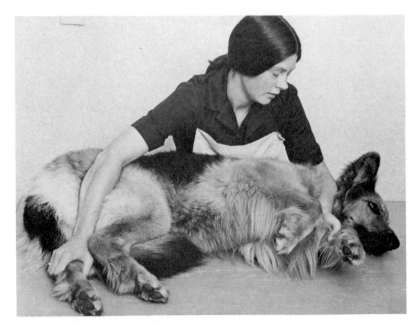

FIG. 3.4.   Holding for examination—method 3.

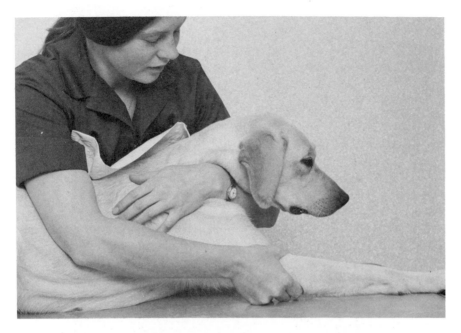

FIG. 3.5. Restraint for intravenous injection in the forelimb.

5. Small and medium-sized dogs may be sat on the knee of a RANA sitting on a chair with all four legs presented to the examiner. The animal's back is placed against the restrainer's chest, and the forelegs are grasped behind the elbow holding the legs in the extended position.

6. The administration of intravenous injections necessitates that the animal be held as still as is possible. Method 2 is recommended as being the best position with the patient in the sitting position. The dog's elbow is grasped in the palm of the right hand and the thumb passed over the radius to compress the vein (Figs. 3.5, 3.6). Once the surgeon has entered the vein the pressure on the vein is released but the leg is still steadied by the hand. Alternatively, a length of rubber tubing is wound around the foreleg above the elbow and the two ends are held with forceps (Fig. 3.7). This raises the vein admirably, and in the small dog does not cover too much of it, whilst allowing the hand to maintain its restraining pressure on the flank and rear quarter. Once the vein has been entered, one end only is released. The tourniquet method is recommended as being preferable to raising the vein with the thumb.

The holding of small dogs by the "scruff" of the neck has little to recommend it and in the presence of an owner is a poor advertisement, apart from the danger of luxating the eyeballs of some breeds.

### The difficult dog

Little has been said regarding the handling of obstreperous and vicious patients, and it will be appreciated that even to administer a sedative the animal must generally be handled and the majority will not take anything hidden in food whilst they are in a strange environment.

Two points are most important: firstly, the patient must not be allowed to escape, and, secondly, that those attending are not

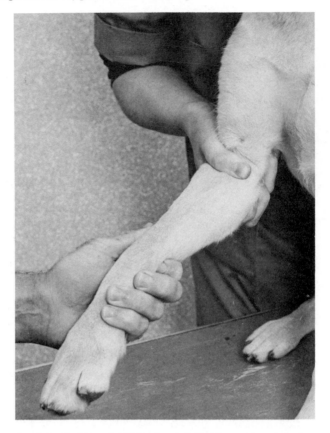

FIG. 3.6.  Position of ANA's thumb before intravenous injection.

injured. Once a muzzle has been applied firmly most of the battle has been won. However, the application of that muzzle may be most hazardous. Should trouble be anticipated it is as well to have the owner affix two strong leads before the animal is admitted. This permits some restraint of the head by two operators pulling in opposing directions whilst a third attempts to apply the muzzle from the rear. Should an approach from behind not be successful the patient may be backed into a wall, and then approached from the front whilst being restrained by two leads pulling in opposite directions. Two muzzles should be applied. The first should be of soft rope or cord, according to the size of the dog, as a tape tends to fold too easily when being dangled in front of the dog. This method is necessary as one may only hold the rope by its ends because the operator's hands will be too close to the animal's jaw if the loop is held. Once the first muzzle has been applied a second tape muzzle may be applied in the routine manner. A leather "box" muzzle may be useful (Fig. 3.8).

The more vicious animals will necessitate resort of the dog catcher (Fig. 3.9). The dog catcher restrains the animal's head and enables it to be kept out of reach of the operator's person whilst an assistant applies the muzzle. It may also be used in conjunction with a lead or noose pulled in the opposite direction. Pressure on the noose should be eased slightly once the

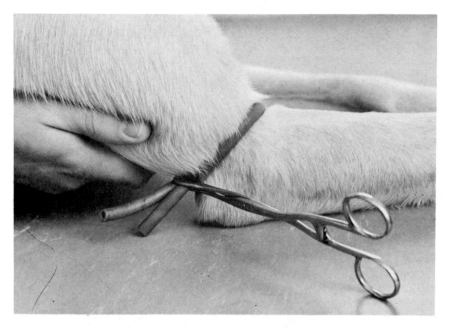

Fig. 3.7.    Alternative method of raising vein.

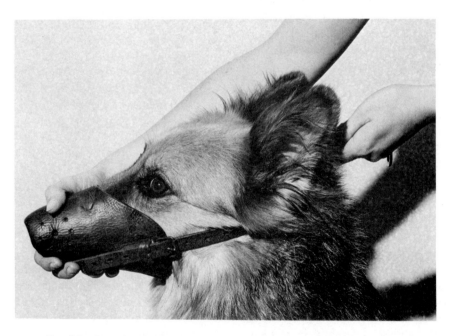

Fig. 3.8.    Use of a leather muzzle on a dog. (This box muzzle has an open end.)

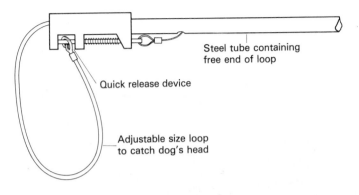

Steel tube containing
free end of loop

Quick release device

Adjustable size loop
to catch dog's head

FIG. 3.9.  The dog catcher.

muzzle has been applied, so as not to cause distress and avoid the danger of choking the patient.

### The Restraint of Cats

In general, cats require a slightly different approach to the dog. A firm, confident attitude is necessary as the cat will often adopt, on the approach of a stranger, an instinctive defensive posture, which looks alarming. This usually collapses once a hand is put confidently on the cat. However, the RANA should normally reassure the animal, before picking it up, by gently stroking the head and talking quietly. A metal cat-catcher with a grasping device will be found useful. The cat can then be placed in a "crush cage".

### Handling

Once the RANA has decided that her patient is reasonably passive, the animal may be lifted by passing the arm over the chest and the hand under the sternum, with the other hand used to lightly grip the scruff of the neck. Alternatively, if the cat is being taken from a cage it may be lifted by grasping both elbows from the front, and when free of the cage it is then tucked

under one arm, with the hand holding the forelegs (Fig. 3.10). However, before a cat is removed from a basket or cage it is essential to ensure that all doors and windows are closed or are escape-proof. There is no more embarrassing situation than reporting to an owner that his pet has been lost, and there is no excuse for this. For the same reason a cat should only be moved from one room to another within a proper basket and not carried loose. Similarly, the animal should be placed in a basket by the owner at reception, and not handed over to the RANA's arms. When a cat is to be removed from a basket the lid should be raised gently and if the animal does not appear to be vicious, the hand is slipped inside to hold the cat before the lid is folded right back.

### Holding for examination and medication

Four methods will be described.

1. The cat is placed on the examination table and one hand is slipped underneath the chin, and, if necessary, the other hand supports the rear (Fig. 3.11).

2. Administration of intravenous injections may be effected in a similar manner to that used for the dog, the left hand holding the head and the right hand

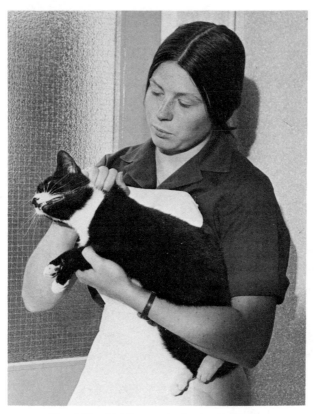

Fig. 3.10.   Holding a cat prior to examination.

holding the far side foreleg or tourniquet, while the cat is held against the RANA's side by the forearm. Although it is common practice for cats to be held by the "scruff", many appear to resent this restraint far more than simply having the head held by a hand under the jaw. The RANA will decide on the most suitable method for the case in hand, as the more obstreperous will require seizing by the "scruff".

3. Should a cat resent examination of parts of the head and attempt to claw the operator's hand, a small towel may be held round the neck in the form of a bib. The cat's claws become caught in the towel when it tries to reach the operator. The method is not intended for a truly vicious animal, but is useful when the cat is a normal patient but unused to having its mouth and ears examined.

4. Cats and kittens are commonly wrapped in a large thick towel when it is desired to administer a local anaesthetic or dress a particular area, the area in question being left exposed. Great care should be taken that adequate ventilation exists via the head end of the roll. The unruly cat may also be restrained inside a towel for intravenous administration, the head and one leg being exposed. The "scruff" is grasped in the left hand and the head is turned upwards whilst the right hand extends the right foreleg and keeps the towel tight enough to restrain the other legs. Pressure is also exerted by the forearm holding the animal into the RANA's side.

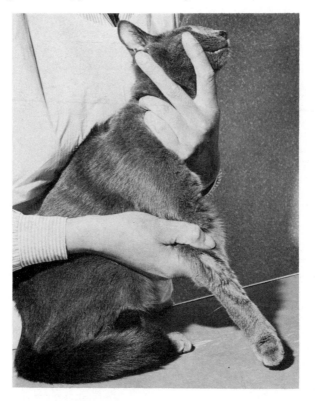

FIG. 3.11.   Holding a cat with hand under chin.

**The difficult cat**

Restraint of a truly vicious cat can present the RANA with a considerable problem as the animal bites quickly and uses all four sets of claws. Even if she is able to grasp the animal by the "scruff" it will still contort itself and succeed in striking with the hindleg claws.

A cat that is proving difficult within a basket or cage may often be restrained by crowding it into a corner with a thick blanket when it may then be grasped by a hand through the blanket. The use of thick garden pruning gloves has much to recommend it when handling the difficult patient. Occasions do arise when it becomes necessary to resort to the use of a catcher.

Whenever a difficult cat is being handled it is most important to ensure that it is kept well away from both the RANA's and the surgeon's face as the truly wild animal will always attempt to inflict injury to the eyes and face.

Resulting from the experience of the use of tongs for handling mink, various patterns have been developed and are now marketed for the catching and restraint of excited and vicious cats (Fig. 3.14). While holding the animals firmly they do not cause any injury or unwarranted distress.

**Restraint by Medication**

Within this section on restraint of the dog and cat, no attempt has been made to deal with restraint by drugs, nor has the administration of medicaments been covered as these points will be dealt with in the appropriate sections elsewhere.

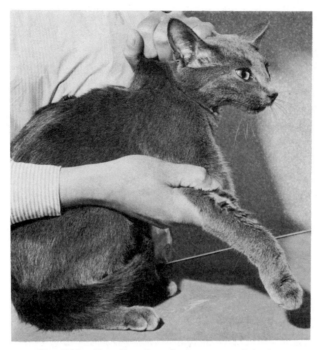

FIG. 3.12.   Restraint of cat for intravenous injection.

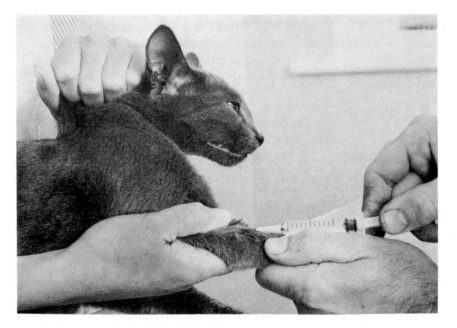

FIG. 3.13.   The intravenous injection of the cat.

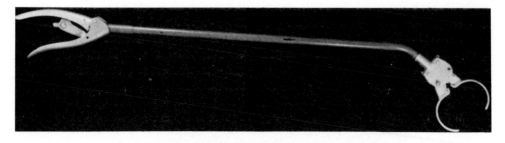

FIG. 3.14.    The cat catcher.

Tranquillizers of various types are now being used more often than hitherto. The advent of the newer phenothiazine derivatives* and the various ataractics, that are safe for cats, has made it possible to subdue vicious and frightened dogs and cats without the necessity of prolonged forceful restraint. This is to be encouraged, but under no circumstances should the RANA take it on herself to administer such a tranquillizer without the expressed instructions of a veterinarian. Given to patients suffering from a particular stress or disease, these drugs can have grave consequences.

*In addition to the phenothiazine derivatives, of which acepromazine is the one of choice, other drugs are now widely used in cats. Ketamine and/or xylazine may be used by intramuscular injection in the cat. The steroid combination ("Saffan") can also be administered by intramuscular injection in the cat for chemical restraint.

## (b) Restraint of Smaller Pets

J. E. COOPER and K. A. APPLEBEE

Species of animal other than dogs and cats are commonly kept as pets and this trend may increase as it becomes more difficult to own a large animal in an urban environment. The types of small pets which may be encountered in veterinary practice include various rodents (for example, mice, rats, guinea pigs, hamsters and gerbils), rabbits, cagebirds, reptiles, amphibians and fish.

It is important that the RANA is able to handle some, if not all, of these species. Proper restraint will facilitate clinical examination and treatment and will also minimize damage both to the animal and handler.

### Mice

Pet mice are generally easy to handle and should be caught and lifted by the base of the tail. However, to allow a proper clinical examination the mouse should be "scruffed". This is performed by allowing the animal to grip on a rough surface e.g. sandpaper, carpet tile or cage lid (Fig. 3.15) and then grasping it by the base of the tail. Using the thumb and forefinger of the free hand, the scruff at the back of the neck is grasped (Fig. 3.16). It is then a simple task to lift the mouse and turn it over, securing the tail between the third and fourth finger (Fig. 3.17). This technique leaves the other hand free for palpation, intramuscular injections etc.

Intravenous injections are most easily given into a lateral tail vein. The mouse is restrained by placing it in a tube which is small enough in diameter to prevent it from turning around. The open end is closed with a stopper or similar device which confines the mouse but allows the tail to protrude. An empty syringe case can be easily adapted for this purpose. The veins may be dilated by placing the tail in warm water or under a lamp prior to injection.

### Rats

Pet rats are usually tame and easy to handle. Rats should not be picked up by the tail, except when briefly removing them from their cage, and then only by the base.

The best method of restraining a rat is to grasp it around the shoulders, with the thumb under the jaw to prevent it biting; the base of the tail can also be held so as to stop the animal scratching with its hind claws (Fig. 3.18). This method is satisfactory for most veterinary procedures, but if tube-feeding is envisaged, it may be necessary to scruff the animal using the procedure described for the mouse.

Generally the main error made when restraining the rat is to hold it far too tightly. Excessive pressure on the trachea can be avoided by ensuring that there is a forelimb between the handler's thumb and the animal's jaw (Fig. 3.18). If the

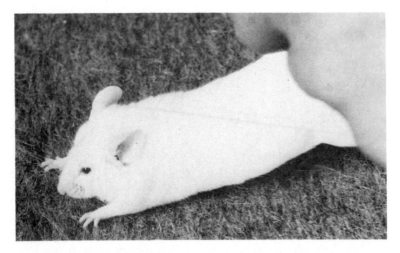

FIG. 3.15.    A mouse is held by the base of the tail. Note how the animal grips the rough surface of the carpet tile.

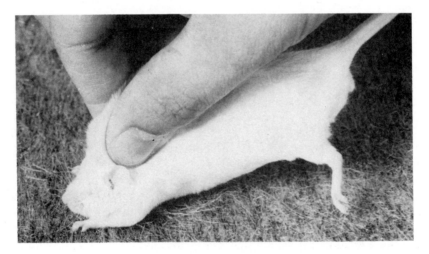

FIG. 3.16.    The scruff is grasped with thumb and forefinger.

animal becomes excited, gentle rocking or talking will help to calm it.

Intravenous injections are given as described for the mouse. However, it may be wise to purchase or make a rat-restrainer. Alternatively the rat can be rolled up in a towel.

### Hamsters

Hamsters are easily frightened and stressed; hence they are more inclined to bite than are tame mice or rats.

To restrain the hamster it is placed on a flat surface. Then gentle pressure is applied using the palm of the hand with the

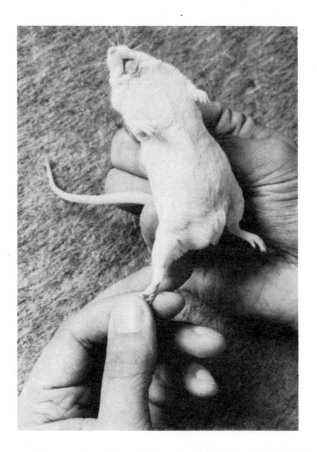

FIG. 3.17.   The mouse is now fully restrained in one hand; the other is left free for examination.

hamster's head facing out between thumb and forefinger. Using all four fingers as well as the thumb, as much as possible of the large amount of loose skin from the neck to the lower back is grasped. The hamster can then be lifted and turned over for examination in a similar way to that described for the mouse.

## Gerbils

Gerbils are nervous animals and can often bite when frightened.

The gerbil must never be picked up by the tail alone as the skin in this area is easily sloughed. The animal should be removed from the cage by gently holding the base of the tail and supporting it on the palm of the other hand. The gerbil is restrained for examination by placing it on a rough surface or cage lid; it is held gently by the base of the tail. Then the animal is scruffed using the thumb and forefinger; it is turned over by securing the tail between the third and fourth finger, as described for the mouse.

## Guinea Pigs

Guinea pigs are probably the most

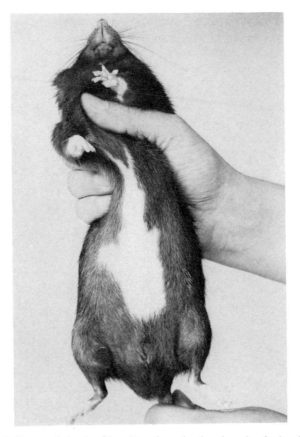

FIG. 3.18.    A rat is held around the shoulders. Note how the thumb under the jaw helps prevent biting.

placid of all smaller pets, rarely biting even when disturbed.

Guinea pigs should be lifted by grasping them around the thorax and supporting the hindlimbs with the other hand (Fig. 3.19). If the guinea pig needs to be more securely restrained—for example, for an injection—the thorax should be held a little tighter and the lower limbs extended by the other hand, with the animal lying horizontally on its back.

### Rabbits

Rabbits, especially the larger strains, can be the most difficult of all the smaller pets to restrain, owing to their size. Injuries to the back and leg due to poor handling are common.

When undergoing clinical examination or prior to handling, rabbits must always be placed on a non-slippery surface e.g. a rubber car mat. If the rabbit is excited the palm of the hand can be placed over its eyes to calm it. It is picked up by grasping the scruff and supporting the lower back with the other hand (Fig. 3.20).

To examine the genitalia and abdomen the rabbit is held by the scruff and the hindquarters rested on the handler's thigh (Fig. 3.21).

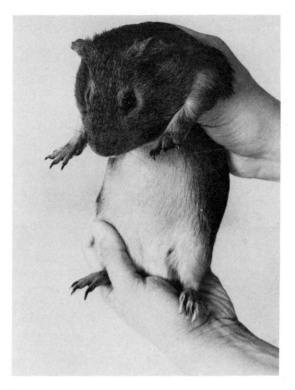

FIG. 3.19. A guinea pig is held around the thorax; one hand supports the animal's hindlimbs.

The incisors are best examined by turning the rabbit on to its back, keeping the forearm holding the scruff in line with the animal's vertebral column, while pushing the hind legs out beyond the handler's body. This technique must be done in one smooth movement; the rabbit will then be totally restrained and one hand will remain free to part the lips (Fig. 3.22).

For an intravenous injection into the marginal ear vein, the rabbit is held with its head away from the handler and its rear end pressed against his body. The rabbit will then feel it is unable to back away; again it is advisable to cover its eyes.

## Other Species

Cagebirds are best grasped in the hand, making sure that the wings are restrained. Gloves or a towel may prove useful for the larger species.

Reptiles vary considerably in their shape, size and temperament. For example, while a land tortoise will rarely attempt to bite, a terrapin frequently does! These reptiles are best grasped by the "shell", with one or both hands. Lizards and small crocodiles should be held with one hand round the shoulders, using the other hand to support the hindquarters. Gloves may be needed for the larger species. Lizards should *never* be held by the tail; it may come off! Snakes often elicit fear or apprehension but most captive specimens will be accustomed to handling and unlikely to bite. Snakes often hold on to a person, rather than the other way round. Thus, for example, a

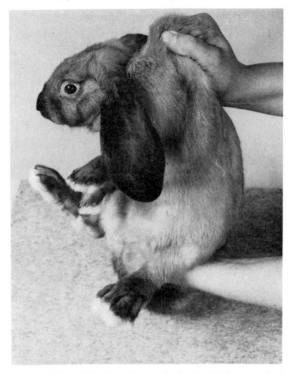

Fig. 3.20.   A rabbit is lifted by the scruff; the hindlimbs must be supported.

small boa constrictor will wrap itself around a RANAs wrist and, so long as the rest of its body is supported, will present few problems. Other, more active, snakes may glide from hand to hand. If detailed examination has to be carried out, or treatment given, it may be necessary to restrain the snake behind the head to prevent it from moving or biting. Gloves will minimize the risk of an injury but will also reduce dexterity. Poisonous snakes may have to be pinned down with a special "snake stick" prior to being picked up; the RANA should leave this procedure to someone more experienced but must be available to assist if required.

Amphibians generally have moist skins and are best handled in a small net or with a wet cloth. They should only be held in the hand for limited periods. Axolotls and other immature amphibians, which breathe through gills, should be treated like fish. Fish can be transported and examined for a short period in a net. Care must be taken to ensure that the surface of the skin does not become dry or damaged.

It may be difficult or unwise to restrain some of the above species for more than a few minutes. Light anaesthesia can then be of assistance and is frequently used to facilitate handling and examining of (for example) parrots, large snakes and fish. Other aids to handling, some of which have been mentioned, include gloves, nets, small cloth bags and a variety of suitable containers—for example, plastic sweet jars, aquaria and boxes.

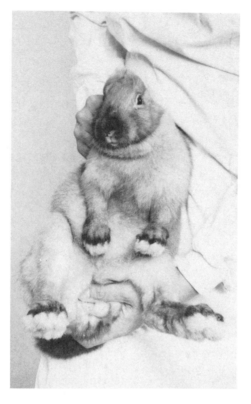

FIG. 3.21.   The rabbit is scruffed and supported for examination.

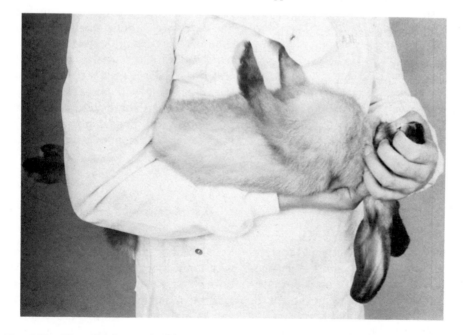

FIG. 3.22.   The rabbit is restrained in order to permit examination and/or clipping of the incisors.

## (c) Smaller Laboratory Animals

ANNE KEELEY

### Introduction

It is impossible in this section to give comprehensive details on the veterinary aspects of nursing the host of different species of small rodents, lagomorphs (rabbits) and small carnivores which are kept. However, the most important factor in the successful treatment of any animal, or giving advice to its owner, is an understanding of the nutrition, husbandry and reproductive physiology of the normal healthy individual. In this section is a table giving brief details of certain normal characteristics of some of the more common smaller mammals (see Table 3.1), only approximations are listed, and certain individuals may show some slight deviation from these average values.

Many of these smaller mammals are routinely maintained as laboratory animals, and details of books on their management in the animal house are given at the end of this section.

The *UFAW Handbook* and the *IAT Manual* have particularly useful illustrated sections on the handling and sexing of several species that are likely to be kept as pets.

### General Considerations

It is important to avoid any undue stress when handling a small animal, particularly if it is already sick. When approaching the cage, no sudden movement or noise should be made, and if, in spite of such precautions, the animal is still ex-

tremely excited, it should be allowed to calm down before being handled.

As rodents tend to rely rather more on their powers of hearing and smell than on their sight and tend to have rather high body temperatures, warmth and quiet are essential factors in their successful nursing.

Many of these small animals can be quite aggressive amongst themselves, and this is particularly true of hamsters, the males of which can be badly bitten by the females. Such fighting amongst the sexes is often lessened if hamsters are kept together from weaning onwards and not introduced to each other when already adult.

Table 3.1 gives some facts on breeding cycles of various small pets, but it should also be appreciated that the majority exhibit a post-partum oestrus, and if the male is kept with the pregnant female, mating will occur within a few hours of the birth of the litter, and another pregnancy will immediately ensue perhaps to the detriment of both animal and owner.

### Environmental Temperature and Caging

Laboratory animals are kept in simple wire-topped boxes without separate nest boxes, and great care is therefore taken to control the temperature and humidity of an animal room within fairly precise limits. When these animals are kept as

TABLE 3.1.    Data on Some Smaller Mammals

| Species | Adult body weight (g) | Approx. life-span (years) | Breeding season | Age when first mated (weeks) | Duration of oestrus cycle (days) | Gestation period (days) | Approx. litter size | Age of weaning (days) | Type of diet (a) | Rectal temperature °C | Respiration rate per minute | Pulse rate per minute |
|---|---|---|---|---|---|---|---|---|---|---|---|---|
| **Mouse** *Mus musculus* | 25–40 | 2–3 | continuous | 6–8 | 4–5 | 19–21 | 6–12 | 21 | A | 37.4 | 84–230 | 120 |
| **Rat** *Rattus norvegicus* | 270–310 | 2–3 | continuous | 10–14 | 4–5 | 21–23 | 6–15 | 21–25 | A | 37.5 | 210 | 260–600 |
| **Golden (Syrian) hamster** *Mesocricetus auratus* | 110–180 | 1½–2 | continuous | 6–8 | 4–5 | 15–16 | 7–9 | 20–25 | B | 36–38 | 33–127 | 300–600 |
| **Chinese hamster** *Cricetulus griseus* | 40–55 | 5–6 | continuous | 8–12 | 4–5 | 20–21 | 3–7 | 20 | B | — | 200 | — |
| **Steppe lemming** *Lagurus lagurus* | 15–25 | 2–3 | continuous | 6–8 | 4–5 | 19–21 | 5–7 | 20 | B | 35.4–41.2 | 250 | 348–4665 |
| **Gerbil** *Meriones unguiculatus* | 40–100 | 5–6 | continuous | 12 | 4–6 | 24 | 6–8 | 21 | B | 38.2–39.4 | 70–120 | 260–600 |
| **Guinea pig (cavy)** *Cavia porcellus* | 850–1000 | 6–7 | continuous | 12 | 16–19 | 59–72 | 3–5 | 21–25 | C | 39–40 | 110–150 | 150–160 |
| **Chinchilla** *Chinchilla lanigera* | 400–600 | 10–12 | November–May | 30–35 | 30–40 | 106–118 | 1–4 | 42–56 | C | 35.5–37.5 | 45–65 | 200–350 |
| **Rabbit** *Oryctolagus cuniculus* | 2000–5000 | 5–6 | continuous, but diminished activity during winter | 25–35 | very prolonged in absence of males. Ovulation only occurs during coitus | 31–32 | 5–10 | 50 | C | 38.5–40 | 38–65 | 135 |
| **Ferret** *Mustela putorius furo* | 750–1000 | 9–10 | March–August | 35–50 | | 42 | 6–8 | 42–56 | D | 38.6 | 40–60 | 216–242 |
| **Mink** *Mustela viso* | 850–1500 | 6–10 | March–August | 40–50 | 7–10 | 39–78(b) | 3–6 | 35–40 | D | 39.0–39.7 | 40–70 | 300–400 |

(a) Refer to appropriate section.    (b) Delayed implantation can occur.

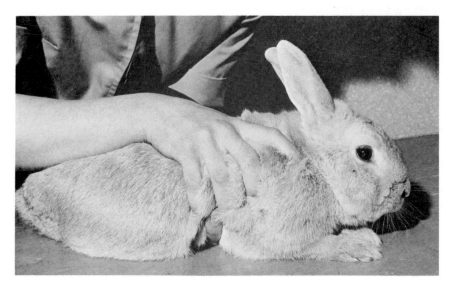

FIG. 3.23.

pets, more elaborate cages with nest-boxes are usually provided, and advice to owners concerning temperatures at which the animals should be kept will be influenced by the type of cage in which the animal is housed. As a general rule, mice, rats, hamsters, lemmings and gerbils require some extra heat in the winter, and should be kept indoors or in a heated shed so that within the nest the temperature is in the region of 22°C (70°F). Lemmings particularly require a nest-box containing loose litter in which they can burrow. Gerbils need hay to chew, otherwise they can injure their noses gnawing at the cage bars, causing a chronic rhinitis and secondary eye infection. Care must be taken with choice of bedding material, in particular Syrian hamsters. For example, if cotton wool or similar is used, it can be eaten and cause constipation or impaction, killing the animal. Wood wool has been known to wind around the limbs or neck of very young pre-weaned rats causing death or loss of limb.

A sudden drop in room temperature during the winter may cause golden hamsters to hibernate, a state easily mistaken for illness or death. The animal will be curled up and feel cold and stiff, with a very slow respiratory rate and heart beat. Gradual warmth will revive the animal, but alternating periods of hibernation can cause adverse physiological effects.

Rabbits, guinea-pigs and chinchillas can be kept out of doors throughout the year as long as well-constructed hutches shield them from the prevailing wind and nesting compartments with plenty of nesting material are provided. The temperature in such nest-boxes should not fall below 16°C (60°F).

Mink and ferrets are well suited to outdoor cages and pens as long as such accommodation is well constructed and weatherproof. The quality of mink pelts will suffer if the animals are not housed outside in open-sided sheds.

### Feeding

Any veterinary establishment that is likely to keep any of these smaller pets for observation, or treatment, should be able to provide a suitable diet. Although pet-shops sell a variety of packaged foods, these are often of doubtful nutritional value. There are commercially prepared and standardized cubed diets available for laboratory animals, which are equally suitable for these domestic pets. Unfortunately these diets are usually sold in 25 kg bags, which may be more diet cubes than are needed to feed a few animals at a time, and could prove an expensive and wasteful purchase. They are available from the usual animal foodstuff compounders.

## Diet A

*For rats and mice*, a specific formula cubed diet is the only source of food necessary. These are based on cereals such as wheat, barley, maize and oats, with added skim milk, fish-meal, bone-flour and soya bean, to a balanced formula, and may be supplemented with vitamins and mineral supplements. Protein levels vary from about 10% for stock animals, to about 22% for breeding animals. If this diet is not available, a suitable substitute can be made by using a mixture of clean broken whole grains, like wheat, barley or oats, and broad bran. This can be fed damp to avoid dust, but must be offered freshly mixed, as a moist feed "sours" quickly. This feed can be supplemented with clean chopped fresh raw greens and carrots.

## Diet B

*For the remainder of small rodents*, the basic ration can consist of mouse and rat cubes supplemented with green food, roots and possibly sunflower seed. Lemmings and gerbils will probably completely satisfy their water requirements from these fresh vegetables. Again, if the cubes are not available, a broken grain and broad bran mixture can be used, as for rats and mice, but with the suggested supplements. Great care must be taken with Syrian (golden) hamsters, as the mucous membranes of their cheek pouches can be damaged by sharp grains like whole oats.

## Diet C

*The basic diet of rabbits, guinea-pigs and chinchillas* is best supplied by a specific formula pelleted diet. These have similar ingredients to those prepared for rats and mice, but are based on grass-meal, and are smaller and green compared with the firmer brown cubes of the rat and mouse diets. The protein levels vary from about 10% to 20% according to whether they are for stock or breeding animals. A specific pelleted diet is prepared for guinea-pigs, which safely combines vitamin C, although it is advisable not to store it for longer than about a month after production. This pellet will be a little more expensive than the standard rabbit pellet, although it can be fed quite safely to rabbits. Again, if the pellets are not available, a broken grain and broad bran mixture can be used, as for rats and mice, but such a diet for guinea-pigs must be supplemented with fresh raw green food, or other source of Vitamin C. An extra source of roughage in the form of good quality hay, is very important in the diet for all three species, and they all enjoy fresh green food and carrots.

## Diet D

*Ferrets and mink* are carnivores, and their staple diet is usually fresh meat and fish. Obviously, care must be taken when feeding raw meat to ensure that the diet is not deficient in vitamins or minerals, particularly calcium, and that feeding utensils are regularly cleaned. If such animals are kept under observation, it would be wise to find out what is normally fed to them.

## Emergency Feeding

The owner could be asked to provide some food for his/her pet. Puppy meal or crushed dog biscuits, crushed cereals, porridge oats, wholemeal brown bread, or baby foods like Farlene or Farex can be used. Ferrets can be offered tinned dog or cat food with brown bread, while guinea-pigs must have fresh green food.

## Sex Determination

It is usually relatively easy to determine the sex of adult animals with well-developed genitalia. Young animals, particularly just after weaning, when they are usually purchased, may provide more of a problem. In most species, one of the most useful criteria is a *comparison of the relative distance between the anus and the urogenital opening* which is greater in the male than in the female.

The scrotal sac is fairly obvious in hamsters, so that the females appear to have a more rounded rump than the males when viewed from a ventral surface. Mice and rats if frightened, often retract their testes, which may cause confusion when sexing these animals. The sex of young mice is determined by the distance between the urogenital opening and anus, and the shape of the urogenital opening, which tends to be rather cone-shaped in females and more spade-shaped or square

in males. Guinea-pigs can be rather difficult to sex, but the penis can be extruded by gentle pressure just anterior to the urogenital opening. This opening in the female has a distinctive Y-shape. Similarly, the penis of rabbits can be extruded, and the vulva is rather slit-shaped, with the labia extending backwards almost to the anus. In adult males, the testes are found either side of the prepuce.

Ferrets have a limited breeding season, and out of season the testes are retracted, and the penis tends to be small and situated rather anteriorly. During the breeding season, the vulval lips of the female become obviously enlarged and elongated, which on cursory examination could be mistaken for two scrotal sacs.

## Some Disease Considerations

It would be impossible, within the limits of a few pages, to summarize all the different diseases to which the animals listed in Table 3.1 are susceptible. Such detailed information can only be obtained from specialist publications. However, there are a few broad concepts which can be briefly discussed and are relevant to the nursing of such species.

Although every group of animals is susceptible to certain specific diseases— for instance, ectromelia or mouse pox only affects mice and myxomatosis is entirely confined to rabbits—rodents and lagomorphs can all be affected with conditions associated with their continually growing incisor teeth. Associated with either insufficient wear on these teeth, due to inadequate exercise or improper food, or to development defects, overgrown incisors and malocclusion defects are relatively common. Similarly, overgrown and distorted claws occur quite frequently, especially in rabbits.

Neoplasia is a relatively common condition of mice, but the type of tumour and the organ affected varies considerably amongst different strains. Rats are particularly susceptible to infectious respiratory disease which although probably is primarily of virus origin is always associated with mycoplasma infections. Rabbits, guinea-pig and chinchillas are particularly susceptible to pseudo-tuberculosis and bacterial respiratory conditions. Organisms associated with these latter respiratory infections include species of *Pasteurella*, *Bordetella* and pneumococci. Although intestinal coccidiosis can affect some of these smaller pets, it can be a particular problem in rabbits which can frequently be affected by a variety of enteric disorders. The soiled perineum, which can result from such diseases or following back injuries from incorrect handling, can be a major problem if the region is not cleaned and treated properly. Flagellates can also cause enteric syndromes in most species, and chinchillas are particularly susceptible to infection with *Giardia* species. Although ectoparasites frequently infect most of these species, the main problem seen clinically will be ear mange of the rabbit.

Both ferrets and mink are highly susceptible to the canine distemper/hard pad complex, and mink are also susceptible to infectious feline viral enteritis (panleucopenia). Great care must therefore be taken to separate such animals from cats and dogs, if being kept in hospital for treatment and observation.

## Recommended Reading

These books all give valuable information on the smaller mammals discussed in Chapter 3:

Buckland, M.D., Hall, L., Mowlem, A. and Whatley, B.F. (1981). *A Guide to Laboratory Animal Technology*. William Heinemann.

Cooper, J.E. (1982). Dealing with non-domesticated species. In *BSAVA Manual of Practice Improvement* edited by P.D. Fry, BSAVA London.

Flecknell, P. (1983). Restraint, anaesthesia and treatment of children's pets. In *Practice* **4**, 85–95.

Inglis, J.K. (1980). *Introduction to Laboratory Animal Science and Technology*. Pergamon Press.

Short, D.J. and Woodnott, D.P. (1969). (Editors) *The IAT Manual of Laboratory Animal Practice and Techniques*. Crosby Lockwood.

Universities Federation for Animal Welfare (1976). *The UFAW Handbook on the Care and Management of Laboratory Animals*. 5th edition. Churchill Livingstone.

(d) Cage Birds

A. T. B. EDNEY

## Introduction

Although small animal veterinary practice is concerned mainly with the treatment of dogs and cats, attention to cage birds makes up a large proportion of the rest of the work of small animal clinicians. Budgerigars, even though they are declining in numbers as household pets, are still the commonest animal which is not a dog or cat presented in small animal practice.

Of the many thousands of avian species in the world, a wide variety are kept as household pets. A good many, if not most of these species, are only free living in other countries, that is they are exotic species.

Types of birds differ from each other just as much as mammalian species vary. Budgerigars are as different from canaries as cats are from dogs.

The majority of cage birds seen by veterinary surgeons are seed eating such as budgerigars and canaries, which normally live on canary seed mixtures.

## General Characteristics of Birds

Birds are more closely related to reptiles than to mammals. Their most obvious characteristic is that they have a covering of feathers modified for flight on most of their body instead of a covering of hair.

In addition to flight feathers those on the body provide insulation which helps to maintain a relatively high body temperature. Budgerigars and canaries normally have a body temperature of about 40°–42°C; some small finches have an even higher temperature in the region of 45°C.

Although birds have no sweat glands there is a **preen** or **uropygial gland** present at the base of the tail. This organ produces the oily secretion used by the bird when preening its feathers.

The beaks of cage birds are modified to adapt to their feeding requirements. Both budgerigars and canaries have to dehusk seed before eating it and have a hard beak usually for this purpose.

The legs of most cage bird species do not have feathers but have a covering of scales. These extend to the toes which are modified to grip the perch. Budgerigars and canaries have three toes to the front and one to the rear. Each has a well-developed claw.

The bones of birds are very light and fragile. The long bones contain air in the cavities which communicate with the respiratory tract. The sternum is enlarged to provide an attachment for the massive muscles used in flight. The extension of the sternum makes abdominal palpation more difficult in birds than most mammals. As birds have no diaphragm, the thoracic and abdominal cavities are not separated. Not only does this affect the signs of disease but is an important

The editor acknowledges the work of D. K. Blackmore who supplied information on Cage Birds and Smaller Mammals in the 2nd Edition (1971).

consideration when handling. Birds can easily die if undue pressure is applied around the body.

Birds breathe through their nostrils or **nares** at the base of the beak. Budgerigars have a fleshy unfeathered structure called the **cere** at the base of the upper mandible. The trachea is similar to that found in mammals but the source of the birds "voice" is the **syrinx** at the lower end of the thorax.

The lungs are small structures close to the vertebral column. The bronchi divide to form an interconnecting series of airways with the air sacs. These are paired structures in the abdomen and thorax. They connect with the air spaces in the long bones in the lower cervical region and within the sternum to increase the oxygen uptake capacity.

The respiratory rate of birds is very much more rapid than in mammals. This is consistent with a higher metabolic rate. In budgerigars the respiratory rate is of the order of 80/100 per minute, canaries vary around 96/144 ventilations per minute.

As in mammalian blood, the blood of birds contains eosinophils, basophils, lymphocytes and monocytes. Unlike mammals the red blood cells of birds have nuclei. There are other differences such as nucleated thrombocytes instead of platelets and cells known as heterophils instead of neurophils. The lymphatic system of birds is much more diffuse except for an accumulation of lymphoid tissue known as the **bursa of fabricius**. This is located around the cloaca, the common digestive and urogenital exit.

The avian digestive tract differs considerably from that of mammals. At the base of the oesophagus a dilation known as the **crop** acts as a storage organ for food. The true glandular stomach is known as the **proventriculus**. As birds do not have teeth, food has to be ground in a much larger muscular organ called the **gizzard**, which harbours grit to assist with the food grinding process. The intestine is relatively short and simple with a duodenum which encloses a pancreas and loops of ileum packed alongside the gizzard. The large intestine is short and opens into the **cloaca**.

The kidneys are in cavities close to the vertebral column. The urine produced is in the form of thick white material mostly made up of uric acid. Urine and faeces are voided together producing typical droppings which are a mixture of black and brown faecal material and white urine. There is no urinary bladder.

The paired testes are always intra-abdominal and are situated near the kidneys. In most hen birds only the left ovary is functional. This sheds ova into a single left oviduct, a complex glandular organ which produces egg white (albumin) and the shell of the egg. It opens on the dorsal surface of the cloaca near the openings of the ureters.

### Sexing and ageing

Male and female adults of some avian species such as Zebra Finches have distinct plumage so the sexes can be differentiated. In many other cases both sexes appear identical, as with canaries. Male budgerigars are easily distinguished by a blue colour to the cere at the base of the beak. Hen budgerigars have a brownish-red colour to this structure.

There is no reliable way of assessing the age of adult birds and it is very difficult to sex immature birds. The timing of feather development is reasonably consistent in budgerigars. The whole process begins around 12 days post-natally when the down feathers begin to cover the body and do so completely after 4 weeks.

Young budgerigars less than 10 weeks

old have horizontal lines of "nest feathers" running across their foreheads giving a barring effect. This gives the impression that the birds have larger darker eyes than adult birds. The "whites" of the eyes are only visible in adult birds.

### Feeding and Management

The most popular pet birds are not surprisingly those which require a simple regime of feeding and management. The psittacine group, which includes budgerigars, parrots and parakeets, is the most widely kept. The other main group kept is made up of passerine birds. These include canaries and finches—birds closely related to the house sparrow. Both groups are seed eaters and are therefore easy to feed on proprietary mixtures.

Budgerigars are normally fed a mixture of canary seed and millet. They also need a dietary source of iodine and this is included as iodised seed, given as a supplement in the form of an iodine nibble or as an addition to the drinking water.

Seed mixtures for canaries are usually made up as a blend such as canary, rape and niger seed and some millet.

Both budgerigars and canaries will eat small amounts of green food. This is best given as an occasional washed lettuce leaf hung in the cage. Both species may be kept occupied with a clean millet spray attached to the bars of the cage.

It is vital to provide grit for seed-eating birds. Most pet shops will provide mixed grit which has soluble and insoluble grit present. The soluble grit provides calcium, the insoluble grit contributes to the action of the gizzard. Pieces of cuttlefish bone are commonly put between the bars of cages for birds to exercise their beaks and act as a source of minerals. It is important to use only cuttlefish bone from a reliable pet

shop and not use pieces washed up on the beach.

A careful note should be kept on the normal feeding regime of any bird which is kept in for observation, as drastic deviations from what the bird is accustomed to may lead to refusal or digestive upsets. Owners should be encouraged to provide food the bird is used to. This is particularly important for the more exotic species, especially omnivorous varieties such as mynah birds and insectivorous or nectar feeders.

Unlike dogs and cats, seed-eating pet birds cannot survive for more than about 48 hours without food. Such birds normally take in around 25% of their body weight daily as food. A continual source of seed should always be available, and the husks which the bird removes should be blown away from the surface of the feeding pot every day so that the bird can reach the whole seed underneath. Birds have been known to starve because an owner thought that a bowl was full of seed when it only contained discarded husks. Dehusking birds such as budgerigars and canaries will not normally eat seed which has had the husk removed, even though it is otherwise wholesome. A medium sized, 45 g budgerigar will normally eat around 10 g of whole seed daily.

Fresh water should always be available for drinking. The standard "Flomatic" type containers can be used to provide water or as seed containers. Budgerigars normally drink about 2–5 ml water daily and canaries proportionately less. A calibrated water container is useful in a hospital cage so that the daily intake can be recorded. Birds with wet droppings or diarrhoea tend to drink much more water to compensate for fluid loss.

Budgerigars or canaries and many other birds admitted for observation and treatment may be kept in a conventional budgerigar breeding cage which is essentially an open-fronted box measuring approximately 60 cm long, 30 cm high and 25 cm deep with a wide front with a wide door and a tray for droppings. The use of a semi-enclosed type of cage helps to prevent birds from becoming frightened by the other activities going on around them.

Large psittacine birds such as parrots continually make use of their powerful beaks and need large robust cages with strongly constructed bars and perches.

All cages should be fitted with perches with enough distance between them to allow flight. The perches should be of sufficient diameter to allow a comfortable grip with the toes and claws without excessive contraction or spreading. It is an advantage to have perches which are ovoid in section rather than round.

A hospital cage is essential if birds are to be admitted regularly. Proprietary cages are available which have thermostatically controlled heating, but it is not difficult to build a cage with a light bulb wired up below it to provide local heat.

It is necessary to have a thermometer incorporated into the cage to achieve the optimum ambient temperature. This is usually around 30°–38°C. Birds which are "fluffed-up" in appearance usually need a higher ambient temperature. A bird which is too hot usually keeps its feathers close to its body, in which case a slightly lower temperature should be aimed for.

Putting "fluffed-up" birds into a relatively high ambient temperature can often get them eating again when they have been off their food. It may be necessary to spread some seed on the floor of the cage as well as in the seed bowls to give the maximum opportunity for the bird to eat.

A bird which is not eating needs energy urgently and should be given 5% dextrose solution by mouth at the rate of 1 ml per half hour.

## Handling Birds

Before any attempt is made to handle cage birds, all doors, windows and any other escape routes must be secure. Fires and fireplaces must be covered and any other hazards removed.

It is much easier to catch a bird in a cage if all the perches and accessories are removed first. Not only does this make it easier to manoeuvre but reduces the chances of the bird injuring itself on the obstructions. Birds must be grasped firmly but gently enveloping the bird to immobilize the wings. Great care must be taken to avoid putting any pressure on the bird's body which can result in shock, cardiac or respiratory arrest (Fig. 3.24).

Most birds will not normally move in the dark and can more easily be caught if the lights in the room are turned off or if the cage is taken into a darkened area such as a large cupboard. Small birds should not be handled any more than is absolutely necessary. A small dark cloth bag with a draw-string can be used if a small bird has to be kept out of a cage for a long period. It will remain quiet and can be easily caught without the undue stress of being continuously handled. Birds may be weighed on a sensitive balance while in such a bag or while rolled up in a paper towel or cloth.

Large psittacines such as parrots can inflict quite severe injuries if badly handled. Even budgerigars, especially hen birds, can give quite a painful nip. Most small finches cause little damage to handlers. If smaller birds are held in the palm of the hand with the head between the thumb and forefinger, bites can usually be avoided. It is useful to have someone to help by offering an inert object such as a pen top for the bird to attack if it proves too lively. Leather gauntlets may be needed to handle large birds, although they tend to restrict the handler's movement.

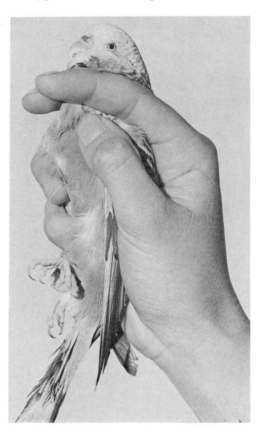

Fig. 3.24.    Holding a budgerigar for examination.

If done carefully and quickly it is often easier to drop a sizeable (say bath size) towel over the bird and grasp the back of its neck with one hand and support the body with the other. Great care must be taken to avoid injuring the bird during this procedure.

In spite of all precautions taken, birds will sometimes escape and have to be caught while flying free in the room. A large net with a padded rim is invaluable for this eventuality.

### Administration of Medicines

**By mouth**

The method of oral dosage depends very much on the type of bird concerned, its food and water requirements and the effect any drug might have on palatability. With larger birds administration of drugs by way of drinking water is only really satisfactory and an accurate dosage achieved if the daily water intake is known.

Pet budgerigars in cages drink about 2–5 ml of water daily; even this may vary considerably. Medicaments in water may be rejected, and as seed is always de-husked, medicine mixed with the seed may be discarded.

Frequently birds require medication when the crop is almost empty, which makes direct injection into the crop difficult. In such cases, **medicaments can be**

**given via a tube** that can be passed from the pharynx directly into the crop. In small birds the beak can be held open by a pair of forceps used as a gag. In the case of budgerigars and other small parakeets, a small blob of solder on the lower arm of the forceps, which fits the concavity of the lower mandible, prevents the gag from slipping out of position. A length of narrowgauge polythene tube with one end pushed over a 15-gauge hypodermic needle with its point removed can now easily be passed into the crop by pushing it over the back of the tongue in a slightly oblique direction from the left to the right of the bird's pharynx. The other end of the tube can now be attached to a syringe by means of the needle, and, in the case of the budgerigar, up to 1 ml of solution injected. A very similar technique can be used for birds as large as a macaw, but using a more robust gag. The ideal instrument for such purposes can be made from a tapered metal rod approximately 23 cm in length, 2 cm in diameter at its thickest point, with a horizontal slit through its length, and a handle at one end (p. 212).

If one of the larger psittacines is approached, it will almost invariably bite the rod at a point dependent on the size of its open mandibles. As soon as the rod has been grasped by the bird, it can be held firmly in place and rotated until a tube can be passed through the slit into the bird's oesophagus in a similar manner to that already described.

## Injections

1. *Subcutaneous.* Subcutaneous injections may be given on the side of the chest, under the wing, or on the dorsal surface of the neck. Care must be taken to ensure the tip of the needle is directed downwards and away from the actual site of the injection in order to prevent seepage from the puncture wound in the rather inelastic avian skin. Up to 1 ml of fluid may be given to the smaller species by this method.

2. *Intraperitoneal injection.* When administering an intraperitoneal injection to a bird, care must be taken not to enter the abdominal air sacs. A short needle should be used and inserted in the midline in the posterior part of the abdomen.

3. *Intramuscular injection.* Intramuscular injections are best made directly into the pectoral muscles, but the plunger of the syringe should be slightly withdrawn before administration of the drug to ensure that a blood-vessel plexus, which occurs in this region, has not been advertently penetrated.

4. *Intravenous injection.* In larger birds the median vein under the wing on the ventral aspect of the humero-radial joint is probably the most accessible point for an intravenous injection. In smaller birds the right jugular vein, approached from the dorsal surface of the neck, is more suitable. Both techniques are facilitated by plucking away the feathers overlying the point of injection. The veins of smaller birds are rather fragile, and a serious haematoma or subcutaneous haemorrhage can occur unless great care is taken.

## Dressings and Limb Immobilization

It is quite common for birds to break the long bones in the leg, the tarsometatarsus, the lower long bone or the tibiotarsus, the long bone just below the femur. This is usually the result of being shut in a door, the cage collapsing or being tipped over. Occasionally the leg may be broken by clumsy handling or even by the bird catching its claws in something unyielding.

It is possible to put an intramedullary pin into a broken tarso-metatarsus of a large bird. Smaller birds need the fracture immobilized with adhesive or cellulose ("Sellotape") tape.

Wing fractures result from similar trauma, particularly flight accidents.

Fractures of the leg may be immobilized with adhesive tape. The limb may be fixed between two squares of tape if the fracture is in the mid-shaft. If the joint needs to be included in the tape applied, the leg must be flexed at as natural an angle as possible.

When taping the wings to the body to immobilize fractures of the humerus or radio-ulna, care must be taken to fix the wings in as near to the natural rest position as possible. A piece of tape is laid down the back of the bird with a broken wing. This is covered at the forward end by an encircling tape placed around the wing tips, fairly well forward. A second circle of tape needs to be placed at the wing tips over the tape running along the back. This arrangement of adhesive tapes allows the bird to balance more effectively.

As budgerigars normally weigh between 35 g and 65 g and canaries considerably less than 50 g any dressings or immobilizing material needs to be light enough for the bird to be able to move around, balance and feed. Cellulose tape is suitable for most cases.

For fractures in birds of 100 g or more such as parrots, large parakeets and mynah birds, other splinting materials such as split matchsticks, a quill or even fine gauge wire may be incorporated into a dressing.

With the exception of psittacine birds, that is parrots, parakeets and budgerigars, birds do not normally interfere unduly with dressings. Psittacines may need to be controlled by applying an "Elizabethan collar" arrangement which can be cut out of thin card cut to size and stapled or stuck together with cellulose tape around the neck. An old playing card is ideal for the purpose. A disc 5–8 cm across is cut out with a central aperture for the neck about 1 cm across. The top of a small plastic detergent bottle serves the same purpose for larger birds, although a leather collar may have to be made for large parrots or macaws.

If skin lacerations are present or surgery is being carried out, feathers around the site should be plucked out rather than clipped or shaved. Feathers normally take 5–6 weeks to grow again after removal. The area can be cleaned and antiseptic solution applied as with mammalian skin.

Haemorrhage is much more critical in birds than with mammals. Birds can only afford to lose a small percentage of their circulating blood before it becomes a serious life-threatening situation. Bleeding from the beak or claws are common occurrences and can be controlled by applying cotton wool soaked in cold water and then dipped in potassium permanganate crystals. The wet crystals are applied with gentle pressure to the bleeding points for a minute or so.

### Surgery and Anaesthesia

Great care must be taken to avoid dangerous heat loss during operative procedure. Some restraint is necessary for most surgery. This can be improvised with adhesive tape, surgical gauze such as "Tubegauz" (Scholl) or with aluminium foil used in cookery ("Bacofoil"). Considerable care is needed to adjust the restraint so that it eliminates movement during surgery but does not suffocate the bird.

Birds which are to be anaesthetized should have food withheld for 2–3 hours, but *not* for more than 12 hours.

The majority of anaesthetic techniques

used in mammals are applicable to birds. Anaesthetic failures are usually associated with heat or blood loss, with excessive excitement prior to induction of anaesthetic, prolonged abnormal postures, particularly those involving extreme abduction of the limbs, a sudden drop in intra-abdominal pressure (such as that associated with removal of a tumour), or the inadvertent introduction of fluid into the air sac.

*Local anaesthetic* should only be considered for large birds or any which are very bad general anaesthetic risks. Procaine derivatives are contraindicated as they are as toxic to many birds as they are to small mammals. Ethyl chloride can be used as a spray for minor interferences of short duration.

Fortunately, the skin on much of the bird's body is poorly equipped with pain receptors, and so many suturing operations can be done without anaesthesia.

*General anaesthesia*—most inhalation anaesthetics used in small animal practice can be applied to birds. Methods range from using a cotton wool pad soaked in ether in a loose-fitting mask, to intubation of large birds using halothane ("Fluothane", ICI).

As the tidal volume of most birds is very small, open-circuit methods are used with volatile anaesthetics.

For small birds the end of the thick corrugated tubing from the anaesthetic apparatus is large enough to act as a mask. Masks of all sizes can be improvised by cutting down old plastic syringe cases of various sizes or fitting a surgical glove over a small mask and cutting a suitable hole for the bird's head.

*Parenteral anaesthetics*—in recent years injectable anaesthetics have become more popular with small animal clinicians dealing with birds. The steroid anaesthetic CT1341 ("Saffan", Glaxovet) has been found to be an effective agent for most birds, particularly budgerigars. Birds of prey may also be anaesthetized successfully with this drug although adverse effects have been observed in a red-tailed hawk.

Birds may be given a dose calculated on the basis of 10 mg/kg body weight which normally means that a budgerigar would receive 0.10–0.12 ml by the intraperitoneal or intramuscular route.

On the other non-volatile anaesthetic agents, sodium pentobarbitone is the most widely used. This is normally given at the rate of 0.05 mg/g body weight (i.e. 5 mg/kg) by intramuscular, intraperitoneal, or the intravenous route in larger quantities.

Some avian anaesthetists favour the use of of a mixture of sodium pentobarbitone, magnesium sulphate and chloral hydrate ("Equithesin-Jensen"), by intramuscular injection.

## The Nursing of Wild Birds

Most small animal practices are presented with injured or orphaned wild birds* at fairly frequent intervals. Although the same principles apply as for cage birds, special considerations are needed for wild birds. They should be handled as little as possible and must not be subjected to bright light since they are more sensitive to noise and human activity generally than domestic animals. Wild birds usually attract a good deal of attention and stimulate interest within the practice with clients. It is important that the temptation to exhibit the bird is firmly

*An excellent leaflet on the "Treatment of sick, orphaned and injured birds" is obtainable by sending a large stamped self-addressed envelope (preferably with a donation) to the Royal Society for the Protection of Birds, The Lodge, Sandy, Bedfordshire, United Kingdom.

resisted and that it is taken away to some quiet corner with subdued light which it can treat more as a refuge than where there are barking dogs and threatening cats.

The first point with orphan birds for the RANA is to establish if they really have been abandoned or their parents are dead. Many birds which are said to have "fallen from the nest" are still being fed by their parents in the normal course of events. These are normally feathered, i.e. fledglings.

Truly orphaned birds are a real challenge to rear. They need very frequent feeding if they are to survive. If the bird is not fully feathered it will lose heat very rapidly if not kept well insulated or on a heated pad at around 30–35°C. The hospital cage previously described is also a useful way of achieving these conditions.

Part of the cage should be covered with a piece of cardboard or similar material to allow the bird to hide away. It is very stressful for birds to be exposed to watchful eyes.

Nestling birds may be fed with a small spatula which can be used to place food in the mouth. Most small birds thrive well on a fairly thick solution of a complete canned dog food (i.e. one of high energy concentration; see manufacturer's product data sheet) made up with a small amount of water to the consistency of a very thick mousse. Birds are much less likely to take food which is too liquid, and inhalation accidents may cause death. The food must be given warm and to begin with it may be necessary to prise open the beak. Once birds associate human presence with food they will exhibit the strong gaping reflex seen in the wild.

Birds must be fed every 2 hours up until late evening and again early in the morning. Between these times they need to be kept in the dark.

**Oiled birds**

Considerable effort has been put into the investigation of the management of sea birds fouled with oil. As more facts accumulate, expert opinion changes.

Space does not allow a detailed description of current thinking on the subject but the main points may be summarized as:

1. All oiled or otherwise injured birds are in a state of shock and need to be approached slowly and handled very carefully.
2. Casualties on the shore should be approached from the seaward direction if possible. They should not be chased. A large (60 cm) net is very useful for catching injured sea birds.
3. Cleaning and rehabilitation should be confined to individuals that are otherwise in good condition, with normal bodyweight and have a bright, alert appearance.
4. Birds that are thin, very dull or have been heavily contaminated internally or externally, are almost certainly better off humanely destroyed.
5. Some species such as geese, surface feeding duck, cormorants and swans are more likely to survive than divers, grebes, sea duck or waders.
6. Sea birds that have been in captivity for 3 weeks or more, are less likely to survive in the wild again.
7. Most oiled birds have some degree of enteritis. Treatment with a kaolin or similar preparation should begin as soon as practicable.
8. All oiled birds should be fed appropriate food e.g. sprats or filleted white fish for sea birds, starter chicken pellets for water fowl.
9. A consistent room temperature of 20°–24°C should be maintained and the bird kept in suitable housing which is draught free. Newspaper or

clean rags, if changed frequently is suitable bedding. Access to small amounts of clean sand, gravel or grit is needed and a few stones provided for perching.

Drinking vessels should not be large enough for the bird to get into and adequate opportunities must be given for the bird to bath itself.

10. A solution of mild washing-up liquid, 100 mls in a gallon of warm (40°C) water is useful to remove oil. The bird's beak should be taped or immobilized with an elastic band, but this must be removed immediately afterwards. All the fluid must be rinsed out with warm water afterwards.

11. Birds should not be released until the plumage is water repellent again. This normally takes 2–3 weeks. Treated birds should be returned to an appropriate location. Near to where they were found if it is not polluted.

Further information is available from the Royal Society for the Protection of Birds, The Lodge, Sandy, Bedfordshire, SG19 2DL, United Kingdom.

An excellent leaflet on the *Care and Handling of Oiled Birds* is obtainable from the RSPCA Wildlife Unit, The Causeway, Horsham, Sussex, RH12 1HG, United Kingdom. Please send a stamped addressed envelope.

Where *large numbers of sea birds have been contaminated with oil* the Oiled Bird Cleaning Unit, Little Creech, Somerset, United Kingdom should be contacted as soon as possible for advice.

## General Points in Summary

A healthy bird usually has sleek plumage, appears bright and alert, and holds its wings close to its body. It will eat regularly and readily. Its droppings normally consist of a black/brown faecal part and a white semi-solid urinary part. Any obvious deviation from the characteristics listed will lead to suspicion of some ailment being the cause. Normal periods of moult will, however, result in the plumage being less sleek and rather threadbare for a few weeks.

An important point about cage birds is their ability to hide illness in the way often seen in zoo animals. That is they make efforts to appear less vulnerable than they really are when ill. This usually means that when birds are presented for attention they are at a more advanced stage of any illness than most dogs and cats would be.

Although many cage birds can be trained to be "finger tame" they cannot tolerate physical contact in the way dogs and cats put up with and mostly enjoy.

Infectious disease is less common in individually housed pet birds than with groups kept in aviaries, particularly where they have contact with wild species.

Budgerigars are remarkably resistant to infectious diseases. Because of this and their general hardiness they survive on average for around 6–7 years.

## (e) Management and Hygiene of Kennels and Catteries

### H. BRIGGS

### Kennel and Cattery Construction

When you are considering the construction of either kennels or catteries there are several basic points to bear in mind affecting both the animals that have to occupy them and the personnel who are responsible for them and for the running of them.

Basically, all kennels and catteries have to have the same requirements, but those used for special purposes, e.g. quarantine, hospitalization, etc., in addition need to incorporate special features. The basic requirements as far as the animals are concerned are to provide warm, comfortable and hygienic accommodation where they can be kept often for long periods of time. As regards the requirements for the personnel responsible, in addition to the above type of accommodation for the animals they require the kennels and catteries to be escape-proof, designed to be easily maintained and cleaned so as to prevent as far as possible disease problems and to be able to be built and run economically.

If new kennels and catteries are to be built in the United Kingdom, before construction can actually begin permission has to be obtained from the local authority, as this body acts as the planning authority for the control and development of land under the Town and Country Planning Act 1971.

Where kennels and catteries are to be used for specific purposes, they will have to conform to standards specified in such laws as the Rabies Act 1974, the Animal Boarding Establishment Act 1963 and the Breeding of Dogs Act 1973.

The regulations and legal requirements for the construction of quarantine kennels are very strict and very definite, and are designed to achieve the ideal accommodation to prevent the dissemination of disease. If this type of accommodation is considered first, it can be used as the general pattern for all other types with modifications incorporated for specific purposes.

Great Britain and Eire are free of Rabies at the present time and a policy of 6 months' quarantine of pet animals imported to the countries is rigidly enforced.

### Quarantine Kennels

The legal requirements relating to the owning and management of this type of kennel need not be gone into in detail. All dogs and cats entering the United Kingdom have to be held for 6 calendar months in official accommodation, which is under the daily supervision of a veterinary surgeon; and the accommodation must be constructed so that escape is impossible, and that no nose or paw contact is possible between two or more animals at any time, except where the animals are in the same unit.

Only animals entering quarantine at the same time and in the same ownership are allowed to share a unit, and that is subject to the agreement of the veterinary super-intendent. A maximum of 3 animals are allowed to share a unit, and they must be of the same species, i.e. dogs or cats. Suitable alternative accommodation must always be available, however, so that animals can be separated if it becomes necessary. Premises should be built in small self-contained groups of units so as to minimize the spread of disease. Special restrictions, in the event of a rabies outbreak or outbreak of other less serious infectious disease are easier in small units.

## Design and construction of quarantine units

The following are some of the require-ments needed.

1. *Every animal* must have accommo-dation designed so that it has direct access to **an individual run**. Communal exercise runs are no longer allowed.

2. *The minimum sizes* of accommoda-tion required for various sized dogs is shown in Table 3.2.

For cats the sleeping compartment plus exercise area must have a total minimum floor area of 1.4 m². The width and length of either must not be less than 0.9 m.

3. *Some form of sleeping bed or bench,* must be provided, for each animal.

4. *Partitions and walls* of both sleeping compartments and exercise runs must extend from the floor level to the roof.

5. *All entrances* to a block or section of units must have double doors. These must open inwards and be self-closing, and thus will be an additional measure against escape. Further to this, the exterior doors must open inwards, but it is still permis-sible for the doors of individual compart-ments to open outwards. All the doors and gates of the premises must be fitted with locks and the premises must always be kept locked when there are no staff on duty. Under no circumstances may the premises have more than two entrance gates, and whilst visitors are on the premises one of these gates must be kept locked, and someone must be on duty the whole time at the other. At least one of the entrances must be large enough to enable a vehicle to enter the quarantine area, as loading and unloading of animals must take place within the premises with the gates locked.

6. *All premises must have a surrounding fence* or wall which will prevent the escape of the dogs or cats in quarantine; it will also prevent other animals from gaining access to the quarantine area. This fence or wall must be a minimum height of 1.8 m. If it is less than 3 m high it must have

TABLE 3.2

| Accommodation areas | Small dog 11.3 kg body weight | Medium-sized dog 11.3–29.5 kg body weight | Large dog 29.5 kg body weight |
|---|---|---|---|
| Sleeping compartment | Not less than 1.1 m² | Not less than 1.5 m² | Not less than 1.5 m² |
| Width and length | Not less than 0.9 m | Not less than 1.2 m | Not less than 1.2 m |
| Adjoining exercise run | Not less than 3.7 m² | Not less than 5.6 m² | Not less than 7.4 m² |
| Width | Not less than 0.9 m | Not less than 1.2 m | Not less than 1.2 m |
| Height of unit | Not less than 1.8 m | Not less than 1.8 m | Not less than 1.8 m |

an additional security feature, namely a wire netting guard 0.6 m wide securely fitted to the top and set at an inward and upward angle of 45 degrees. In addition, the base of the fence must be secure against the escape of animals by digging and there should be a minimum distance of 1.22 m between this fence and any buildings within the compound. In winter, snow, and during the rest of the year, any other materials, must not be allowed to accumulate against the wall or fence or on the wire guard so as to weaken, lower or damage it.

7. *Washing facilities* and suitable protective clothing for all the staff must be provided so that proper disinfection can take place before they leave the premises.

8. *Suitable building materials must be used in construction.*

Obviously all buildings, partitions and fences must be well built and well maintained and, in addition, they must be built of materials approved by the licensing authority.

External walls of compartments are best built of a cavity brickwork, i.e. two rows of bricks with a cavity between them. Apart from security, this cavity is important when heating is being considered, as it helps in insulation and thus in the prevention of heat loss from the building. Concrete or concrete blocks are also suitable, but wood must not be used for walls, floors, partitions and doors of sleeping compartments under any circumstance unless it is covered with a durable, smooth and impervious material. The reasons for this are that it is easily chewed, therefore not escape-proof. The crevices in it are ideal sites for fleas to lay their eggs and it is a material which cannot be adequately disinfected. The interior surfaces of the walls of the sleeping compartments must be covered with a smooth, hard, impervious material to a height of not less than 1.22 m. Usually these requirements are met by plastering the walls with a sand cement skin and then painting over this, but other materials, e.g. stainless steel, aluminium sheeting or some form of laminated plastic finish, e.g. "Formica", can be used.

Most people agree that dogs in quarantine are more contented when they can see what is going on around them, and this must be borne in mind in any building programme. It is legally required that for small and medium-sized dogs the first 0.457 m, and for large dogs the first 0.609 m of height of the partitions of exercise runs, must be of a smooth, hard, impervious material, and here, again, metal concrete and brick are considered suitable. Above these heights it is suggested that see-through materials which are nose- and paw-proof are better than solid ones. For this reason if the upper section is made of wire, and this is allowed, it must be a double fence with a space between the two parts which will thus ensure that two animals in adjoining runs cannot make contact with each other.

The regulations for cat accommodation are slightly different. Here the walls of compartments, and where there are outside runs, the dividing partitions of adjoining runs must be constructed from a solid material for the entire height. Under circumstances where wire-mesh could be used, the size of the mesh must not be greater than 2.5 cm$^2$ and not less than 165 WG.

9. *The surface of exercise runs* should be impervious and constructed so that adequate drainage is provided and in such a way to ensure that urine is prevented from passing from one run to another. The drainage system will have to be approved by the local authority, and will have to be rodent proof also. Although owners often complain about not having (and occupants would probably prefer) grass runs, these are usually not considered suitable

as they soon become unsatisfactory through constant use or in wet weather. If such a grass run is approved and its surface then deteriorates, the authorized use of the run, as well as the sleeping compartment, would be suspended until the condition again becomes satisfactory.

**General management of quarantine premises**

1. *All staff must be instructed* on the dangers of rabies to themselves, the seriousness of the situation if the disease entered the United Kingdom, and on the precautions to be taken to prevent possible cross-infection between the animals.

2. *The quarantine premises must be run as a completely separate unit* where the owners of quarantine kennels also keep non-imported animals, e.g. boarding, breeding or hospitalization cases on the same site.

3. *Fire hazard.* Proper provision must be made for the protection and security of the animals, and there should be easy access to fire-fighting equipment, e.g. fire extinguishers, fire blankets, etc. In addition other precautions should be taken to prevent fires. Care should be taken in the storage of bedding and newspaper because of the risk of spontaneous combustion. All electrical cables should be protected and switches boxed in. No smoking should be allowed at any time in any part of the premises by anyone.

4. *Animals have to be vaccinated against rabies at the owner's expense.* Depending on the vaccine used, this consists of one or two doses. The initial dose should be given on the day of arrival, and if the two dose course is used, the second, 28 days later. The full course of vaccination, as given in the manufacturer's instructions, should be carried out. If for any reason postponement of vaccination has to take place, e.g.

because the animal is ill, permission for this has to be obtained from a divisional veterinary officer of the Ministry of Agriculture, Fisheries and Food. Vaccination must be carried out by the veterinary surgeon in charge. Under no circumstances can he delegate this to nongraduate staff, and if for some reason a deputy is required for him, this must be another veterinary surgeon.

5. *An animal must be kept to one unit* throughout its stay in the premises unless for some reason the veterinary surgeon in charge first gives permission for its move to another.

6. (a) *All occupants of units must be clearly identified* by cards on the unit giving a brief description of the animal, its import licence number, the country from which it has come and the date of its arrival in the United Kingdom. (b) If the veterinary surgeon in charge has authorized the movement of an animal from one unit to another, a record must be kept of this movement, and must be kept until 12 months after the animal has been released from quarantine. (c) A detailed case history must be kept of each animal in quarantine and this must be kept for 12 months after the animal has been released from quarantine. The details in it should include a full description of the animal and dates of vaccination. Further details regarding the name of the vaccine used and its batch number must also be recorded. Any illnesses, treatments, or incidents in which the animal is concerned at any time during the period it is in quarantine must be recorded, however trivial or minor they may seem at the time. The entries must be made immediately and the record cards kept up to date at all times. They have to be available also for inspection by any authorized person at any time.

7. *Cleanliness of kennels and exercise areas is important.* The veterinary surgeon will advise on a suitable disinfectant, and

this product, and no other, must always be used. It is also important that it is used exactly as instructed, as contrary to popular belief the efficiency is not increased with the concentration beyond a certain maximum. It is also essential that the floors of units and passageways must be kept clean, as dry as possible and free from vermin at all times. The veterinary surgeon will also probably remind staff from time to time that no disinfectant can be fully effective unless the area is thoroughly cleaned before it is used.

Food preparation rooms and all utensils used should always be kept in a clean and hygienic condition and should be disinfected each day. Bedding must also be kept in a clean and hygienic condition. If owners provide proprietary beds, blankets or cushions, or, if they are provided by the management, they should be allocated to that one animal for the whole period it is in quarantine. It is preferable then to dispose of them, ideally by burning, but if they are to be released with the animal, they must be thoroughly cleansed and disinfected before they are released. An incinerator, or some other means, which is acceptable as satisfactory by the authorizing authority, must be available for the disposal of faeces, carcasses, clippings, uneaten food and other waste.

8. *A visitor may only visit his own animal.* For the first 14 days after its first rabies vaccination, i.e. the first 2 weeks the arrival is in quarantine, it cannot have visitors unless there is some specific reason which the veterinary surgeon in charge feels necessitates it. If this occurs he will obtain special authorization for visitors from the Ministry of Agriculture, Fisheries and Food. An animal can only be visited in its own unit or exercise run. At all times the visitors must be attended by the veterinary surgeon or a representative for him whom he has authorized previously; unless, as often happens, the visitors

request, or agree to, being locked in with their animal. If this happens, the key is kept by a member of the staff of the premises, and an agreement reached as to the length of the visiting period. An official book must always be available and must be signed by the visitor on each of his visits. In addition to his signature, his address must be recorded and also the date of the visit. Rules regarding visitors should be given to each visitor on his first visit and in addition should be prominently displayed on the actual premises.

9. *Animals must be transported* by an authorized carrying agent from either the airport or dock, and only certain companies are authorized for importing of animals to the quarantine area. This must be in a special vehicle and container which has previously been inspected by and then approved by the authorizing authority.

## Hospital kennels

Here the requirements are somewhat different to those for quarantine kennels because the animals are usually ill and are being kept confined for only short periods of time until they are well enough to return home.

The same basic principles apply, but, in addition, methods for providing supplementary heat to individual animals and for the administration of special treatments may be required.

It is an advantage to have an oxygen kennel, which can be useful for so many types of case and is easy to construct, as all that is required is a cage which is airtight, has a supply of oxygen to the interior, and the front either being of glass or some form of viewing panel being provided.

A **whelping kennel** also is useful and can be used for other purposes with the whelping box removed when not in use for the purpose for which it is designed, e.g. hospitalization of giant breeds. The whelping kennel should have a viewing panel where an attendant can observe the animal without her realizing that she is being watched, and have a removable roof so that the animal can be approached from above or for an infra-red lamp to be provided for supplementary heating.

Metabolic Cages are being introduced into some veterinary hospitals nowadays. They are necessary if e.g. accurate measurement is required of urine passed over a given period of time. For reasons relating to their use they have to be smaller and less comfortable than ordinary hospital kennels. For this reason patients are only kept in them for the minimum amount of time that is required for the tests to be carried out. If they are only to be used for very simple metabolic tests as given in the example above a monitoring cage can be made in the practice from an ordinary hospital cage by inserting a wire mesh floor with catchment tray underneath.

Basically, in a hospital a number of small wards are preferable to one large one, and they should be located as near the operating theatre as possible and, conversely, be as far away from the reception and examination or consulting rooms as possible.

A small **isolation ward** is essential in all hospitals for the use of an animal which develops clinical signs of an infective disease, e.g. canine distemper whilst being hospitalized for another purpose. This isolation ward should be completely self-contained. On some occasions, however, it is more practical to make one small ward an isolation area if a disease problem occurs there than to move animals out. This is, however, a controversial point and depends on both individual situations and personnel. Each ward or kennel area

should in addition to having accommodation for the patients have also an examination table, sink unit and storage space.

Cages should be on one side only of the ward in an attempt to prevent the spread of infections, and both cats and dogs can be housed in the same ward. This is often more desirable than having comparatively large numbers of cats housed together when there is always a risk of outbreaks of airborne respiratory infections.

## Cages

There are two main types available which are suitable for most types of patient, either of a walk-in or locker type. There are advantages and disadvantages of each, and often the available space is an important factor in deciding which method to use; and sometimes a combination of both types is the best solution.

*Locker types.* These are the most economical to run in terms of floor space, and one of the most usual arrangements is a three-tier system with cages for large dogs on floor level, medium-sized cages which can be used for dogs or cats in the middle row, and a third tier of small cages for cats. There are several disadvantages of this type of system, perhaps drainage being the most serious. As far as management and daily running is concerned, handling of bad-tempered or nervous animals, certainly in the top and sometimes in the middle tiers can be difficult.

If this system is decided upon, cages of the following sizes prove adequate:

|        | Width (cm) | Depth (cm) | Height (cm) |
|--------|-----------|-----------|------------|
| Large  | 130       | 100       | 60         |
| Medium | 85        | 75        | 55         |
| Small  | 60        | 65        | 45         |

*Walk-in types.* These are considered more desirable by many owners, but they are much less economical in the fact that far fewer animals can be accommodated in the same space as when using locker types. Drainage is, however, much more satisfactory as they can be designed so that all materials drain to outside the cage. If they are used they should be of a minimum size of 140 cm by 100 cm.

In constructing hospital kennels it is important that they are escape-proof, but it is not as essential that they are paw- and nose-proof as in quarantine kennels, although it is desirable: and ease of cleaning and nursing may be more important considerations.

Again wood should be avoided in construction for the reasons given previously, and whatever material is used, if at all possible all corners should be coved, i.e. rounded, to facilitate easy cleaning. If a tier system is used, often the bottom tier is built of different materials, from those above. For the bottom tier, or walk-in cages, solid walls of brick, cement or cement blocks are ideal if cement-rendered or plastered and then painted. The best type of paint to use depends on the type of wall, but it should be remembered that gloss paints tend to show up all irregularities and defects in the plaster. Obviously any paints containing lead should not be used because of the danger of poisoning the animals if licked or chewed. As regards colour schemes, light colours are best as they can reflect light and so cut down the cost of artificial lighting. Both dark and bright colours should be avoided.

The middle and top tiers can be made of fibre glass or stainless steel. If individual cages are used for the middle and upper tiers, they have the advantage that they can be moved for easy cleaning or other purposes, but if so must be mounted in a wooden frame for stability. There are arguments for and against tilting the cages in these tiers to assist in drainage.

*The doors of all cages,* regardless of type, must be very well constructed, as they are in constant use and are the means of escape for the occupant. The most suitable are made of stainless steel and with a stainless steel mesh front. Double handles or bolts to each door are advisable, and should be so designed and positioned so that paws cannot be put through the mesh and the bolts opened. It is also desirable that the construction is such that a padlock could be fitted to these handles on occasions, as this is sometimes the only way of preventing animals opening doors. The mesh should be no bigger than 1.5 cm by 1.5 cm.

## Runs

It is absolutely essential to have some runs where the patients can be put several times daily so that they can urinate and defecate and whilst their cages are being cleaned out. It is essential that these runs are cleaned out thoroughly and often, and for this reason should therefore have a surface which can be cleaned with a hosepipe. Concrete is possibly the most suitable material and the one most often used. It is also essential that there is a good drainage system connected with the runs. These runs need not be very large but should be a minimum size of 180 cm by 120 cm. In a veterinary hospital it is often more convenient to have them actually constructed within the wards themselves as outside runs can be unsatisfactory for several reasons—escape, noise nuisance if they are situated in an urban area, and are also undesirable for ill patients in unfavourable weather conditions. It is desirable to have one run for every eight dog cages. Perhaps the most important disadvantage of indoor runs is the fact that house-trained animals are reluctant to use them.

### Heating, ventilation and soundproofing

It is absolutely essential in hospital kennels that heating and ventilation is adequate. Soundproofing is desirable and in urban areas essential.

Efficient ventilation is not necessarily expensive and some means of forced ventilation is necessary in wards or kennel blocks to remove unpleasant smells. A simple Vent-axia fan is often adequate. Ducted ventilation is very good and can be comparatively easily installed even in converted buildings which have high ceilings. The ducts can be placed below this high ceiling, and then concealed by building a new false ceiling below them which has a second function in reducing heat loss from the building. At least ten changes of air are required per hour. What ever method is used some means of sound proofing all inlets and outlets must be undertaken, and also ensuring that they are escape proof.

If the building is properly insulated, e.g. made of cavity brickwork, this cuts down on heat loss from inside and makes heating much easier. Double glazing of windows and doors, and also reducing the number of windows to a minimum, cuts down both heat loss and also decreases nuisance, as it cuts down loss of noise. Double glazing of windows and doors is also helpful as an additional escape-proof measure. If windows are not double-glazed they should be covered with a layer of wire mesh as an additional escape-proof method.

Sound proofing has become a necessity in an urban area. Unfortunately, if walls, floors or ceilings are made of concrete, sound echoes from them. This problem can be overcome quite easily by covering the interior walls of the building with peg-board or hard-board and placing wadding between this and the concrete. This wadding also acts as an insulating material and helps in heat loss.

The type of heating system decided upon depends somewhat on the type of building being used, whether it is an old building which has been altered or one being newly constructed. Whatever method is selected it must fulfil the requirements that it can be easily regulated for the building in general and, in addition, for each individual cage. In new kennels, under-floor central heating is often installed, but conventional central heating of any of the recognized types is quite adequate; and a thermostat and easy means of regulation should be incorporated in the system.

Adequate electricity points should be fitted so that infra-red lamps can be provided for supplementary heating, or possibly heating pads, in addition to use for electric fan heaters in an emergency and various instruments, e.g. clippers, driers, etc.

A general rule if a new building is being constructed is always to install as many electricity points as possible, and probably more than you think you will need at that stage. Obviously, all cables must be enclosed for safety, and if possible all switches boxed in. As has already been stated, supplementary heating to individual cages can be provided by fan heaters, infra-red heaters and radiant heaters. You should, however, always remember that with both radiant and infra-red heaters the intensity of heat produced is very great near them, and they should always be positioned so that there is no danger of burning the patient or causing damage to the structure of the building.

## Bedding

Some form of this will be necessary for each patient. There are various types available, all with advantages and disadvantages. Blankets are favoured by owners; they provide warmth and comfort, but in a hospital they involve a considerable amount of work for the staff to keep them constantly clean and hygienic. They are also chewable, and in some cases can cause problems in addition to the ones for which the animal is being hospitalized. Some Siamese cats have a strange propensity for eating wool, and certainly this material should not be used for them. Straw is warm, but is often a source of ectoparasites; it is also difficult to handle and difficult to keep the premises tidy if it is used. Some kennels use wood wool, but this has become increasingly more costly to use for bedding. Other materials used include sawdust, peat and "vet bed"—this is very useful for paraplegic patients or ones suffering from warfarin poisoning. Perhaps the most suitable material for general purposes is newspaper. This is readily available everywhere, is cheap, very absorbable, easily disposed of, and is very warm. The disadvantage of the material is that the print will sometimes stain the coats of white or light-coloured animals.

Most cats will need providing with a litter tray, but in some circumstances, e.g. certain orthopaedic cases, they are contraindicated. The trays can be of metal or plastic, so they can be easily disinfected, but metal has the disadvantage, unless stainless steel is used, that it rusts very quickly. Many people use cardboard boxes as they can be disposed of after use, and it is also possible to purchase special disposable containers. The litter itself can be of various types, possibly one of the proprietary ones being the most suitable, possessing a deodorant as well as being highly absorbent. Other materials such as screwed-up pieces of newspaper, sawdust, peat, and soil can be, and are, also used.

## General cleaning of hospital kennels and ancillary facilities

This is obviously a very important job and not just a menial task as sometimes thought. Good kennel hygiene and maintenance are most important in disease control and prevention. It is a task often delegated to a RANA or ANA trainee, and one which is much more responsible than it seems at first. All urine and faeces should be removed from each cage as soon as possible after it has been passed and disposed of adequately, preferably by being burnt. It should be remembered, and junior staff instructed, that both urine and faeces are sources of potential illness, both to other animals and humans, e.g. worm eggs from faeces and possibly leptospirosis organisms from urine. It is therefore essential in addition to thoroughly disinfecting the surface of runs, floors of cages, also to do the fences, the posts and walls of the cages, etc., where dogs could have urinated. **All cages must be thoroughly cleaned out at least once a day**; and it is most important that the animal remains in the same cage throughout its stay. Whilst its cage is being cleaned out it can either be put in the exercise run or, in the case of a cat, in a carrying box. If it remains in its own cage, if by any chance some disease should develop, especially skin disease, there is less risk of other animals in the unit developing problems, so this procedure can be considered another disease-prevention one.

Once an animal has been discharged the individual cage must be even more thoroughly disinfected and if the unit is not constantly fully occupied, cages should be used in rotation so that routinely a cage remains empty after a patient has been discharged. It is even more important for this if the cage has housed an infectious patient, where special disinfection will be required and probably carried out several times. Various proprietary disinfectants are available, and should always be used at the recommended dilution only; they are not as some people think more efficient if more concentrated, in fact sometimes they are less so. Some people recommend that the only effective means of disinfection following a ringworm infection is the use of a blowlamp. It must be remembered though that these can only be used on non-inflammable surfaces, and should always be used with very great care. It should also be borne in mind that some cats are very sensitive to even minute traces of disinfectant and can get unpleasant skin reactions if they come into contact with them. As a result all cages after disinfection should be thoroughly rinsed with plain water to ensure that all traces of disinfectant are removed. All cages must be allowed to thoroughly dry after cleaning before being used again.

All passages between cages and floors should be kept scrupulously clean at all times, and dirt and dust not allowed to collect on any ledges, as if this occurs it is an ideal place for fleas to lay their eggs and ringworm spores to lodge.

Precautions must be taken to keep the whole area free of flies, but animals, especially cats, are susceptible to certain types of fly-killer, and care must be taken in the selection and use of fly-killer.

All feeding dishes must be thoroughly cleaned and disinfected after each meal. Once the animal has been discharged, they should then be disposed of or be sterilized before being used by another animal. The kitchen and any other preparation areas must be thoroughly cleaned after each meal. All bulk supplies of biscuits, etc., should be kept in airtight rat- and mouse-proof containers. If fresh food is used it should be kept in a deep freeze or refrigerator, and if tinned food is used the tins opened only as required. If some food remains in the tin it should then be transferred to a plastic airtight container or some other covered container and stored in the refrigerator until the next meal.

All waste food should be removed from the unit and disposed of after each meal. Apart from doing this for hygienic reasons, it is a good preventative measure against vermin. If vermin are suspected, adequate measures must be taken for their elimination, and it must always be remembered that many proprietary products available for their destruction are also toxic to dogs and cats; so if used must be placed so that patients have no access to them.

## Boarding kennels and catteries

Boarding kennels and catteries need to be similar in design to the previous types but with various modifications since here normally healthy animals are being housed for comparatively short periods of time. These establishments come under the legislation contained in the Animal Boarding Establishments Act 1963. This means that the owner has to obtain a licence from the local authority, and the premises have to be inspected annually by the licensing authority and conform to certain standards laid down in the Act. Most of the points have already been covered in the previous sections, but, briefly, they are as stated in the Act:

1. Animals must be kept in accommodation that is adequate in construction and size. As regards size and general structure, these requirements are basically

the same as required for quarantine kennels.

2. Adequate exercise facilities should be provided. Again the requirements are similar to those for quarantine kennels except there is no need for double nose- and paw-proof fences. Again grass is not allowed except in paddocks large enough to prevent them getting in an unsuitable condition, and even so, the entrance and the inside perimeter should be paved. For cats, if they are in cages of less than 1.4 m² in floor area, they must have access to an escape-proof run. Many boarding catteries are now of the chalet type construction, however, where each cat has its own individual run and free access to it. An inspector can only ascertain that animals are having exercise by enquiry from the owner and other staff and observation of the kennels and exercise areas.

3. All sleeping compartments must be kept at an adequate temperature. They should be designed to prevent overheating in summer, and so that the temperature never drops below 7°C in the winter.

4. Lighting and ventilation should be adequate and the construction such that draught and damp are excluded, and be suitable for proper working by the staff in the units, and for the observation and the comfort of the animals.

5. All animals must be provided with adequate food. This is difficult to interpret in the legislation, but general basic principles regarding feeding should be followed.

6. Each animal must be provided with its own individual supply of drinking water, i.e. a bowl in each kennel, and not communal ones in the exercise runs; and fresh water should be available for the animal all the time.

7. Every animal has to be provided with a bed or sleeping area where it can lie down in comfort. Some kennels allow owners to supply the animal's own bed, others provide them. The bedding must always be kept clean and dry and any of the types mentioned earlier can be used.

8. Whilst animals are being boarded, someone must always be resident at the premises, and all animals must be visited at suitable intervals. Suitable intervals are interpreted as intervals of less than 4 hours except from 18.00 hours to 08.00 hours, but obviously they must be checked at least once, and more frequently if any potential problems are likely, between these times. Again the term resident is difficult to interpret, but it is not considered adequate that the place is locked up at 18.00 hours until the following morning. Someone should live either on the premises or near enough that they can be quickly there in case of emergency. If they do not actually live on or adjacent to the premises, their name, address and telephone number must be prominently displayed at the entrance to the premises, and this information must also be given to the local police and fire brigade.

9. Cats must always be provided with a sanitary tray. There are no exceptions to this as here we are housing healthy animals.

10. Disposal of all waste materials, food, bedding and faeces have to be done in a manner approved by the local authority.

11. Again the regulations regarding the storage of the food are similar, in rat- and mouse-proof containers, or a freezer or refrigeration.

12. Flies must be kept under control.

13. Reasonable precautions must be taken to prevent and control the spread of infectious and contagious disease, and must include the provision of isolation facilities. These are the same precautions you would take in a veterinary hospital.

14. Adequate precautions must be

taken to prevent fires, and suitable equipment should be available should one occur, to fight them.

15. A register must be kept, which should be available to all members of the staff, containing a description of the animals boarded, and also giving the date of arrival and departure of each. This must always be available for inspection by a representative of the local authority.

16. All reasonable precautions should be taken to avoid the animals escaping, but also to avoid people illegally visiting them. It is a good idea to keep a guard dog as a deterrent, but also geese have a similar effect, and the noise they make when being disturbed acts as a good means of warning. The other escape-proof precautions are again similar to those which would be used in a veterinary hospital.

17. Obviously, proper washing and toilet facilities have to be provided for staff, and these should also be available for owners of the animals being boarded, if necessary.

18. Finally, once the licence has been granted, a copy of it must be suitably displayed so that the public can see it in a prominent position in the establishment; the reception area is often a good place for it.

## General kennel and cattery management

This work may be the responsibility of a RANA. It is an important job, and the following guidelines, if routinely carried out, will greatly increase the efficiency of the establishment, the impression given to the owners of the animals, and lessen the possibility of disease occurring on the premises:

1. *All vaccination certificates should be checked* on arrival before the animal is admitted to ensure that they are up to date.

2. *Special cards should be available* and on these at the time of admittance should be recorded the following information:

(a) The owner's name, address and telephone number.
(b) A contacting address and telephone number in case of emergency if the owner is going away on holiday or is out at work during the day.
(c) Name of animal.
(d) Species of animal.
(e) Breed of animal.
(f) Colour of animal.
(g) Age of animal.
(h) Sex of animal and if neutered.
(i) Any peculiarities in behaviour of significance of the animal.
(j) Any belongings, e.g. collar, lead, toys, carrying box, which are going to be kept. It is advisable that these are kept to a minimum for many reasons; where appropriate these should be clearly labelled.
(k) The date of entry and, if known, the date the animal will be released.

3. *Obtain details of the diet normally fed to the animal,* and these, together with the normal routine of feeding times, the availability of water normally, and the routine regarding exercising, should all be recorded on the cards used in (2). If the owner specifies peculiarities, this is of great importance for dainty eaters, but more especially for geriatric animals.

4. *Before the owner leaves, ensure that he has signed any necessary forms,* e.g. consent for anaesthetic to be given, or for veterinary assistance to be sought should the animal become ill whilst being boarded.

5. *Check the animal for any visible signs of illness* unless being admitted for medi-

cal reasons, and also for the presence of ectoparasites and endoparasites.

6. *Once the animal has been admitted, observe its behaviour* thoroughly for the first few hours or days, then if changes subsequently occur they can be immediately noted as abnormal.

7. *Always work to a routine in the kennels or cattery;* be tidy, observe high standards of hygiene there and also personal hygiene.

8. *On arrival each morning, carry out a general check of the animals in the establishment,* and then, once it has been assessed that there are no urgent problems, each animal should be checked individually.

9. *The individual check* will depend on the reason for which the animal is being kept. If for hospitalization, many more will be needed than if for boarding. All should, however, be checked to see if:

(a) They have urinated or defecated, and if so if it is normal. These details should be recorded on either the cards used in (2) or special cards.

(b) If food has been kept in the cage overnight, records should also be made if all, some or none of this has been eaten. Although many people do not believe in leaving food with animals overnight because of possible problems, e.g. gastric torsion in large dogs, many animals, especially cats and also if they are inclined to be finicky feeders, will eat it then.

(c) Any development of signs of illness, bed sores or skin troubles.

10. *Routine cleaning of accommodation* should then be carried out, and it should always be remembered, as previously stated, that one cage or kennel should be kept for one animal during its stay, and whilst being cleaned out, it should be put either into an exercise run or carrying box, not another cage or kennel.

11. *Fresh faeces and urine should then be removed from each cage or kennel,* as soon as possible after it has been passed, throughout the day.

12. *If hospitalized cases are in the kennel or cattery,* then treatments as requested by the veterinary surgeon in charge of the case should be carried out, all procedures performed recorded, and any changes in the animal reported to the veterinary surgeon. At this stage routine nursing procedures of cleaning the eyes, nostrils and other natural orifices, can be carried out.

13. *Each day, every animal, unless there is some specific reason to contraindicate it,* e.g. skin trouble or warfarin poisoning, *should be groomed.*

14. *Separate grooming equipment should be kept for every animal,* but if this is not possible, frequent thorough disinfections of it must take place.

15. *Always feed small meals.* Often animals in confinement eat less, even if offered the normal amount, but they certainly need less, as in these circumstances they have a much lower metabolic rate. If the animal eats all it is given, it can then be offered a little more, but if it does not, it avoids waste as under no circumstance must any food left by one animal be offered to any other.

16. *Throughout each working day, periodically check the animals,* as emergencies can develop. It is also amazing how sensitive you become to a cat sneezing, or a dog coughing, if you are working conscientiously.

17. *Before leaving at night, again make a general check of each animal,* make sure its accommodation is clean and that it is comfortable.

18. *Ensure you lock the premises on leaving* and that heating and ventilation is correct.

### Control of Infection in the Boarding Cattery

The following procedures should be considered essential when preventing respiratory infection in cats:

1. Vaccination of cats before entry into the cattery.
2. Individual housing.
3. Solid-sided houses or a gap of at least 1.2 m between each pen.
4. Disinfect hands, boots, feedbowls, etc. Use two sets of feed bowls and litter trays so that one set can be left to soak in a suitable disinfectant solution.
5. Minimal contact between cats.
6. Feed and clean out cats in the same order each day. Deal with any suspected flu carriers last of all.
7. Reduce the concentration of the virus in the environment: allow plenty of fresh air to circulate, regular air changes with clean and dry conditions inside the cattery are best.

### Grooming

All animals coats, regardless of species, need daily grooming. Although many will attempt to do this themselves when well, they will stop doing so when they are ill. Self-grooming can also cause problems, e.g. furballs in long-haired cats.

Grooming is necessary for many reasons. Firstly, it gives the animal a sense of well being; secondly it aids cleanliness, and the presence of ectoparasites when they are cared for or other skin conditions become apparent immediately; thirdly it stimulates the sebaceous glands of the skin to produce secretions; fourthly, it accustoms the animal to regular handling; and fifthly it prevents various skin conditions occurring, e.g. matting of fur.

General basic principles can be applied to all species and under most situations, but special grooming methods are needed for certain breeds of both dogs and cats if they are to be shown, and also special precautions must be taken with animals which are ill, either with surgical wounds or skin conditions. It is obvious with short-haired breeds, irrespective of species, the time to be spent will be less than with a long-haired one, and whereas only a few minutes daily is necessary for a short-haired one, half an hour may be necessary for a long haired one.

A good basic grooming kit is essential and should include brushes, combs and a piece of chamois leather or nylon tights, or a piece of velvet material. The type of brush required varies considerably. For a long-haired cat it is essential that it should not have harsh wire bristles that will pull the coat out. Each animal should have its own grooming kit in a hospital, or the equipment should be sterilized between use on each patient; as grooming equipment is a great potential risk in the transmission of infectious skin disease, e.g. ringworm. For this reason, brushes with natural bristles and steel combs are preferred to nylon or plastic ones, which can warp or otherwise be damaged when being sterilized.

Dead hair on all species can be loosened and removed by finger-tip massaging with the hand, and this should be done as the hair causes irritation to the animal if it is not removed. It is important that all parts of the animal are brushed and combed and care taken with long-coated animals to ensure that the fur is kept free from tangles and matts. Once the coat has been thoroughly brushed and combed, the coat can be improved by polishing with the chamois leather, nylon or velvet.

In addition to general coat care, all discharges from the eyes and nose should be cleaned with cotton wool, soaked with sterile water or saline. The external ear orifices can be gently wiped clean as for the eyes and nose, but if there appears to be excessive dirt present, a veterinary surgeon should be consulted, as it could indicate the presence of the mite, *Otodectes cynotis,* or other ear problems. The perineum region should also be cleaned and any urinary or other discharges cleaned. It may also be necessary to keep the hair or fur in this area clipped short to prevent soiling.

**Cutting of claws and beaks**

In many animals this is never necessary, but in others it can be done for medical reasons, cosmetic reasons or to prevent the animal from causing damage to the owner's property. For medical reasons it is carried out when the claws become too long, then become curved, causing difficulty in movement, or so long as to be ingrowing into the pads. Claws tend to grow excessively long in all dogs that are only exercised on soft ground, in dogs insufficiently exercised, in light-boned dogs, in old animals with abnormal gaits, e.g. due to arthritis, and in these only some of their claws are worn down, and in patients with disease conditions of the feet, legs or nails, e.g. a fungal infection of the nail or a broken toe.

Cutting a dog's nails is a task which the RANA should undertake with care. If the nails are white or light coloured it is comparatively easy to see the blood vessel or "quick". It is important that this is not cut into as pain and haemorrhage will occur. There are various types of nail clippers, either of the scissor or guillotine type available; it is essential that these are sharp and only used for the purpose for which they were designed. If the nail is black or dark coloured, an estimation must be made of the position of the quick; this is done by applying slight pressure

with the cutters to the nail and the animal's reaction noted. If in the "quick" a pain response will be evoked, and the clippers should be removed a little further down the claw before the cut is made. Special attention should always be made to the dew-claws. These, as they do not touch the ground, do not wear down, and usually need more frequent attention than the main claws. The structure of the claw in the cat is somewhat different. Here the claws are retractable. It is unnecessary to cut cat claws except in very aged animals and in cats that damage furnishings. Claws of all other small mammalian pets need cutting from time to time, chiefly because of the methods of husbandry in domesticity. Rabbits' claws can be very long and cause problems in walking. The general principles regarding clipping apply.

If inadvertently the "quick" is cut into, in any species, the haemorrhage can be controlled by such substances as ferric chloride solution applied on a cotton bud, friar's balsam, or silver nitrate applied as a caustic pencil with care.

The budgerigar's beak and claws may need frequent trimming because of the bird's domestic conditions. The same principles apply to the claws as described above. If one of the perches is replaced by a bough of apple wood of irregular diameter, this will often prevent the claws from overgrowing. With the beak, care again has to be taken, not to cut the longitudinal-running blood vessel, and if possible the shape of the beak should be maintained by making two cuts at right angles to each other rather than one right across. The beak can sometimes overgrow because of disease, about which the veterinary surgeon should be consulted, or because of lack of use, and this can often be overcome by supplying the bird with a piece of cuttle fish or hardwood in the cage.

### Disposal of Waste

Within the veterinary practice, the disposal of waste involves the disposal of many types of materials, carcasses, surgical waste, pathological and laboratory waste, sharp articles, (e.g. needles or knife blades), drugs, domestic waste, and office waste.

Probably the most efficient way of getting rid of all types is a private incinerator, but at present only a few practices have one. There is also legislation contained in the Health and Safety at Work Act, and the Control of Pollution Act, which controls adequate disposal of waste in the United Kingdom, so care has to be exercised in any disposal. This legislation is being constantly updated so it is essential that practices are aware of the present requirements.

#### Carcasses

Local authorities in the United Kingdom are responsible for the disposal of pet carcasses but not for their collection from the practice premises. Carcasses should be stored in strong polythene bags, certainly not transparent, and the neck of the bag securely tied to exclude flies and the escape of smells. They should ideally be removed from the premises immediately, but this is not always possible. A special cool area should be set aside or a refrigerated container should be available, which can be easily disinfected and situated away from other buildings and without access to unauthorized persons, animals and free from infestation by rodents and insects. It must also be accessible to collection vehicles, who may call after normal working hours. Many local authorities will allow carcasses to be burnt in the public incinerator, but unfortunately, this is not always possible. Bodies of animals may be buried in the ground

depending on local facilities and regulations. There are firms who will collect carcasses to use for recycling for tallow and bone meal, and these can be a convenient method of disposal for a practice if a reputable firm can be contacted. It is most undesirable for one of these lorries to arrive when clients are about and can see them.

Private cremation is becoming more and more popular, and although expensive is an excellent method of disposal.

#### Surgical Waste

This includes both tissues and organs removed at operation and also blood-stained dressings, swabs, etc. It should be disposed of by incineration after packing in strong polythene bags and securing the bags tightly.

#### Pathological and Laboratory Waste

Much of the waste in this category could be a potential human health hazard and should be treated with great care. All bacteriological culture plates should be decontaminated before disposal, and again the best method of disposal is incineration after storing in secure plastic bags.

#### Drugs

Small amounts of solid medicants and small volumes of injectable substances should be incinerated. Small amounts of liquid should be emptied from their containers, and then flushed down the toilet or down the sink, followed by large quantities of cold water. If large quantities of fluid are to be disposed of advice should be sought. If the drugs are controlled by the Misuse of Drugs Act 1971, special methods will have to be used and prior advice sought (pp. 428–9). Again solid dose products are best incinerated except where it is not recommended by the manufacturer.

### Sharp Articles

This includes syringes, needles, razor or knife blades, in addition to drug containers. Syringes should always be cleaned, separated from their needles and the nozzles destroyed before disposal; they should then be packed in rigid containers and sealed or destroyed by special crushing apparatus which can be purchased. Needles should be broken from their hubs and then incinerated. Nowadays it is possible to obtain special sharps disposal containers and the suppliers organize a regular collection and replacement service.

### Domestic Waste

This is collected free in the United Kingdom by the local authority, but care should be taken that it is not contaminated with practice refuse of any type.

### Office Waste

To maintain the ethics of the practice, if records are to be discarded, they should be torn into small pieces or shredded before being burnt.

(f) Nutrition and Feeding

R. S. ANDERSON

An animal is what it eats.

Apart from the short but important period of foetal development, the entire animal body of bones, muscle, blood, viscera, brains, hair, teeth, eyes and ears has originated as ingested food. Even during the foetal period the tissues have developed indirectly from the food of the mother. When broken down to its basic components—protein, fat, carbohydrate, vitamins and minerals—an animal and its food are basically the same. Indeed, in nature they often are the same, since the bodies of small animals provide a balanced source of nutrients for their predators.

There is, of course, one fundamental difference between an animal and its food—life. The animal is living and the food is dead (although perhaps only recently) and the study of nutrition is an important aspect of understanding how the remarkable transition from the dead food to the living animal tissue takes place.

### Determination of Nutritional Requirements

#### Nutritional balance

There is relatively little change in the body size and composition of a dog over its adult lifetime of 10–15 years, and yet a 14 kg (30 lb) dog will in about 20 days, consume its own body weight in food (wet weight) and, if water intake is also included, will consume in 10 years an amount equal to 300 times its own weight, or 4200 kg (4 tons).

Since the nutrients which make up this substantial quantity of food approximate only roughly to the needs of the body, it is a remarkable feat to maintain body composition relatively constant or "in balance" during this period of time. Only by varying the proportion of nutrients absorbed and excreted from the food is the constancy or balance of the body's components maintained. The detailed consideration of nutritional balance is usually applied to single nutrients such as calcium and water, but it may also be applied to energy. Balance measurements can only be made under carefully controlled experimental conditions, where it is possible to quantify accurately the total daily intake and output of the nutrient under investigation.

It is from this type of experiment that data are accumulated on the minimum daily requirements of some individual nutrients, particularly protein and minerals. When the intake of any nutrient is equal to the rate of excretion, balance is maintained and the minimum daily requirements are being supplied. This is not to say that it is the self-same elements being excreted as are ingested; many such substances in the body, for instance calcium and phosphorus in bones or iron in blood, are constantly being mobilized and replaced even in adult animals. So, in practice the recommended daily allowances for a given nutrient are usually greater than the minimum daily requirement to allow a safety margin and permit individual variation.

### Growth trials

It is not sufficient for a growing puppy to be merely "in balance" for any nutrient. In addition to the requirement for maintaining existing tissues it must transform a proportion of its food into new living tissue and each day more nutrient must go in as food than comes out as excreta, thus creating a net positive balance. Because of these nutrient requirements, the growing animal is much more sensitive and vulnerable to an inadequate or imbalanced diet, and this sensitivity has been used more than any other technique to establish nutrient requirements of dogs and cats. By including a nutrient at several levels in an otherwise adequate diet and feeding to matched groups of growing pups, minimum and recommended levels can be established based on the relative growth rate of each group. An unresolved problem posed by this technique is—What is the *optimum* growth rate of puppies? There is some good experimental evidence that **maximum growth rate is not always compatible with optimum skeletal development** in Great Danes (p. 200), and in laboratory animals maximum growth rate is associated with a curtailed life expectancy.

### Other techniques

Balance and growth experiments are not usually used for determining the metabolic needs of some nutrients such as vitamins, some trace elements and essential fatty acids. Vitamin requirements have been determined by the progressive elimination of the vitamin from the diet until a metabolic and/or clinical abnormality is demonstrated, the diet is then supplemented to a level at which the abnormality is resolved.

The use of radioactively labelled nutrients and the study of the biochemical pathways in which the nutrient participates are other valuable techniques in establishing the requirements for essential dietary components.

### Nutritional Requirements

As food and water provide the basic raw materials from which the dog builds, maintains and repairs its body structure and function, it is important to examine the basic components of these raw materials.

### Water

Water is the most important single nutrient of the diet. **A deficiency of water will cause disease and death** more quickly than deficiency of any other nutrient. Dogs which have had access to water but no food have survived in reasonable health for much longer than when food and no water were available, and the restriction of water quickly affects both the intake and digestibility of the food. Water is by far the largest component of the body (approximately 75% of the fat-free body weight) and it is also subject to the most sensitive control mechanisms (p. 16). A diagrammatic representation of the various routes by which water balance is maintained is shown in Fig. 3.25.

A knowledge and awareness of some of the factors affecting water balance is one

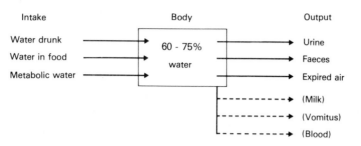

Fig. 3.25. Water intake and loss from the body.

of the most practical and important aspects of the feeding and care of the healthy and, in particular, the sick animal.

### Intake of Water

#### Water Drunk

Thirst and drinking are the most important mechanisms for regulating fluid balance and, with few exceptions, drinking water should always be available.

The amount of water required as drinking water is, however, very variable depending on the availability of water in the food and variations in water loss from the body.

#### Water in the food

The water content of food materials may vary from 70–80% in raw meat to 5–10% in dry biscuit. If water is mixed in with the food during preparation, the final water content may be greater than 80%, and in some greyhound kennels no drinking water is provided, there being sufficient in the food to meet their daily requirements.

Under most conditions, however, dogs and cats do not appear to receive sufficient water from their food to meet requirements. Thus assuming that a dog has a daily water requirement of 1000 ml/day it could obtain approximately 75% of this amount from a wet food (canned dog food) and require about only 250 ml as drinking water. If fed dry biscuit, however, it would have to meet almost all its requirements from drinking water, thus it would need **four times as much drinking water**.

#### Metabolic Water

When protein, fat and carbohydrate are completely broken down in the body, the hydrogen in each organic molecule combines with oxygen to form water by the process of oxidation. The complete oxidation of 100 g of protein, fat or carbohydrate yields 40, 107 or 55 g of water respectively. In general, about 100 g of this water of oxidation or metabolic water is produced for every 1000 kcal of energy metabolized, and under normal conditions will provide about 10% of the animal's water requirements. In desert conditions, however, small mammals have developed physiological and behavioural mechanisms which permit them to meet their entire water requirements from the oxidative water of their dry food.

*Output of Water*

## Urine

The kidneys regulate water output in addition to their other regulatory functions. When water intake is reduced relative to output, water reabsorption is increased in the kidney tubules, thus conserving water and maintaining water balance. There is, however, a limit to the amount of water which the kidneys can reabsorb, as the waste products of metabolism must be excreted by the kidneys in a fluid medium (urine). This minimum (or obligatory) urine production continues even under conditions of extreme dehydration.

In kidney disease, the capacity to reabsorb water from the urine is impaired and the kidneys are unable to respond adequately to the needs of the body to conserve water. Similarly in diabetes insipidus and mellitus, urinary water losses may be excessive and balance can only be maintained by increased water intake.

## Faeces

Water losses in normal faeces are relatively small and only when diarrhoea is profuse and continuous does faecal water loss become a significant factor in water balance.

## Expired Air

Respiratory water loss is continuous and obligatory and in the dog represents an essential aspect of temperature regulation. At high environmental temperatures, panting is the most important mechanism of heat loss, since little or no sweating takes place. If unable to compensate for the rapid loss of respiratory water, the heat-stressed dog rapidly becomes dehydrated, body temperature rises rapidly and death ensues. If heat stress is unavoidable, access to drinking water is essential.

Panting and respiratory water loss is a much less well-developed regulatory response in the cat than in the dog. Although some sweating occurs through the pads, the main response in the cat to high environmental temperature is *increased salivation and licking of the fur, with resultant evaporative cooling from the surface of the body.*

## Milk, Vomitus, Blood

Milk production by the nursing bitch requires a substantial increase in water turnover and is significantly impaired if water is restricted.

Water losses from chronic vomiting and/or haemorrhage may present an urgent need for fluid replacement, but the parenteral route is usually preferred under these conditions.

## *Water requirement*

Individual requirements for drinking water vary according to the type of food, environmental temperature, amount of exercise and physiological state. These variations in requirement are best met by permitting free access to drinking water at all times—or at least three times per day.

Because of this variability and the ease with which drinking water can be supplied, there is little practical need to quantify the requirements for water. However, water intake has been measured under laboratory conditions for both dogs and cats and the values obtained are shown in Table 3.3.

Thus a 14 kg dog will normally need about 1 litre of water per day and a 3 kg cat about 230 ml/day derived from food and water. Virtually all of this water must be obtained from drinking water if the

TABLE 3.3. *Estimated water requirements of dogs and cats in temperate conditions*

|  | Dog | Cat |
|---|---|---|
| Total water intake in food and water (excluding metabolic water): |  |  |
| ml/kg body weight | 70–80 | 70–80 |
| ml/g of food (dry matter) | 4 | 4 |

food is dry, whereas only 25% of these amounts is required as drinking water if the food has an average water content of 75% (p. 183).

The cat adapts its water intake less accurately and completely than the dog to changes in the water content of the food. The failure of some cats to drink sufficient water when receiving dry food is a possible factor in the development of stones in the urinary bladder.

### Energy

One of the fundamental characteristics of the living animal is the constant expenditure of energy for the maintenance of life. Even sleeping dogs use energy for life processes such as circulation, respiration and the maintenance of body temperature. The basal energy expenditure is called the **basal metabolic rate** (BMR).

In practice additional energy is used for activity, digestion, growth, reproduction and control of body temperature. Because of these large variables there are large variations in energy requirements between individuals and in the same individual from day to day.

*Hunger and appetite.* The need to replace energy used is the most important factor in regulating food requirements and intake. An animal will actively seek out food sources in response to a variety of signals and physiological mechanisms which indicate that it requires "refuelling". Hunger and appetite are stimulated by a decrease in the level of blood glucose, free plasma amino acids, by contractions of the empty stomach and by other physiological and biochemical stimuli as yet poorly defined. For dogs and cats meal time conditioning and competing for food also play an important part in stimulating food intake.

The control of food intake is via a nerve centre in the hypothalamus which regulates eating behaviour in response to these various stimuli, among the most important of which is decreasing blood glucose levels. Glucose is an essential—if not the only—fuel for the central nervous system and, as the blood glucose level falls, there is increased activity of the hypothalamic hunger centre, which is associated with the sensation of hunger and a stimulus to feeding activity. This sensation and activity is depressed by a variety of other stimuli which include gastric distension and the increasing blood glucose level which occurs after a meal.

*Energy sources.* For the normal healthy animal, the only source of energy is the food which it eats. (The unconscious or inappetent animal may be "refuelled" by the parenteral administration of glucose or dextrose solutions.)

The food components which supply energy are protein, fat and carbohydrate. (Although vitamins and minerals do not supply energy, their absence or deficiency in the diet may interfere with energy utilization.)

Energy is needed and utilized as thermal (heat), chemical and mechanical energy in the animal body. The energy units in food are expressed as kilocalories (kcal) or kilojoules (kJ) (1 kcal = 4.2 kJ).

TABLE 3.4. *Factors by which protein, fat and carbohydrate (g per 100 g of food) should be multiplied to obtain metabolizable energy (kJ/100 g)\* or (kcal/100 g)*

|  | Conversion factor | |
|---|---|---|
|  | kJ | kcal |
| Protein | 17 | 4 |
| Fat | 37 | 9 |
| Carbohydrate | 16 | 4 |

\*Multiply conversion by 10 for kJ/kg.

When protein, fat or carbohydrate are completely burned, they each produce a characteristic amount of energy in the form of heat. This is called the **gross energy** and provides an indication of the energy content in food. In practice, however, when an animal converts these fuels to energy it does not break them down so completely, some being excreted as unutilized energy in the faeces and urine. The energy which the animal actually derives from its food—the **metabolizable energy** —is, therefore, obtained by measuring the total energy of the faeces and urine for several days and subtracting this value from the gross energy of the food eaten during the same period. Thus: Metabolizable energy = gross energy (food) − energy in faeces and urine. For practical purposes, the metabolizable energy can be calculated by applying energy conversion factors to the protein, fat and carbohydrate values of the food (Table 3.4).

The actual metabolizable energy content of dog and cat foods depends on several factors, the most important of which are its fat content and its water content. The metabolizable energy of the three main categories of dog and cat foods is shown in Table 3.7 (p. 196).

*Energy requirements.* The metabolizable energy requirements of adult dogs and cats are shown in Tables 3.9 and 3.10 (p. 198). Growing puppies and kittens require 2–3 times as much as adult animals of the same weight. Lactating bitches and queens and working dogs may require up to three times the maintenance requirement.

**Protein**

The place of protein and cooked or raw meat in the diet of dogs and cats has received more attention than most other nutrients. Protein and meat are occasionally regarded as synonymous, thus upholding the traditional view that meat is a dietary essential and the higher the meat content the better the diet. In fact there are many useful protein sources other than meat, and dogs are able to maintain good health on vegetable proteins alone. There is, however, growing evidence that the cat, in addition to requiring a relatively greater proportion of dietary protein than the dog, needs at least some food materials of animal origin for the maintenance of health.

All the basic food materials (animal matter, cereals and vegetables) commonly fed to dogs and cats contain protein and, apart from the quantitative differences in the protein content of these materials, the main difference is in quality due to a number of factors.

*Amino acids.* All proteins of biological origin are composed of twenty primary units called amino acids arranged in varying sequences. Ten of these amino acids are essential in the diet to provide for growth, metabolism and replacement of the animal's own tissue proteins. These **essential amino acids** are histidine, isoleucine, leucine, lysine, methionine, phenylalanine, threonine, tryptophan, valine and arginine. The proportion and availability of these amino acids in dietary proteins affect their usefulness for incorporation into the animal's tissue proteins. If the proportion is ideal the protein is said to have a **high biological value**, i.e. it can be used efficiently by the body. Egg protein is considered to have the highest biological value and is given a value of 100. The proteins of meat, liver, kidneys and milk all have a high biological value, whereas plant proteins from such as the soya bean and other legumes and from cereals, although of lower biological value, nevertheless are useful protein sources.

*Digestibility.* The digestibility of protein is another important aspect of its nutritional value. Not only must the requisite amino acids be contained in the dietary protein, they must be available for absorption after the process of digestion. Thus although whole skin, hair, feathers, horns and hooves are all proteinaceous materials, they have a low digestibility and therefore a low biological value.

Excessive heat also lowers the biological value of proteins, as in some meat meals based on low-grade materials and subjected to prolonged high temperature during processing.

*Functions.* Proteins in the diet supply the amino acids needed for the growth in puppies and kittens and also those needed for maintenance of adult tissues. The amounts needed for growth are much greater than for maintenance, and a diet inadequate in protein will affect growth rate of the young animal much more quickly than it will show as weight loss and tissue wastage in the adult. In the adult, injury or surgical operation causes increased protein loss (as urinary nitrogen) as part of the general tissue breakdown in association with injury.

In addition to tissue growth, protein serves many other essential functions such an enhancement of metabolic reactions (enzymes), the transportation of oxygen in the blood (haemoglobin) and the protection of the body against infection (antibodies).

*Protein deficiency.* If the amount or quality of the dietary protein is insufficient to meet the animal's needs, then protein deficiency results. Because of its high dietary protein requirement for growth, the effects of deficiency are most obvious in impaired growth of the young animal. Weight loss, depressed appetite, poor coat condition, decreased plasma protein and haemoglobin levels, and increased susceptibility to toxic and infective agents are all associated with protein deficiency.

*Taurine.* Some years ago it was noticed that cats given casein only as a protein source developed a progressive central retinal degeneration leading to eventual blindness. Further work has shown that the cat, unlike other animals, is unable to synthesize an amino acid, taurine, which is concentrated in the retina of the eye and is necessary for its normal health.

Foods of animal origin all contain taurine, and under normal dietary conditions cats should receive sufficient for their requirements. If, however, the protein in the cat's diet is largely of vegetable origin, there may be insufficient taurine intake and retinal degeneration may occur.

*Protein requirements.* The amount of protein required depends on the quality of protein in the food and the physiological or clinical status of the animal. The recommended amount for an adult dog is 4.8 g/kg body weight per day. The recommendation for the growing puppy and kitten or lactating bitch or queen is two to three times this amount, but, because food consumption is also two to three times greater, this higher protein intake can be attained without protein supplementation provided that the diet contains a sufficient quantity of good quality protein in the first place.

*Recommended allowance of protein per 100 g of diet (dry basis)*:
　　Dog, 22%　　Cat, 28%

## Fat

*Dietary source.* The main dietary source of fat is animal fat from the tissues of mammals, fish or poultry. Vegetable oils such as corn, soya bean, safflower or cottonseed also provide fat which is readily accepted and easily incorporated into the food.

*Essential fatty acids.* A minimum amount of dietary fat is necessary in order to supply the **essential fatty acids** (EFAs) for normal growth, skin health and the synthesis of certain compounds (prostaglandins) vital to many metabolic functions including reproduction. The essential fatty acids are linoleic, linolenic and arachidonic acid, and they are found in the structural fat of animal tissues and in vegetable oils.

*Digestibility.* Fat is highly digestible by healthy dogs and cats. More than 90% of ingested animal and vegetable fat is absorbed, and levels up to 40% of the dietary dry matter have been fed successfully to dogs for long periods.

Absorption is markedly impaired in pancreatic insufficiency in which there is inadequate secretion of pancreatic lipase to break down the fat in the food to glycerol for absorption. Undigested and unabsorbed fat thus appears in the faeces, which are voluminous, grey and fatty in appearance.

*Function.* Apart from supplying the essential fatty acids, fat acts as a concentrated and palatable source of energy in food. Its presence is also necessary as a carrier of the fat soluble vitamins A, D, E and K.

Fatty food exposed to air will, however, undergo oxidation and become rancid unless the food contains anti-oxidants such as vitamin E or betahydroxytoluene. Rancid fat may destroy other nutrients such as vitamin A and E and the essential fatty acids, and the prolonged feeding of foods containing rancid fat has been associated with the development of skin lesions, impaired reproduction and muscular dystrophy in dogs.

*Deficiency.* In the dog, the EFAs can be substituted for each other within the tissues; thus if any one of the EFAs is present in sufficient amounts, the requirements for all the EFAs will be met. Where an absolute deficiency occurs on a very low fat diet, puppies show impaired growth, dry, coarse hair and scurfy skin which later develops into raw areas susceptible to infection and slow to heal.

In cats the EFAs are probably not all interconvertible in the tissues, and in practice this means that cats may have a specific requirement for EFAs of animal origin; thus animal fat rather than vegetable oils are essential as a dietary fat source for the cat.

*Fat requirement.* The minimum level of dietary fat depends on concentration of essential fatty acids. Assuming that the fat source is mainly of animal origin, the following is the recommended allowance.

*Recommended allowance of fat per 100 g of diet (dry basis)*:
　　Dog, 5%　　Cat, 9%

## Carbohydrate

Carbohydrate is probably not an essential nutrient for dogs and cats and they will remain in good health for long periods on diets containing no carbohydrate. It is, however, a readily available and economical energy source for the dog and may, therefore, be included in any dietary regime.

*Dietary source.* Carbohydrate is most readily provided as part of the diet when given as the cereal starch of dog biscuits and meals, or other carbohydrate-rich sources such as potatoes and rice. Animal matter contains little or no carbohydrate.

Because of their low water content, biscuits and meals have a relatively high energy content (330–350 kcal per 100 g) and it is, therefore, simple and convenient to manipulate a dog's energy intake by increasing or decreasing the proportion of carbohydrate as biscuit, potato, rice, etc., in the diet. As in fat supplementation, when an excessive (more than 40% dry weight) proportion of the diet is carbohydrate, there is a risk that sufficient quantities of other essential nutrients will be displaced with impairment of the balance and quality of the diet.

Supplementation of the cat's diet with carbohydrate as biscuit or meal is less common than in the dog, but canned and dry cat foods containing carbohydrate as cereal provide a satisfactory diet for the cat.

In general the carbohydrate-rich foods are less palatable than the animal protein and fat rich foods. The addition of small amounts of animal protein and fat to cereal-based dog foods markedly improves palatability, and complete dry cereal-based dog foods invariably contain a substantial component of added animal protein and fat.

*Digestibility.* Carbohydrate as cereal starch and as simple sugars such as glucose, sucrose and dextrose-maltrose is highly digestible by both dogs and cats. Lactose (milk sugar) is usually well tolerated by puppies and kittens but adult animals may develop diarrhoea if substantial amounts are suddenly introduced to the diet. Individual animals may be intolerant of even small amounts of dietary lactose.

Raw uncooked starch may cause diarrhoea and flatulence due to fermentation of undigested starch granules in the large intestine.

Vegetable fibre is usually present in the cereal-based foods. Although not available as an energy source (since dogs and cats do not secrete the necessary cellulase enzyme to break down vegetable fibre), vegetable fibre probably aids digestion of other nutrients by promoting peristaltic movements. It also contributes to the production of well-formed stools—often an important consideration in kennel management.

*Function.* The main function of carbohydrate is to provide a source of energy. After digestion in the intestine, the main end-product—glucose—may be used directly as an energy source or it may be stored in muscle or liver as glycogen or converted into fat and stored in adipose (fatty) tissue.

*Deficiency.* Although dogs and cats do not require carbohydrate and so deficiency does not occur, the absence of dietary carbohydrate results in the utilization of dietary protein and fat as an energy source; thus carbohydrate "spares" these nutrients, particularly protein, for their essential function in tissue growth and metabolism.

## Vitamins

Vitamins are substances needed in minute amounts for many of the body's vital functions. With the exception of vitamin C, dogs and cats require the same vitamins as man, A, D, E, and K (the fat soluble vitamins) and the B complex (water soluble). These vitamins occur in various proportions in animal, cereal and vegetable foods, and a mixed diet of muscle meat, organ meat (liver or kidney) and cereal or potato is unlikely to be vitamin deficient unless cooked for an excessive period.

calcium and phosphorus may be a factor in abnormal bone formation, enlarged joints and reluctance to move in growing puppies, particularly of the giant breeds.

Hypervitaminosis A occurs not infrequently in cats fed largely or exclusively on fresh liver. The main effect is fusion of spinal vertebrae and bony outgrowths on limb and other bones resulting in a progressive impairment of normal movement.

### Vitamin A

*Dietary source.* Liver, kidney and milk are good sources of vitamin A and, while green vegetables and carrots contain no preformed vitamin A, they contain a precursor, **carotene**, which can be converted to vitamin A by the dog but not by the cat.

*Function.* Vitamin A is essential for the production of visual pigments in the retina which are necessary for vision in dim light. It is also important to the maintenance of the health and integrity of skin and other epithelial surfaces, growth of bone and teeth, and normal kidney function.

*Deficiency.* Deficiency is slow to develop in the normal adult dog which stores vitamin A in its liver, kidneys and fat. In young dogs a vitamin A deficient diet causes poor growth, eye and skin lesions, and bone abnormalities. Deficiency is more likely where the diet has a very low fat content.

In cats, deficiency is unlikely on most normal diets, or in cats which have an opportunity to catch small animals and birds. Vitamin A deficient diets are associated with a variety of eye and epithelial lesions with increased susceptibility to secondary infections.

*Hypervitaminosis A.* Excessive supplementation of a diet already rich in protein,

*Recommended allowance of vitamin A per 100 g of diet (dry basis):*
   Dog, 500 IU      Cat, 1000 IU
IU = international units.

### Vitamin D

*Dietary source.* Vitamin D is formed in the body in response to sunlight. Dietary sources are fish-liver oils, egg yolk, milk, butter and cheese.

*Function.* Vitamin D is a vital factor in the absorption of calcium and phosphorus from the intestine, the maintenance of calcium and phosphorus levels in the blood and bone and tooth formation (by affecting the mineralization and demineralization of tissues).

*Deficiency.* Vitamin D deficiency is most unlikely in adult dogs and cats, and even in puppies and kittens the effects of a vitamin D deficiency are only likely if the diet is deficient or severely imbalanced with respect to calcium and phosphorus. Under such conditions, rickets—complicated by decalcification of the bone—occurs.

*Hypervitaminosis D.* Over-dosage with vitamin D supplements such as the fish-liver oils can cause retarded growth, bone and tooth malformation and calcification of soft tissues such as lungs and kidneys.

*Recommended allowance of vitamin D per 100 g of diet (dry basis)*:

Dog, 50 IU     Cat, 1000 IU

## Vitamin E

*Dietary source.* Vitamin E occurs in several forms (known in their purified form as tocopherols) and is present in many foods such as egg yolk, cereal grains, milk and vegetable oils.

*Function.* Vitamin E has an antioxidant effect both in foods and in the body. It thus prevents oxidative rancidity of fats and the destruction of vitamin A in foods and also protects cell membranes from oxidative changes. Dietary requirements are directly related to the content of polyunsaturated fatty acids in the diet.

*Deficiency.* In dogs fed vitamin E deficient diets, muscular dystrophy and impaired reproduction which responded to vitamin E supplementation has been reported. In cats diets containing high levels of polyunsaturated fats from tuna fish have been associated with pain and inflammatory changes in muscle (myositis) and fat (steatitis) which respond to vitamin E therapy.

*Hypervitaminosis E.* Hypervitaminosis has not been reported in dogs or cats.

*Recommended allowance of vitamin E per 100 g of diet (dry basis)*:

Dog, 5 IU     Cat, 8 IU

## Vitamin K

Vitamin K is an important factor in the normal clotting of blood and has proved useful when clotting is impaired after ingestion of rat poisons containing Warfarin (p. 550). In normal animals, a dietary source is probably not required as it is synthesized by the intestinal bacteria.

## The Vitamin B Group

The B group of vitamins are water soluble and, because their stores in the body do not last as long as the fat-soluble vitamins, occasional cases of deficiency occur. Several members of the B group are quite thermolabile (i.e. readily destroyed by heating), thus food which is heated severely or for a long period may have some of the B vitamin destroyed.

The functions and sources of the B vitamins are shown in Table 3.5.

As Table 3.5 shows, meats, eggs, cereals and yeast are a good source of most of the B vitamins; thus an uncomplicated clinical case of deficiency of a single vitamin is unlikely.

*Thiamin deficiency* has occurred in dogs and cats fed on large quantities of raw fish which contains an enzyme thiaminase which destroys the naturally occurring vitamins. In most canned foods the constituents are supplemented with thiamin before processing in a sufficient amount to offset the losses during cooking and sterilization in the can.

*Black tongue* (nicotinic acid deficiency) is now uncommon, though it used to occur occasionally in shepherd dogs living on a diet of flaked maize and little or no supplementary meat or milk.

While raw egg white contains a substance (avidin) known to destroy biotin, there is little or no evidence that biotin deficiency occurs clinically. For allowances see Table 3.6.

## Vitamin C

Dogs and cats do not require a dietary source of vitamin C though, as in man, claims have been made that large doses prevent or control virus diseases such as canine distemper and kennel cough. A number of controlled studies have, however, failed to demonstrate any effect on

TABLE 3.5.    *The functions and dietary sources of the vitamin B complex*

| Vitamin | Source | Function | Deficiency |
|---------|--------|----------|------------|
| **Thiamin** ($B_1$) | Meat (especially pork, cereals, yeast) | Carbohydrate and protein metabolism | Loss of appetite weakness, spasticity, heart failure and death |
| **Riboflavin** ($B_2$) | Organ meats, eggs, yeast, cereals | Growth and skin condition | Unlikely under most conditions |
| **Pantothenic Acid** | Organ meats, eggs, cereals | Growth, skin condition | Unlikely |
| **Niacin** | Organ meats, eggs, cereals, yeasts | Health of mouth tissues | Ulceration of mouth and tongue, salivation bloody diarrhoea (black tongue) |
| **Pyridoxine** ($B_6$) | Organ meats, eggs, cereals, fish, yeast | Protein metabolism, blood formation, growth | Unlikely under most conditions |
| **Folic acid** | Organ meats, yeast | Normal blood, facial growth | Unlikely |
| **Biotin** | Organ meats, egg yolk, milk, yeast | Normal growth, healthy skin | May occur with excessive feeding of egg white. Poor growth |
| **$B_{12}$** | Muscle meats, milk, liver | Normal blood | Unlikely |
| **Choline** | Organ meats, eggs, yeast | Protein metabolism | Unlikely |

TABLE 3.6.    *Recommended allowance of vitamins of the B complex per 100 g of diet (dry basis)*

| | Dog (mg) | Cat (mg) |
|---|---|---|
| Thiamin | 0.1 | 0.5 |
| Riboflavin | 0.2 | 0.5 |
| Pantothenic acid | 1.0 | 1.0 |
| Niacin | 1.1 | 4.5 |
| Pyridoxine | 0.1 | 0.4 |
| Folic acid | 0.02 | 0.1 |
| Biotin | 0.01 | 0.005 |
| Vitamin $B_{12}$ | 0.002 | 0.002 |
| Choline | 120 | 200 |

these conditions. Vitamin C has been implicated in skeletal scurvy in dogs and also advocated for treatment of hip dysplasia, though evidence of its value in the latter condition is not convincing.

## Minerals

Minerals are inorganic chemical elements which serve a number of essential structural, metabolic and osmotic functions in the body, particularly during growth and reproduction.

### Calcium and Phosphorus

*Source.* For the young puppy or kitten, its mother's milk provides the required dietary calcium and phosphorus during the first few weeks of life. From weaning onwards the food must supply their increasing requirements in a readily available form. Cows milk and milk substitutes usually supply a continuing source during the transition to solid food, and sparing use can be made of bone meal or calcium supplements.

Foods recommended specifically for growing puppies and kittens and many other standard canned, semi-moist or complete dry foods will supply calcium and phosphorus in sufficient amounts for growth.

The source in these foods is ground bone, bone meal, or calcium phosphate. If fresh foods based on meat and vegetables are fed, the diet must be supplemented with a calcium and phosphorus source such as milk, bone meal, egg shells or a proprietary mineral supplement. **Muscle meat is grossly deficient in calcium** and a growing puppy would have to consume about five times its own weight of meat each day in order to obtain its calcium requirements. About 2 g of raw bone per 100 g of muscle meat is necessary to provide a satisfactory level of calcium and phosphorus intake.

To ensure adequate absorption from the intestines, calcium and phosphorus should be present in approximately equal quantities. A **calcium:phosphorus ratio of 1:1 to 1.4:1** is satisfactory for both dogs and cats (the ratio in meat is 1:20).

*Function.* Calcium and phosphorus play an essential structural role in the formation of bones and teeth in the young animal and in maintaining their health and integrity in adult life. The lactating bitch and queen have a particularly high calcium and phosphorus requirement to replace the tissue stores which are mobilized for milk secretion.

The complex mechanisms of normal blood clotting, nerve transmission and muscular contraction are all dependent on an adequate supply of calcium in the blood.

*Deficiency.* A dietary deficiency or imbalance of calcium and phosphorus is most likely in growing animals—particularly large or giant dog breeds fed on a predominantly meat diet without adequate calcium supplementation. The main signs are poor growth, misshapen long bones, enlarged and painful joints, reluctance to move and even spontaneous fractures. In adult animals, signs of deficiency are much slower to develop because of the relatively slower rate of calcium exchange in bones. However, the lactating bitch or queen may develop acute calcium deficiency if she is unable to maintain her blood calcium levels in response to the rapid calcium losses in the milk.

The low blood calcium results in abnormal neuro-muscular function and sustained muscular contraction or hypocalcaemic tetany (p. 666) (milk fever). In canine nephritis, excessive losses of phosphorus in the urine may result in bone demineralization which may be particularly obvious in the jawbones, with recession of alveolar bone and slackening of the teeth (p. 507).

*Requirements.* Although the amount of calcium required during growth, pregnancy and lactation is much greater than for adult maintenance, there are several mechanisms which increase its availability. The percentage of dietary **calcium retained varies from 40% to 70%** in a diet containing 0.6% calcium and is higher in the growing than in the adult animal. Furthermore, the amount of food, and therefore, the amount of calcium ingested, is greater by a factor of 2 or 3 in the growing and lactating animal than in an adult of the same weight.

*Recommended allowance of calcium and phosphorus per 100 g of diet (dry basis):*
    Dog, 1.1 g calcium
          0.9 g phosphorus
    Cat, 0.1 g calcium
          0.8 g phosphorus

## Iron

*Source.* Iron is found in a readily available form in liver, muscle meat, heart and soya beans. Spinach, blood, wheat and oats are also useful sources.

*Function.* Most of the iron in the body is present in the blood where it plays an essential role in the formation and function of haemoglobin. It is also present in the myoglobin of the muscles and is stored in bone marrow, liver and spleen.

*Deficiency.* Because of its essential role in haemoglobin formation, iron deficiency is usually manifest as anaemia. In the dog and cat, however, dietary iron deficiency is rare, as the normal food materials contain an abundant supply. Anaemia, may, however, occur due to chronic intestinal bleeding or heavy intestinal or skin parasitism in which the iron deficiency is secondary to impaired absorption or increased losses.

*Recommended allowance per 100 g of diet (dry basis):*
    Dog, 6 mg     Cat, 10 mg

## Sodium

*Sources.* Sodium is present in all naturally occurring foodstuffs and in all proprietary foods.

*Function.* Sodium is the main inorganic constituent of extracellular fluid and is essential for normal fluid and electrolyte balance and for cardiovascular function.

*Deficiency.* Dietary deficiency is unlikely as sodium is widely available in natural foodstuffs and is usually present in proprietary dog and cat foods at 1–2% dry weight. In sodium depletion the main signs are fatigue, decrease in blood pressure and haemoconcentration (high haematocrit values).

## Toxicity

Dogs and cats will readily tolerate sodium chloride levels of 3–4% (dry weight) in the diet, but water intake increases in proportion to salt intake. Drinking of large quantities of sea water and subsequent deprivation of drinking water have, however, caused death by salt poisoning in dogs.

*Recommended allowance (as sodium chloride) per 100 g of diet (dry basis):*
    Dog, 1.1%     Cat, 0.5%

## Other minerals

Dogs and cats have a dietary requirement for potassium, magnesium, copper, manganese, zinc, iodine, selenium, fluorine and probably other trace elements such as molybdenum, tin, silicon, nickel, vanadium and chromium, and theoretically a dietary deficiency of any one or more of these elements is possible. It is, however, unlikely as these elements occur naturally in most foodstuffs in sufficient quantities to meet requirements. The recommended allowances in the diets are given below.

*Recommended allowance per 100 g of diet (dry basis):*

|  | Dog | Cat |
| --- | --- | --- |
| Potassium (g) | 0.6 | 0.3 |
| Magnesium (g) | 0.04 | 0.05 |
| Copper (mg) | 0.7 | 0.5 |
| Manganese (mg) | 0.5 | 1.0 |
| Zinc (mg) | 5.0 | 3.0 |
| Iodine (mg) | 0.2 | 0.1 |
| Selenium (mg) | 0.01 | 0.01 |

## Foods

Increased controls over human food hygiene, such as the Meat (Sterilization) Regulations 1969, have reduced, if not abolished, the once general availability of cheap meat which, though unfit for human consumption, could be sold for dogs and cats. Even if such sources again became available, it is doubtful if the modern housewife would be willing to prepare such material in her kitchen. Furthermore, the amount of waste or scrap food from the household has decreased with the increasing use of convenience foods.

These changes have resulted in a progressive increase in the proportion of commercially prepared foods in the diet of pet animals, though a substantial amount (approximately 50%) of the total food intake of dogs in the United Kingdom is met from other sources.

### Homemade food

Dogs can be fed nutritious and highly palatable homemade diets if the owner is prepared to expend the necessary time, money and care. It would be inappropriate to give a selection of detailed canine recipes in this book, but a few guiding principles may be given.

*Protein.* Scrap meat from the butcher tends to have a high fat content, so a significant amount of trimming of fat may be necessary. Scrap fish and liver may be hard to come by in sufficient amounts, but are excellent protein sources. Eggs and cheese are also well accepted and useful protein sources, but milk powder can only be used in limited quantities without provoking diarrhoea (p. 532). Beans and peas make a useful contribution but have a relatively low palatability and a well-merited reputation for causing flatulence.

*Fat.* Though readily available from the butcher and an excellent energy source, a high fat diet will reduce the intake of other nutrients and must therefore be used sparingly, particularly for growing and lactating animals.

*Carbohydrate.* Dogs will readily accept carbohydrate-rich foods such as bread, boiled potatoes, rice and pasta, though their bland taste usually requires enhancement with other material of animal origin to increase palatability. Bread and potatoes make some contribution to protein intake, while that of the others is relatively low. Thus their proportion of the total diet must be restricted.

*Vitamins.* **Most vitamins will be supplied by a mixed diet** of meat, liver, fish, eggs, milk and cereals. Prolonged cooking will, however, destroy some vitamins, notably vitamin A and some of the B complex. The cooking water should be fed with the other constituents to preserve the vitamins and minerals which are leached into it.

*Minerals.* Natural sources of calcium and phosphorus include milk or milk powder, cheese, whole eggs, sterilized bone meal and ground bone. Other minerals will be provided in sufficiency by a mixed diet of the nutrients so far listed.

Green and root vegetables provide a useful and relatively cheap source of vitamins, protein and vegetable fibre. The palatability of these materials to dogs and cats is, however, generally low, and the general **acceptability of the meal may be depressed** if included in large amounts.

### Commercial foods

Commercial foods for dogs and cats are available in three basic forms: canned, semi-moist and dry. Frozen foods and sausages are also available but are much less common than the others.

The main characteristics of the canned,

TABLE 3.7.

|  | Canned | Semi-moist | Dry |
|---|---|---|---|
| **Appearance** | Soft, meaty | Firmer, like minced meat or chunks of raw meat | Hard, particulate, various shapes and colours |
| **Smell** | Meaty or fishy | Little | Little |
| **Food Ingredients** | Meat and meat byproducts, fish, cereal, vegetable protein, bone, blood, vitamins and minerals | Meat, poultry or fish meals, cereals, fat, dry milk, soya<br>Vitamins and minerals | Cereals, meat, poultry or fish meals, fat, dry milk<br>Vitamins and minerals |
| **Preservation** | Heat-sterilized sealed containers | Humectants propylene glycol, glycerol, sugar | Too dry for bacterial growth |
| **Palatability** | + + + | + + | + |
| **Cost per kJ** | + + + | + + | + |
| **Nutritional completeness** | Most meet the nutritional requirements of the adult<br>Some meet nutritional requirements for growth and reproduction | | |
| **Typical analysis** | | | |
| Moisture (%) | 75 | 25 | 8 |
| Protein (%) | 8 | 19 | 21 |
| Fat (%) | 4 | 9 | 8 |
| Carbohydrate (%) | 12 | 40 | 55 |
| Calcium (%) | 0.4 | 0.8 | 1.1 |
| Phosphorus (%) | 0.3 | 0.8 | 0.9 |
| Energy: | | | |
| kJ/kg | 3780 | 13,020 | 15,120 |
| kcal/per 100 g | 90 | 310 | 360 |

semi-moist and dry foods are shown in Table 3.7.

## Nutritional Characteristics of Prepared Foods

A wide variety of commercial prepared foods is available to the dog and cat owner, and his choice will be influenced by his own subjective assessment of the food's colour, texture, smell and price, the reputation of the manufacturer and the reaction of his or her pet to the food.

An increasing amount of information is being included on the labels, and it always pays to read it. Some foods are formulated to meet nutritional requirements when fed on their own without any other supplementary food (complete foods); others are designed to be fed with other foods.

*Complete foods.* If the manufacturer claims that the food meets all the nutritional requirements of the dog or cat it means that **the nutrient content of the product by analysis will meet the known nutrient requirements of the animals** for which it is intended. In addition, some manufacturers will have carried out practical feeding trials maintaining adults and possibly growing or reproducing animals over long periods.

*Canned foods.* The canned foods are distinguished from the semi-moist and dry by their higher palatability, moist and meaty texture and the presence of cooked, fresh, raw materials. They may or may not contain cereal. The presence of cereal gives a higher energy content and usually alters the texture to a more loaf-like appearance.

The canned foods for dogs, which do not contain cereal, should be mixed with a biscuit or other carbohydrate source,

TABLE 3.8. *Comparative protein levels (wet and dry (a) basis)*

| | Canned | | Semi-moist | Dry |
|---|---|---|---|---|
| | No cereal | With cereal | | |
| Protein (% wet matter) | 9 | 8 | 19 | 21 |
| Protein (% dry matter) | 50 | 32 | 25 | 23 |

(a) Dry matter (DM) content of food = 100—moisture content (%)
Thus DM content of canned food = $(100 - 75)\%$
$$= 25\%$$

Therefore protein content (% DM) $= 8 \times \dfrac{100}{25}$
for canned food with cereals
$$= 32\%$$

otherwise their relatively higher protein content is used wastefully as an energy source (instead of its more important function in protein metabolism). The protein content of canned foods is greater than other foods in relation to its other nutrients—as shown by expressing the values in Table 3.7 on a dry-weight basis (Table 3.8).

Canned foods for cats are also formulated with or without cereal, but because of the cats' higher protein requirement it is justifiable to feed products containing no added cereal on their own.

*Semi-moist foods.* Specialized processing and the inclusion of **humectants** such as propylene glycol, glycerol, sorbitol, butane-diol or sugars permit these foods to be preserved at a higher moisture content (20–25%) and a softer texture than dry foods and without the necessity of processing at a high temperature and packing in sealed cans.

Nutritionally they are often formulated to provide all nutrient requirements without other supplementary foods. Because of their higher calorie and lower water content they require to be fed in smaller amounts than canned foods—and both dogs and cats will require more drinking water.

*Dry foods.* Prepared by baking or expanding under heat, dry foods may be formulated as complete foods for dogs or cats or as supplementary foods to be added to meat. The complete dry foods have a substantial amount of animal protein as meat, fish or poultry meals and have added fat, vitamins and minerals to meet nutritional requirements and may be fed dry or moistened with warm water or milk (particularly for puppies or kittens). The biscuits or meals are predominantly cereal, though there may be some added protein or minerals, and are designed to provide an economical energy source when mixed with meat or canned meat.

### Principles of feeding the adult dog and cat

*Time of feeding.* The integration of the animal's feeding time into the domestic arrangements requires thought. It should be **at a time convenient to its owners** when they are least likely to be hurried or have to change or delay the process. Feeding is one of the highlights of the pet animal's day and should be treated as such. Feeding should never be too late in the day, thus allowing several hours before the animal is shut up at night. As ingestion of the main meal causes increased peristalsis and is also associated with increased fluid intake, the need to defaecate and urinate

TABLE 3.9.    *Guide to the daily food requirements for maintenance of dogs of different weights*

| Weight of dog | | ME required | | Canned(a) (kg/dog) | Semi-moist(a) (kg/dog) | Dry(a) (kg/dog) |
|---|---|---|---|---|---|---|
| kg | lb | kJ/day | kcal/day | | | |
| 2.3 | 5 | 1,033 | 247 | 0.21 | 0.08 | 0.07 |
| 4.5 | 10 | 1,707 | 408 | 0.35 | 0.13 | 0.11 |
| 6.8 | 15 | 2,326 | 556 | 0.48 | 0.18 | 0.15 |
| 9.1 | 20 | 2,895 | 692 | 0.60 | 0.22 | 0.19 |
| 13.6 | 30 | 3,912 | 935 | 0.81 | 0.30 | 0.26 |
| 22.7 | 50 | 5,744 | 1,373 | 1.19 | 0.44 | 0.38 |
| 31.8 | 70 | 7,347 | 1,768 | 1.54 | 0.57 | 0.49 |
| 49.8 | 110 | 10,355 | 2,475 | 2.15 | 0.80 | 0.69 |

(a) Assuming the metabolizable energy values on Table 3.7 in the analysis.

TABLE 3.10.    *Guide to the daily food requirements for maintenance of the adult cat*

| | Weight of cat | | ME required kJ/day | Canned(a) (g/cat) | Semi-moist(b) (g/cat) | Dry(c) (g/cat) |
|---|---|---|---|---|---|---|
| | kg | lb | | | | |
| Inactive | 2.2–4.5 | 5–10 | 604–1318 | 154–315 | 49–100 | 43–88 |
| Active | 2.2–4.5 | 5–10 | 782–1598 | 187–382 | 59–121 | 52–10 |

(a) ME = 4,200 kJ/kg (100 kcal per 100 g).
(b) ME = 13,230 kJ/kg (315 kcal per 100 g).
(c) ME = 15,120 kJ/kg (360 kcal per 100 g).

during the following three or four hours should be recognized and sufficient opportunity given.

*Quantity of feed.* The estimated daily food requirements for dogs and cats are shown in Tables 3.9 and 3.10. There are, however, very large individual variations even between dogs of the same size under similar conditions. The only real monitor of food requirements is **the condition and behaviour of the animal.** Most owners err on the liberal side as manifested by the high level of obesity in the canine population. No opportunity should be lost to advise owners to reduce food intake when fat animals are presented for whatever reason. Where an owner is genuinely giving a small amount of food, then the likelihood is that the animal is augmenting its rations from other sources—a more difficult problem to solve.

Food which is left in the bowl after the meal should invariably be removed and no more presented until the next meal— and then in reduced quantity. Between-meal snack feeding is to be deplored as it leads usually to obesity and the social disadvantage of a "begging" animal.

In changing from one category of food, say canned, to another, say semi-moist, the relatively greater (×3) energy density of the latter must be realized in reduction of the quantity offered, and the change-over brought about by stages over two or three days.

*Frequency of feeding.* Adult dogs and cats will satisfactorily maintain health and body weight on one meal per day. Two or more meals can, however, be fed provided this does not result in increasing the total daily intake and provided the principles in the section "Time of feeding" (p. 197) are followed. **Increased feeding frequency** can be a successful way of increasing the body weight of animals that are too thin.

*Water.* Water should always be available during the day, particularly at meal times, and particularly with dry foods. The amount required depends on the moisture content of the food and other factors such as exercise and ambient temperature.

*Hygiene.* Food bowls should be washed thoroughly between meals, but not at the same time, and ideally not in the same place as the family dishes.

*Multiple feeding.* While competition with another animal at mealtime may be a wonderful cure for anorexia, arrangements for feeding of several animals should be such that the weaker is not threatened by the stronger, faster eaters.

*Food temperature.* Very cold food is much less palatable than food at room temperature or, better, blood heat. An inappetant or convalescent animal is often **encouraged to eat by warm food**, and the practice of feeding food straight from the refrigerator is to be avoided.

*Table scraps.* Consumption of food remains from the family table is a traditional function of the family pet. It would indeed be wasteful to discard material of this nature which has some food value for a dog or cat. These should not, however, be given at any time other than the animal's normal meal time and should be incorporated into his other food. Bearing in mind that the scrap food is probably the least acceptable and nutritious of the human food, the proportion given should as a general rule be not greater than 25% on a regular basis.

*Bones.* There is a lack of general agreement about the value and safety of bones for dogs. Large marrow bones present no hazard as potential foreign bodies. However, dogs and cats which are accustomed to getting a wide variety of bones will rarely suffer harm from most bones with the possible exception of chop bones and some chicken bones. Undoubtedly the marrow bone is thoroughly enjoyed and contributes protein, fat, calcium, phosphorus and dental health to the dog's nutritional status and well-being. One disadvantage of the bone is that it may be defended with unusual ferocity—and it is advisable to accustom the young puppy to having a bone removed and any objection firmly discouraged. The growls of a six-week-old pup can be amusing but those of a two-year-old less so, particularly if it is a Great Dane.

*Grass.* Most dogs chew grass occasionally, some regularly. For some it is a preamble to vomiting, but by no means always. The reasons for grass eating are not clear, though it may be in response to **a need for the vegetable fibre** which is a regular component of the wild dog's diet. It is not a cause for concern unless the grass has just been treated with a herbicide.

*Coprophagia.* Like grass eating, no clear cause has been established for faeces eating. It is, of course, normal behaviour for the bitch with puppies, and licking of the puppy's perianal region is an important stimulus for evacuation of its bowels and bladder. It is particularly prevalent in animals confined in kennels or small yards, which suggests that it may well be a behavioural **response to boredom** rather than a dietary or nutritional phenomenon.

### Feeding the growing puppy or kitten

The nutritional requirements of growing puppies or kittens are **two to three times those of an adult** of the same weight. Furthermore, it is during growth that the basic structure of the hard and soft tissue is formed and the genetic potential in terms of conformation and size is realized. If feeding is incorrect, poor conformation

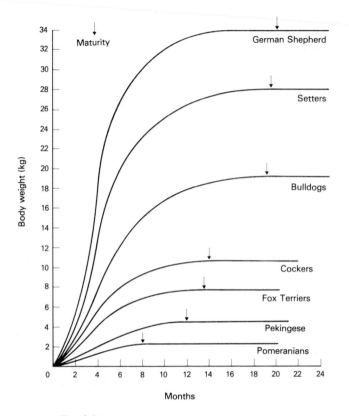

Fig. 3.26.    Average growth of various dog breeds.

will result no matter how good the parentage, and conversely there is no nutritional regime which will develop good conformation or characteristics if the genetic potential is not there.

The growth curves of some common breeds of dogs are shown in Fig. 3.26.

One question which is unresolved is whether maximum growth rate can be equated with optimum conformation and health. Work with Great Danes suggested that a high consumption of a protein, mineral and vitamin-rich diet caused abnormal bone development and unwillingness to move about freely, compared to littermates fed a more restricted amount of the same diet. Work with laboratory rodents has shown that animals on diets which supported maximum growth rate had a shorter life expectancy than those fed for lower growth rates.

*General principles.* This higher nutritional requirement of the growing animal does not necessarily mean a need for special foods. Given the right basic food of adequate palatability and the opportunity to eat throughout the day, the puppy will obtain its extra nutrient requirements simply by eating two or three times as much as an adult of the same weight.

The young puppy recently taken from its mother should initially be fed four times during a 16-hour period each day. There are no rigid guidelines for the reduction in frequency with age, and it will be found that the need and desire for one of these feeds and then another decreases as the pup begins to consume a greater proportion of its needs at each meal.

By 3 months three meals per day, and by 6 months two meals per day is probably enough. Only when the animal has stopped growing is it reasonable to reduce frequency to one meal per day.

Commercial foods which are recommended for puppies provide a reliable way of feeding a growing puppy. Homemade diets can also be fed with good results but some experience is necessary or should be sought to ensure that the balance of protein, fat, vitamins and minerals is right.

The informed breeder will usually be happy to give advice and an indication of what **the previous dietary regime** has been. While it may not be possible to follow the previous regime, specialist advice of this nature can be very useful.

Variety of foods, while not essential, adds to an animal's interest in its food and gives the owner experience in the relative palatability characteristics and value for money of a wide range of foods.

*Ad libitum* feeding of puppies is more widely practised in the United States than in the United Kingdom and is more appropriate to the use of dry and semi-moist foods than canned. Such feeding may result in obesity, is a less-controlled situation than meal feeding and dispenses with the mutually rewarding nature of the meal-time occasion for owner and dog.

## Supplements

Milk or milk replacers are useful supplements for growing puppies, though cow's milk may in a few puppies cause diarrhoea if given in large amounts. Even if milk is given, it is not a substitute for water, which should always be available.

Vitamin B supplements such as yeast tablets may be given—particularly as a reward during training—but vitamin and mineral supplements are unnecessary and, if given in excess, potentially harmful if a balanced diet is being given.

## Feeding the pregnant bitch

There are relatively few special nutritional or feeding requirements of the bitch during gestation. The following are, however, some general principles which should be followed.

Body weight at mating should be stable at the desired weight for the breed. Provided that a balanced diet is being used, the normal feeding and exercising regime should be continued during the first 6 weeks of pregnancy. While occasional sickness may occur, the diet should not be changed unless food intake decreases. Body condition and weight should show little change and any tendency to obesity be controlled.

During the last two or three weeks of gestation, food intake may be increased slowly by **augmenting the protein** or meaty component of the diet. If the bitch has previously been receiving one meal per day, the increase is best achieved by introducing a second small meal, since the greater volume occupied by the uterus and its contents restricts space in the abdomen. The amount of extra food at this time depends on the breed and the number of foetuses—thus a maiden bitch with only a few foetuses will require a smaller increase in food than a bitch likely to have eight or ten puppies. During the last week or so the food should be appetizing, nutritious, non-bulky and readily digestible.

The bitch may go off her food in the last day or so of gestation, but can often be tempted by small quantities of an appetizing food rather than the usual larger meals. It is, of course, important that water be constantly available. Complete commercial foods of good quality, whether canned, semi-moist or dry, are quite satisfactory throughout gestation, though it is probably more likely for the bitch to lay down fat on the semi-moist and dry foods if fed *ad libitum.*

### Feeding the bitch and puppies

After parturition the bitch should be offered frequent small meals with plenty of fluid for a day or so while the uterus involutes, but gradually be returned to her balanced diet. Food requirement and intake will quickly increase if sufficient opportunity and appetizing food is given. It is important to realize that by the time the pups are about 3 weeks old the bitch may require at least **three times her maintenance ration** in order to provide for her litter and retain her own condition. Any sudden decrease in food intake during early lactation should be immediately noticed as it may be the first sign of milk fever or eclampsia due to a decrease in blood calcium, mastitis (inflammation of the mammary gland) or metritis (inflammation of the womb), and immediate veterinary attention is indicated.

If the litter is large, hand-feeding may be used to supplement the bitch's milk supply. Commercial milk substitutes are readily obtainable or a home made substitute can be made from a blend of 8 fluid oz (1 cup) of a 50/50 mixture of milk and cream, 1 yolk of egg. This mixture can be stored in the refrigerator for up to 2 days, sufficient only for each meal being removed and warmed to blood heat immediately prior to feeding. All, or only a selected few, of the puppies can be supplemented depending on their apparent hunger. The well fed and the hungry pups are easily distinguished, the well fed being

placid, quiet and sleepy after feeding, while the hungry one remains awake restless and whimpering (p. 671).

**Weaning** should begin at about 3 weeks when the bitch begins to tire of the puppies' constant demands for milk. The puppies can then be offered small amounts of a good quality commercial puppy food prepared to the manufacturer's instruction or any complete food mixed with a little boiled warm water or warm milk in the form of a gruel. Healthy pups need little teaching or encouragement to start feeding, but the backward puppy should be given some assistance if the competition is strong. Weaning is usually complete at 5–6 weeks when the pups are able to eat and drink satisfactorily. As the puppies grow older the consistency of the food can be made firmer and the quantity steadily increased.

Following the peak of her lactation at about 3 weeks after parturition, the bitch's food intake can be slowly reduced. If she is below her usual weight, she should be kept on a fairly high plane of nutrition with a liberal protein and mineral intake for a few weeks until she has regained her normal weight. Yeast tablets may well improve this recovery. Loss of weight and condition during lactation can, however, be prevented if sufficient of a balanced diet is fed three or four times a day.

### Feeding orphaned puppies

The rearing of very young puppies by hand requires special feeding, care and conditions.

Apart from food, a primary requirement for young puppies reared away from the bitch is warmth. The recommended air temperature for new-born puppies is 29–32°C. This temperature should be maintained for the first 5 days after whelping. The following week the temper-

TABLE 3.11.   *Composition of milk of cow and dog*

|  | Bitch | Cow |
|---|---|---|
| Protein (g per 100 g) | 7.1 | 3.4 |
| Fat (g per 100 g) | 8.3 | 3.7 |
| Lactose (g per 100 g) | 3.8 | 4.8 |
| Energy: kJ/kg | 5082 | 2720 |
| (kcal per 100 g) | 121 | 65 |
| Calcium (mg per 100 g) | 230 | 120 |
| Phosphorus (mg per 100 g) | 160 | 95 |

ature may be reduced to 27°C and during the fourth to sixth weeks reduced further to 24°C.

Cow's milk alone is unsuitable for puppies as it contains too much lactose and too little protein, fat, calcium and phosphorus relative to bitches' milk (Table 3.11).

The easiest, but not necessarily the cheapest solution, is to use one of the proprietary bitch's milk substitutes which are available. However, a satisfactory home-made recipe can be made up such as that described previously (p. 202) or a more complex mixture of:

800 ml whole cow's milk
200 ml cream (12% fat)
1 egg yolk
6 oz white steamed bone meal
30000 IU vitamin A
500 IU vitamin D

This is mixed together with a beater, adding 4 g of citric acid for acidification. The mixture is fed at blood temperature six times a day for 3 weeks; then five times a day until the puppies begin eating solid or semi-solid foods. The mixture contributes about 1 kcal/g. The amount required by a 5-day-old puppy weighing 680 g is about 90 g/day.

Puppies may be fed from a doll-sized bottle and nipple or an eye dropper. Alternatively, puppies can be successfully reared by feeding through a stomach tube using a human male urethral catheter or an infant feeding tube (No. 8 size French) (p. 670).

## Feeding the working dog

The main difference between the working dog—guide dog, police dog, sheep dog, army dog, sledge dog—and the pet dog is the expenditure of and therefore the requirement for energy. Although energy is obtained from the protein, fat and carbohydrate components of the food, the most economical way to provide the additional energy is by increasing the proportion of carbohydrate and/or fat in the diet. There is no evidence that the protein needs of a dog doing hard exercise are any greater than for maintenance.

It is not uncommon for dogs to lose weight under hard working conditions despite being offered increased amounts of food. While some weight loss may be acceptable or desirable, it may progress so that the dog's condition, fitness and performance are impaired. In such cases weight loss may be arrested or reversed by:

*Increasing the frequency of feeding.* A dog only fed once a day, particularly after a hard day's work, may be too fatigued to eat sufficient to maintain body weight.

*Increasing the palatability of the food.* If, despite weight loss, the dog will not eat the increased amount of food offered, palatability can be increased by offering a different food, moistening or even warming the food. While the addition of a more meaty component is not a requirement, it may provoke the required increase in total food intake by increased palatability.

*Increasing the energy density of the food.* If the food, though palatable and adequate for maintenance, has a low calorie content, then the dog may be unable to accommodate the increased amount needed to offset his increased energy requirement. Energy intake can be increased by adding fat or changing to a food with a more concentrated energy content.

### Feeding the ailing or convalescent dog

Little work has been done on clinical nutrition in dogs and the following are general comments which may be applicable to a number of conditions.

*Inappetence.* Loss of appetite may be the first or only sign of the onset of disease. Provided that the cause is not simply unappetizing food, effort should be directed at diagnosing the underlying cause rather than coaxing the animal to eat.

*Vomiting and diarrhoea.* Both vomiting and diarrhoea are usually grounds for withholding all food for at least 24 hours until a diagnosis has been made or the condition has cleared. Reintroduction of food should be slow and in small frequent meals rather than an immediate return to the normal regime (p. 531).

*Post-operative feeding.* After any operation involving anaesthesia, small meals of palatable and digestible food should be given on the following day—but certainly not until all anaesthetic effects have worn off. Liquid or semi-liquid foods are preferable for several days after gastrointestinal surgery.

*Convalescence.* After a prolonged illness, particularly with sustained antibiotic therapy, protein and vitamin supplements may well be indicated to aid recovery of condition and body weight. Proprietary convalescent diets are available and have been used successfully with hospitalized dogs.

*Diabetes mellitus.* The essential principle is to balance energy expenditure, energy intake and insulin dosage. Feeding of a good proprietary complete canned food is a good way of ensuring a constant energy intake. Several meals spaced throughout the day are better than one meal a day. Semi-moist foods, or any foods containing sugars, are contraindicated.

*Obesity.* By far the commonest disease of nutritional origin affecting dogs in Britain, obesity is often difficult to treat. The main problem is in convincing the owner to treat it seriously. The basic action is to reduce the dog's total calorie intake so that it loses weight. The diet should be completely changed no matter what the previous regime, and a diet of low calorie density substituted. Proprietary products for weight reduction are beneficial not only in reducing the dog's calorie intake but in convincing the owner that the condition is treatable and worth treating.

*Chronic nephritis.* One of the causes of malaise and sickness in chronic nephritis is the failure of the kidneys to excrete the end products of protein metabolism, resulting in uraemia. Clinical improvement can be obtained by reducing total protein intake either by feeding a proprietary low protein diet or by formulating a home-made diet with the lowest protein levels which are compatible with the maintenance of body weight and condition.

If there are substantial protein losses via the kidney, a higher compromise level of protein intake may have to be attained in order to prevent protein depletion, muscle wastage and increased susceptibility to other disease processes.

## (g) Genetics and Animal Breeding

SUSAN LONG

Genetics is the science of heredity, the study of how characteristics or traits are transmitted from parents to offspring in both plants and animals. The modern science of genetics began when Gregor Mendel, a monk living in Czechoslovakia at the turn of the last century, discovered that some characteristics were transmitted from parents to offspring in a predictable manner by means of genetic material called genes. These were the hereditary characteristics. In order to understand how genes are responsible for hereditary characteristics it is first necessary to understand the processes involved in cell division.

### Cell Division

A cell consists of a nucleus surrounded by cytoplasm. It is the structures within the nucleus which control the cell and the most important of these are the *chromosomes*. Chromosomes are composed of chromatin fibres held together at the *centromere* and these fibres contain the genetic material which form the *genes*. Chromosomes are only individually visible under the microscope when the cell is dividing, because in the non-dividing or *interphase* cell their fibres are elongated and form a confused network. Each species of animal and plant has a specific number of chromosomes. For example, all domestic dogs have 78 chromosomes, whilst the domestic cat has 38 chromosomes. Two of the chromosomes are the

*sex chromosomes* and are called either the X or the Y. A female mammal has two X chromosomes, whilst a male mammal has one X and one Y chromosome. The remaining chromosomes are called the *autosomes*. The autosomes are composed of pairs of chromosomes which are alike. Because of their similarity they are called *homologous* chromosomes from the Greek word *homo* meaning "same". The dog, therefore, has 38 homologous pairs of autosomal chromosomes and two sex chromosomes, giving a total of 78.

Cells normally divide by a process of *mitosis* (Fig. 3.27). This begins with the disappearance of the nuclear membrane. Each chromosome then splits into two identical fibres, called chromatids, which are held together at the centromere. The chromosomes arrange themselves so that their centromeres are in a line along the centre of the cell. The chromatids then pull apart from their partners until the centromere splits and the separated chromatids move to opposite sides of the cell. Meanwhile, the cytoplasm begins to divide. The nuclear membrane reforms around the chromosomes and the cell is completely divided. The result is two new cells with the same number of chromosomes as the original cell.

A different type of cell division occurs in the testis and ovaries when the germ cells or gametes, i.e. spermatozoa and ova, are formed. This type of cell division is called *meiosis* (Fig. 3.28). It begins as in mitosis with the formation of chromatids but then each chromosome aligns with its

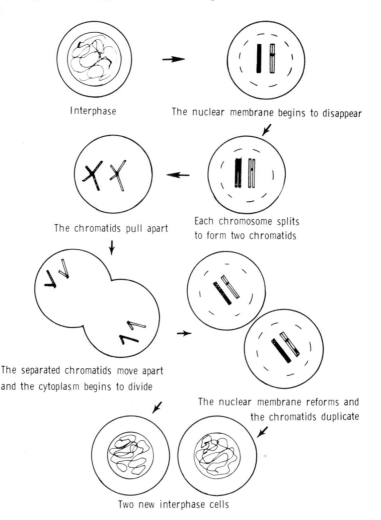

Interphase

The nuclear membrane begins to disappear

The chromatids pull apart

Each chromosome splits to form two chromatids

The separated chromatids move apart and the cytoplasm begins to divide

The nuclear membrane reforms and the chromatids duplicate

Two new interphase cells

FIG. 3.27.    Diagrammatic representation of a mitotic division of a cell.

homologous partner. The four chromatids become entwined and exchange segments. This is called *crossing-over*. Crossing-over may occur at any point along the length of a chromosome and at more than one point. Once crossing-over is finished the chromosomes move apart and the cellular cytoplasm divides. However, the nuclear membrane does not reform because each cell immediately divides again by a mitotic division. The result is four new cells each with only half the number of chromosomes of the original cell. These are the sperm or ova. When a sperm fertilizes an ovum the result is a fertilized egg called a *zygote* which has the full number of chromosomes. In this way the new individual inherits the genetic material from each parent but with some variation because of the crossing-over. Thus offspring resemble their parents and yet are different from them.

## The Inheritance of a Pair of Genes

As it has been stated, genes are located

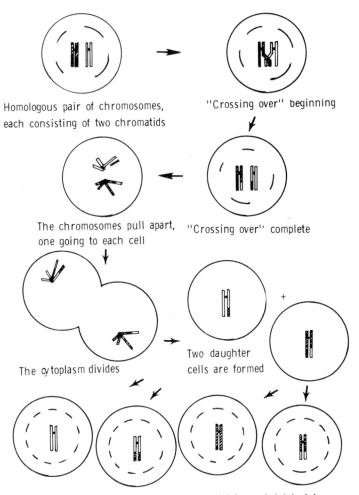

Homologous pair of chromosomes,
each consisting of two chromatids

"Crossing over" beginning

The chromosomes pull apart,
one going to each cell

"Crossing over" complete

The cytoplasm divides

Two daughter
cells are formed

Each daughter then divides by a mitotic division.   A total of four
gametes are produced from one original cell

Fig. 3.28.   Diagrammatic representation of a meiotic division of a cell.

on the chromosome. Each gene has its own allocated place on a particular chromosome. This place is called the *gene locus.* Since an individual inherits one chromosome of each pair of homologous chromosomes from each parent, it follows that he receives two of any particular gene. In this way genes are considered to occur in pairs. A gene at any given locus may have more than one form. All genes that can occupy the same gene locus are called **alleles** or *allelomorphs.* Those genes which can suppress the effect of the allelomorphic partner are called *dominant* genes. They are denoted by a capital letter, e.g. B for black. Those genes whose effects are masked by their partners are called *recessive* genes. These are denoted by a small letter, e.g. b for liver colour. Sometimes alleles are not completely dominant or recessive. In this situation they are said to show incomplete dominance, and the effect produced is a mixture of each. An animal can only carry two alleles from any allelic series because each chromosome only has one partner—its homologue. An animal is said to be *homozygous* for a gene when both allelomorphic partners are identical, e.g. BB. When the two partners are dissimilar, e.g. Bb, then the animal is said to be *heterozygous* for a gene. The genetic make-up of an animal, which it receives from its parents, is said to be its *genotype*. The outward appearance of the animal is said to be its *phenotype*. The phenotype of an animal is obvious, but the genotype may be different from the phenotype because of the presence of recessive genes.

In order to understand the inheritance of genes it is important to know the first law of genetics which states: "Genes exist which influence characteristics. They exist in pairs and retain their identity from generation to generation". In the formation of gametes each gene separates from its partner so that the gamete has only one of each pair of genes. This law is demonstrated in Fig. 3.29.

## Identification of a Recessive—the "Back-cross"

Animals homozygous for a particular pair of genes will always breed true. In the example in Fig. 3.29, the black-spotted dog BB will always have black offspring. However, heterozygous black-spotted dogs Bb will produce some liver-spotted offspring if mated to another animal homozygous for the b gene. This type of mating is the *back-cross to the recessive* and it is used to identify a recessive gene in an individual whose phenotype is the same as an animal homozygous for a dominant gene (Fig. 3.30).

One example of a recessive gene which has a deleterious effect is that for peripheral progressive retinal atrophy (PRA). This is a condition seen in *inter alia* Poodles, Cocker Spaniels and Irish Setters, where there is progressive loss of vision due to a reduction in the blood supply to the retina. It is caused by a simple autosomal recessive gene, s. Animals which are homozygous for this gene (ss) suffer from the clinical condition. Conversely, animals which do not have this gene (SS) are not affected and cannot pass the condition to their offspring. However, heterozygous animals (Ss) are unaffected themselves but they carry the gene and can pass it to their offspring. By using the backcross to the homozygous recessive animal (Fig. 3.30) heterozygous animals can be identified and removed from the breeding popula-

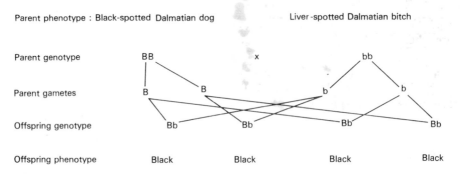

| Parent phenotype : Black-spotted Dalmatian dog | | | Liver-spotted Dalmatian bitch | |
|---|---|---|---|---|
| Parent genotype | BB | x | | bb |
| Parent gametes | B | B | b | b |
| Offspring genotype | Bb | Bb | Bb | Bb |
| Offspring phenotype | Black | Black | Black | Black |

FIG. 3.29.   Diagram of first law of genetics.

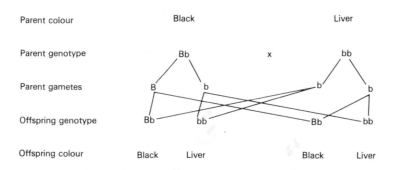

FIG. 3.30.   Diagram of identification of recessive gene.

tion. In this way the condition eventually can be eliminated altogether.

### Sex-linked Genes

Sex-linked genes are genes located on the sex chromosomes. The Y chromosome carries very few genes so that most examples are for genes on the X chromosome. The female, with two X chromosomes, can carry two alleles of a gene but the male, with only one X, can carry only one allele.

One important disease that is controlled by a sex-linked gene is haemophilia. This condition is manifested by very poor clotting of the blood so that even minor abrasions or bruises result in massive bleeding. The normal gene H is located on the X chromosome and its allele h, which causes haemophilia is a recessive. It follows therefore that a male, carrying the gene ($x^h$Y) will always be affected by the disease whereas a female may either be an unaffected carrier ($X^HX^h$) or suffer from haemophilia herself ($x^hx^h$). The homozygous condition is often lethal but some affected females have been known.

*A sex-limited gene*, by contrast, is one whose expression is limited to one sex. Such genes are not located on the sex chromosomes. For example, a gene controlling the volume of milk produced by a lactating female can be carried by the male as well as the female, but its effect can only be seen in the female.

### The Inheritance of More than One Pair of Genes

Animals obviously have a large number of genes controlling various factors. However, each pair of genes is inherited without being influenced by the presence of other genes. This is the second law of genetics, called the law of independent assortment, which states that "each pair of genes separate in the gamete independently of every other pair".

There are, however, a few exceptions to this law; for example, *Linkage*. Two pairs of genes are said to be linked when they occur on the same chromosome. They are even more closely linked when the occur close together on the same chromosome. At meiosis, closely linked genes tend to take part in the same cross-over event and so do not assort independently.

### Epistasis

Some genes affect the expression of other genes although they do not influence segregation at meiosis. When the genes are alleles they are said to be dominant but when they are not alleles they are said to be epistatic. This is seen in albino animals which are homozygous for a recessive gene, c. This prevents coat colour being expressed. A cc animal will be albino, irrespective of any other coat colour genes it may possess.

## Multifactorial Inheritance and the Influence of Environment

Most of the characteristics considered so far have been influenced by one gene or its alleles. However, a more common phenomenon is that a characteristic will be influenced by a number of genes, and a variation in any one gene will cause a slight variation in the characteristic or even a failure of expression of that characteristic. Furthermore, the degree to which the genes can be expressed will depend on the environment. For example, the size of a dog will depend upon the genes he possesses but also on the amount and type of food available. Characteristics that are governed in this way are difficult to influence by selective breeding. One genetic disease of this type is hip dysplasia seen in, for example, German Shepherd dogs and Labradors. This condition is caused by a number of genes inter-reacting with themselves and the environment and it is almost impossible to accurately identify carrier animals. For this reason it has not yet been possible to control the condition in affected breeds, a situation in marked contrast to that of PRA (see p. 208).

## Mutation

It has been previously stated, in the first law of genetics, that genes retain their identity from one generation to another. There are some exceptions to this rule. On some very rare occasions genes fail to duplicate themselves exactly and there is a slight mistake in their structure. This is called mutation. Most instances of mutation cause the gene to fail to function and this is incompatible with the normal development and survival of an individual. These are called lethal mutations. However, a small number of mutations are beneficial in that they convey some competitive advantage to the animal carrying the new gene. Mutations are important since they provide another means whereby offspring can differ from their parents.

## Breed Variations

Selection for various characters by careful breeding has caused the development of a number of different breeds of both cats and dogs. It has been so extensive in the dog that there are now six *breed groups* recognized by the English Kennel Club. These are hounds, gundogs, terriers, utility dogs, working dogs and toys. Cats have not undergone such intensive selection and are usually divided into long- and short-hair breeds. However, there is considerable variation in body size, length of head and of course coat colour. The variation in coat colour has been brought about because of the number of alleles for this characteristic. For example, the Siamese form of pigmentation is due to a gene $c^s$, which produces little pigmentation on the body with marked pigmentation on the points, i.e. those areas of the body with slightly lower temperatures. The Burmese coloration is due to a gene $c^b$, which is an allele of $c^s$. The $c^b$ gene is incompletely dominant to $c^s$ with the result that the first cross between a Burmese and Siamese results in an animal which shows slightly darker points than a Burmese but is not so pale bodied as a Siamese. In the United States such a cross is known as a Tonkanese.

One method of selecting for specific characteristics is by *inbreeding*. This involves the mating of individuals more closely related than animals chosen from the population at random. It usually implies very close relationship, for example, parent to offspring or brother to sister. Inbreeding has the advantage of rapidly increasing the homozygosity of the offspring and desired characteristics become fixed. However, it has the disadvantage of also producing homozygosity for undesirable characteristics. *Line breeding* is a form of inbreeding but the animals are not so closely related. It involves mating within a certain family, or line, and maintains a relationship with a particular ancestor. It has the advantage of preserving some desirable characteristics without too quickly increasing the number of undesirable ones.

By contrast to these two systems, *outbreeding* involves the breeding of individuals less closely related than mates chosen at random from a population. It increases heterozygosity and introduces new genes into the population. This type of cross conveys some superiority on the heterozygote which is said to show *heterosis* or *hybrid vigour*.

Genic strength!

## Deformities and Malformations

Any deviation from the normal anatomy is described as a malformation or deformity. These can arise during foetal development or be acquired during life. If they are present at birth they may be either an inherited defect or a congenital abnormality.

**Inherited defects** are caused by genes acquired from the parents. These genes are likely to be passed on by the affected individual to any offspring. The common inherited malformations are as follows:

*Common inherited conditions in the dog:*
Cryptorchidism
Entropion
Hip dysplasia
Hernia
Merle syndrome
Patella luxation
Polydactyly
Progressive retinal atrophy (PRA)

*Common inherited conditions in cats:*
Cryptorchidism
Polydactyly
Spina bifida in *Manx* cats

**Congenital abnormalities,** in contrast, are not inherited from the parents but occur because of a failure of normal foetal development. This failure may be due to the influence of environmental factors or to chemical agents. Such agents, which cause maldevelopment of the foetus, are called teratogenic agents or teratogens. The sort of abnormalities they may cause may be similar to, or indeed identical with, inherited disorders. It is, therefore, very important to be able to distinguish between an inherited abnormality and a congenitally acquired abnormality. Differentiation is based on careful examination of the case history and is often difficult.

Deformaties acquired during life, such as a bent leg following poor healing after a fracture, are never passed to offspring. Some genetic abnormalities are not apparent at birth and only manifest themselves when the animal is older, e.g. PRA. These abnormalities can be passed to the offspring at any time.

## Summary

It has been demonstrated that hereditary characteristics can be transferred from parents to offspring by means of genes which are located on the chromosome. In general, genes retain their identity from one generation to another and each pair of genes separate in the gamete independently from every other pair. However, because of crossing over during formation of gametes and because of the occurrence of mutations, no two individuals are exactly the same.

## Further Reading

ARNALL, L.K. and KEYMER, I.F. (1975) *Bird Diseases,* Baillière Tindall, London.

BLACKMORE, D.K. and LUCAS, J.F. (1965) A simple method for the accurate oral administration of drugs to budgerigars. *J. Small Anim. Pract.* **6,** 27–29.

COWIE, A.F. (1976) *Manual of the Care and Treatment of Children's and Exotic Pets.* BSAVA, London. (Supplemented 1979).

PETRAK, M.L. (1969) *Diseases of Cage and Aviary Birds.* Lea and Febiger, Philadelphia.

PFAFFENBERGER *et al.* (1976) *Guide Dogs for the Blind: Their Selection, Development and Training,* Elsevier, Amsterdam.

ROBINSON, R. (1977) *Genetics for Cat Breeders,* 2nd edn. Pergamon Press, Oxford.

ROBINSON, R. (1982) *Genetics for Dog Breeders.* Pergamon Press, Oxford.

WHITE, K. (1977) *Dogs: Their Mating, Whelping and Weaning.* K and R Books, Leicester.

# CHAPTER 4

# First Aid

S. HISCOCK

First aid is the immediate treatment of injured animals or those suffering from sudden illness.

It is the only situation in which a lay person may examine and give simple treatment to an animal in order to achieve the three principles of first aid:

1. **To preserve life.**
2. **To prevent suffering.**
3. **To prevent the condition of the patient deteriorating.**

Many first aid cases will be seen by the animal nurse at the surgery when the veterinary surgeon is not instantly available, and may be divided into:

(a) Life-threatening emergencies requiring immediate action by the owner at home and the nurse at the surgery e.g. unconsciousness, severe haemorrhage.

(b) Emergencies requiring immediate action at the surgery but where life is not imminently threatened e.g. fractures, wounds such as cut feet, tails, ears, etc. and accidents where internal injury may be suspected.

(c) Minor emergencies where telephone advice to the owner can alleviate suffering e.g. insect stings, minor burns, accidental intake of poisons.

When dealing with the emergency, there are four cardinal rules:

The editor acknowledges the work of Dr F. G. Startup who supplied information for this chapter in previous editions.

1. **Don't panic.**
2. **Maintain the airway.**
3. **Control the haemorrhage.**
4. **Contact the veterinary surgeon as soon as possible.**

**Phone calls**

In most cases, the owner of the animal will ring the surgery often in a state of distress to get help. It must be remembered that animals are usually very precious to their owners—emotionally, financially or both. Therefore the owner is rarely able to judge the severity of the illness or injury and questioning by the nurse may seem a time-wasting delay. However, history taking over the phone is very important, so that advice on immediate first aid can be given and correct preparations be made to receive the animal at the surgery. Bearing these points in mind, the nurse should remain calm but sympathetic and patient, ask specific questions clearly and concisely and advise on first aid measures which may be used to preserve the life of the patient until professional help can be given. "Second-hand" phone conversations are frustrating and lead to inaccuracy, so it is always best to speak to the owner direct to ascertain:

1. The name and the address of the owner, and phone number if possible.

2. The exact location of the animal if injured or taken ill away from home.

3. The age, sex and breed of the patient.

4. The nature of the injury e.g. scalding due to a household accident, burns from a house fire, road accident.

5. The extent or degree or injury—the appearance of the animal and posture of its body, severity of haemorrhage and wounds, ability to breathe freely, etc.

### Recognition of Major Injuries

History taking and a routine examination are essential to diagnose the extent of the injury. Only when the diagnosis has been made can treatment be commenced. However, the diagnosis must always be provisional, pending the veterinary surgeon's attendance on the case. When there is doubt as to the severity of the injury, the worst should be assumed and the patient treated accordingly.

### History taking

It is very important to obtain a full and correct case history. Failure to do so may result in false assumptions being made and wrong conclusions being drawn. Questions should be asked as to the previous health and treatment (if any) of the patient before the accident or illness e.g. is the patient a previously diagnosed diabetic, has she recently had pups, is a lameness due to chronic arthritis or an acute sprain?

### Routine examination

Firstly, the general condition and bearing of the patient should be assessed. This is of paramount importance in evaluating the overall condition of the animal and severity of its injuries.

The unconscious patient must always be treated as a serious case, but conscious patients can be more difficult to assess. The animal which is withdrawn, lies still and seems afraid to move, staring out on the world with blank unfocused eyes is a patient likely to be in serious trouble. The animal which follows the movement of human hands with its eyes and responds normally to human voice or touch is less likely to be suffering from life-threatening injuries.

The character and rate of the respiration should also be taken into account. Shallow, rapid respiration can denote shock or pain. Laboured deep respiration may be due to an airway obstruction or collapsed lungs.

Having ensured an unobstructed airway and controlled any severe haemorrhage, the patient should then be examined from nose to tail tip to ensure that no area of the body is left unchecked. The first aider must be able to appreciate any possible complications which may underlie a seemingly simple wound e.g. broken bones, penetration of thoracic or abdominal cavities etc. Forewarned is forearmed, and the mere suspension that there may be a serious complication can help the nurse to alleviate suffering, preserve life, and prevent the situation deteriorating.

### Examination

*Nose.* Note any haemorrhage (*epistaxis*) and whether it comes from one or both nostrils. Note any swellings which may suggest fracture of the nasal bones.

*Mouth.* Carefully open the mouth, if possible, to examine the bony structures for signs of fracture: splitting of the hard palate down its centre, jaw fractures.

Check for signs of haemorrhage and locate its source e.g. gums, tongue, palate etc. If no injuries are apparent, the blood may have been coughed up from the lungs or issued from wounds in the throat area.

If the gums or lips are not darkly pigmented, test the **capillary refill** by pressing the mucosa to blanch it (see Haemorrhage).

*Eyes. Eyeball.* Check for bruising to the sclera or conjunctiva. Note any injuries to the eyeball, prolapse of the eyeball or abnormal movement e.g. *nystagmus* (involuntary flicking movement of the eyeball from side to side).

*Pupils.* Note the size of the pupil in each eye and check for response to light. Brain damaged patients often show a difference in the size of the two pupils.

*Eyelids.* Check the palpebral reflex and examine the colour of the conjunctival mucosa for an indication of anaemia (pale pink or white), jaundice (yellow) or cyanosis (mauve colour).

*Skull.* Look for signs of depressed fractures, swelling, pain or crepitus.

*Ears.* Examine for signs of haemorrhage from the ear canal as this can occur with brain damage.

*Limbs.* Palpate all limbs for signs of swelling or pain. In cases of suspected deformity, it is useful to compare the injured leg with its normal partner. If a fracture is suspected, treat it as such pending diagnosis by the veterinary surgeon.

Record the way the limb is held and note any seeming paralysis—**flaccid** when the muscles are totally relaxed or **spastic** when the muscles are contracted to fix the limb rigidly in extension or flexion.

*Rib Cage.* Gently palpate for signs of fractured ribs, and listen to any wounds to detect a "hiss" sound on inspiration which indicates penetration of the pleural cavity.

*Abdomen.* Palpation of the abdomen is a skilled procedure and can cause considerable harm if attempted by the inexperienced. This procedure should not therefore be attempted. Haemorrhage from the penis or bruising of the abdominal wall should be noted.

*Spine.* Note any obvious deformities in the spinal column and gently palpate to detect any gross abnormalities. The spinal column is covered by large muscle trunks and severe spinal fractures are not always obvious. Always assume a fracture is present if there is any doubt.

*Pelvis.* Gently palpate the pelvic bones for signs of instability pain, crepitus and deformity.

*Perineal Region.* This should be examined for evidence of haemorrhage from skin wounds and from internal organs, e.g. the bladder.

In cases of paralysis, it is useful to note the presence or absence of the anal ring reflex by watching for anal sphincter contraction when a thermometer is inserted into the anus.

*Tail.* Observe the signs of voluntary movement e.g. correct carriage of the tail, wagging etc.

*General Body Surface.* Note any matting of the fur which may indicate an underlying wound. If in doubt as to the severity of the wound, assume the worst and treat accordingly. If foreign bodies are present, removal may be attempted unless they are embedded. Dislodging embedded foreign bodies may provoke more serious injury and must therefore be avoided.

Following the examination and first aid treatment of the animal, **make notes of the findings and mark the time of the examination.** Brain injuries in particular can rapidly deteriorate or improve over short periods of time, and it is vital to chart the course of events as accurately as possible.

When the examination and treatment are completed at the surgery, the animal should be made comfortable in a warm, quiet, darkened room, kennel or basket where it may feel secure. Direct heat, alcohol and other such stimulants should not be supplied to the shocked patient as this causes vasodilation of the blood vessels on the body surface. These blood vessels are "non essential" in cases of shock, and should be constricted. Dilation will result in an enlargement of the volume of the circulatory system "pipework" which has to be filled by the circulating blood. Enlarging this volume will cause a drop in the overall blood pressure. Vasodilation in the skin will also be more likely to restart haemorrhages from surface wounds. However, the body heat of the patient should be conserved by laying the animal on an insulated surface e.g. thick blankets, *"Vetbeds"*, polystyrene "bean bags" and covering the patient with further insulation to prevent heat loss from the body.

If a veterinary surgeon is not immediately available and there are no apparent contraindications to offering fluids (e.g. vomiting, unconsciousness), the patient should be offered a small drink. The ideal is a mixture of salt and bicarbonate to guard against the effects of shock. Half a teaspoonful of salt and half a teaspoonful of bicarbonate of soda to two pints of water is recommended. 25–100 ml should be offered every 30 minutes, depending on the size of the patient. (p. 315).

Constant observation of the patient is essential to continually reassess the condition, and any change in condition should be noted on kennel charts and case records.

**As soon as possible, veterinary assistance should be obtained, and the fully comprehensive notes should be handed to the veterinary surgeon in charge of the case.**

## Handling and Transport of Injured Animals

Unless life is endangered by falling masonry, fire, poisonous atmosphere etc., accident victims should be given a brief examination before attempting to move the animal so that injuries can be adequately protected.

In order to carry out this examination, the patient must first be restrained and it must be remembered that these animals are frightened and shocked, so the "softlee softlee catchee monkee" approach is usually necessary. Slow deliberate movements by humans accompanied by the continuous gentle reassurance of the human voice can do much to calm the anxious patient.

*Cats.* Shocked and injured cats are not usually aggressive when approached. Observe the animal closely whilst extending the hand to stroke under the chin. If this is permitted, slide the hand around the face to stroke the neck and then gently grasp the scruff. The animal is now restrained to allow an examination to be made. If the animal reacts aggressively when approached, do not persist in the attempt as this may only provoke an attack or make the cat try to escape. In these cases an inverted box or basket should be gently lowered over the cat to confine it, and a thin piece of hardboard or cardboard slid slowly under the inverted box so that the cat comes to lie on it. The whole may then be lifted and made secure for transport to the surgery.

*Dogs.* Frightened injured dogs are much more inclined to "have a go" at an approaching human, especially if it is a stranger. Even the dog's owner may get bitten if the normally placid pet is in pain from its injuries. If there is any indication of aggressiveness, try to drop a looped lead, arranged to form a running noose, over the dog's head. Many dogs immediately feel more secure if they are on a lead with a human in control but may still bite. A muzzle should therefore be tied in place before handling *unless the dog is dyspnoeic or the muzzle is injured.*

Once the animal is under control and the brief examination has been carried out, the airway is unobstructed and the haemorrhage is controlled, the patient should be restrained until transport can be arranged to move it to the surgery or until the veterinary surgeon can attend the animal. The animal should be allowed to assume the position which it finds most comfortable. Most injured animals will lie on the injured side which distresses the owners, but the patient should not be interfered with if comfortable. The owners should be asked to stay with the animal to reassure and comfort it.

### Transport to the surgery

*The aim*—to remove the injured animal to the surgery with minimal discomfort to the patient and without disturbing any dressings applied to the patient.

There are two groups of animals:

(1) *Ambulatory*—the dog which can rise to its feet and able to walk or just limp slowly. Often these dogs may be transpor-

ted less painfully if they are allowed to move themselves rather than submitting to the restrictions of being carried. Gentle encouragement should be used to lead the animal to the transport vehicle but assistance may be given to help the patient climb into the van or car.

(2) *Non ambulatory* (a) *Lifting in the owner's arms.* Small dogs and cats may be held firmly round the neck with one hand (taking care not to obstruct the breathing), whilst the other hand and arm are slid around the hindquarters and under the spine to "scoop" the body up, supporting the weight along the length of the forearm. (Fig. 4.1).

Medium-sized dogs may be lifted with one arm encircling the front of the sternum, the other around the back of the pelvis to support the hindquarters. The animal is then held against the handler's chest to support the trunk. If possible, the injured side should be held next to the handler's chest (Fig. 4.2).

Large heavy dogs should be lifted by two or more people. One person stands at the shoulder with one arm curled round under the dog's neck, holding the head against the handler's shoulder to control it. The second arm is passed under the thorax, just behind the front legs. The second person stands by the hindquarters

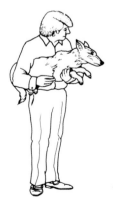

FIG. 4.1.

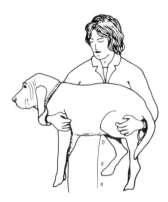

FIG. 4.2.

and places one arm under the abdomen just in front of the hind legs and the other around under the pelvis. Remember always to lift the heavy dog with an almost straight back using your bent knees to provide most of the lifting effort. Always ask for help if the dog seems too heavy for you.

None of these methods should be used in cases of suspected spinal fracture, and the last method must not be used in cases of suspected abdominal or thoracic injury.

(b) *Boxes and Baskets.* These are suitable for cats and small dogs. Types range from wire, wicker or wooden cages to cardboard boxes, laundry baskets, washing baskets etc! There are three important criteria:—

(i) The basket should be escape-proof—cardboard boxes, etc. should have a lid firmly secured on the open top.

(ii) Ventilation must be adequate. Meshwork sides are safer than solid wall boxes.

(iii) It should be possible to constantly observe the patient. Wire baskets and plastic laundry baskets are best for this.

(c) *Stretchers.* Stretchers should always be used to transport patients with suspected spinal factures who are too large to fit into boxes or baskets. They are also the easiest way to transport dogs whose in-juries are too severe to allow manhandling.

The principle is to have a flat, rigid object, which is big and strong enough to support the animal in lateral recumbancy, yet small enough to fit into the transport vehicle. Stretchers can be made from:

(i) Wood/hardboard sheets—very good for small or medium-sized dogs.

(ii) Wire mesh or plastic coated fencing wire. This may only be used if there are two handlers to stretch the wire taut when lifting the animal so that the wire provides a firm support.

(iii) Sacks/coats mounted on wooden poles as described for human patients (See First Aid, Junior Manual, British Red Cross Society).

(iv) Blankets—Offer little support for injured spines but may be slid underneath the patient easily. (Fig. 4.3).

**Transferring the patient to the stretcher**

1. Place the stretcher close to the patient's back as it lies on the ground.

2. Apply a tape muzzle to the conscious patient if possible as these animals often may be in pain and could bite when handled.

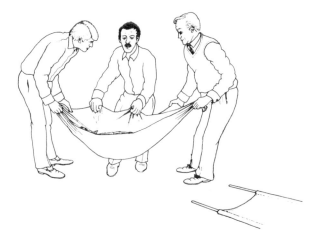

FIG. 4.3.

3. Either (a) roll the patient half on to its chest and push the stretcher underneath the animal as far as possible, before allowing the animal to collapse back on to its side and thus on to the stretcher. Several people should help in this movement to try to move the animal as a unit to avoid any twisting of the spine if a spinal injury is suspected.

Or (b) grasp the skin along the back at several points—above the scapula, midway along the back and above the pelvis. The patient may now be pulled the short distance on to the stretcher. This is particularly useful in cases of fractured limbs as it does not involve twisting the body or limbs. A tape muzzle is strongly advised for this procedure.

### Arrival at the surgery

When a patient is admitted, the animal should be examined as previously described, the history taken, and veterinary assistance obtained. The nurse may prevent any delays by preparing dressings, drips, transfusions, instruments, anaesthetic machine and operating theatre in readiness for any further treatment which may be necessary. Notes on any history should be left for the veterinary surgeon to refer to. When several casualties arrive at the same time, it may be necessary to individually identify each accident victim to avoid errors in treatment. Labels can be attached to dog's collars or identity bands fixed on the front or back leg of each animal.

### Haemorrhage

Haemorrhage is bleeding from any part of the body and is usually caused by injury, but may also occur when blood vessels are affected by disease. It must be regarded as serious, for a sudden or severe loss of blood may result in death. Even a slight haemorrhage which continues over a long period may result in loss of blood which jeopardizes the life of the patient. Haemorrhages are classified as:

*Arterial Haemorrhage.* This is the most serious form of haemorrhage. Blood from an artery is bright red and issues from the wound in spurts which synchronize with the heart beat. The force behind each spurt will depend on the size of the artery that has been severed. If the wound is large, the blood issues from the side of the wound nearest the heart. Usually a definite bleeding point can be detected.

*Venous Haemorrhage.* This is slightly less serious than arterial haemorrhage and may be easier to control, since the force is never so great as with arterial haemorrhage. Rapid blood loss will occur if a large vein is damaged.

Blood from a vein is darker in colour than arterial blood and issues from the wound in a steady stream. The force varies according to the size of the vessel damaged. In cases of a large wound, the blood will issue from the side farthest from the heart. A definite bleeding point is visible.

*Capillary Haemorrhage.* This type of bleeding occurs from damaged capillaries, and occurs in all wounds, since the fragile capillary wall is easily damaged.

The blood escapes from multiple, pinpoint sources in the tissues and oozes from the wound with very little force. No definite bleeding points are visible.

*Mixed Haemorrhage.* The arteries and veins of the body usually lie very close to one another, so often all three types of blood vessel are injured at the same time. When an artery and vein are severed at the same time, the haemorrhage may be so great that the characteristics of arterial haemorrhage are not detectable.

Haemorrhage may also be classified according to the time when blood loss occurs:

**Primary Haemorrhage.** This occurs as the immediate result of damage to the blood vessel wall.

**Reactionary Haemorrhage.** The primary haemorrhage will cause a drop in blood pressure, which may be sufficient to allow a blood clot to form around the damaged blood vessel and seal it. Occasionally, the blood pressure rises within 24 hours of the primary haemorrhage and displaces the clot so that the haemorrhage recurs.

**Secondary Haemorrhage.** This is haemorrhage which recurs from the damaged vessel because bacteria have contaminated the wound and destroyed the blood clot and the new repair tissue. It may occur any time after the first 24 hours but is usually seen at 3–10 days following the injury.

When the blood escapes on to the surface, it is termed *external haemorrhage.* It may come from open wounds or escape from regions such as the nose, ear, mouth, stomach linings, bowels, urinary tract or uterus.

If the blood is lost into the tissues or into a cavity such as the thoracic or abdominal cavity, it cannot be seen and is termed *internal haemorrhage.* Such haemorrhage occurs when an internal organ is damaged, such as lungs, liver or spleen, or if there is disease e.g. Warfarin poisoning, or if there is severe bruising. It is very difficult to detect, but usually causes swelling of the tissues (bruising) or a distended cavity e.g. abdomen, joints.

**Recognition and general signs**

The type of haemorrhage is recognized by its characteristics as described above.

The general signs will vary according to the amount of blood lost and the rate at which the loss occurred.

In cases of severe haemorrhage, there is pallor of the visible mucous membranes i.e. the gums, inside the lips, the conjunctiva. The colour may vary from very pale pink to almost white. The inside of the mouth feels cold, and if the gum is pressed to squeeze out the blood from the capillaries, the pink colour will only return very slowly as the capillaries refill with blood. This is called testing the *capillary refill*—in an animal with normal blood pressure, the refill occurs rapidly within 1 to 2 seconds of the pressure being removed from the gum, but when the blood pressure is lowered, the refill can take up to 5 seconds.

The patient is withdrawn, dull and listless, and will sometimes show a desire for water. There is an increased rate of respiration which rises markedly if the animal struggles in any way. The pulse is very rapid and may be so feeble that it cannot be felt.

The skin of the legs and tail feel cold as the cutaneous blood vessels constrict to divert the circulating blood to the vital organs.

If the haemorrhage continues, the brain will suffer a decreased blood supply and become *hypoxic* (short of oxygen). The animal will then become restless, gasping for breath, and stagger as it moves. Finally, convulsions set in, followed by collapse and death.

**Natural arrest of haemorrhage**

Four factors tend to stop initial bleeding:

(a) *The Retraction of Cut Ends* of arteries, arterioles and large veins due to the elastic nature of their walls. When the cut ends recoil, the elastic tissues contract and bunch up the end of the vessel. This closes or reduces the size of the aperture through which blood is flowing. Tearing of the vessel produces a better recoil as the vessel is stretched before it breaks. Therefore a lacerated wound bleeds less than an incised wound.

A lessening of blood flow allows a clot to form more rapidly to completely seal the blood vessel.

(b) *Fall In Blood Pressure.* Loss of blood will result in a lowered blood pressure so that less blood reaches the affected vessel and there is less pressure to force it out of the cut end of the vessel.

(c) *Back Pressure.* Internal haemorrhage will eventually fill the cavity (e.g.

abdomen) or distend the surrounding tissues (bruising) until the lowered blood pressure *in* the severed vessel is equal to the pressure of the fluid *surrounding* the severed vessel.

When the pressures are equal, no further blood can escape from the damaged blood vessel.

(d) *The Clotting of the Blood.* Clotting takes place in the wound and within the around the cut end of the vessel. The clot acts as a plug and prevents further blood loss (p. 9).

When haemorrhage has been arrested, the body will repair the damaged vessel. If this is not possible (e.g. in complete severence of a vessel, where the two ends have recoiled away from each other) the vessel will become permanently sealed. The flow of blood will be re-directed via other vessels, which enlarge to cope with the increased flow. New vessels will develop to re-establish the natural circulation.

This by-pass system works well unless all arteries supplying a part of the body are severed. The circulation cannot then be re-established in time to prevent the tissues dying, as is often seen in crushing injuries to the tail and digits.

**First aid treatments of haemorrhage**

A number of methods can be used to stop bleeding:

(a) *Direct Digital Pressure.* Direct pressure on a wound, particularly over a bleeding point, is both quick and effective and needs no equipment other than a finger and thumb. It is best to try pinching the wound edges together so that there is no further bacterial contamination of the wound by asterile hands. If the wound is too severe for this to be effective, the hands should again be washed, or a piece of clean, non-fluffy material placed over the wound before direct digital pressure is applied to the bleeding points in the wound itself.

Care must be taken, if the presence of a foreign body is suspected, not to push this deeper into the wound. In the presence of underlying fractures, care must be taken not to cause any further displacement of the fragments.

(b) *Pad and Pressure Bandage.* A pad of gauze swabs, or gauze overlaid by cotton wool is applied to the wound and bandaged firmly in position. If the bleeding continues, a second pad may be bandaged over the first; it is best not to remove the first dressing or the blood clots will be disturbed to restart the haemorrhage. Deep wounds may need to be packed with sterile gauze before the pressure pad is applied.

Where there is an embedded protruding foreign body, or shallow underlying fracture, a ring pad should be used so that the foreign body is not driven deeper into the tissues and the fracture is not complicated or displaced. (Fig. 4.4).

If internal bleeding is suspected, a crepe bandage may be applied firmly to effectively increase the back pressure in the affected tissues. Blood loss is quickly controlled and there should be minimal swelling of the tissues.

(c) *Pressure Points.* A site in the body where it is possible to press an artery against a bone is called a pressure point. The pressure of the artery against the bone prevents the flow of blood along the vessel and escaping from the wound further down the leg or tail. The method is limited to three points in the dog and cat.

1. THE BRACHIAL ARTERY as it runs down the medial shaft of the humerus and swings cranially behind the fleshy brachialis muscle. The pulse can clearly be felt in the distal third of the humerus. Pressure applied to this vessel will arrest arterial haemorrhage from below the elbow.

2. THE FEMORAL ARTERY as it passes obliquely over the proximal third of the femur on the medial aspect of the thigh. It lies just in front of the small taut pectineus muscle, and pressure applied to this vessel will arrest arterial haemorrhage from below the stifle.

3. THE COCCYGEAL ARTERY as it passes backwards along the underside of the tail. Pressure at the root of the tail where the pulse can easily be felt will arrest arterial haemorrhage from the rest of the tail.

(d) *Tourniquet.* This appliance stops bleeding by constricting the main arteries supplying blood to a wound on a limb or a tail. Correct application of this method is essential, and the tourniquet should only be used in cases where there is severe haemorrhage that cannot be controlled by other methods e.g. limbs that have been severed. Many forms of tourniquet are available, the usual one consisting of a flat elastic bandage with a fastening clip. In an emergency, a length of strong bandage or material, a piece of rubber tubing or a narrow belt can be effectively applied. String or rope are not good materials to use as they dig in and cause severe tissue damage at the point of application.

The tourniquet is fixed firmly round the limb or tail, a few inches above the wound. It should be adjusted so that the pressure is just sufficient to stop the haemorrhage. This is achieved by adjusting the clip of the conventional tourniquet. With less conventional tourniquets, a half-hitch is tied firmly on to the skin and then a stick or rod tied over the half-hitch. Twisting this stick will thus twist with tourniquet and gradually tighten it (Figs 4.5, 4.6).

However, it must be remembered that a tourniquet will also cut the circulation to all the tissues of the limb or tail so that they will start to die from the moment the tourniquet is applied. Therefore a

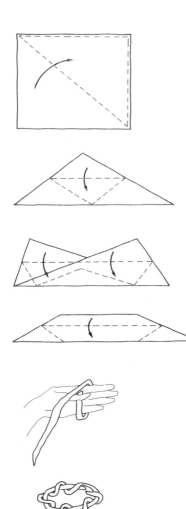

**STEP 1**

Take a clean tea-towel, headscarf, or any material 3' square or oblong.

Fold diagonally.

**STEP 2**

Fold point down onto diagonal fold.

If cloth is oblong, fold both points down.

**STEP 3**

Fold in half again to create a narrow band.

**STEP 4**

Hold one end of the band between ball of thumb and palm of hand. Make a loop around the fingers.

**STEP 5**

Remove the loop from the fingers and wind the long free end tightly around the loop. Tuck in the end to make a compact ring.

FIG. 4.4.
Step 1 Take a clean tea-towel, headscarf, or any material 3' square or oblong. Fold diagonally.
Step 2 Fold point down on to diagonal fold. If cloth is oblong, fold both points down.
Step 3 Fold in half again to create a narrow band.
Step 4 Hold one end of the band between ball of thumb and palm of hand. Make a loop around the fingers.
Step 5 Remove the loop from the fingers and wind the long free end tightly around the loop. Tuck in the end to make a compact ring.

tourniquet should NEVER be left in place for more than 15 minutes before being released for at least 1 minute to allow blood to circulate to revive these tissues.

When removed, the tourniquet should be slackened off slowly, and any further bleeding controlled, if possible, by pressure bandages. If it is found necessary to replace the tourniquet it should be applied a little further towards the wound to allow the tissues at the original site to recover from the effects of the constriction.

At no time should a tourniquet be covered with a dressing and no animal should be returned to a kennel with a tourniquet in place.

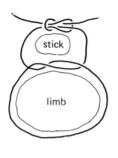

FIG. 4.5.

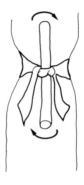

FIG. 4.6.

**Observation of the patient**

Once the haemorrhage has been controlled, the patient must be constantly and carefully observed in case of recurrence. Dressings must be inspected frequently, and the general condition of the patient checked.

The animal should be kept quiet and confined, whilst body heat is conserved with blankets. No direct forms of heat should be given—this will only dilate the cutaneous blood vessels so that blood is directed away from vital organs to flow through the skin. Provided there are no contra-indications e.g. vomiting, severe mouth or throat injury, small volumes of fluid (25–100 ml.) may be offered at 30 minutes intervals. Oral Hartman's Solution (lactated Ringers Solution) will help to guard against the effects of blood loss and shock, but plain water will suffice if Hartman's is not available. Alcohol should *not* be given as this also dilates cutaneous blood vessels.

**Wounds**

A wound is an injury in which there is a forcible break in the continuity of the soft tissues.

Wounds are classified as:
(a) Open—when the injury causes a break in the covering of the body surface i.e. skin or mucous membranes. These wounds can be seen and blood loss evaluated.

(b) Closed—when the injury does not penetrate the thickness of the skin to cause a break in the body covering. This category includes anything from minor bruising to serious damage to internal organs e.g. rupture of the liver. The wounds cannot be seen and blood loss is difficult to evaluate.

**Main types of open wounds**

*ABRASION*—This is the name given to a graze and is a wound which is caused by rubbing off the top layers of skin. Since the wound does not penetrate the entire skin thickness, this is not a true open wound, but is superficial and has thus been included here for completeness. The cause is usually a glancing blow or road accidents where the animal is dragged along the ground. The wound is superficial and the haemorrhage consists of capillary bleeding, so these wounds, though very painful and often contaminated, are rarely serious. Some veterinary authorites refer to these as "scrub wounds".

Healing of the abrasion takes place under the scab formed by coagulation and drying of the serum exuded from the damaged area after the bleeding has ceased. Abrasions should be gently but thoroughly cleaned whilst still fresh to prevent a contaminated wound becoming an infected one.

*INCISED WOUNDS*—An incised wound, usually caused by sharp cutting instruments such as knives or broken glass, is one in which the edges are clean cut and clearly defined. The edges of the wound will usually gape, especially on movement, but small incised wounds may remain closed, particularly in cats.

Incised wounds usually bleed freely as there is little elastic recoil from the cut ends of the blood vessels to allow natural arrest of haemorrhage. Such wounds often penetrate deeply to damage underlying structures such as nerves, tendons. The incised wound tends to heal quickly if the edges are held together, leaving little scar.

*LACERATED WOUNDS*—There are the commonest type of wounds encountered in small animals, and are usually caused by road accidents, dog fights, tearing by barbed wire etc.

The wounds are irregular in shape, with jagged, uneven edges, and often considerable loss of skin. The severity of the wound depends on how deeply the wound penetrates, but often underlying muscle, tendons, ligaments and even bones may be affected. Haemorrhage, even from large wounds, is often surprisingly little as the ragged tearing of the blood vessels causes good elastic recoil and natural control of haemorrhage. There is, however, considerable risk of infection from ingrained dirt, saliva and bacterial contamination.

Healing is slow and there is usually considerable risk of extensive scar formation.

*AVULSED WOUNDS*—In some lacerated wounds, especially those resulting from dog fights, large areas of skin and underlying tissues are torn away from the body as a loose flap. These are known as avulsed wounds.

*PUNCTURE WOUNDS*—These are produced by blows from sharp pointed instruments such as nails, stakes, thorns, fish hooks, and also, commonly, from teeth in bite wounds. The actual skin wound may be quite small but this will often lead to a long narrow track which penetrates deeply into the underlying tissues. Infection in such wounds is common, for bacteria may be carried deep into the tissues at the time of injury. The small skin wound usually heals rapidly, trapping infection in the tissues and an abscess will form. Bleeding from puncture wounds is often small and **such wounds are liable to be overlooked**. In animals covered with hairy coats the only sign of such a wound may be a small tuft of matted, bloodstained fur over the site of the wound.

In some cases, the cause of the wound may be seen projecting from the surface, but in others, the damaging foreign body may be hidden below the surface. Bullets can penetrate right through the body, leaving wounds both at the point of entrance and exit, air gun slugs and shot gun pellets usually remain in the depths of the puncture wound.

*CONTUSED WOUNDS*—A contused wound, which may be incised, lacerated etc, is one in which there is **bruising** (p. 228).

**Complications**

A wound will often be associated with damage to other structures in the vicinity such as blood vessels, nerves, tendons and an underlying fracture may be present. Foreign bodies may be present in the depths of the wound. Grit and dirt usually contaminate road accident wounds, and hair is commonly found buried deeply in gunshot wounds and bite injuries.

The three main dangers of wounds are haemorrhage, shock and sepsis. The healing of wounds is hindered by bacteria, which, being present on the skin and on objects causing the injury, will gain access to the wound. In the first instance, these germs are not very numerous, and are present only on the surface of the injured tissues. Such a wound is called a **contaminated wound**.

Some bacteria present may be of a type harmful to living tissues. If they are a virulent type, and the wound is not treated correctly or the natural body defence mechanisms are poor, these bacteria will invade the tissues around the wound and multiply. Such a wound is an **infected wound** and will exhibit the usual signs of inflammation, become unhealthy in appearance, and may discharge pus.

### Healing of wounds

Wounds usually heal by one of two methods—*first intention* healing or *granulation*.

**First Intention**—The edges of the wound are not widely separated, and are held together by blood clots. New blood vessels grow into these clots from the sides of the wound, carrying with them the healing components which will produce the fibrous scar tissue to tie the wound edges permanently together. Epithelial cells quickly spread across the narrow scar and start producing a new skin layer over the scar tissue (Fig. 4.7).

Providing there is no sepsis to interfere with the healing process, healing will be complete in 5 to 10 days.

First intention healing can only take place in incised wounds where the edges remain closely together. This may be achieved by stitching or bandaging whilst the healing takes place.

**Granulation**—This is a far slower process as the wound edges are widely separated. Clusters of cells are produced on the exposed tissue of the wound and multiply rapidly to form granulation tissue which eventually will cover the entire wound area. Granulation tissue is moist, bright red tissue, with a bubbly, uneven surface. It is easily damaged and bleeds if disturbed, as it has a very rich blood supply. The tissue grows up towards the skin surface level, filling the gap between the wound edges. When it is level with the skin surface, new epithelial cells spread across the top to complete the healing process. However, as large areas may need to be covered, this may take weeks to complete (Fig. 4.8).

Granulation tissue usually heals lacerated, avulsed and infected wounds, and the repair process may take several weeks.

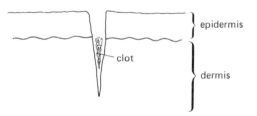

FIG. 4.7.

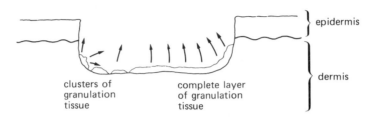

clusters of granulation tissue

complete layer of granulation tissue

epidermis

dermis

Fig. 4.8.

## Factors delaying wound healing

*Movement*—If the wound edges move against each other, the delicate healing tissues are continually destroyed and need to reform. Injuries over joints will take longer to heal than injuries where skin movement is minimal.

*Infection*—Bacteria in the wound will cause death of the healing tissues so that healing is delayed.

*Disturbance in circulation.* Heavily contused wounds may take longer to heal as the local circulation to the wound edges is impaired. Avulsed wounds may result in large flaps of skin which lose their blood supply.

*Self-trauma*—Continual licking of the wound will cause movement, possibly infection and damage to the healing tissues.

## Treatment of open wounds

The objects of treatment are to arrest haemorrhage, to treat shock and to prevent sepsis. The first two are the most important, and it is sometimes preferable to delay the treatment against infection until the general condition of the patient has improved.

(a) *Remove any dressings applied by the owner.* All instruments used in treating the wound should be sterilized if possible, and the first aider must ensure personal cleanliness to prevent further contamination of the wound.

(b) *Remove the cause of the injury* where this is possible, particularly if it is likely to cause further damage. Traps, fish hooks etc. may be removed, but deeply penetrating foreign bodies should be left alone. Glass fragments can be triangular, with only the tip showing above the skin, and attempts to remove this will cause the animal pain, and it may only serve to drive the glass deeper into the tissues. Stakes penetrating the chest wall may have entered the thoracic cavity or ruptured a large blood vessel. To remove these foreign bodies may cause a pneumothorax or disturb clots formed around the blood vessel to restart a serious haemorrhage.

Such penetrating foreign bodies should be cut down till they just protrude above the skin surface, and a ring pad dressing applied over the whole wound.

(c) *Immediate steps must be taken to control any severe haemorrhage.* Blood that has clotted should never be removed by the person applying first aid as this will invariably restart the haemorrhage.

(d) *Contaminating foreign bodies* e.g. dirty hair, in the depths of the wound should be removed if possible.

(e) *The hair around the wound should be clipped carefully.* Cream or ointment may be smeared on to the fur surrounding the injury so that it sticks together in clumps and when clipped or cut away, the fur will fall from the body as a piece. This avoids contaminating the wound with multiple, individual hairs.

The wound should be cleansed thoroughly with a suitable antiseptic solution (p. 404). Antiseptics destroy or hinder the growth of micro-organisms, but must be used at the exact strength recommended by the manufacturers. Higher concentrations may have a harmful effect on the body tissues. The cleansing of the wound should be gentle but thorough, making sure that the antiseptic penetrates into the depths of the wound, but taking care that the wound is not further contaminated by dirt derived from the skin. The chief value of bathing is mechanical i.e. to wash away dirt and bacteria.

(f) A suitable dressing should now be applied preferably of sterile gauze overlain by cotton wool and bandage. Cotton wool must never be applied directly to the wound as it will stick to the wound and the wisps will be hard to remove.

If the wound is heavily contaminated an antiseptic cream may be used, particularly in those cases where application of a dressing is not possible. Ointments should be avoided as they are difficult to remove at subsequent surgery.

(g) Treatment for shock especially fluid therapy should be commenced at an early stage. (p. 224).

**Main types of closed wounds**

*CONTUSION*—A contusion or bruise is produced by a blow with a blunt instrument, causing rupture of small blood vessels below the surface of the skin and a varying degree of damage to the soft tissues beneath. Heat, pain and swelling will be exhibited, and, in animals with white skin, discoloration which is first red, and later purple, fading to yellow will be present. Deep bruising of muscles will cause a swelling which often increases in size as it heals. This severe bruising remains painful for a period of weeks until healing is complete. Treatment consists of cold compresses and firm bandaging to limit swelling in the early stages. If the swelling has already developed, hot compresses will relieve pain.

*HAEMATOMA*—If blood is lost under the skin in greater quantities than in a contusion, a rounded swelling called a haematoma is formed. Unlike an abscess, this swelling is soft, usually painless and cool to the touch. In time, the blood clots and the clots contract over a period of weeks to become hard and knobbly. Haematomas are commonly seen affecting the earflaps of dogs and cats, and are frequently caused by violent head shaking.

Treatment will be as for contusions, but surgical interference will often be required. (p. 591).

**Reptile bites**

The only indigenous venomous snake in Britain is the adder, (*Vipera berus*) and, although cats are rarely bitten, snake bites can be a problem in the dog. The adder has a characteristic dark "V" or "X" marking on the head, and dark zig-zag markings along the length of its body. It is commonly found basking on warm sunny days on dry well-drained heathland. When disturbed, it may strike and therefore bites are usually inflicted on the head or neck of the sniffing dog.

*Clinical Signs*

Following the bite, the tissues swell rapidly and to such an extent that the two fang marks are rarely visible. The swelling is very painful and oedematous, and may be serious if it affects the mouth or throat area to cause narrowing or blockage of the airway. The patient is often dull and depressed, but may show signs of great distress, and may, on occasion, collapse.

*Treatment*

Antivenom for adder bites, cortico-steroids, antihistamines and diuretics are all used in the treatment of these wounds.* The assistance of a veterinary surgeon should be obtained as soon as possible. The animal should be kept as still as possible. The area of the bite should be washed thoroughly with soap and water, but not scrubbed as this will massage the poison into the tissues. Cold compresses may be applied in an attempt to limit the swelling.

Mention might be made here of poisoning by the Common Toad, which secretes toxic venom on to its body surface.

Dogs mouthing toads may show signs of excessive salivation, and occasionally, some distress. If part of the toad has been eaten, nervous signs may be shown, and may require treatment with atropine or corticosteroids.

**Wasp and bee stings**

*Clinical Signs*

Stings by these insects are common in the dog, usually in the mouth or around the lips, but occasionally on the feet. Stings in the mouth may cause consider-able swelling, excessive salivation and discomfort. The dog will often paw at the mouth and if the swelling is marked, a veterinary surgeon should be con-tacted. Some animals develop a severe allergic reaction to the sting and may collapse, with pale, cold mucous mem-branes.

*Treatment*

In event of collapse, the animal should be given first aid for shock, and the assistance of a veterinary surgeon ob-tained as soon as possible.

Wasps rarely leave the sting behind, but bees invariably do. In all cases, the area should be examined to see if the poison sacs remain. If visible, the stings should be carefully removed with tweezers or for-ceps, taking care to grasp the poison sac by the neck, close to its entry point to the skin. If the actual sac is grasped, it will contract to pump more poison into the animal's tissues, making the situation even worse.

Stings inside the mouth should be washed with an alkaline solution; either one dessertspoon of bicarbonate of soda to one pint of water or one table-spoon household ammonia to half a pint of water. If available, blue-bag could be used and held on to the affected area. If nothing else is available, soap and water will alleviate the pain.

Stings outside the mouth should be swabbed generously with surgical spirit or the above solutions.†

**Burns and Scalds**

A burn is an injury to the body caused by dry heat, such as a fire or a piece of hot material. A scald is an injury caused by the effect of moist heat, such as boiling water, tar or oil. Other varieties of burns are caused by certain chemicals, excessive cold (frostbite, cryosurgery) radiation or electric currents.

The distinction between burns and scalds is not of practical interest, for the

---

*As infection after a bite is often a problem, it is likely an antibiotic will need to be injected as well. Specific antivenom for foreign snakes kept in Britain are held by regional hospitals, for humans who suffer snake bites.

†Calcium and vitamin D tablets have been used to control the swelling after bee stings. The effect depends on cell permeability. The discovery of the value of this treatment was made by Dr Thompson, a beekeeper in Kent, about 50 years ago.

signs and principles of treatment are the same in each case. It is more important to identify the cause of the injury, whether caused by heat or cold, physical or chemical agents. Injury from radiation would be self evident.

## Classification

Burns vary greatly both in the area of the body surface affected and in depth. Classification used to be by degrees according to the depth of the burn, but now they are simply classified as:

(a) Superficial—penetrating no deeper than the skin surface (1st and 2nd degree burns).

(b) Deep—penetrating through the skin thickness into the tissues beneath (3rd, 4th, 5th and 6th degree burns).

## Clinical signs

In cases of heat burns, the signs are immediately apparent, but it may take several hours or even days before the symptoms are seen in cases of cold or chemical burns. Heat, cold or chemicals cause tissue damage and inflammation in the affected area. Blood vessels dilate and the area becomes reddened (only seen in unpigmented, white skin). Fluid is released from the blood vessels into the tissues and onto the skin surface so that the tissues swell and the surface becomes moist. Blisters are rarely seen in animals.

The hair is burnt off or, in the case of scalds, matted together by the fluid, which then evaporates, leaving the area covered by a thick crust of hair and dried fluids. Hair follicles in the area are usually destroyed so that the fur falls out after a few days.

Pain is variable, but as a rule, deep burns are less painful than large superficial ones. This is because the deep burn destroys the sensitive nerve endings, which the superficial burn leaves intact.

Surface tissues are destroyed in deep burns and dry out to become leathery and totally insensitive in the days following the injury.

## Complications

The degree of shock is very severe in cases of extensive burning and is caused by pain, tissue damage and infection. Tissue death and wound infection release toxins which are absorbed into the blood and may cause a toxaemia or septicaemia. The combination of shock and toxaemia or septicaemia may be severe enough to cause the death of the animal.

Local complications can include sepsis if the wound is infected and contracture due to shrinking of the skin associated with scar formation.

## Treatment

(a) *Extensive burns or scalds* e.g., domestic fires and accidents at work places. These burns and scalds are extremely painful and animals resent interference. All cases of extensive burns of scalds should be treated by a veterinary surgeon as soon as possible. In many cases, a suitable narcotic or general anaesthetic will be needed before local treatment may be carried out. Inhaled smoke or fumes may be a further problem (p. 263).

First aid measures must be to prevent and limit shock by keeping the animal warm, ensuring rest and offering small volumes of fluid. Warmth may be provided by blankets and shielding from draughts. Direct heat e.g. lamps will cause considerable pain in the damaged areas. Splinting can be used to limit movement if there are severe burns to the limbs, but must be used in such a way so that no pressure is applied to the damaged area.

(b) *Less extensive wounds* e.g., kitchen accidents. The most important first aid measure is to cool the affected area. This immediately decreases the pain and the heat in the tissues, so fewer cells die and less damage is done by the burn or scald. Flushing the burnt area with cold running water may be possible or ice cubes could be used. Scalds are best treated with copious volumes of cold water. If caused by a water-soluble fluid, e.g., boiling milk or jam, plain cold water will remove the fluid and cool the tissue. If caused by fat or oil, the fat must first be removed or it will congeal in the coat, sealing in the heat. Detergent solution should be poured on to the area to loosen the fat, followed by cold water washes to remove the detergent and cool the tissues.

**Dressings**

Burns and scalds are sterile wounds as the initial heat destroys the bacteria on the skin surface. Therefore the wound should be gently cleaned with sterile saline to remove any loose or charred remnants of hair before a dressing is applied. In long haired animals, fur covering a scalded area should be clipped away if possible. Burns are dressed with dry, sterile dressings, and paraffin tulle is used in the case of scalds. However, it must be remembered that these wounds are extremely painful and thorough cleansing may be possible only under a general anaesthetic when strict aseptic precautions can be observed.

**Electrical burns**

Burns are seen in pups that chew through electrical cables and also in cases of electrocution of animals.

*Clinical Signs*

Burns are seen at the points where the current flows into and out of the body. The pup which chews a wire may have red inflamed areas on the lips, gums or tongue, but the electrocuted animal can show burns to very different parts of the body, e.g. nose, chest, paws. The burns resemble heat burns and the cause of the injury is often all too apparent.

*Treatment*

**Do not touch an electrocuted animal until the electricity supply has been disconnected**—See later for treatment of unconscious animals (p. 264).

Minor burns may be alleviated by cold compresses, but corticosteroids may be needed in cases of more extensive burns.

**Chemical burns**

*Clinical Signs*

These burns also resemble a heat burn, but may take several hours to develop.

*Treatment*

Copious volumes of water should be used to wash the chemical off the skin. A mild detergent may be used to ensure complete removal of the chemical.

If the chemical is a known alkali e.g. caustic soda, or quicklime, an acid solution should be prepared (by mixing equal quantities of household vinegar and water) and used to wash away the chemical. If the burn is caused by a known acid, a concentrated solution of bicarbonate of soda or washing soda should be used.

Paraffin, petrol and sump oil should also be removed from the coat, as they can cause extensive inflammation and are highly toxic, especially to cats. Heavy duty cleaner e.g. Swarfega, or cooking oil should be smeared on the affected area, worked well in and then washed off with detergent and copious volumes of water.

Lumps of tar in furry feet can be clipped away with scissors or loosened by smearing the area liberally with butter and bandaging the dressing in place overnight. The following day, the tar may be removed by detergent washes.

### Fractures

A fracture is said to have occurred when a bone is broken. The nature of the injury may vary from a crack to a complete break, but the condition is still technically a fracture. *Fragments* are the pieces of bone that are formed as the result of a fracture. They are often sharp and jagged and thus likely to cause further damage to the adjacent tissues. The fragments may be displaced due to muscular spasm.

### Causes of fracture

*Direct violence*—When a bone fractures at the place to which violence is applied, the fracture is termed "direct". This is the commonest cause of fractures and may be seen as the result of severe blows, street accidents, gunshot wounds etc.

*Indirect violence*—When a bone fractures at some distance from the area where the force is applied, the fracture is termed "indirect". Jumping over a cliff on to the feet and sustaining a fracture of the radius and ulna is an example.

*Muscular action*—Sometimes the extreme force of muscular action is sufficient to break a bone. This is seen particularly in racing greyhounds.

*Spontaneous fracture*—Occasionally a bone will be broken without the application of violence. This is a spontaneous or pathological fracture and is due to some existing bone disease which weakens the bone structure.

### Varieties of fracture

*Simple Fractures* are ones in which the bone is broken but there is no communicating wound between the fracture site and the skin or mucous membranes.

*Compound Fractures* are ones in which the bone is broken and the skin or mucous membrane is punctured so that air can gain access to the fragments. Such access may be obtained either through a surface wound or, in the case of fractured ribs, through tearing the pleura and penetration of the lung. These fractures carry a risk of sepsis entering via the wounds.

Fractures may also be classified as:
*Incomplete Fractures.* These fractures do not extend through the complete width of the bone shaft.

(i) Greenstick fractures occur in young animals with immature bones which are softer and more supple. The bone bends on impact and is cracked on one side only, as a green twig of a plant will break if bent (p. 580).

(ii) Fissured fractures are ones in which the bone cortex is cracked but the bone fragments are not separated.

*Complete Fractures.* These fractures occur across the entire width of the bone and are described as:

(i) Transverse—one where the fracture line runs at right-angles to the bone cortex.

(ii) Oblique—one where the fracture line runs at an oblique angle across the bone shaft.

(iii) Spiral—one where the fracture line curls spirally around the bone cortex. This is a common type of fracture of the humerus.

(iv) Comminuted—one where the bone is broken into more than two fragments.

The bone fragments may be displaced by force or movement and are described as:

(i) *Depressed fracture*—This can occur when a bone surrounding a cavity is fractured and the fragments displaced inwards. For example, the bones of the cranium may be depressed into the cranial cavity, injuring the brain.

(ii) *Overriding*—This commonly occurs when the muscles surrounding the fracture site contract, and the fragments displace and override each other.

(iii) *Distracted*—The opposite to overriding. Muscular contraction in this case pulls the fragments apart, e.g. the olecranon process of the ulna is pulled away from the elbow joint fracture by the action of the triceps muscle.

(iv) *Impacted*—One in which the broken ends are driven into one another.

In addition to these classifications, a fracture is said to be **complicated** when there is damage to important structures or organs around the fracture site, e.g. blood vessels, nerves, joints, spinal cord, lungs, heart etc.

Finally, a **multiple** fracture is said to have occurred when the bone is fractured in two or more places with an appreciable distance between the sites of the fracture.

## General signs of fracture

(a) *Pain* at or near the site of the fracture. The severity of the pain depends upon the amount of movement which can occur between the bone fragments, and how much the fragments rub against each other. Incomplete fractures are less painful than complete fractures, as the fragments scarcely move. Overriding and distracted fractures tend to be less painful because the broken ends do not grate on each other. It must be remembered that pain increases shock and gentle handling is essential to avoid increasing the pain.

(b) *Swelling* makes its appearance soon after the accident due to the haemorrhage from the bruised muscles and soft tissues surrounding the fracture site. This haemorrhage will be worsened if the sharp fragments are allowed to move freely following the accident and cause more soft tissue damage.

(c) *Loss of function* which may be partial or complete. There is always some limitation of use after a bone has been fractured.

(d) *Deformity of the limb*—This may not be obvious unless the fragments are displaced. Comparison with the opposite side of the animal's body may help to detect slight deformities. The leg will be shortened in overriding fractures or a sharp edge or bump may be palpated on the bone surface.

(e) *Unnatural mobility*—This is usually noted in fractures of the limb long bones. Movement may be noticed at the fracture site.

(f) *Crepitus*—A grating sound may be heard or felt when the broken ends move against one another. This, and unnatural mobility, should not be looked for by the person giving first aid, but, if noticed during the course of an examination, give positive evidence of the presence of a fracture.

The last two signs will not be detected in incomplete fractures, and it must not be expected that all the above signs will be found in every case. If there is any reason to suspect a fracture, the injury should be treated as such pending diagnosis by a veterinary surgeon.

## First aid treatment

The principle of treatment for a fracture

is to minimize the movement of the fracture fragments. If this can be done, there will be minimal damage to the soft tissues by the fragments thus preventing a simple fracture becoming complicated or compound and minimizing the pain experienced by the animal. In cases of compound fractures, additional objectives are to arrest haemorrhage and prevent sepsis.

*Treatment*

(a) The first criterion is to handle the broken bone as little as possible. Under no circumstances should resetting of the limb or reduction of the fracture be attempted.

(b) Support for the fracture should be applied as soon as possible to limit movement and prevent further damage. However, if this is impossible without a struggle, splinting should be abandoned as provoking the animal to thrash around will do the animal more harm than the splint will do good. Such animals are best kept still, warm and comfortable until professional help is available, or until the animal has calmed down and will allow a splint to be applied without a struggle.

(i) Bandaging—the affected part is bandaged firmly to unaffected parts of the body, using the healthy body as a splint. This technique is used for the scapula which can be bound against the rib cage, or single fractured metacarpals, metatarsals or digits which may be bound to adjoining unaffected bones of the same foot, by bandaging the foot. Such support will also decrease the amount of swelling following the fracture and thus minimize the pain (p. 293).

(ii) Splinting—a splint is an appliance which restricts the movement of an injured part, and may be anything from a rolled-up magazine to a plaster of paris splint. They are only of value if used on certain bones when professional help may be delayed for some time or if the animal has to be moved some distance e.g. on to a stretcher prior to transporting to the surgery. A splint should then be applied when possible, taking care to avoid pressure at the fracture site by fastening it only above and below the injured area if possible.

(c) Haemorrhage in a compound fracture should be controlled by applying a dressing if possible. Digital pressure must only be used with care as this could displace the fragments and cause complications. The ring pad dressing is very useful here, as, when applied *around* the fracture site, no pressure is applied *to* the fracture site by the dressing. Cleansing of the wound should not be attempted for fear of introducing further infection into the fracture site.

**The value of splints in first aid**

If a splint is used, it should be *rigid* so that it will not bend and allow movement of the injured part; *smooth* so that there are no projections which can dig into the underlying tissues of the patient; *conforming* so that it holds the injured part firmly in position, does not allow movement and is comfortable for the patient.

Many materials have been used depending on the initiative of the person at the scene of the accident and the size of the patient! Broom handles, rolled-up newspapers and magazines, ice-lolly sticks, wire coat hangers have all played a part. More conventional splinting materials are listed below:

(a) *Wooden splints*—straight pieces of wood of varying length may be employed.

(b) *Metal splints*—preformed splints, made of tin or aluminium are available. Malleable aluminium splinting of varying width, backed by foam (Zimmer Splints) are very useful and can easily be bent to conform to the shape of the leg.

(c) *Plastic*—recent developments have produced varying diameters of plastic gutter splints, lined by foam, which may be snapped off at the desired length.

(d) *Plaster or resin*—roller bandages made of coarse material and impregnated with plaster of paris or resin are commonly used in fracture treatment. The bandage should not encase the limb—this is beyond the scope of first aid—but may be used as a slab to form a gutter splint on one side of leg only. For this purpose, a bandage is soaked in water, wrung out, unrolled on a smooth surface and folded several times on itself to form a slab of the desired length. This is then moulded upon the affected limb and secured in position by an ordinary roller bandage, used wet. The plaster will set hard and form a good splint. This splinting should not be used on a compound fracture as, at best, any wound dressings will become saturated, and at worst, the wound will be contaminated by plaster of paris.

(e) *Inflatable airbags* in the form of tubes could be used around a limb if a suitable size can be found to immobilize a broken leg. A range of such appliances have been used in human first aid but there may be a risk of obstructing the circulation if the bags are too tight.

### Application of splints

Splinting in the dog and cat is restricted to the bones and joints below the elbow and stifle joints. Above these joints the bones are surrounded by large muscle masses and it is impossible to apply a simple effective splint to these areas.

The splint must be long enough to immobilize the joints above and below the fractured bone. The splint should be made as smooth as possible and any sharp edges must be cut away or padded. If possible the splint should be moulded to fit the shape of the limb.

The limb itself is covered in a layer of orthopaedic wool or cotton wool thick enough to prevent the hard splint from pressing on the skin and causing damage or discomfort. The splint is then applied to the limb and bandaged firmly in place to immobilize the limb. Where possible, the bandaging should not encircle the limb at the actual fracture site for fear of causing complications. The foot should be left uncovered if possible so that it can be examined frequently to ensure the circulation is not impeded by too tight a splint. Tight bandages may obstruct the venous return up the leg and the foot will swell. More seriously, the foot may become swollen, cold and clammy if both arterial and venous flow are obstructed by over-tight dressings. Such dressings must be removed immediately and replaced by looser bandaging.

The patient should also be constantly observed for signs of discomfort, usually indicated by biting at the splint. If this occurs, the dressings should be checked, and if the animal persists in attacking the splint, the dressings should be removed and replaced.

### Recognition of a healing fracture

For the initial 2 weeks after the fracture has been immobilized, the swelling subsides and becomes firmer and more distinct (fibrous callus). p. 581.

The pain subsides, but direct digital pressure on the fracture site or movement of the fracture site still causes acute pain. The animal is still very lame and may not weight bear on the affected limb, although it will often touch the toes to the ground when standing still.

The fibrous callus gradually hardens as

the bony callus is formed. The pain declines further as the repair becomes firmer and more permanent, but there is still tenderness at the fracture site 4 weeks after the fracture occurred. The animal will weight bear but usually still favours the leg and is not sound. There is no movement of the fracture site at this stage.

After 4 to 6 weeks, the bony callus strengthens and the animal becomes sound as the spongy bone is replaced by lamellar bone. By 8 to 16 weeks, the animal is back to normal although the bony callus is still palpable on the bone's surface. This may never disappear completely, but will decrease in size gradually over the following months.

### Principles of fracture fixation

Prevent fragments moving at fracture site. Movement breaks down the weak fibrous callus and so delays healing.

The ends of the fragments should be held together as closely as possible. This means that the callus does not have to bridge a large gap, and the smaller the gap, the smaller the callus. The smaller the callus, the more rapidly it is formed and the more rapidly the bone heals.

The fragments should be reduced to restore the normal bone anatomy as closely as possible. If the fragments are replaced, then there are no missing pieces to create gaps in the cortex which must be bridged by the callus.

### Common Sites of Fracture

### Fractures of the skull

Fractures to the upper part of the skull are usually due to direct violence—e.g. a kick by a horse, road accident, blow to the head. Fractures to the base of the skull are usually due to indirect violence—e.g. a blow to the jaw or side of the head, or a fall on to the nose.

(a) **Frontal and nasal bones.** Serious injury to the cranium will usually cause unconsciousness or death. There may be haemorrhage from the nose and there can be much swelling at the site of the fracture. Less serious fractures will cause bleeding from the nose and/or mouth, and possibly may cause vomiting if much blood has been swallowed. There is rarely loss of consciousness as the frontal sinuses protect the cranium from a frontal blow.

(b) **Bones of the orbit.** Fractures here may cause the eyeball to prolapse, but almost certainly will bruise the sclera of the eye. The eye may seem to bulge in the socket if there is haemorrhage behind the eyeball.

(c) **Base of the skull.** Fractures of the hard palate may be seen if the mouth is opened. Other fractures will show little visible evidence, but haemorrhage from the ears, nose or mouth may indicate the presence of a skull fracture. The animal may be unconscious.

All cases of fractured skulls must be handled with care as the situation may easily be complicated by clumsy handling. There is always a danger that the patient's condition may deteriorate and the animal must be constantly observed for changes in its condition.—See "Unconsciousness".

### Fractures of the lower jaw

The common sites of fracture of the mandible are:

(a) *At the mandibular symphysis*—which is not a true fracture, but a separation of the fibrous joint holding the two halves of the mandible together. Less frequently, a piece of bone carrying some of the incisor teeth may be completely detached from the mandible, although this fragment usually remains supported by the soft tissue of the gums.

(b) *Just below the temporomandibular* jaw joint, on the side of the face near the base of the ear.

(c) In the middle of the *horizontal ramus,* in the area of the premolar teeth.

The most noticeable signs of fracture of the lower jaw are excessive movement, deformity, irregularity of teeth and often the loss of power to move the jaw freely. Crepitus and haemorrhage from the gums are often present.

*Treatment*

Wounds and haemorrhage should be dealt with in the normal manner. Some support may be given by applying a wide tape muzzle, as used in restraint, but this must not be tied too tightly and must *never* be used if there is a fracture to the nasal bones as well as the lower jaw. Fractures of the symphysis rarely need support, but, if there is much movement between the bones, a flat bandage may be tied around the lower jaw just behind the canine teeth.

**Fracture of the scapula**

Although uncommon, these fractures are usually a result of direct force, but may be overlooked, particularly if other bones of the limb are fractured at the same time.

Fractures of the scapula, which are usually simple, rarely cause displacement, as the bone is encased in muscle which tends to hold the fragments in place. There is usually little evidence of swelling or haemorrhage. Lameness will be exhibited and there may be some dropping of the shoulder. Pain is variable but not usually marked unless the shoulder joint is involved in the fracture. Crepitus is rarely present.

Support may be given by applying a spica, binding the scapula to the side of the chest.

**Fracture of the humerus**

(a) *Upper third of humerus*—fractures here are uncommon and usually seen in young animals (less than 9 months old). They usually occur because indirect force has been applied to the limb and the fracture occurs through the growth plate of the bone. There is pain, swelling and deformity of the shoulder region, and the shoulder joint is usually held flexed.

(b) *Mid-shift fractures*—this is a common fracture and can be transverse, oblique, spiral or comminuted. It is usually caused by direct force, and pain, swelling and crepitus are usually present. This fracture can be or become complicated as the radial nerve lies very close to the midshaft of the humerus. The limb is held with the shoulder flexed and the other joints fully or partly extended, the toes of the foot often just brushing on the floor. If the radial nerve is damaged the limb may trail on the ground as the paralyzed muscles cannot flex the shoulder joint.

(c) *Lower third of humerus*—fractures in this area may involve the elbow joint and can be due to direct violence or indirect force such as jumping down from a height. The fractures may be simple, but are often comminuted. Pain and crepitus are usually present and the area may be swollen. Lameness varies in degree depending upon the actual site of the fracture. The limb is held with the shoulder flexed, elbow extended.

*Treatment*

Splinting of the humerus is impossible and, although the spica could be used for the upper third fractures, confinement to limit limb movement is the most practical form of first aid.

## Fracture of radius and ulna

In most cases, both bones are fractured, but occasionally only one may be affected. This is the second most common site for fractures seen in the dog and cat.

Most fractures are due to direct force, but indirect force e.g. jumping from a height can cause fractures, especially in the toy breeds of dog. The fractures are usually in the lower two thirds of the bones and are oblique, transverse or comminuted and may occasionally be compound. Pain and crepitus are usually present though the degree of swelling is very variable. The animal will hop around, with the shoulder and elbow joints flexed.

### Treatment

This area may be usefully immobilized by a splint, but the patient should still be confined to avoid undue movement.

## Fractures of the pelvis

Fractures of the pelvis are almost always multiple and can affect any or all three of the pelvic bones. Compound fractures are rare, as the pelvis is covered by thick muscles. Separation of the pelvic symphysis can occur in young animals but separation of the sacroiliac joint may happen in any age of animal, usually associated with other pelvic fractures. Fractures of the pelvis should always be considered in cats brought in after road accidents because they can easily be overlooked.

The cause is usually a direct blow as received in road accidents, but indirect fractures occur elsewhere in the pelvis as the girdle is twisted by the blow, or the head of the femur may be punched through the acetabulum.

Deformity is a common finding in these fractures and is best judged by gently palpating the iliac crests (anterior points of the pelvis), the tuber ischii (the caudal point of the pelvis) and comparing the two sides of the pelvis to see if either side is shortened or displaced in any way. Pain and crepitus are variable depending on the severity of the fracture. If the acetabulum is involved, the fractures are very painful. If there is little displacement of the fragments e.g. separation of pelvic symphysis, the animal will still be able to walk. If only one side of the pelvis is affected, the animal may be severely lame on that side, but able to move around. If both sides are affected, the patient is unable to stand. Severe pelvic fractures are very, very painful. An X-ray examination will usually be necessary to assess the damage.

### Treatment

General nursing care and minimal movement are the only measures which can be adopted. It is important to note the colour and amount of any urine or faeces passed.

## Fractures of the femur

(a) *Head and neck*—Young animals under 9 months of age may fracture the femoral neck along the growth plate as a result of indirect violence. The signs are similar to a dislocated hip in that the greater trochanter of the femur is usually displaced in relation to the iliac crest and tuber ischii. There is often pain on manipulation, some swelling and the leg is shorter than the opposite leg. The limb is carried in flexion.

(b) *Shaft fractures*—These are the commonest fractures encountered in the dog and cat, and usually result from the direct trauma of a road accident! Fractures are more common in the middle and lower third and are often comminuted. Owing to the large muscle masses, compound fractures are rare, but there is always some bruising and swelling of the muscles. The limb often appears shortened as the fragments usually override each other. Pain is variable—if crepitus is absent, the fracture is not so painful and a cat may even attempt to use the leg. Unnatural mobility in these cases is obvious. Usually, the hip is held in flexion whilst the rest of the leg hangs limply.

(c) *Low shaft fractures*—Again, such fractures are usually a problem in young animals and may often involve the stifle joint as the fractures occur across the distal growth plate. The cause may be direct or indirect violence, and the fractures are usually simple and transverse although compound fractures can occur especially as the result of road accidents. The fractures are frequently overridden, but not always very swollen or painful, and crepitus is not evident in many cases. The limb is usually held flexed, often with the toes just touching the ground.

*Treatment*

There is little possibility of effectively splinting these fractures. Rest and confinement are the most important requirements to limit movement at the fracture site.

**Fractures of the tibia and fibula**

As with the front leg, most fractures affect both bones.

In young muscular dogs e.g. greyhounds, distracted fractures can occur if the muscular action pulls the tibial crest away from the main bone. In other cases, fractures of the growth plate separate off the entire epiphysis, usually as a result of direct force.

Pain is not marked in the former case and there is little swelling, but the latter cases are more painful.

Midshift fractures can occur in any age of animal and are usually due to direct violence. It is also a common site for greenstick fractures in the young. Fractures are usually simple oblique, transverse or comminuted. Compound fractures do occur as the sharp bone fragments penetrate the skin which directly overlies them. The fractures are painful on manipulation although the swelling is not great. The hip and stifle are held in flexion, whilst the rest of the leg dangles—the degree of deformity depends upon the fracture.

In many cases of severe lacerated wounds to the hock following road accidents, the lower end of the tibia or fibula may be rubbed away, allowing the hock to dislocate (p. 242).

*Treatment*

Immobilization of the fracture may be achieved by splinting the leg.

**Fractures of the carpus and tarsus**

These fractures are uncommon except in the racing greyhound. All usual signs of fracture may be present except that normal mobility of the joint may be restricted by muscular contraction.

*Treatment*

Bandaging will immobilize the joint and minimize swelling.

### Fractures of the metacarpals and metatarsals

Fracture of these bones is usually due to direct violence experienced by crushing injuries. One or more bones may be affected, and, depending on the severity of the injuries, varying degrees of swelling and pain will be exhibited—single fractures may only cause lameness; multiple fractures cause the limb to be carried.

*Treatment*

A wide splint should be applied to the back of the injured paw to support the fracture.

### Fracture of the bones of the digits

These are usually due to direct violence and are commonly compound following road accidents. Racing greyhounds and whippets often suffer simple fractures of digits as do pet animals that may be trodden on. Support may be afforded by bandaging.

### Fracture of the ribs

Fracture of the ribs and sternum are uncommon but may escape detection, especially when only one rib is involved. The ribs are closely bound to each other by muscles and ligaments so that, unless a number of ribs are fractured, displacement is not usually marked. Any deformity may be obvious or discovered by gentle palpation.

The fracture may be complicated by fragments which pierce the pleura or even the lungs. Should this happen, the escaping air will fill the pleural cavity creating a **pneumothorax** and lung collapse (p. 503). Air may also penetrate the tissues of the thoracic wall and come to lie under the skin causing **subcutaneous emphysema.** This gives the skin a crackly, spongy feeling when palpated, and a note should always be made when this is observed. If a blood vessel is penetrated, haemorrhage into the chest (**haemothorax**) will occur and may also collapse the lungs if severe enough. Severe damage to the chest cavity may therefore result in acute signs such as cyanosis, increased respiratory rate and the coughing up of bright red, frothy blood.

*Treatment*

Where there is no internal injury, rest is all that is necessary. General principles must be applied in all cases where there is evidence of internal damage to counter the respiratory distress.

### Fracture of the spine

Direct trauma is usually the cause of vertebral column fractures, e.g. road accidents, heavy weights falling on the animal's back. Occasionally indirect force may be the cause—the dog which hits a stationary object head-on whilst running at full speed may fracture its back as a result of indirect violence.

Fractures are almost always complicated by dislocations of the vertebrae which causes deformity of the spinal canal, damage to the spinal cord and possible paralysis. Uncomplicated fractures of the spine are very uncommon.

(a) *Fractures of the cervical region* may result in immediate death, but severence of the spinal cord in this area will lead to **quadriplegia** (paralysis of all four legs). **Hemiplegia** (paralysis of one side of the body only) is rarely seen but may occur if the spinal cord is only damaged on one side of the cervical region.

(b) *Fractures of the thoracolumbar region* are the most common spinal fractures, and, in most cases, the animal is *paraplegic* (hind legs paralysed). Many cases also show rigid extension of the forelegs and flexion of the hind legs, with the back arched at the fracture site. It is important to realize that the spinal cord may continue to function perfectly above and below the site of the injury. Thus limb withdrawal reflexes in response to pain (e.g. pinching the toes) are often unaffected, as they are a local reflex arc and do not require input from the brain. However, conscious proprioception (realization) of pain stimulus may be absent in the areas *caudal* to the spinal injury if the nerve impulses are unable to pass to the brain.

(c) *Fracture of the sacrum* is a relatively common finding in cats following a blow to the hindquarters. This fracture is often associated with a fractured pelvis but may occur alone. In these cases, the animal can stand but the tail is limp and floppy and there is no pain sensation. The bladder and rectum/anus are often paralysed as a complication of these injuries, but the control may return after 3 to 4 weeks.

### Treatment

All spinal fractures are intensely painful and patients must be handled with great care. Euthanasia will often be necessary in these cases and the animal must be kept as comfortable as possible pending the arrival of the veterinary surgeon. Animals should be carried on a rigid board and the spine never twisted when the patient is handled.

### Dislocations

A dislocation is a persistent displacement of the articular surfaces of the bones which form a joint. A total dislocation or **luxation** occurs when the articular surfaces no longer have any contact with each other. A partial dislocation or **subluxation** occurs when the bones are displaced, but the articular surfaces still remain in partial contact.

Luxations may be:

*Compound*—the dislocation is associated with a skin wound over the joint. This type of luxation may occur in conjunction with lacerated wounds of the hock or carpus following road accidents.

*Fracture luxations*—the dislocation is associated with a fracture of the bones of the joint.

Luxations are described as being medial when the distal bone in the joint comes to lie medially to the proximal bone of the joint; lateral when the distal bone is displaced lateral to the proximal bone. Dorsal or ventral are terms used to describe dislocations which occur in joints in the horizontal plane of the body, (e.g. hip, spine) and some luxations may also be termed anterior or posterior.

### Causes of joint luxation

Luxations can be:

*Congenital* when the animal is born with a deformed joint. These are always chronic dislocations.

*Acquired* as a result of direct or indirect violence. These dislocations can become recurrent or chronic if the ligaments and joint capsule are damaged, or degenerate so that they can no longer hold the joint surfaces in place.

### General signs

*Loss of function of the limb.*

*Deformity*—usually obvious as the limb may be anglulated or shorter than its partner.

*Limited movement of the joint.*

*Pain on manipulation of the joint*—much less in the chronic case.

*Swelling of the joint.*

*Crepitus may be noticed,* but it is much less obvious than between the ends of broken bones and is due to the cartilaginous surface rubbing on bone.

### Treatment of luxations

No attempt should be made to reduce the dislocation, nor to apply splints or bandages. The patient should be rested in a confined space and cold compresses may be applied to reduce swelling.

### Common sites of luxations

### Luxation of the Mandible

This occurs less frequently than fractures, and usually it is caused by indirect force, such as chewing on large solid objects, or pulling against an object e.g. a lead held firmly by the owner. Luxations are almost always anterior.

The mouth is usually held open, with the lower jaw protruding if both joints are affected, or twisted to one side if only one joint is affected (the jaw twists to the opposite side to the luxation). The patient may or may not be able to close the mouth and may drool saliva. The eyes may appear to bulge slightly.

### Luxation of the Shoulder

Acquired luxations are rare as strong muscles surround the joint, but may occur following a severe blow to the humerus.

The leg is held on flexion, and the joint is swollen and painful. The animal is acutely lame.

### Luxation of the Elbow

Acquired luxations occur as a result of a direct blow to the side of the flexed joint. Indirect force applied to the lower limb when the joint is flexed may also cause a dislocation. Fracture dislocations usually occur due to direct violence and involve fractures of the distal humerus or proximal ulna.

The limb is held in flexion, often with the elbow rotated outwards. Deformity of the joint is obvious, and there is usually much pain and swelling surrounding the joint. This luxation is even more painful if a fracture is involved.

### Luxation of the Lower Limbs

Compound luxations and subluxations of the lower limbs are relatively common in conjunction with lacerated wounds to carpus, hock, metacarpal and metatarsal regions following road accidents. The ligaments which support these joints may be completely worn away by the abrasive road surface. Occasionally, luxations are seen in racing dogs due to indirect trauma and the tibial tarsal joint is the one more usually affected. Subluxations or luxations of the carpus may occur in dogs which have fallen from a height.

Grotesque deformity of the limb is often seen following luxations received in road accidents, when the tibia or radius may actually project from the skin wound. In other cases, the limb is held in flexion and the paw angled medially or laterally depending on the luxation. Pain and marked swelling are present.

### Luxation of the Hip Joint

This is the joint most commonly dislocated in the dog and cat. Subluxations rarely occur, but fracture dislocations are seen from time to time, and vary from a small bone chip fractured off the femoral head to severe fractures of the acetabulum.

These dislocations are usually due to indirect force such as a blow to the femur when the leg is rotated inwards. These cases commonly occur following a road accident. Other cases are caused by falling on to the extended limb or wrenching the joint if the hind foot remains trapped as the animal jumps from a height. Luxations are usually anterior and dorsal.

The limb is held in flexion, and the stifle rotated outwards. There may be some swelling, although this is often not apparent, but the joint is very painful on manipulation. If the dislocation is anterio-dorsal, the greater trochanter can be felt riding higher and further forward in relation to the pelvic bones than the normal joint.

### Luxation of the Patella

The majority of luxations are congenital, and seen in small breeds of dogs, especially Yorkshire Terriers and Poodles. The patella usually luxates medially.

In early life the pup may suddenly pull up when running and cry out, holding the leg flexed. The patella soon reduces and the dog is often perfectly sound and running around after a few minutes.

Extending and flexing the dogs limb whilst rubbing the inside (medial) stifle may help the patella to return to its correct place.

Acquired luxations usually occur due to indirect force, such as the animal turning at speed. In these case, the joint is often swollen and painful and the patella can be palpated either medially or laterally to the femur. The leg is held flexed, but, if gently extended, the patella might well slip back into place. Occasionally gentle massaging

may be necessary to encourage the patella to move into its correct position.

### Luxation of the Stifle

Dislocation of this joint (other than patella luxation) is not common, and will only occur when the ligaments are ruptured due to direct force. Subluxation of the joint is more common, following **rupture of the cruciate ligaments**. Indirect force is usually responsible, such as twisting the limb whilst running at speed.

The leg is carried in flexion although the toes often just touch the ground when the animal stands at rest. The joint may not be very swollen, and the limb is not deformed, nor is it very painful unless firmly handled (which should not be attempted).

### Luxation of the Vertebrae

The luxations are usually associated with fractures and the signs are identical to those described under "Spinal Fractures". Toy dogs can have a subluxation of the atlanto-axial joint, which can result in sudden quadriplegia with no history of accident or trauma.

### Sprains

Sprain is the term used to describe damage to the tissues surrounding a joint as a result of violence which forces the joint too far in one direction. Ligaments and other tissues are stretched or torn and the synovial membrane may also be damaged. The joints most likely to be affected are the shoulder, stifle, carpus and tarsus.

### Signs of sprain

*Pain*, which is more severe when the joint is moved.

*Swelling*, which develops shortly after the injury is sustained and is due to bleeding from damaged tissues and inflammation of the synovial membrane.

*Loss of power*, which is not so severe as in a fracture or dislocation injury.

*Tenderness on palpation.*

### Diagnosis of sprain

The degree of swelling can make it impossible to locate exactly which structures are painful, and an X-ray may be necessary to rule out the possibility of a fracture or dislocation. Pain is increased by moving the joint in a direction which stretches the damaged tissues, whereas fractures which occur around the joint are painful if the joint is moved in any direction. There is no distortion of the limbs as seen with dislocations, and the joint moves freely.

If there is any uncertainty as to the type of damage sustained, the injury should always be treated as if a fracture were present.

### Treatment of sprains

The affected joint must be rested as far as is possible, and the swelling minimized or prevented by applying a pressure bandage. Layers of cotton wool wrapped around the joint and bound firmly in place by crepe bandage will enforce rest and minimize the swelling. Cold compresses do not relieve pain or prevent swelling to the same degree.

### Strains

A strain is the stretching or *tearing of a muscle,* usually as a result of a sudden wrench, particularly in the racing dog. (It is more common in greyhounds running on sand surfaces rather than dogs that race over grass).

### Signs of Strain

Lameness follows the straining of a limb muscle and there is loss of power, tenderness and swelling of the affected muscle. Further exercise is impossible when the dog pulls up.

### Treatment

Rest must be enforced and, if necessary, a splint may be applied. Heat applications, in the form of hot compresses or electric heating pads can be applied to alleviate pain and help speed recovery. The recovery may take a long time.

### Ruptured tendons

This is a form of severe strain or injury in which the tendon is either partially or completely torn as a result of sudden violence. Wounds to the distal limbs should always be checked to find out if the tendons are damaged. The tendons may also rupture due to indirect violence e.g. twisting the leg can rupture the Achilles tendon.

### Signs of Ruptured Tendons

The tendons of the metacarpus and metatarsus are commonly damaged in lacerated wounds to these areas, and the claws may stick up rather than curve neatly down to the ground. This injury also occurs in the racing dog due to indirect force (the so-called "knocked-up toe").

In some cases, the Achilles tendon may be severely damaged and the animal will show a peculiar lameness, being unable to extend the hock, and so walking with the metatarsus on the ground (like a kangaroo). The Achilles tendon may appear slack, and the ruptured ends are usually palpable through the skin.

*Treatment*

Any wounds should be dressed and the limb placed in a splint and kept as still as possible to prevent the cut ends of the tendon separating further from one another.

### Injuries to the Thorax

Any wounds on the thoracic wall must always be treated with caution since it may not be obvious how deeply the injury penetrates.

The causes of such wounds may be road accidents, severe bites, staking accidents, gunshot wounds etc., and the danger is always that the wound may have penetrated the pleural cavity to create an **open pneumothorax** (air in the pleural cavity). As the animal inhales, air is sucked into the pleural cavity through the wound so the negative pressure in the pleural cavity is destroyed, and the lungs will gradually collapse. Fractured ribs may also cause a pneumothorax if the sharp ends of the fragments pierce the lungs to allow air to escape into the pleural cavity from the lung spaces. This is called a **closed pneumothorax,** as there is no wound leading from the body surface to the pleural cavity. Finally, if a blood vessel is damaged in the thorax and the blood collects in the pleural cavity, the condition is termed **haemothorax**. If the bleeding is severe, this will also cause lung collapse.

*Signs*

Thoracic wounds causing an open pneumothorax often "hiss" on inspiration as the air is drawn in through the wound. Patients with closed pneumothorax may have subcutaneous emphysema over the chest wall (p. 503).

Animals with collapsed lungs show increasing "air hunger" as the situation deteriorates (p. 263).

*Treatment*

The wounds should be carefully cleaned, taking care that no fluid is drawn into the pleural cavity. **Penetrating foreign bodies should not be removed** as this may lead to sudden lung collapse and death. Instead, the protruding portion should be cut off close to the skin and a ring pad dressing used to protect the remaining portion from being pushed deeper into the wound. The torn tissues may be folded back over the injury to seal the hole and a lint or gauze pad placed over the wound and bound on to the thorax to keep the tissues in position. If the "hissing" noise can still be heard after the tissues are folded down, an airtight dressing such as polythene or cling film should be placed over the wound before the lint and bandage are applied.

All patients should be encouraged to rest as much as possible and should be allowed to breathe oxygen if there is evidence of "air hunger" (p. 264).

### Injury to the Abdomen

Injuries to abdominal wall are caused by similar accidents to those damaging the thoracic wall. Wheels of vehicles may pass over the abdomen causing severe crushing injuries. It must also be remembered that many surgical operations involve incising the abdominal wall.

*Signs*

As with the thoracic injury, abdominal wounds must be treated cautiously as it can be difficult to appreciate the severity of the wound.

If there has been penetration of the abdominal cavity, part of the contents (particularly the lacy fat of the omentum) can escape and protrude from the wound. Therefore, fatty tags on the surface of the wound may be cause for concern and reassessment of the injuries.

Occasionally, no external wound is seen and yet the muscles of the abdominal wall are torn to allow abdominal organs to escape from the peritoneal cavity. Such injuries are common following crushing of the abdomen e.g. in road accidents etc.

The most serious of this type of injury is the **diaphragmatic hernia**, or rupture when the muscular diaphragm is torn, and liver, stomach and intestines can enter the chest to collapse the lungs. Other serious injuries can occur in the inguinal region. The empty bladder may escape through a small muscle tear and then become trapped outside the muscular abdominal wall as it fills with urine over a period of hours.

Any organs trapped outside the peritoneal cavity may gradually swell if the venous blood return from the organs is cut off or reduced. The organs then become very painful, swollen and inflamed. The arterial blood supply may also be reduced and the tissues start to die. This is then termed a **strangulated hernia**, and will cause severe illness.

*Treatment*

In cases where abdominal viscera protrude through an open wound, the hair should be clipped away in the normal manner, but no antiseptics used in case irritant chemicals penetrate the peritoneal cavity. The protruding viscera should be washed with warmed sterile saline to remove any grit or dirt and an attempt made to gently replace them into the peritoneal cavity. No force should be applied and it is easiest to restrain the animal in such a position that the wounded side of the abdomen lies uppermost so that gravity assists the replacement. However, if there is any difficulty in breathing, the animal should not be forced to lie on its side or its back as this could prove fatal.

If it is impossible to replace the viscera, they must be kept warm, moist and undamaged by a covering of sterile swabs soaked in sterile saline and bandaged firmly but gently in place by a crepe bandage encircling the abdomen. Many-tailed bandages may also be used to keep the swabs in position and to avoid damage to the viscera. The viscera should be inspected every 15 minutes to renew the dampened swabs and check that the bandaging has not interfered with the circulation to the protruding viscera. The animal must be constantly observed to prevent it tampering with the dressings as animals can inflict severe damage to protruding viscera. Loops of small or large intestine may be literally eaten away.

The patient should be confined, made comfortable and treated for shock. Veterinary assistance must be sought as soon as possible so that strangulation can be treated or avoided.

## Injuries to the Alimentary Tract

### The mouth

Pieces of stick or bone sometimes become wedged transversely across the roof of the mouth between the molar teeth. Portions of soft bone may become wedged on or between the teeth. Needles are occasionally found embedded in the tongue and fish-hooks may penetrate the lips or tongue. Dogs playing with sticks occasionally "run on to" the stick, which can cause extensive lacerations, especially to the underside of the tongue and pharynx. Fragments of wood may break off and lodge in the wound. Curious cats and dogs may get their heads or noses wedged into discarded food tins etc.

*Signs*

Foreign bodies in the mouth usually cause profuse salivation and continuous movements of the jaws and tongue as the animal tries to dislodge the problem. Animals usually paw frantically at the sides of the mouth or rub their face on the ground, in an attempt to remove the foreign body.

*Treatment*

Removal of foreign bodies should be attempted cautiously, as the animal will often resent handling of the mouth, and general anaesthesia may be required. If the foreign body does not dislodge easily, excessive force should not be applied as the object may have penetrated the tissues more deeply than it appears. **No attempt should be made to pull out a fish-hook.** Because of its barbed end, the shaft should be pushed still further into the tissues until the barb comes out through a second puncture. The shaft of the hook is then cut through and the two halves removed independently. (p. 592).

### Pharynx and oesophagus

Foreign bodies may often lodge in the pharynx, and the most serious of these is the partly swallowed ball which lodges just behind the tongue on top of the larynx, being just too large to pass down the oesophagus. Dogs suffering this problem may become rapidly asphyxiated and collapse.

Cats eating grass frequently get a blade of grass stuck in the pharynx as they try to swallow it. Sewing needles are occasionally found embedded in the walls of the pharynx or come to lie across the pharynx of young animals. In many cases a length of cotton thread remains attached to the needle and this should not be removed as it serves as a valuable guide to locate and, in some cases, remove the needle. The bones which are usually incriminated are either fish bones or rough irregular bones such as chop bones or chicken bones, where the projections prevent them from being swallowed. Inflammation of the pharynx as a result of trauma, stings etc. can also cause severe problems if the walls of the pharynx become swollen.

*Signs*

A cat with a pharyngeal foreign body will often sit patiently, refusing to eat or drink, or gulping convulsively when swallowing. Dogs with foreign bodies in the pharynx or oesophagus show more distress, retching and gagging and frequently gulping. Food is not normally taken, but, if it is, and the obstruction is complete, the food will be regurgitated almost immediately. All affected animals will salivate if swallowing is too painful.

When the walls of the pharynx are

swollen or a foreign body partially obstructs the pharynx, the breathing is usually noisy and the animal may show evidence of "air hunger" (see asphyxia). Total obstruction results in rapid asphyxiation, collapse and death.

*Treatment*

With the animal held firmly, the mouth should be opened as far as possible to inspect the throat. Pharyngeal foreign bodies are rarely removable without an anaesthetic, as they are usually lodged beyond reach, but it may be possible to carefully attempt removal of a foreign body with fingers or forceps if it can be seen clearly. A thread should not be pulled, but traced to determine if it is attached to a needle/fish-hook etc. If this is so, and the needle cannot be dislodged, the two ends of the thread should be tied together to prevent unthreading of the needle. If a fish-hook is involved, the line should not be tampered with for fear of worsening the injury.

Foreign bodies which obstruct the airway will kill animals very quickly, and **must be removed or held to one side to allow air to pass** down the trachea. A small endotracheal tube may be passed down the trachea alongside the foreign body to maintain the airway in the asphyxiated unconscious patient. The patient must be closely observed as these animals gain consciousness very rapidly and the endotracheal tube may need to be removed so as not to compound the problem by the inhalation of a chewed-off endotracheal tube. Should unconsciousness return, the patient must be intubated again with all speed. A loose fitting face mask may be improvised but if this upsets the animal, do not persist in trying to use it.

Removal of smooth pharyngeal foreign bodies, such as the ball, may be attempted using the *Heimlich manoeuvre* as applied to animals. The animal should be suspended upside down if possible and a sharp punch administered to the abdominal wall just above the xiphisternum, angled downwards towards the diaphragm.

This should stimulate the animal to cough and the smooth foreign body will often be dislodged and fall to the floor. If the dog is too large to suspend by the rear legs, the hindquarters should be raised as much as possible and the head allowed to hang down before the blow is administered. The procedure may be repeated four times, but if not successful after this time, attempts should be discontinued for fear of causing internal injury, and the theatre should be prepared for an emergency operation. First aid workers also refer to this Heimlich manoeuvre as the "abdominal thrust" since it suggests the technique used in removing a foreign body.

**Stomach**

(a) *Foreign Bodies.* Many objects may be swallowed and lodge in the stomach. They usually cause little trouble except occasional vomiting. Sharp objects may injure the stomach wall and cause haematemesis (see b.)

*Treatment*

If a foreign body is suspected, all food and water should be withheld until a veterinary surgeon is consulted.

(b) *Haematemesis or Vomiting Blood.* This may occur if the stomach lining has been damaged (e.g. by a sharp foreign body, a blow to the abdomen) or inflamed (e.g. by infections which cause persistent vomiting). Certain poisons also cause hae-matemesis (e.g. Warfarin). Ingested blood (e.g. from licking haemorrhaging wounds or metritis discharges) may be commonly vomited.

## Signs

Fresh blood appears bright red or gives a pinkish tinge to the vomit. Blood which has remained in the stomach for any length of time is brown in colour and resembles coffee grounds as it is partially digested.

## Treatment

The animal should be kept quiet and treated for shock. In some cases, great thirst may be exhibited, but no food or fluid should be given by mouth. A piece of ice placed on a flannel in a dish so that the water formed as the ice melts is absorbed and cannot be taken, may be given to the animal to lick.

(c) *Gastric Dilation and Torsion.* This is an extremely serious condition, almost always seen in large, deep-chested dogs, but dilations occasionally occur in elderly small dogs. Death may occur unless the first aider is prepared to take certain emergency measures.

## Signs

Restlessness, and signs of discomfort are usually first seen several hours after feeding. The dog tries to eat grass and attempts to vomit without success. In some cases, gas may be belched up, and the owner usually notices a swelling of the anterior abdomen, which also pushes out the posterior rib cage. Breathing becomes laboured as the swelling enlarges and the condition becomes more painful. The dog collapses gradually into lateral recumbancy, when the gas-filled stomach can be clearly seen to bulge on the left side, just behind the rib cage. Gentle tapping on the abdominal wall with finger-tips produces a hollow, drum-like sound. If untreated, the dog will become unconscious and the stomach will rupture and the animal will soon die.

## Treatment

The patient must be kept quiet and treated for shock. The condition is acutely painful and the animal must be handled very gently and with care. **Veterinary assistance must be sought immediately**, but, if the dog is collapsed and uncon-scious and veterinary help is delayed, an attempt may be made to pass a stomach tube once the airway has been maintained by intubating with a cuffed endotracheal tube.

The stomach tube is first measured against the outside of the patient, laying the tube on the dog so that it follows the course of the oesophagus down the neck, through the thorax to the posterior edge of the thorax. A mark is made on the tube where it lies level with the canine tooth. This precaution ensures that the operator knows how far to pass the tube in order to position one end inside the stomach. (Fig. 4.9).

The blunted end of the stomach tube is then lubricated and passed down the oesophagus. When the cardiac sphincter of the stomach is reached, there will be some resistance, but gentle pressure may overcome this. If not, **do not persist** in the attempt to enter the stomach. The sto-mach may have twisted on itself and force will only rupture the oesophagus.

If stomach tubing is unsuccessful, the gas may be allowed to escape by using a wide bore (G 16) intravenous needle to pierce the left abdominal wall at the point

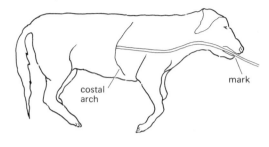

FIG. 4.9.

of maximum distension. *This procedure must only be performed with the knowledge and consent of the veterinary surgeon.* It must only be attempted if the patient has become unconscious and as an emergency measure, to save the dog's life. The skin is clipped and prepared for surgery. The large bore needle is **inserted at right angles to the skin at the point of maximum distension.** As soon as the stomach is entered, a gust of gas will escape, and the pressure will gradually reduce. The needle hub must be held in position, pressed against the skin at right angles as the abdomen slowly deflates. The dog should then be treated for shock.

In all cases, surgery will be necessary, and the nurse should prepare the theatre accordingly.

**Intestine**

(a) *Obstruction.* The small intestine can become blocked by foreign bodies similar to those found in the stomach, or by portions of intestine which "telescope" into one another (*intussusception*).

*Signs*

Many foreign bodies cause partial or complete obstruction, occasionally resulting in acute abdominal pain and persistent vomiting which, if the obstruction is complete, is often brown, foul-smelling faecal vomit. Once the foreign body passes through into the large intestine, the signs disappear, as the large bowel has a far greater diameter and the foreign body no longer causes an obstruction.

*Treatment*

No useful first aid is possible beyond making the patient comfortable. Frequently, radiographs must be taken and surgical intervention is necessary. Any suspected case should be referred to a veterinary surgeon at once, and intravenous fluids may be prepared for administration.

(b) *Infection.* Infection by canine parvovirus will cause acute, continual vomiting and possibly collapse, especially in young, unvaccinated animals. The vomit may be clear, bile stained or tinged with blood and the owner may report that bloody and foul-smelling diarrhoea is also being passed.

*Treatment*

Isolate these patients and contact the veterinary surgeon as soon as possible. Lactated Ringer's Solution (Hartman's Solution) may be prepared for intravenous administration.

## Rectum and anus

(a) *Prolapse of the Rectum.* A protrusion of the rectum through the anal opening may involve only the mucosal rectal lining or the entire thickness of the wall is included in the prolapse.

The condition is more commonly seen in young puppies or kittens, and is often associated with conditions producing diarrhoea and tenesmus (straining to pass faeces). It is also seen in hamsters and can be quite severe.

*Signs*

A reddish mass protrudes from the anus, which is covered with mucous membrane and often coated with thick mucus. It is frequently congested and may dry out or ulcerate if not replaced. There are times when it may be difficult to distinguish this mass from a prolapse of the vagina in the female.

*Treatment*

The protrusion should be bathed in warm saline (0.9% solution is least irritant) and lubricated with liquid paraffin. Gentle pressure may then be applied to ease it back into place—a finger-and-thumb "pinching" movement on the end of the protrusion is usually the most successful, but may not work if the protrusion is severe and involves the entire thickness of the rectal wall. Many cases will require surgical treatment either to reduce the prolapse or to prevent further prolapse at a future date. An analgesic suppository may be inserted to prevent straining until further treatment can be carried out.

(b) *Anal Foreign Bodies.* Sharp pieces of bone or small pieces of bone impacted into a mass may become lodged in the posterior rectum and anus. Pins, safety pins or needles may also lodge across the rectum or anus, or penetrate their walls.

*Signs*

The animal may show constant irritation by persistently licking the anus. Constant straining is a sign of the non-penetrating foreign bodies, whereas the sharp foreign body will cause the animal to cry out when it strains to pass faeces.

*Treatment*

Any foreign body in the anus should be removed very carefully to avoid further damage and prevent pain. The area should be lubricated with liquid paraffin and the bone may then be removed with fingers or forceps, if it is not too firmly lodged. If a thread is found hanging from the anus, a search should be made to discover the other free end, and the two ends tied together. Gentle pulling may remove the needle, but no force must be applied. If the foreign body cannot easily be removed, the animal should be referred to a veterinary surgeon.

(c) *Impacted Anal Sacs.* Blockage of the ducts of the anal sacs and subsequent impaction may lead to abscess formation. Such an abscess will usually break to the outside of the rim of the anus.

*Signs*

The animal shows initial irritation of the area, but, as the abscess forms, the area is swollen and the skin becomes reddened, shiny and very painful. The abscess soon bursts to the relief of the patient.

*Treatment*

Matted hair should be clipped away from the area and the wound washed with mild antiseptic solution. Hot fomentations may speed the pointing of the abscess in the earlier stages—a pad of cotton wool moistened with hot water can be held against the perinaeum.

## Injuries to the Respiratory Tract

### Epistaxis

Epistaxis, or bleeding from the nose, usually arises from the vascular turbinate mucosa and is not, in itself, a serious haemorrhage. Most cases occur following a direct blow to the nasal bones and this rarely causes any problems, but occasionally epistaxis is associated with severe skull fractures. Other cases are caused by haemorrhaging nasal tumours, or, more commonly, persistent sneezing.

*Treatment*

The animal should be rested as much as possible. Cold compresses applied to the nose will help to control the haemorrhage, but in some cases, adrenalin swabs may be needed to treat the condition.

### Foreign bodies in the nose

Grass seeds, grass blades and occasionally wooden splinters can gain access to the nose of the dog and cat. It is not uncommon to find that a blade of grass will work its way forward down the cat's nose from the pharynx.

*Signs*

Nasal foreign bodies give rise to violent sneezing and rubbing of the side of the nose with fore-paws. Epistaxis may be induced by sneezing and there is often a purulent nasal discharge present.

*Treatment*

The foreign body will sometimes be visible at the nostrils, and may be carefully removed. On other occasions, nothing is visible and the advice of the veterinary surgeon must be sought.

### Injury to the larynx

*Signs*

Wounds or blows to the laryngeal region may produce rapid swelling of the tissues which, in turn, will lead to difficulty in breathing and asphyxia in extreme cases. Any wound penetrating the larynx will allow air to escape and haemorrhage is likely to be frothy in nature as the blood is mixed with air.

*Treatment*

Asphyxia, haemorrhage and wounds should be treated as described elsewhere in the text. Care must be taken when cleansing the wound that no fluid is allowed to enter the air passages.

### Injury to the trachea

The trachea may be injured in street accidents, fights or by strangulation. It may be lacerated by barbed wire or incised if the animal falls through glass.

*Signs*

The tissues of the neck may be swollen and painful and breathing is often harsh and noisy or the animal is dyspnoeic. Any wound penetrating the trachea allows air to be sucked in and blown out of the wound during respiration. Subcutaneous emphysema may develop around these injuries.

*Treatment*

Treatment is as outlined for injuries to the larynx.

## Injury to the lungs

Lungs may be injured by indirect violence such as a blow to the chest which causes multiple minor haemorrhages into the lung tissues, or by direct violence such as a displaced fractured rib, penetrating gunshot wounds or staking injuries.

*Signs*

External wounds and haemorrhage may or may not be present in both cases, but animals are usually shocked and breathing is often painful and difficult. Bleeding from the lungs (**haemoptysis**) may be present, in which case bright red, frothy blood is coughed up. These injuries may be complicated by a haemothorax or a pneumothorax.

*Treatment*

Lung injuries must always be regarded as serious. Rest is essential and the animal should be allowed to assume the position which if finds most comfortable. Wounds, haemorrhage and shock should be treated as discussed elsewhere and additional oxygen supplied (p. 579).

# Injuries to the Urogenital System

## Kidney

Crushing injuries of the abdomen which rupture the kidney result in instant death. Less severe trauma may bruise the kidney tissue and result in **haematuria** or blood in the urine.

## Bladder

Rupture of the bladder is also seen following crushing injuries to the abdomen when the bladder was full of urine. The animal is pale and shocked, and occasionally a small drop of blood-stained urine is seen at the vulva or prepuce. If the bladder is simply bruised or inflamed, the animal shows **dysuria** (difficulty in passing urine), **polyuria** (passing urine at frequent intervals) and haematuria in many cases. This is usually observed when there is a bacterial bladder infection or if bladder stones are present, but haematuria is also commonly seen in cases of pelvic injuries (p. 238).

## Urethra

*Signs*

Occasionally wounds may involve the male urethra as it runs through the penis, and this may also result in dysuria and haematuria.

**Anuria** (absence of passing urine) or the passing of small volumes of urine may be reported if the urethra of the male is blocked by small stones which have been washed out of the bladder to lodge firmly in the narrow part of urethra as it passes through the os penis. The animal will make frequent attempts to urinate and may succeed in passing a few drops. However, as more urine is produced by the kidneys, the bladder becomes distended. The animal is very distressed and cries in pain. As the condition progresses, the patient will collapse and eventually the bladder may rupture. Palpation of the abdomen must not be attempted, but the hard, spherical shape of the bladder is sometimes felt in the posterior abdomen whilst moving the patient.

*Treatment*

There is no specific first aid treatment for any of the above conditions and the animal should be made as comfortable as possible and treated for shock, pending the arrival of the veterinary surgeon. Surgical intervention is usually necessary and the theatre should be prepared.
Note—Care must be taken when examining a bitch to ensure that the normal bleeding of the oestrous cycle is not confused with haematuria.

**Paraphimosis**

This occurs in the male dog when the erect penis becomes too engorged to slide back into the prepuce.

*Signs*

The penis is very swollen and reddened, and the prepucial opening appears to cut into the engorged tissues.

*Treatment*

Cold compresses and ice packs will markedly decrease the blood flow to the penis and allow it to slip back into the prepuce. Pinching the skin just in front of the scrotum also will often cause the swollen penis to reduce rapidly in size. Liquid paraffin, K–Y jelly etc. may be used to lubricate the penis if the tissues

have become dry and tacky. If these procedures are not successful, the penis should be kept moist and veterinary assistance sought, as it might be necessary to surgically enlarge the prepucial opening.

## Injuries to the Eye

### Examination of the eye

The eye is a delicate and sensitive organ, so examination and treatment must be carried out gently and carefully.

It is best to examine the animal in a dimly-lit or darkened room, as the patient is more likely to open the eye. For detailed examination, an auroscope head or torch may be used to illuminate the eye itself.

The lids may be easily examined for evidence of injury and may be opened gently and everted slightly to allow examination of the conjunctiva and nictitating membrane (third eyelid). Whilst examining the eye, note any discharges of fluid, their appearance and quantity. Clear fluid escaping could indicate a ruptured eyeball; purulent discharges may be evidence of a foreign body.

*Signs*

Whatever the cause of pain in the eye, the clinical signs are similar:
The eyelids are screwed up against the light and the patient may seek to hide away in dark corners.
Tear production is increased and may overflow the eyelids.
The sclera and conjunctiva are often reddened and inflamed.
The animal may rub the eye with a fore paw, or rub its head against furniture etc.

## Eyelid

Wounds to the eyelid are seen following road accidents, fights etc. Allergic reactions, insect stings etc. may produce severe oedema of the eyelid conjunctiva so that it becomes like a pink cushion, bulging out when the eyelids are open. Grass seeds and other foreign bodies may become lodged in the conjunctiva or beneath the nictitating membrane.

### Signs

All conditions exhibit a varying degree of pain and discomfort, although foreign bodies in the eye cause the greatest pain, and may cause a purulent ocular discharge.

### Treatment

Any wounds should be cleansed with care to ensure that irritant antiseptic solutions are not washed into the eye.

Non-penetrating foreign bodies should be removed wherever possible. Large foreign bodies (e.g. grass seeds) may be grasped manually and removed, but smaller ones (e.g. grit) should be flushed into one corner of the eye using warmed sterile saline solution. Once lying on the sclera or lid conjunctiva, the culprit can be removed more easily and safely as the tissues are far less sensitive than the cornea, and more robust. A piece of moistened lint or fine paint brush is used to lift the foreign body from the eye surface.

If the foreign body does not move when saline is flushed across the eye, it must be assumed to have penetrated the eyeball, and should not be disturbed. Veterinary advice must be sought immediately.

## Eyeball

The eyeball is well protected by the bony orbit and the eyelids. However, fracture of the orbital bones can produce severe bruising of the eye and blows to the eye can cause haemorrhage within the eye, despite the protective eyelids.

### Signs

Affected animals show signs of pain and bruising of the bulbar conjunctiva over the sclera (seen as a bright red blood blister) may often indicate that the eye has received a blow.

**Prolapse of the eyeball** is most commonly seen in short-nosed breeds which have a very shallow bony orbit and protruberant eyes. The prolapse usually occurs as the result of a road accident or after a fight. The eyeball quickly becomes inflamed and congested as the eyelids close behind it. The cornea rapidly dries and other damage to the eyeball can occur as it is now totally unprotected.

### Treatment

The prolapsed eyeball is the only condition where specific first aid measures may be applied. The eyeball must be replaced as soon as possible because the dry cornea will soon become ulcerated and the optic nerve may suffer permanent damage. Liquid paraffin, olive oil, or, preferably, "false tears" (e.g. methyl cellulose preparations) should be used to lubricate the eyeball, and an attempt made to gently draw the lids out and over the eyeball. No force should be used and, if the attempt is unsuccessful, the cornea should be kept well moistened with sterile saline or "false tears" until a veterinary surgeon can attend the case. The animal must be constantly observed to ensure that it does not cause any further damage to the eye, and should be treated for shock and made as comfortable as possible.

### Cornea

Non-penetrating wounds (ulcers) may be caused by foreign bodies in the eye, or sharp objects such as cats' claws, thorns etc. Penetrating wounds occur as the result of more serious injury received in fights, road accidents etc. and may be complicated by injury to, or prolapse of, the internal structures of the eye, particularly the vascular iris. Any pressure on the eyeball results in a gush of clear or bloodstained watery fluid escaping from the eye (aqueous humour).

The cornea may also be damaged by scalding fluids, paint, acid or alkali splashing onto its surface.

*Signs*

The cornea is extremely sensitive and any injury causes squinting, blinking and excessive tear production. There is often a bluish or white tinge to the cornea at the site of the injury.

*Treatment*

Splashing of the eye should immediately be treated by repeatedly flushing the eye surface. Sterile saline or contact lens solutions should be used, but tap water can be used in an emergency in the home. Bicarbonate solutions may be applied to neutralize acid splashes and vinegar solutions for alkali damage, but **thorough flushing of the eye** is what really counts. Cold liquid paraffin should be used in hot fat splashes to avoid the fat congealing on the cornea. Penetration wounds of the eyeball should be disturbed as little as possible to avoid aqueous humour loss. The cornea may be cleansed by sterile saline and a sterile gauze pad fixed loosely in position over the eye by adhesive plaster, pending veterinary attendance.

Following first aid measures, the animal should be confined in a darkened room or kennel to alleviate discomfort, but steps must be taken to ensure that the wounded eye is not disturbed (e.g. by fitting an Elizabethan collar).

### Injuries to the Ear

### Injuries to the ear flap

*Signs*

The ears are frequently a site of injury following road accidents, or more often, from fights and bites. Wounds of the ear bleed freely and may cause shaking of the head and irritation. Scratching at the ear will increase the haemorrhage, and may even enlarge the wound.

*Treatment*

Wounds to the ear flap should be treated by normal methods, but care must be taken when clipping the fur that the ear flap itself is not cut. It is usually necessary to bandage the ear flap by folding it back to lie over the top of the head, and fixing it with a bandage which encircles the head. Large wounds may require surgical treatment later.

### Foreign bodies in the ear

*Signs*

Grass seeds commonly gain access to the ear canal and travel downwards to lie up against the ear drum. The animal will show intense irritation and pain, holding the head to one side, shaking its head violently and rubbing the ear with a forepaw, or along the ground.

### Treatment

The foreign body, if visible, should be gently removed with forceps. If this is not possible, olive oil or liquid paraffin may be poured into the ear. No attempt should be made to probe the ear, but veterinary attention should be awaited. No food must be given as a general anaesthetic will usually be needed before any foreign body can be removed from the depths of the ear canal.

### Collapse

Collapse is the commonest emergency reported by owners and covers a multitude of situations. The cause of the collapse must first be discovered so that the correct first aid procedures may be carried out. Careful questioning over the phone can help to distinguish whether the type of collapse is a real emergency or not.

Collapse can be divided into three classes (Table 4.1) which may be due to a variety of causes. It is not a static condition in many cases—the patient may deteriorate and die or rapidly improve to assume normal health. Constant observation is vital to detect changes in the patient's condition.

### Examination of the Unconscious Patient

Loss of consciousness occurs when the brain is affected so that the animal is unable to respond normally to external stimuli. In most instances, the brain is depressed and the patient becomes comatose, but in some cases the brain is very active and the body is violently affected as in epileptiform convulsions. In all cases a history is essential, and inquiry should be made to ascertain possible injuries that have been inflicted, the mode of onset of unconsciousness, the possibility of previous attacks of a similar nature and the previous medical history of the patient.

The patient must then be examined as described at the beginning of this chapter, paying particular attention to:

(a) *The position of the eye in the socket*—Cases of unconsciousness may mimic the planes of anaesthesia, and experience in judging the depth of anaesthesia can usefully be applied to assess the degree of central nervous system depression of the unconscious patient. Evidence of **nystagmus** (rapid involuntary side-to-side or up and down movement of the eyeball) or **strabismus** (squint) should be noted.

(b) *Palpebral reflex*—or, if absent, the *corneal reflex*. The cornea is easily damaged so this reflex should only be tested by touching a wisp of moist cotton wool onto the cornea and this is sufficient to make the eyelids blink. The cornea is so sensitive that this is one of the last reflexes to be lost as the animal loses its fight for life. However, it should be remembered that, in some cases of head trauma where the motor nerves of the eyelid muscles are damaged, the animal will be unable to respond and may not necessarily be dying.

(c) *Pupil size*—compare the pupil size of both eyes.

(d) *Pupillary light reflex*—a torch can be used as a source of bright light. Both pupils should constrict equally.

(e) *Depth of unconsciousness* as assessed above (a). In *stupor,* the animal can be roused with difficulty and pupillary and palpebral reflexes are present. In *coma,* the animal cannot be roused, the pupils are usually dilated and the eye reflexes are often absent.

TABLE 4.1.

| Class | Cause | |
|---|---|---|
| Conscious collapse | Partial oxygen deprivation | —e.g. following lung collapse, obstruction of the respiratory tract |
| | Circulatory problems | —anaemia e.g. following haemorrhage<br>—shock e.g. following road accidents<br>—"stroke"<br>—thrombosis of iliac or brachial artery. |
| | Abdominal catastrophies | —e.g. gastric torsion<br>urethral obstruction<br>bladder rupture |
| | Central nervous system conditions | —e.g. inner ear inflammation<br>disc protrusion |
| | Locomotor conditions | —e.g. arthritis, fractured bones<br>muscle wasting |
| | Drugs | —e.g. ACP, owner's medication |
| Spastic (rigid) unconscious collapse | Epileptic convulsions | |
| | Metabolic dysfunction | —e.g. uraemic fits, eclampsia |
| | Physical causes | —electrocution |
| | Chemical poisonings | —e.g. strychnine, slug bait |
| Flaccid (relaxed) unconscious collapse | Oxygen deprivation | —Asphyxia |
| | Metabolic dysfunction | —e.g. diabetes mellitus |
| | Central nervous system injury | —e.g. trauma following road accidents etc |
| | Chemical poisoning | |
| | Physical causes | —e.g. heat stroke |
| | Death | |

(f) *Odour of the breath*—certain poisons impart a characteristic odour to the breath, but more commonly, the smell of pear drops (acetone) is detected in cases of diabetes mellitus, and the smell of urine may be noticed in uraemic animals.

(g) *Convulsions*—violent irregular involuntary movements of the body. The time of onset and duration should be noted.

(h) *Rigidity*—involuntary spasm of muscles to appear stiff and firm should be noted, including the area involved.

(i) *Paralysis*—the muscles are relaxed in the paralysed area but the animal may struggle to move.

(j) *Incontinence*—note should be made as to any leakage of urine or faeces and whether passive or active (e.g. urination during an epileptiform convulsions).

## General care and resuscitation procedures

*Maintaining the airway*

If the animal is dyspnoeic but conscious, the airway should be cleared as much as possible.

Tight collars should be removed and the mouth examined to ensure that there is no obstruction at the back of the throat. However, it is most important that these animals are allowed to rest as much as possible, so attempts to examine the mouth should be abandoned if they cause distress. Asphyxia cases are hypoxic (that is, the blood does not contain as much oxygen as normal) to some degree and struggling will only increase the body's demand for oxygen, so that the hypoxia becomes more severe and the patient's condition deteriorates.

The animal should be encouraged to breathe oxygen or oxygen-enriched air to correct the hypoxia. Small dogs and cats can be placed in wire baskets, which in turn are placed in large plastic bags which may be inflated with oxygen to create a small oxygen tent. "Gas out" boxes (used in some veterinary surgeries for anaesthetising recalcitrant cats) can be used as oxygen tents if connected to an oxygen-only anaesthetic machine. Larger dogs must be encouraged to lie still and a stream of oxygen is directed at the nostrils. Forcing the dog's head into the mask will only distress the animal and worsen the problem. However, a plastic bag may be used to create a light flexible mask funnelling oxygen to the face. Some animals may allow a nasal cathether to be inserted into the nostrils, especially if only semi-conscious.

If the animal is unconscious but trying to breathe, the head and neck are extended and the tongue pulled out to clear the airway. The throat should be examined for signs of obstruction e.g. blood, mucus etc. (see p. 248 for Heimlich manoeuvre to remove pharyngeal foreign bodies). Fluids should be swabbed away and the trachea intubated. The cuff should be inflated to avoid inhalation of fluids. The animal can then be connected to an oxygen-only anaesthetic machine, but should be carefully observed as many of these cases regain consciousness rapidly.

*Artificial Respiration*

If respiratory movements have ceased, the **lungs must be mechanically inflated** if the patient is to continue to live.

*Non-intubated patients* should be laid on their side, the head and neck extended, tongue pulled out and the forelegs pulled forwards. The palm of the hand is laid flat on the chest wall just behind the mass of the triceps muscle of the foreleg. Firm steady pressure is applied and then released and the elastic rib cage springs back, drawing air into the lungs. **The pressure is reapplied every 1–2 seconds.**

This procedure must *not* be used in cases where any damage to the thoracic wall is suspected, as fractured ribs could easily pierce the lungs or heart during compression of the thorax. In these cases **"mouth to nose" resuscitation** should be used if no intubation facilities are to hand. The patient's nose is grasped in the left hand and the right hand is used to ensure an airtight seam along the lips once the tongue has been pulled forwards. Blowing down the nose should inflate the lungs, but care must be taken not to over-inflate the lungs. Gentle puffs are best blown in at one second intervals.

*Intubated patients* should be connected to an oxygen supply from a closed-circuit anaesthetic machine and **the rebreathing bag used to inflate the lungs.** Only very gentle pressure may be needed at frequent intervals to mimic panting respiration—i.e. approximately 120 breaths per minute, 2 breaths a second. Massive inflation of the lungs (equivalent to drawing a deep breath) can over-inflate the lungs causing damage to the lung alveoli and possibly driving the lungs against the sharp fragments of broken ribs. This panting form of artificial respiration can be so effective that it is possible to "rest" the respiration for 5 seconds in every 15 seconds to see if the breathing has restarted. However, if there is any sign of cyanosis, the respiration should be maintained continuously.

If no anaesthetic machine is available immediately, the animal should be intubated and the lungs inflated by blowing down the tube to mimic the panting movements. Carbon dioxide in your exhaled breath may stimulate the dog to breathe.

Artificial respiration is continued until the animal starts to breathe on its own, (which may take up to an hour or more) or until death has intervened.

### Cardiac Massage

The heart of an apparently dead animal may be stimulated by rhythmical compression at half a second intervals, simultaneously applied on either side of the rib cage over the area of the heart (ribs 3–6). Artificial respiration must also be maintained and for this reason, it is necessary to have two operators.

*Control any haemorrhage*—in the severely wounded animal, see earlier.

### Conserve Heat

These animals are in a state of shock and should not be allowed to lose heat. (p. 216)

### Administration of Fluids

Fluids by mouth should never be given to an unconscious animal unless the trachea is intubated with an inflated cuffed tube and a stomach tube is passed. The only indication for such measures is the hypoglycaemic diabetic patient, when glucose solution should be given via the stomach tube.

### Further Observation

When the patient has been stabilized and made comfortable, the most important point is to maintain constant, keen observation. This will help to avoid potential disasters, and enables a thorough, complete case history to be tabled for referral to the attending Veterinary Surgeon.

### Signs of death

*Absence of respiratory movements.*

*Absence of a heart beat* for 3 minutes as detected by palpation of the chest for the apex beat, and listening to the chest with a stethoscope.

*Loss of the corneal reflex.*

*Dilation of the pupil and loss of light reflex.*

*Glazing of the cornea.*

*Body cooling* and rigor mortis. After the muscles have relaxed, they gradually stiffen due to chemical changes in the muscle cells. Rigor mortis usually takes about 12 hours to set in throughout the body, but the rate is variable depending on the room temperature, cause of death and physical condition of the animal. The cooling of the body also takes several hours, again depending on the room temperature.

Rigor mortis will pass off after several days as decay sets in.

### Specific causes and treatment of unconciousness

Primary cases include those in which the patient becomes unconscious as an immediate result of injury or dysfunction of the nervous system itself. Secondary cases include those where the metabolism or function of the other body systems is upset, which then results in a loss of consciousness.

| Primary causes of loss of consciousness |
|---|

(a) Epilepsy
(b) Direct trauma to the brain
(c) Chemical causes—Poisons

Secondary causes
(a) Asphyxia
(b) Metabolic disturbances—hypoglycaemia in diabetic animals
       —hypocalcaemia in eclampsia
       —uraemia in kidney failure
       —cardiac failure
(c) Circulatory disturbances—strokes
       —shock
(d) Physical causes—Electrocution
       —Heat stroke
       —Hypothermia

## Primary causes

### Epilepsy

*Signs*

Clinical signs vary from animal to animal. The condition is more common in dogs than cats and is usually seen in young animals, especially if inclined to nervousness (primary fits) or the old animal (secondary fits following brain damage from diseases such as distemper).

Before the fit commences, the animal often becomes restless and may be unusually affectionate, continually seeking reassurance from the owner. Occasionally the dog will become hysterical, barking and rushing madly around before succumbing to the fit. The fit itself will usually happen suddenly. The animal collapses on to its side and goes into violent convulsions. The legs are extended, the head pulled back, neck extended, and there is involuntary champing of the jaws, which churns the saliva into a foaming froth around the lips. The eyes are open and stare fixedly. The respiratory rate is much increased and defaecation and urination are common during severe fits. Most convulsions subside after 5–10 minutes, but occasionally the dog will remain in a fit for hours, relaxing from one attack only to start shaking with the next fit (p. 515).

Following an attack, the dog will usually rise and wander aimlessly and unsteadily about, looking dazed and confused. Soon it will recognize the owner and although very tired, will be back to normal.

Often, the fit is not so severe as described above and the animal simply wanders around, staring fixedly and unable to settle. This is the least severe form of fit, and it is as well to remember that epileptic fits can vary in severity from this mild form to the most severe "grand mal" fit.

*Treatment*

Whatever the cause of the attack, the treatment remains the same. These attacks represent vast overactivity of the central nervous system 'circuits' and any extra stimulus will usually only worsen the situation and prolong the fit. The owners should be advised to contain the dog in a darkened (no visual stimulus) quiet (no auditory stimulus) room and remain in the room with the dog, but not to touch it (minimal tactile stimulus) unless the dog threatens to injure itself. Above all, **the owners must remain calm**, and any member of the family who threatens to become hysterical should not be allowed to stay with the dog. As the fits are often of short duration, it is best to leave the dog in the house to avoid stimulating it any further, but should the fit persist or should the owner be unable to cope with the situation the dog may be brought to the surgery where the dog should be confined to a dark, quiet kennel and observed, until the animal can be attended by the veterinary surgeon. When the dog is recovering from the fit, reassurance may be given if the dog seeks it, but no attempt should be made to prevent the restlessness as this may simply spark off another fit. Similar advice should be given in the case of the very mild epileptic dog.

Finally **the possibility of rabies** must always be considered in cases of unusual nervous signs in the dog and cat, although the likelihood of this lethal disease manifesting itself in the household pet in the UK is still mercifully remote.

### Direct Trauma

*Cause*

A blow to the head as sustained in a road accident or following a kick from a horse etc. may result in unconsciousness because pressure is exerted on the delicate cerebral hemispheres. Depressed fractures of the cranium will obviously cause such pressure and damage but concussion is frequently seen without any fracture being present. In such cases it is due to intracranial haemorrhage or oedematous swelling in the meninges overlying the hemispheres, or in the nervous tissue itself. As the entire cranium is formed by bone, any swelling must press inwards on to the brain itself.

*Signs*

The signs are very variable, ranging from a slightly dazed animal to the comatose patient, depending on the degree of injury. There may be haemorrhage from the ears, nose or mouth, vomiting, incontinence, paralysis, but all patients will be badly shocked. Breathing is slow and shallow, the body feels cold and the mucus membranes are pale.

In mild cases of concussion, the eye reflexes are usually present; in severe cases, the pupils may be unequally dilated, and vary in their reaction to light. Palpebral and corneal reflexes may be absent and the eyes may show nystagmus or strabismus. In the most severe cases, the pupils are dilated and all eye reflexes are absent.

The unconscious patient is usually flaccidly collapsed, but occasionally there may be spasmodic muscular shivering.

*Treatment*

Gentle palpation of the skull will reveal the presence of any fracture. **Constant assessment of the eye reflexes and degree of depression of the nervous system is essential.** Reflexes should be checked every 15 minutes, and the time and observations fully noted on the kennel chart. The airway must be maintained and action taken to conserve heat and minimize the shock, by confining the animal to a quiet warm darkened kennel. Constant monitoring of these patients is an important part of the animal nurse's duties (p. 643).

*Poisons*

Poisons should be considered in unconscious animals if no other cause is apparent.

*Signs*

The effects of poisons are very variable, depending upon the poison ingested. See p. 544–8. Specific treatments may be necessary.

If owners suspect that the animal has been poisoned, ask them to bring the packets which contained the chemical to the surgery, or ring the corporation involved to enquire what rat poison/weed killer had been used. Non-specific complaints against neighbours putting out poison should be regarded with scepticism but any vomit produced should be kept, in case of pending court actions.

## Secondary causes

*Asphyxia*

Asphyxia or suffocation results from any failure to oxygenate the blood.

*Causes*

*Partial or total airway obstruction* —Pharyngeal foreign bodies, swelling of the pharyngeal walls, collapsed trachea as seen in cases of strangulation etc.

*Interference with respiratory movements*—Paralysis of the respiratory muscles by poisons such as strychnine, scoline, or nervous damage. Crushing injuries prevent normal respiratory movement.

*Interference with oxygenation of the blood*—Fluid in the alveolar spaces prevents the air entering these structures where the blood can be oxygenated. Drowning accidents, bleeding from the lungs, paraquat poisoning, congestive heart failure may all cause asphyxiation. Carbon monoxide poisoning from car exhaust fumes will also suffocate the animal as the red blood cells combine with the carbon monoxide in preference to

oxygen, so that the oxygen content of the blood is severely reduced. Inhalation of noxious fumes from house fires may result in oxygen starvation because there is little oxygen contained in the gases inhaled (most of the oxygen has been "used up" by the flames) and the gases may be irritant which provokes inflammation of the respiratory tract, and fluid release into the alveolar spaces.

Animals that survive house fires but have inhaled smoke or fumes may be expected to develop bronchitis 48 hours after the incident. The nurse should anticipate this complication.

*Pleural cavity problems*—pneumothorax, haemothorax and diaphragmatic hernia will all cause lung collapse. Fluid pleurisy is quite common in the cat and may produce collapse and asphyxia.

*Signs*

Partial asphyxia occurs when small supplies of oxygen manage to reach the lungs and oxygenate the blood, but the patients are always hypoxic, and often in great distress, exhibiting **air hunger**. The respiratory movements are strenuous and exaggerated, the animal literally gasping for breath. The respiratory rate is increased (**tachypnoea**) and the animal will often lie in sternal recumbency with its neck extended and often mouth-breathing. Initially, the patient tends to sit very still and rest, but as the oxygen blood levels fall, the animal becomes **hyperaesthetic** (excitable), reacting with abnormal violence to any stimulus, and throwing itself around in an uncontrollable manner until unconsciousness intervenes. Death will soon follow.

Cyanosis is seen, and occurs rapidly in cases of airway obstruction, but more slowly in other cases. The mucosa changes from pink to mauve, and, unless rapid action is taken, the animal will die. Carbon monoxide is the exception to the cyanosis rule. The blood remains a brilliant cherry red despite the fact that there is very little oxygen in the blood stream. This is because the blood corpuscles carrying the carbon monoxide maintain the same colour as the corpuscles carrying oxygen.

### Treatment

Oxygenation is vital in all these cases, and providing pure oxygen for the animal to breathe means that the small volume of gas reaching the alveolar spaces is at least pure life-giving oxygen instead of the mere 20% present in inhaled air (pp. 258/9).

The cause of the problem must be removed if possible. Fluid in the alveolar spaces as the result of drowning accidents must be drained out immediately. Any weed etc. in the mouth should be removed and the animal held up by the hind legs if possible and swung round so that the fluid drains from the lungs. If the animal is too big, it must be laid on as steep a slope as possible and artificial respiration applied to encourage oxygenation and drainage of the chest. Once the animal has been resuscitated, it should be dried, and kept warm. Direct heat may be applied in these circumstances and warm fluids should be given by mouth.

### Metabolic Disturbances

*Hypoglycaemic coma.* Hypoglycaemia occurs in the diagnosed diabetic animal when there is an imbalance between the insulin given and the glucose available. Too much insulin removes the soluble circulating glucose and converts it to glycogen in the liver. The animal becomes hypoglycaemic (low levels of blood glucose) and the metabolism slows down.

The common causes are:

(i) mistake in measuring the dose when too much insulin is given, usually by the inexperienced owner or "dog sitter".

(ii) the correct dose given, but the animal refused to eat its meal.

### Signs

The time of onset depends upon the type of insulin used but usually the signs occur about 10 hours post injection. The animal first becomes dull and lethargic, but then has difficulty in moving and is ataxic (incoordinated). The mouth and body feel cold to the touch and the patient soon collapses into unconsciousness. Death soon follows (p. 524–6).

### Treatment

Glucose solution should be administered immediately the first signs are seen. One or more tablespoonful should be given by mouth, but, if glucose is not available, honey should be used instead. If neither of these is available, sugar water can be given, but this has the disadvantage that the dissaccharide of sugar must be digested first to release the glucose molecule, and this may not happen quickly enough to arrest the onset of the diabetic coma. If the patient is unconscious, the owners should bring the animal to the surgery immediately for an intravenous injection of glucose. The injection should be prepared ready for administration by the veterinary surgeon and a glucose solution may also be prepared for oral administration by stomach tube.

*Hypocalcaemia.* Lack of circulating calcium ions causes malfunctions of the nervous and muscular tissue. The problem of eclampsia is usually seen in lactating bitches with large litters when the pups are 2–3 weeks old, but it has also been seen in cats nursing kittens. The demand by the rapidly growing offspring for milk is enormous and drains the calcium from the mother's body. To meet this demand, the bitch must either take in calcium from the diet or reabsorb calcium from her bones. The latter is a slow process so that, unless enough calcium is given in the diet to cope with the demand, the bitch or queen will soon become deficient in circulating calcium ions and show signs of eclampsia.

### Signs

Initially, the bitch is restless and will not settle. She pants a lot and starts to shiver. This progresses to collapse and a hyperaesthetic animal, which jumps and twitches at the slightest sound. She soon becomes unconscious, and, in the last stages, the twitching will cease. Death soon follows unless treatment is given.

### Treatment

Calcium given by mouth is not effective as it is poorly absorbed. Intravenous calcium must be injected, and syringes should be prepared (usually with 10% calcium solution) ready for injecting when the veterinary surgeon can attend the case (p. 666).

No further sucking should be allowed by the pups as this will drain yet more calcium from the system.

*Uraemia.* Uraemic fits are usually seen in old dogs with chronic kidney failure and are due to a build up of toxic substances (especially phosphates) in the bloodstream which would normally be excreted by the kidneys. There is a long-standing history of polydypsia and weight loss in most cases, culminating in vomiting, anorexia and lethargy, and, in the last stages, epileptiform convulsions.

### Treatment

Euthanasia is usually necessary and the animal should be made comfortable and treated as an epileptic pending diagnosis by the veterinary surgeon.

### Circulatory Disturbances

*Cardiac failure.* Cardiac failure is usually seen in the older animal although acute heart failure does occur in association with parvovirus infection at a very young age. This is very rarely seen, as pups are now protected by the immunity of the mother.

### Signs

The animal may have been reluctant to exercise for some months and owners often report coughing on exertion, which becomes more severe as the condition advances. The animal may become cyanosed and collapse after unexpected exercise, but spontaneous revival sometimes occurs. In other cases, there is no heart beat when the dog is presented at the surgery.

### Treatment

If there is no heart beat, cardiac massage should be applied as soon as possible. However, these cases rarely respond unless they are presented to the surgery within minutes of collapse.

If the heart is still beating, oxygen therapy should be given, for the animal is almost certainly hypoxic to some degree.

*Strokes.* This condition also affects the older animal and is caused by a disturbance in the circulation to the area of the brain concerned with balance and coordination. However, in more serious cases, larger areas of the brain are affected with wide-reaching consequences.

*Signs*

All affected animals have some degree of nystagmus. Mildly affected patients may also have a marked head-tilt but more severe cases show in-coordination and a stumbling gait. Some animals are unable to stand and the most severely affected lose consciousness altogether.

*Treatment*

The patient should be reassured and calmed if conscious. Limiting the movement helps to make the animal feel more secure. Unconscious animals should be kept under constant surveillance and the airway maintained. Diuretics and corticosteroids may help these cases, but complete recovery is rare.

*Shock*—See p. 577–8.

*Physical Causes*

*Electrocution.* Electrocution occurs when a high voltage passes through the animal's body. If the line of conduction passes through the animals heart, the result is instantaneous cardiac arrest.

*Signs*

The animal is found collapsed by the source of the problem, but it may not be obvious exactly what has happened. Most cases occur because of electrical faults in everyday equipment and the most extraordinary things can happen. The wire mesh of the exercise runs of a kennels became "live" following an electrical fault and all the dogs in that block were electrocuted. A more gruesome story is the dog which urinated on a lamp post and electrocuted himself because the lamp post was "live", which goes to show that water in any form is a marvellous conductor of electricity.

*Treatment*

**SWITCH OFF THE ELECTRICITY SUPPLY** before touching the animal—the animal may well be electrically "live" though clinically dead. If the mains switch cannot quickly be located, *use a dry wooden pole* (remember that water conducts electricity) to push the animal well away from any object which may be electrically active. The animal should be given cardiac massage if no heart beat can be felt, and the airway of the unconscious animal must be maintained.

*Heat Stroke.* The cause is usually over exposure to heat, classically seen in the short-nosed breeds left in a closed car in the full sun. However, hairy dogs which have undergone considerable exercise or become very excited may suffer if the weather is humid and warm.

*Signs*

Initially, the animal is distressed, panting excessively and restless. As the situation worsens and the body temperature increases, the animal starts to become cyanosed, drools copious volumes of saliva and becomes unsteady of its feet. If the body temperature continues to climb, the animal will collapse, become comatose and soon dies. The body feels burning hot and the rectal temperature is off the scale.

*Treatment*

Cool the animal immediately using hose pipe, buckets of water, blankets and towels in cold water, ice packs, etc. Intravenous drips may be chilled before administration (p. 578). The airway should be maintained, saliva swabbed away from the unconscious patient, and oxygen given at the first signs of cyanosis. The rectal temperature should be checked every 15 minutes to avoid overdoing the cooling of the body. As soon as the temperature has fallen to 102°F, the animal should be dried off and placed in a cool kennel with access to cold water to drink. The temperature must be checked every 30 minutes to ensure that it is not allowed to rise again.

*Hypothermia.* Hypothermia is a common problem of the very small and the very young. Small mammals and birds readily suffer hypothermia and young puppies and kittens, with little or no temperature regulation are helpless if warmth is not given.

*Signs*

The animals become sleepy, lethargic and do not bother to feed. Movements become weaker and the patient will become comatose. The body feels cold to the touch (p. 579).

*Treatment*

Direct warmth must be applied, preferably with some form of temperature regulation. Hospital cages are ideal for anything from birds to young puppies as they may be thermostatically controlled. Heat lamps have to be used with caution as the young kitten or puppy is unable to move away easily from the heat and can become burnt. Hot water bottles are good, but must be constantly replenished.

Suggested temperatures for pups and kittens for revival:

0–7 days—85°F
7–14 days—80°F

**Further Reading**

1. Bush, B.M. (1982) *The Dog Care Question and Answer Book*, Orbis Publishing Ltd. London.
2. Kirk, Robert (1978) *First Aid for Pets*, Pelham Books.
3. Playfair, As. (1972) British Red Cross Society's *First Aid, Junior Manual*, E.P. Publishing Ltd.
4. West, Geoffrey (1979) *All About your Dog's Health*, Pelham Books.

# CHAPTER 5

# The Theory and Practice of Nursing—I

(a) Ethical Aspects

A. R. W. PORTER

The Veterinary Surgeons Act of 1966 provides that "no individual shall practise or hold himself out as practising or as being prepared to practise veterinary surgery unless he is registered in the register of veterinary surgeons or the supplementary veterinary register". Since qualification as a RANA does not entitle one to be listed in either register, it follows that a RANA is no more entitled to perform any act of veterinary surgery than any other lay person. Proposals have been made for a review of The Veterinary Surgeons Act 1966. It is possible that this will lead to the status of the RANA being more clearly defined than at present.

This is not to discount the training which a RANA receives. To quote the *Guide to Professional Conduct* issued by the Royal College of Veterinary Surgeons to its members, RANAs are trained personnel "who carry out nursing duties or assist veterinarians more competently, more expeditiously and with less explanation of what is required than untrained staff". Through their training they should, for example, be able competently to assist veterinarians in radiological examinations and the administration of anaesthetics, carry out side-room tests and so on. This does not, however, alter the fact that

RANAs are still lay persons in the context of the Veterinary Surgeons Act.

This statement of the general position still leaves two questions to be answered. First of all are there *any* acts of veterinary surgery which may be carried out by lay persons in spite of the general ruling set out above? And, secondly, What constitutes an act of veterinary surgery?

The answer to the first question is that the Veterinary Surgeons Act (and the subordinate legislation made thereunder) does allow certain classes of people who are not registered veterinarians to perform particular acts of veterinary surgery in certain circumstances. Dotors, dentists, physiotherapists and farmers all have special provision made for them within very closely prescribed limits. The ordinary citizen is also given the right by Schedule 3 of the Act to treat his own animals and this right is extended to the employee of the owner or any other member of the owner's household. In addition, anyone over the age of 18 years may carry out certain operations such as the docking of the tail of a dog or the amputation of its dew claws, provided that in each case this is done before the dog's eyes are open. But the general dispensation given to lay persons (and therefore to RANAs) which is of the greatest practical

269

importance is the provision in Schedule 3 of the Act whereby it is permissible for lay persons to render first aid, in an emergency, for the purpose of saving life or relieving pain. This plainly gives a RANA the right to administer first aid to an animal when there is no veterinary surgeon available. The question is, however, often posed—What is first aid? To this there can be no precise answer since the first-aid measures appropriate to different cases will vary enormously. But the wording of the appropriate part of the Schedule goes some way towards providing guidance by making it plain that the treatment given to the animal must:

(a) *be given in an emergency* (this means among other things that the RANA should not administer first aid if there is a veterinary surgeon available to treat the animal);

(b) *be given only if it is necessary to do so in order to save the animal's life or to relieve its pain* (thus if the animal's life is not in danger and it is not in pain, it is not permissible for a RANA to administer even first-aid treatment).

In addition one can say that the plain implication of the words "first aid" is that the treatment is given only as an interim measure until a veterinarian can take over. It is therefore not intended that this provision should be used as a cloak to enable RANAs or any other lay persons to deal completely and finally with any case.

The second question as to what is veterinary surgery is largely answered by Section 27 of the Veterinary Surgeons Act. This states that the term "veterinary surgery" includes:

(a) the diagnosis of diseases in, and injuries to, animals including tests performed on animals for diagnostic purposes;

(b) the giving of advice based upon such diagnosis;

(c) the medical or surgical treatment of animals;

(d) the performance of surgical operations on animals.

Even although this will cover the great majority of cases in which a RANA may be wondering whether what she is going to do constitutes an act of veterinary surgery or not, this definition can be amplified a little. There are obviously some procedures which do not amount to veterinary surgery, e.g. the removal of sutures and the replacement of dressings, the cutting of nails and beaks unless performed for the relief of a pathological condition, and the scaling of teeth carried out for cosmetic or prophylactic purposes. It follows that there can be no objection to RANAs carrying out such procedures, particularly if they are carried out on the orders of a veterinary surgeon so that there can be no suggestion that there is an element of diagnosis in the RANA's actions.

At the other end of the scale there are a number of procedures which would appear to be acts of veterinary surgery and which a RANA may still be asked by a veterinary surgeon to carry out in assisting him, for example, in an operation. Although the courts alone can decide whether or not a particular act amounts to veterinary surgery, the view taken by the Royal College of Veterinary Surgeons is that in such cases it is unlikely that the RANA would be deemed to be breaking the law *provided* what was done was carried out in the form of assistance to the veterinary surgeon under his immediate and personal supervision so that the act is really the act of the veterinary surgeon and the RANA is, in a sense, his "other pair of hands".

These guidelines should enable RANAs to avoid running foul of the law relating to the practice of veterinary surgery, but in any cases of doubts the invariable rule for any RANA should be to consult the employing veterinary surgeon who can himself consult the Royal College of Veterinary Surgeons if necessary.

## (b) Practice Organization

### I.O. KNAPP

One of the most valuable assets of any veterinary practice is the favourable impression that a client receives on a visit to the premises or from the telephone call made to the practice.

This impression is usually gained by talking to or meeting the RANA in the practice. Hence it is very important that the RANA should be efficient in practice reception work, answering the telephone, taking case histories, case recording and admitting and discharging patients.

**1. Reception.** One of the most responsible duties is receiving clients. The RANA's manner, therefore, while not lacking in dignity, should be pleasant and welcoming and her voice warm and friendly.

(a) *Personal appearance.* The RANA should maintain a very high standard of personal appearance and cleanliness. She should be neat, tidy and clean at all times. She should have an efficient manner, be understanding but firm and patient as owners may often be upset or fussy about their pets.

(b) *The reception room.* This should be kept clean and tidy. Ashtrays should be emptied and magazines tidy. Unpleasant animal odours should be dealt with.

(c) *The RANA should have a knowledge*

*The contribution of B. Rose is acknowledged in compiling some of the information for the 3rd edition.

of the practice's policy relating to routine work such as vaccination, spaying and worming in order to deal with owners' inquiries. Remember the following DO's and DONT's:

### DO's

(i) Be kind and patient.
(ii) Be polite, smart and efficient.
(iii) Be sympathetic and understanding. In fact DO be perfect.

### DONT's

(i) Show obvious fear of an animal.
(ii) Panic.
(iii) Show annoyance with a client.
(iv) Leave a client "dangling" on the end of a telephone.
(v) Send an animal out dirty or blood stained.

**2. Telephone answering.** The telephone today plays an important part in veterinary practice. It is therefore essential that the RANA is able to use the telephone efficiently and also to convey a good impression of the practice every time she receives or makes a call. A practice is often judged by the telephone manner of the staff.

(a) *Speak directly into the mouthpiece* in an even, pleasant tone. Speak clearly. Be brief but courteous.

(b) *Always answer the telephone promptly* by giving the number or name of the practice.

(c) *Always ask who is speaking* and if possible deal with the call. Never put a call through to your employer before you know that he is willing to take it, thus shielding him from unwelcome calls. It is often possible on asking who is calling and determining the reason for the call for the RANA to deal with the call without transferring it. If it is necessary to transfer the call to the veterinary surgeon it is useful to be able to give him some details first as it can be embarrassing if he cannot recall the essential details of a case. A client's confidence may be shaken if he does not immediately remember the case.

(d) *Give advice in an informed and firm manner* but if in any doubt consult the veterinary surgeon.

(e) *If necessary ask the client to telephone again* or otherwise obtain a telephone number so that you can call back.

(f) *If in any doubt* as to whether the animal needs treatment ask the client to *bring it into the surgery for examination.*

(g) *Make appointments for clients* for consultation or surgery.

(h) *If domiciliary visits are undertaken* by the practice, make sure to obtain the full postal address and suitable directions from the client. Spell the name.

(i) *Be prepared to give clear advice on first aid.*

**3. History taking.** Note:
(a) *Client's name, address, telephone number, date.*
(b) *Species, breed, sex, age and reason for visit.*
(c) *Outline of the condition to be examined.*
(d) *A brief note of the owner's observations of the accident or the illness shown by his animal.*

(e) *Details of previous illnesses/vaccinations.*
(f) *If necessary administer first aid until the veterinary surgeon arrives.* When taking a history write clearly, neatly and briefly. It is often possible to use abbreviations or write in note form, e.g. R.T.A. = road traffic accident, T.C.A. = To come again, # = fracture.
(g) *Obtain the signature of the owner on a standard consent form.*

**4. Case recording.** It is easy to see that hospital records are extremely important in the business operation of a veterinary practice for providing information about income and expenses. Medical records are also important to the veterinary surgeon for providing a history of previous treatments as it is impossible to recall in each case what treatment an animal has received. The patient's card should be retained in a filing system. Whether you are making entries in the records or filing them you should strive to be accurate. Inaccurate records are worse than no records, while the best records are useless if you cannot find them.

When samples have been examined or other tests carried out, the laboratory or X-ray report should be attached to the case card or details entered on the card.

### Admission and Discharge of Animals

1. Ideally, the admissions area will be separate from the central thoroughfare and close to the hospital cages.

2. Admission times can be staggered to relieve congestion and allow time with the owner.

3. The client's impression of a veterinary practice is important. The nurse

should introduce herself and welcome the client the moment he arrives in the admissions area, encouraging his questions as well as informing him fully of the treatment his pet will receive while it is hospitalized.

4. The owner may wish to speak to the veterinary surgeon in charge of the case or inspect the premises where the animal is to be housed. There should be a clear practice policy on these matters.

5. The nurse should take down the routine details and ask any question relevant to the type of condition for which the animal is being hospitalized. For example:

Fasting—when did the animal last eat any solid food?

Fluid intake.

Medication given—as prescribed by veterinary surgeon or any home remedies.

Eating habits, especially in the more unusual species of pet.

Bowel motion.

Urination.

Vaccination status.

Oestrus phase: in the case of a bitch, ask if neutered or when was the last season.

Temperament.

Any abnormalities the owner may have noticed.

In the case of a whelping bitch the owner should be asked how long the bitch has been whelping, the length of interval between puppies, etc., and the previous whelping experiences of the bitch. If the animal is to have abdominal surgery or X-rays, the nurse should inquire if it has recently passed urine or faeces.

6. The admissions nurse must check the details on the case record:

Name and address of owner.

Telephone number at home and work.

Details of the animal: name, age, etc.

Ensure there has been no change in these since the client last attended the practice.

She must see that the relevant forms are signed if this is the routine procedure.

If a child has brought the animal to the surgery, the permission of the parents must be obtained before the animal is admitted for surgery or treatment.

The nurse must also note the items left with the patient, such as a bed and feeding bowls, collar or lead.

7. It is best to ask the owner to leave the room before his dog is taken to the hospital kennels. This saves him the distress of seeing the dog dragged away from him. It may be preferable to carry a small dog or allow the owner to take the dog to the hospital cage himself.

8. Collars and leads must be firmly secured and a check chain will eliminate the possibility of escape during transfer to the kennels. Cats must be carried in containers at all times when out of doors. There is nothing more distressing for the owner or embarrassing for the practice than to have to report than an animal has escaped. Escaper's must be labelled so that staff are warned to be extra careful, as should aggressive animals in the hospital.

9. Some owners will wish to wait with the animal while the pre-medicant injection is given. In some cases a pre-medicant is contraindicated, for example:

(a) When a pre-medicant has already been given by the owner.

(b) Breed idiosyncrasy to promazines or other drugs.

(c) When barium studies are to be performed (slows intestinal tract). Acetyl promazine is considered safe to use before contrast radiography.

(d) In shocked animals (lowers blood pressure further).

(e) In hypertensive disease.

(f) In animals that are likely to require heavy analgesia after surgery.

10. The cage must be labelled clearly with the hospital record and any other relevant charts, such as a record of fluid balance. The name of the owner, a description of the animal and the reason for admission are essential requirements.

11. Care must be taken when allocating space, i.e. dogs are best kept away from cats and cats from birds and small mammals. Nocturnal species will require daytime seclusion. Infectious cases must be isolated and barrier nursed.

12. During the admission procedure the nurse must continually reassure the patient; there are very few animals which enter hospital showing no signs of anxiety.

13. The nurse should note any physical or behavioural abnormalities on admission:

(a) Activity level: ability to walk;
lying or sitting;
abnormal     position
causing distress;

(b) Mental state: anxiety;
bright/dull;
nervous/placid.

(c) Level of consciousness.

(d) Colour: pallor, jaundice, cyanosis.

(e) Nutritional state: obese, dehydrated, oedematous.

(f) Deformity: joint deformity, weakness of limbs, unusual swellings.

(g) Skin and coat: lesions, bruises, wounds, rash, parasites, bed sores.

(h) Respiration: dyspnoea, noisy respirations, coughing, sneezing.

(i) Eyes: jaundice, inflammation, discharge.

(j) Nose: wet, dry and crusted, discharge.

(k) Pain: on movement, at rest.

(l) Retching or vomiting.

14. It is best if animals are arranged to be admitted at least 2 hours before surgical procedures, etc., are performed; they become acclimatized to their new and strange environment; routine blood samples can be taken and body temperature can be measured at rest.

### Discharging Animals from Hospital

1. It is of no use discharging an animal that has been intensively nursed, until it has reached a stage within the capabilities of the owner. If, for example, the patient's fluid balance is unstable, it is best that it remains hospitalized.

2. The value of early discharge should be considered when an animal is obviously missing its owner and home or the owner has good nursing experience.

3. Sometimes it is preferable to hospitalize an animal for an extra day if it is likely to be in a more acceptable state for the owner to take home. This may apply to a bitch that has undergone ovariohysterectomy, for example. The owner will be relieved to see that his pet has been returned to him in a similar condition to when it was admitted.

4. In some cases written instructions must be given to the owner, e.g., when an animal has been admitted to hospital for diabetic stabilization or digitalization, or if the owner is hard of hearing or has difficulty in grasping instructions.

5. Medications must be prepared in containers along with the animal's belongings which must be clean and dry.

6. Transport arrangements must be

made if the animal is unfit to walk and care should be taken to see that it is kept warm during its journey home.

7. By staggering the time that animals are discharged, the nurse will have time to give the owner full instructions regarding after care at home and to answer his questions. The owner must feel that he is welcome to telephone the surgery for advice if he is at all concerned. The client's final impression of the hospital will be like his first, a lasting one. If he can see that his pet has been returned to him clean, well-groomed and comfortable he will be assured it has received the best possible care during its stay.

8. Make an appointment for a return visit if necessary. Make sure everything left with the patient is returned. Do not forget to make arrangements for paying the account.

*Editor:* The title Veterinary Nurse was approved for use in September 1984 by the RCVS and is likely to supersede the RANA title that has been in common use for the last 20 years.

(c) Observation and Care of Patients

E. M. CARR and D. P. McHUGH

## Observation of the Patient

One of the most important roles of the animal nurse is the day to day care and observation of patients. It is a field in which she is specifically trained to recognize the normal and abnormal states of the animals under her care. A good nurse should have the ability to recognize the changes which may occur and be aware of their importance in relation to disease patterns and their treatment. She should record her findings and report them to the veterinary surgeon in charge of the case and act on instructions given.

## Normal Appearance of the Dog and Cat

Close observation is necessary to assess what is normal and what is abnormal for each individual patient. It must be taken into account that the animal may be distressed by being in a strange environment and may need a little time to settle. For this reason it is advisable for one nurse to be responsible for the daily care of a particular animal so that she will become familiar with the appearance and behaviour of that patient. It will also give the animal a chance to get to know and trust the person who is looking after him.

A healthy dog will appear bright eyed, alert and interested in what is going on around him. He should react to stimuli such as a lead being rattled or a can of food being opened, and will usually be pleased to see people. He should be keen to exercise and be able to walk and run freely etc.

Behavioural patterns will vary with age, breed and temperament. Puppies for example will alternate periods of playing with periods of sleeping, whilst most older dogs will be content with regular exercise and longer sleeping periods. Some dogs when confined to a kennel develop a "guarding" instinct at first, but once out of their kennels will become more friendly.

A dog should be interested in food when offered and should eat and drink without difficulty. The actual quantities of food and water consumed will vary with the individual, but it is wise to ask the owner this information and type of food fed before admitting the patient to the hospital.

When taken out, it is normal for a male dog to urinate frequently to "mark" out territory; the bitch however may be content with emptying her bladder 2–3 times daily. Urine should be passed without difficulty or discomfort and it should be pale yellow and clear in colour; quantity will vary with the individual. Faeces are normally passed once or twice daily, but again there are individual variations and

The editor acknowledges the work of C. O'Hagan who supplied information on this topic for the 3rd Edition (1980).

in puppies they are usually passed more frequently. Firm faeces should be passed without undue straining and should be brown in colour.

On examination the coat should be clear and glossy, with no evidence of alopecia. The skin should feel supple and be free from scabs and parasites. The body should be well covered with flesh without showing signs of obesity. This should not be confused with the pot-bellied appearance which may be seen with abdominal fluid or an abdominal mass.

The eyes, ears and nose should be clean and free from discharges or swellings. The mucous membranes should be pink and moist. The external genitalia should also be free from swellings and discharge although during oestrus and after parturition it is normal for the bitch's vulva to be swollen and to have a clear or blood-stained discharge.

Temperature, pulse and respiration should be within the normal range. Respiratory movements should be apparent, but not laboured. There should not normally be any respiratory sounds or panting when the dog is at rest although most of the brachycephalic breeds do exhibit some respiratory noise.

It is often difficult to assess the normal appearance and behaviour of the cat under hospital conditions. Away from familiar surroundings they tend to become introverted or occasionally aggressive and may refuse food and drink. Under normal circumstances the cat will show an interest in food and drink although in general they are fussier eaters than dogs and may refuse food for several days. It is sensible to have asked the owner what the cat is normally fed. A cat's urination and defaecation pattern may be disturbed by hospitalization and the cat may totally refuse to use the litter tray provided.

The coat should be clean and glossy and a healthy cat will pay particular attention to washing and cleaning himself. Cats are usually content to sleep a lot of the time, but should be aware of what is going on around them and respond to being stroked or handled. Kittens like puppies will show alternating periods of sleep and play. Purring should not be confused with "snuffling" or wheezing which may be seen with upper respiratory tract infections. Like the dog there should be no signs of discharge from eyes, nose, ears and mouth. Temperature, pulse and respiration should be within the normal range.

## Appearance and Implications of Abnormalities in the Dog and Cat

The ability to detect abnormalities in animals undergoing hospitalization can only be gained with experience. An ill animal will usually exhibit signs which may not be obvious to an untrained person but which a nurse should recognize. Certain conditions show specific symptoms and an experienced nurse will know what signs to look for and realize their significance.

All abnormalities or changing clinical signs should be recorded no matter how minor they may seem, because to the veterinary surgeon they may take on more relevance. With other subsequent findings these may be very important in the diagnosis and treatment of the patient. This is particularly important in hospital kennels where the nursing staff must be constantly on the look out for developing signs of infectious diseases such as feline respiratory disease or canine parvovirus, which may not have been apparent at the time of admission.

Often the first sign that a dog is unwell is a change in behaviour—a normally happy, lively dog becomes dull and miserable. He may be disinterested in food and drink or may have developed an excessive thirst or voracious appetite. He will be disinclined to move or adopt an unusual posture. A closer examination should then be made to see whether other symptoms are exhibited. It is not always easy to assess whether an animal is in pain as different breeds and individuals have different pain thresholds. Restlessness, crying, trembling, panting and an elevated temperature are all possible signs of an animal in pain.

There may be a discharge from the eyes or nose; coughing or sneezing and possibly changes in the respiratory pattern. The temperature may be elevated or subnormal, the pulse rate and character may change. The mucous membranes can become pale, jaundiced or even cyanosed and they may feel dry and tacky. Vomiting and diarrhoea may be observed or conversely, constipation and tenesmus may occur. There might be excessive salivation and retching. Halitosis can be a feature of dental problems or a sign of nephritis when there will be a distinct uraemic smell. A "sweet" smell may be evident with ketoacidosis in cases of diabetes mellitus.

Polydipsia (an increased thirst) which is usually accompanied by polyuria (increased urine production) may be evident, although sometimes a decreased fluid intake and oliguria (decreased urine production) may be noticed. If a change in the drinking/urination pattern is suspected then fluid intake and output should be measured. There may be difficulty (dysuria) or a total inability (anuria) to pass urine, which must be dealt with promptly to avoid an emergency situation arising. Urine may appear blood stained or change from its normal pale yellow colour and become turbid—both of which should be reported.

Cats show many of the same abnormal signs as dogs, but some of them tend to be more marked. An unwell cat or one that is in pain can look almost moribund. The coat quickly takes on a "staring" appearance and the cat will cease to wash and clean itself. The third eyelids often become prominent. Cats tend to try and hide or sit and stare—they will be disinclined to move and generally get upset if disturbed.

Although it is important to be familiar with the aetiology of the common disorders, it is more important that the nurse is able to differentiate between signs of health and disease and to understand their significance.

Some of the common signs which the nurse should report to the veterinary surgeon are listed below. The important observations and common causes are also included:—

## Vomiting

1. *When it occurs in relation to feeding.*
2. *How often it occurs and the quantity produced.*
3. *Content e.g. blood, mucus, food, bile.*
4. *How ill the animal seems, if at all.*
5. *Accompanying signs.*
6. *Type:*

    *Vomiting* starts with salivation and nausea and is followed by active abdominal contractions which result in the expulsion of vomitus.

    *Regurgitation* is a passive process which results in the expulsion of undigested food from the oesophagus.

    *Projectile vomiting* is the violent ejection of stomach contents without nausea or retching.

    Gagging or retching is often mistaken for vomiting as a small amount of mucus is expelled.

*Common causes*: Ingestion of irritants such as decaying food and rubbish, or poisons; presence of foreign bodies or furballs; viral infections e.g. distemper, parvovirus, hepatitis; bacterial infections e.g. leptospirosis; metabolic disturbances e.g. nephritis, diabetes mellitus, pancreatitis, pyometra; abdominal tumours, endoparasites (especially puppies), reaction to drugs; travel sickness.

Additionally in cats, feline infectious enteritis, feline infectious peritonitis.

## Diarrhoea

This is the frequent passage of soft to liquid motions.

1. *Note colour and smell.*
2. *How often it occurs.*
3. *Evidence of straining.*
4. *Presence of blood, mucus etc.*

*Common causes*: Change in diet; bacterial infection such as leptospirosis; viral infection such as canine parvovirus, the early stages of distemper, hepatitis; feline infectious enteritis; pancreatic insufficiency, intussusception, tumours and endoparasites.

## Constipation

This is the infrequent or difficult evacuation of faeces.

*Common causes*: Dietary—especially after eating bones; fur balls in cats; prostatic hypertrophy; pelvic deformities; impacted anal glands; tumours; perineal hernia.

## Ocular discharge

1. *Whether unilateral or bilateral discharge.*
2. *Whether clear, purulent, bloodstained.*
3. *Whether the animal appears ill or not.*

*Common causes*: Various eye conditions; presence of a foreign body e.g. a grass seed; canine distemper; feline upper respiratory tract infections; trauma.

## Nasal discharge

1. *Whether unilateral or bilateral discharge.*
2. *Whether clear, purulent or bloodstained.*
3. *Whether the animal appears ill or not.*
4. *Whether accompanied by sneezing.*

*Common causes*: Distemper; upper respiratory tract infections in cats; chronic rhinitis or sinusitis; aspergillosis; foreign bodies e.g. grass seeds; tumours, which may cause distortion of facial outline.

## Aural discharge

1. *Whether unilateral or bilateral discharge.*
2. *Whether clear, purulent or bloodstained.*
3. *Whether the animal appears ill or not.*

*Common causes*: Presence of foreign bodies, ear mites, polyps; bacterial/fungal infection.

## Coughing

1. *When it occurs i.e. after excitement, exercise or at night.*
2. *Whether dry or productive and what is brought up.*
3. *Whether the animal is distressed.*
4. *Whether there are any other signs e.g. cyanosis.*

*Common causes*: Bacterial and viral infections such as distemper, kennel cough, pneumonia; congestive heart failure, chronic bronchitis; presence of foreign bodies, tumours, parasites e.g. *Filaroides osleri*, and roundworms in puppies and kittens.

## Polydipsia/Polyuria

1. *A fluid intake/output chart should be kept as an accurate record.*
2. *Whether drinking follows exercise.*
3. *Other accompanying signs.*
4. *Whether the animal is continent or incontinent.*

*Common causes*: Nephritis, pyometra, diabetes mellitus, Cushings syndrome, diabetes insipidus, salty diet, drug induced especially following corticosteroid therapy.

## Vaginal discharges

1. *Colour.*
2. *Consistency.*
3. *Is the animal ill?*
4. *Is there any vulval swelling?*
5. *Is the animal known to be pregnant?*

*Common causes*: Pro-oestrus, parturition, abortion, metritis.

## Convulsions

1. *Duration and frequency of seizures.*
2. *Description of seizures.*
3. *Behaviour prior to seizures.*
4. *Attitude after seizures.*
5. *Pupil constriction/dilatation/equal size. Nystagmus.*
6. *Presence of generalized illness.*

*Common causes*: Canine distemper; encephalitis, hydrocephalus, epilepsy, poisoning, storage diseases, brain tumours, uraemia, liver disorders, hypoglycaemia or hyperglycaemia.

## Changes in temperature

An elevated temperature (pyrexia) is usually associated with infectious diseases, pain, excitement, convulsions or heatstroke.

A subnormal temperature is seen in circulatory collapse and sometimes in puppies, kittens and anaesthetized animals who are unable to regulate their body temperature. Artificial heating may be necessary for these patients to prevent hypothermia occurring.

## Changes in the colour of mucous membranes

Mucous membranes should be examined in daylight as artificial lighting and coloured walls may affect their appearance.

If icterus (jaundiced mucous membranes) is present, note the severity and presence of accompanying signs. Common causes are leptospirosis, liver disease and autoimmune haemolytic anaemia.

Pallor of the mucous membranes occurs when there has been blood loss i.e. internal or external haemorrhage in circulatory collapse. It also results from destruction of red blood cells as in feline infectious anaemia and autoimmune haemolytic anaemia, and failure to produce red blood cells as in aplastic anaemia.

If cyanosis of the mucous membranes occurs the nurse should check for any obvious airway obstruction, other accompanying signs and note whether it is continuous or intermittent. Cyanosis may be caused by a reduced airway, depression of rate or depth of breathing or reduction of the effective size of the lungs.

## Changes in posture

An animal that is in pain or discomfort will assume a position in which it is most comfortable. With abdominal discomfort an animal may adopt a "tucked up" appearance or assume a "praying" position. A dyspnoeic animal will be unwilling to lie down and may prefer to sit up or even stand with elbows abducted.

Animals with spinal lesions especially cervical disc lesions will show unwillingness to change position. When walking the neck is held stiffly and the head moved as little as possible.

## Gait

1. *Which limb(s) is affected.*
2. *Degree of lameness.*
3. *Whether lameness increases or improves after exercise.*
4. *Signs of swelling.*
5. *Whether the leg is carried in an unusual way.*
6. *Whether the head carriage is normal.*
*Common causes*: Musculo-skeletal abnormalities, spinal lesions, neurological conditions and viral infections.

## Temperature, Pulse and Respiration

### Temperature

Body temperature is of importance both as evidence of good health and as one of the basic signs of illness. In hospitalized patients the temperature should be routinely taken twice daily and if abnormal, should be taken every 4 hours. Patients undergoing intensive care and paediatric cases should have their temperature taken every half hour.

### Chart of normal temperatures

| Dog | Cat |
|---|---|
| 38.3–38.7°C | 38.0–38.5°C |
| (100.9–101.7°F) | (100.4–101.6°F) |

Guinea Pig 39–40°C (102.2–104°F)
Rabbit 38.5–40°C (101.5–104.2°F)
Rat 37.5°C (99.9°F)
Hamster 36–38°C (98–101°F)

## Types of thermometer, their care, use and storage

The mercury thermometer is the type most commonly used in veterinary medicine. It consists of a bulb containing mercury and an evacuated glass capillary tube which has a kink near its junction with the bulb. When the temperature rises, the mercury expands and travels up the capillary tube. The kink in the tube prevents the mercury contracting when the temperature drops, so that when the thermometer is removed from the patient to be read the mercury level will not drop until it is shaken down.

The temperature is read from the calibrated scale along the glass tube. This may be in degrees Celsius (°C) or Fahrenheit (°F). Although degrees Celsius is now the standard unit for measurement of temperature, the nurse should be familiar with both. A Fahrenheit reading may be converted to Celsius by use of the formula:

$$°C = (°F - 32) \times 5/9$$

The bulb of the thermometer should be of the stubby type and the scale should go several degrees above and below the normal range. Special clinical thermometers are available which record very low body temperatures.

Electronic thermometers are also available which contain thermistor probes which are connected to a monitor from which the temperature is read. These probes are designed for both oesophageal and rectal use. Some are also available for recording skin temperature as well.

### To take the temperature

1. *The animal is suitably restrained* (in the cat this may take two people).
2. *The thermometer is shaken down* to return the mercury to the bulb and the end lubricated with K–Y jelly, vaseline or mild soap.

3. *The thermometer is gently inserted into the rectum* with a rotating action. The cat has an internal anal sphincter which may prevent insertion of the thermometer, but gentle pressure on the anus will usually result in relaxation of this muscle.

4. *The thermometer is held with the bulb well into the rectum for the specified time* (usually 30 seconds) after which it is removed and wiped with cotton wool.

5. *It is then held horizontally and rotated until the mercury can be seen and the temperature read off against the scale.*

6. *The thermometer is rinsed in cold water,* replaced in its container and the temperature recorded on the patient's chart.

7. *Unusually high or low temperatures should be repeated* to eliminate the possibility of error and the veterinary surgeon notified.

Thermometers should be stored in a jar containing an antiseptic solution such as cetrimide or chlorhexidine. The bottom of the container should be padded with cotton wool to prevent the thermometer being broken. Hot water should not be used to clean thermometers as it will cause the mercury to expand and the glass to break. When transported, the thermometer should be placed in the case provided by the manufacturer. Probes for electronic thermometers should be cleaned with an antiseptic solution and then stored in the case with the monitor.

**Pulse**

The pulse can be described as the local rhythmic expansion of an artery, which can be felt with the finger, corresponding to each contraction of the left ventricle of the heart. It may be felt in any artery sufficiently near the surface of the body. In the dog and cat the most common site for taking the pulse is the femoral artery where it crosses the medial aspect of the femur at about midshaft. Other sites include the anterior aspect of the hock, the digital artery on the volar aspect of the forepaw and the lingual artery on the underside of the tongue in anaesthetized dogs.

The rate and character of the pulse should be recorded as they reflect the ability of the heart to pump blood round the body.

The pulse varies according to the state of the animal's health, being faster in fevers and slower and weaker in debilitating diseases. During exercise it increases greatly, but in health it subsides rapidly soon afterwards. During sleep and unconsciousness it is slower.

**The normal pulse** rate at rest is 70–160 beats per minute in dogs (up to 180 in toy breeds), and 110–180 beats per minute in cats. It should be strong, easily felt and have an even rhythm. **Sinus arrhythmia** is characterized by an irregular pulse that is correlated with respiration. When the animal breathes in, the pulse rate increases; when it breathes out, the rate decreases. With sinus arrhythmia, the pulse is regularly irregular and this is seen in normal animals.

*A weak, thready pulse* is seen in shock and diminished cardiac output.

*A strong jerky pulse* is seen in patients with valvular insufficiency and some congenital heart defects.

*A pulse deficit* occurs when there are more heart beats than there are femoral pulses and occurs when severe arrhythmias are present.

**Respiration**

The respiratory rate should be recorded when the animal is at rest and not panting. It is normally between 10 and 30 breaths per minute (20 at rest). The depth, rhythm and type should also be recorded and is more important clinically than the rate.

*An increased respiratory rate* (tachypnoea) may be caused by heat, exercise, pain, poisons e.g. paraquat, nervous excitement and structural changes in the lungs. A decreased respiratory rate may result from hypnotic or narcotic poisoning or metabolic alkalosis.

*The rhythm* of respiration may be varied voluntarily or involuntarily (as with nervous excitement). Prolonged respiration may be caused by bronchial or pulmonary disease. In **Cheyne-Stokes respiration** there are periods of rapid, deep breathing, which then become shallower and are followed by a period of apnoea. The cycle is then repeated. It is seen in severe illness and toxaemia and is usually terminal.

*Thoraco-abdominal respiration* is seen in normal cats and dogs. Abnormal respiration may be purely thoracic—resulting from paralysis of the diaphragm or abdominal pressure e.g. ascites; or abdominal—caused by pain in the thorax, pleuritis or paralysis of the intercostal muscles.

Many terms are used to describe respiratory patterns, some of which are useful to know:

*Apnoea*—cessation of breathing.

*Tachypnoea*—increased respiratory rate.

*Dyspnoea*—difficult breathing. There is usually an increased rate and depth. It may be inspiratory, expiratory or mixed.

*Inspiratory dyspnoea*—breathing is through the mouth. The head and neck are extended. The ribs are rolled forward and elevated and the elbows are abducted. It may be caused for example by tumour, obstruction or stenosis of the respiratory tract.

*Expiratory dyspnoea*—inspiration is normal and expiration is prolonged and forced. It may be caused by chronic emphysema bronchitis or pleural adhesions.

*Mixed dyspnoea*—is a combination of inspiratory and expiratory dyspnoea. It is seen in severe respiratory diseases e.g. pneumonia, pneumothorax, hydrothorax, pyothorax or chylothorax.

## Daily Nursing Routine

It is important in the care of in-patients that there is a daily routine which should be adhered to as far as possible. If there are enough nurses available then a weekly rota system should be employed with one person assigned to large dogs, one to small dogs and one to cats. The advantage of this is that slight changes which take place from day to day will be obvious to someone who is familiar with the case, but which might not be noticed by a different nurse.

The importance of noting and recording abnormalities has already been mentioned. This is usually done at the beginning of the morning when the kennel is cleaned and the animal examined and exercised. A daily record chart should be kept on the kennel to monitor the patient's progress and other relevant details about the case.

Examples of the types of charts are given in Figs. 5.1 and 5.2. Before the animal is taken out of its kennel or cage, a mental note should be made of the general appearance of the patient and the state of its kennel and bedding.

Temperature, pulse and respiration should then be taken and recorded. Details of food and water intake, passage of urine, faeces and vomit should be noted. Any abnormal signs such as evidence of haemorrhage should be reported.

The wounds of animals which have undergone surgery should be checked for evidence of interference, infection and

| CASE No. | NAME |
|---|---|
| OWNERS NAME | SPECIES |
| ADDRESS | BREED |
| | SEX |
| | AGE |
| | WEIGHT |
| TEL. No. | ADMITTED |
| WORK | DISCHARGED |
| HOME | |
| VETERINARY SURGEON i/c | |
| REASON FOR ADMISSION | |
| INSTRUCTIONS | |

FIG. 5.1.

breakdown. Plaster casts and bandages should also be examined and may require attention.

### Kennel Cleaning

Soiled bedding should be removed, the kennel washed down with disinfectant, rinsed and the bedding replaced. The most suitable type of bedding for hospital kennels is newspaper because it is absorbent, insulating, cheap and readily available. It is easily disposed of, does not contaminate wounds and provides a good background for observation of abnormal features e.g. colour of urine, haemorrhage etc., PVC covered foam beds and blankets can be provided for extra comfort. Vetbed, a synthetic, washable sheepskin blanket is ideal for this purpose. Litter trays should be provided for cats.

### Feeding

This should be done at the same time each day and will depend on the practice or hospital's daily routine. Puppies, kittens and giant breeds of dog will require feeding more often, as will certain other cases. A variety of different types of food should be available to meet individual requirements and preferences.

### Exercise

Most hospital in-patients will require some form of exercise 2–3 times daily unless their illness or injury necessitates cage rest. Exercise runs should be available to allow patients a little more freedom and help prevent boredom. Dogs should always be put into exercise runs individually to prevent the risk of fighting

| DATE | DAY °F | am | pm | am | pm | am | pm | am | pm | am | pm | am | pm | am | pm | am | pm | am | pm | am | pm | °C |
|---|---|---|---|---|---|---|---|---|---|---|---|---|---|---|---|---|---|---|---|---|---|---|---|

Temperature scale: 108 107 106 105 104 103 102 101 100 99 98 97 (°F) — 42 41 40 39 38 37 36 (°C)

Respiration Pulse scale: 180 170 160 150 140 130 120 110 100 90 80 70 60 50 40 30 20 10

FOOD

DRINK

URINE

FAECES

VOMIT

TREATMENT

| Drug (Approved) Name | | | | | | | | | | | | | | | | | | | | | | |
|---|---|---|---|---|---|---|---|---|---|---|---|---|---|---|---|---|---|---|---|---|---|---|
| Dose | Frequency | Route | am | pm | am | pm | am | pm | am | pm | am | pm | am | pm | am | pm | am | pm | am | pm | am | pm |
| Signature & Date | | | | | | | | | | | | | | | | | | | | | | |
| Drug (Approved) Name | | | | | | | | | | | | | | | | | | | | | | |
| Dose | Frequency | Route | am | pm | am | pm | am | pm | am | pm | am | pm | am | pm | am | pm | am | pm | am | pm | am | pm |
| Signature & Date | | | | | | | | | | | | | | | | | | | | | | |
| Drug (Approved) Name | | | | | | | | | | | | | | | | | | | | | | |
| Dose | Frequency | Route | am | pm | am | pm | am | pm | am | pm | am | pm | am | pm | am | pm | am | pm | am | pm | am | pm |
| Signature & Date | | | | | | | | | | | | | | | | | | | | | | |

FIG. 5.2.

and injury. Most orthopaedic cases will be restricted to lead exercise during hospitalization. Patients with visual problems or following ophthalmic surgery should not be put into exercise runs where they may injure themselves.

Ideally, an enclosed exercise area should be provided for cats, but this is not always feasible and most cats are content to remain in their kennels.

## Care of the soiled patient

As part of the general care of patients, the nurse will usually be responsible for the cleaning and management of soiled patients. Hospitalized animals may become soiled with urine and faeces simply because they are confined to a kennel and their usual routine has been disturbed. More often though it is because they are unable to move as a result of injuries or general debilitation. They may also become soiled by bedding, vomitus, blood and discharges from suppurating wounds.

To try and keep patients clean, it is important to give them plenty of opportunity to urinate and defaecate outside and to replace bedding as soon as it becomes soiled. Cats should be provided with litter trays which should be changed regularly. The use of a fur fabric such as "Vetbed" is very useful as it allows urine to soak through to the bedding underneath whilst the top remains dry.

Soiled patients should be cleaned as soon as possible and as often as necessary to prevent problems such as urine scald or wound contamination. Dogs can be bathed using a mild shampoo or one of the surgical scrub solutions such as "Pevidine" or "Hibiscrub" (these are preferable if the patient has a surgical wound). They should then be dried with a hairdrier or towel and the coat combed or brushed. A little talcum powder can be used to help dry them completely.

If bathing is not feasible, the soiled areas should be washed with a mild antiseptic solution, then dried and the coat brushed and combed. In long haired dogs it may be necessary to clip matted hair especially around the anus.

Cats usually require less cleaning and grooming than dogs. Cats are particular about cleaning themselves and the majority of them are short-haired. Long haired cats however, will require regular grooming to prevent the coat becoming matted and again, it may be necessary to trim hair around the anus in cats with diarrhoea. Cats with injuries to the mouth, such as a fractured jaw, will not be able to clean themselves. They tend to salivate excessively and become very soiled on the chest and front paws. They may be bathed if amenable, but usually, washing of the soiled area with an antiseptic solution will have to suffice. This may have to be repeated daily until the cat can manage to clean itself. Oil on the coats of animals that have been involved in road traffic accidents can be cleaned off using a mild detergent or "Swarfega".

Obviously all patients must be clean and well groomed when they are returned to their owners, as this is a reflection of the care that their animal has received during hospitalization. No blood should be left on an animal's skin at the time of discharge after surgery.

## Care of the recumbent patient

A recumbent animal will be unable to rise and may lie in the same position for long period of time. This will include patients recovering from anaesthesia, paraplegic animals, those with multiple injuries and severely debilitated animals. There are various problems which need to be dealt with:

### 1. *Urination and Defaecation*

Wherever possible, recumbent animals should be taken outside and given the opportunity to urinate and defaecate. They may need to be assisted or carried and will benefit from the fresh air and change of environment. Animals who are either unable to pass urine or are unable to move may require catheterization to empty the bladder. In bitches an indwelling Foley catheter may be left in place and a urine collection bag attached. This has the advantage of allowing observation and measurement of urine output. It may be necessary to flush the catheter with sterile fluid from time to time to ensure patency. Male dogs usually require catheterization 2–3 times daily as a suitable indwelling catheter is not available. Cats' bladders can usually be emptied manually although it is sometimes necessary to catheterize them (p. 333).

Recumbent animals may be faecally incontinent, in which case they should be cleaned as soon as possible. Constipation may occur in recumbent animals and laxatives or an enema given to relieve this.

## 2. Bedsores

These may occur over pressure points and bony prominences in animals that are recumbent for any length of time. They can be difficult to treat and steps should be taken to prevent them occurring. Turning the animal every 4 hours and the use of PVC covered foam beds and Vetbed for the patient to lie on, will help to alleviate this problem. If bedsores do occur, the ulcerated areas should be cleaned with a mild antiseptic solution and dried thoroughly. Cream such as zinc and castor oil can be applied to protect the lesions.

## 3. Hypostatic Pneumonia

This may occur if the animal remains lying on the same side for long periods so it is important to turn a recumbent animal every 4 hours.

## 4. Feeding and Drinking

A recumbent animal may not be able to reach its food and water so help will be needed to encourage eating and drinking. Hand feeding may be necessary.

## 5. Body Temperature

Recumbent patients, especially severely debilitated animals, will become cold very easily so blankets should be used to keep them warm. Electric heating pads and hot water bottles can also be used. Aluminium foil or plastic "bubble" wrapping have also been used to retain body heat.

Recumbent cats can often become quite distressed if they are unable to clean themselves and will benefit from brushing and combing. They should be assisted getting up and time should be spent encouraging them to do so.

## 6. Physiotherapy

Some paralysed animals will benefit from physiotherapy. Gentle massage and exercise of the limbs may help to prevent joint stiffness, improve circulation and maintain muscle tone. Percussing the chest with cupped hands may help bronchial mucus to be coughed up.

### Care of the vomiting animal

Some of the causes of vomiting have already been discussed, but for the purpose of nursing, vomiting patients may be divided into 2 categories. There are those suffering from metabolic disorders such as nephritis, or diabetes mellitus, which may be very ill, recumbent and are usually anorexia. The second group are those who are vomiting because of a mechanical or functional disorder such as megaoesophagus or pyloric stenosis. These animals often appear well in themselves, are willing to eat, but vomit or regurgitate soon afterwards.

Animals in the first group will usually require the most care and attention. Repetitive vomiting will soon lead to dehydration and loss of electrolytes (especially if accompanied by diarrhoea). For this reason, vomiting should always be reported to the veterinary surgeon. Food will usually be withheld if there is repeated vomiting. Fluid replacement with oral preparations such as Lectade or Ionaid which contain glucose and electrolytes, or intravenous fluid therapy may be required to counteract the fluid imbalance. It is better to offer very small amounts of fluid every half hour than to leave a large quantity of fluid in the kennel, as the intake of large amounts will often lead to vomiting. The animal may need encouragement to take the fluid and if necessary it can be syringed into the mouth. Care should be taken to avoid inhalation of vomit or fluid which might lead to pneumonia or even asphyxiation. Soiled bedding should be replaced as often as necessary and the animal kept clean. The vomiting patient will benefit from having his face and mouth wiped with moist cotton wool.

The nursing of animals in the second group will be concerned mainly with finding a suitable method of feeding whereby vomiting or regurgitation do not occur. This will usually be a question of trial and error for each individual case. Sometimes the feeding of semi-solid foods such as Minced Morsels, or feeding the animal from a height, e.g. a step or raised stool will overcome the problem. Often it is necessary to feed very small amounts of fluids or liquidized foods, several times daily. As with all vomiting animals, there is a risk of inhalation pneumonia, which must be avoided if possible.

## Care of the weakly or premature animal

Most of the instructions already given for the care of the recumbent patient will apply to the weakly patient. A lot of time will be needed to encourage them to eat and drink and it may be necessary to experiment with different types of food to try and find something that they will eat. It may be necessary to hand or force feed very weak patients. If possible they should be taken outside to urinate and defaecate. They may need help to walk e.g. using a towel under the abdomen to support the hindlegs. Attention must be paid to keeping them warm, dry and clean, and the eyes, nose and mouth should be cleaned each day. They will also benefit from regular grooming.

Premature puppies and kittens are very demanding, and will require constant attention if they are to survive. They have less control of their body temperature and need to be kept in a constant environment (30°C, 86°F) thus some form of artificial heating will be necessary. An incubator is ideal and will make nursing easier (p. 668), but failing this an infra-red lamp may be used. Heating pads and hot water bottles can be used but must be wrapped in blankets or towels to avoid burning the skin. A thermometer should be kept in the box to record the temperature.

Orphaned puppies and kittens will need feeding every 2 hours during the day and every 4 hours during the night. There are several proprietary milk substitutes available e.g. Welpi, Lactol or Cimicat. These should be warmed and given by syringe or dropper. An alternative method of feeding is by stomach tube if they are unwilling or unable to suckle (p. 670).

The external genitalia should be gently massaged to encourage urination and defaecation. The puppies and kittens should be weighed daily to check progress.

## Forced feeding

The indications for forced or hand feeding are:

1. The animal who is reluctant to eat because of a debilitating condition.

2. The animal who cannot eat because of physical inability e.g. a fractured jaw or oral ulceration.

3. Following oral surgery when the surgeon does not want the patient to have food by mouth.

Much time will be needed to try and encourage anorexic animals to eat. Very often the presence of someone to encourage and generally make a fuss of them works wonders, particularly with cats. Cats with respiratory problems who are unable to smell their food will usually refuse to eat, but can often be tempted by using highly scented foods such as pilchards.

A variety of different foods should be offered in small quantities. It may be helpful to actually put small pieces of food into the back of the mouth and encourage the animal to swallow. Fresh food should be offered each time and warming it will make it more appetizing. Cooked fish, chicken and scrambled eggs are all useful foods to offer. The addition of Marmite or Brand's essence may tempt the animal.

The patient who is unwilling or unable to eat may need to be force fed using a syringe. Small quantities should be offered and care taken to avoid fluid entering the trachea and lungs. Baby foods, soups, milk, Complan and other liquidized foods can be given in this way. The patient's mouth, chest and paws will usually need cleaning afterwards.

If these methods fail it may be necessary to administer liquidized foods by a naso-gastric or oro-gastric tube. This is usually only possible in very weak patients as animals often resent the introduction of the tube. Care must be taken to ensure that the tube does not go into the trachea and lead to asphyxiation. Repeated stomach tubing can lead to ulceration of the oesophagus and stomach.

An alternative to using a stomach tube is the insertion of a **pharyngostomy tube**. This is a plastic or rubber tube which is surgically implanted through the pharyngeal wall and passed into the oesophagus and stomach. As it bypasses the mouth, the pharyngostomy tube is sometimes used following oral surgery. It should not however be used if the animal shows any signs of vomiting. Liquidized foods may then be administered directly to the animal without resentment or the risk of inhalation pneumonia which can be associated with other methods of forced feeding. Between 20–100 ml. of fluid may be offered in 4–8 meals per day depending on size of animal. Before and after each meal the tube should be flushed with warm water to prevent it becoming blocked. A cap is placed over the end in-between meals. The skin around the tube should be cleaned daily and a little vaseline applied to prevent excoriation of the skin. If necessary, a pharyngostomy tube can remain *in situ* for several weeks.

## Intensive care nursing

Candidates for intensive care nursing are those who would almost certainly die without it. These will include animals who have undergone thoracic or airway surgery, those with chest injuries, poisoning cases and other comatose patients. They will need constant undivided attention, during which time the patient will be closely monitored and a written record kept. This will enable subtle changes to be detected so that corrective treatment can be given at an early stage.

Temperature, pulse and respiration rates should be taken every 15 minutes.

Central venous pressure may be measured if a jugular catheter is being used. The patient will probably be given an intravenous infusion or transfusion and the fluid input and output should be measured. Nursing may also include the management of chest drains and tracheostomy tubes, both of which need constant attention.

**An emergency box should be readily available,** containing endotracheal tubes, a laryngoscope and drugs which the veterinary surgeon might need when dealing with emergencies.

Useful drugs include:
Adrenaline 1 ml amps 1:1,000
(dilute to 1:10,000 with sterile water)
Calcium Chloride 10% Sol. 10 ml amps.
Lignocaine 2% 10 ml amps.
Atropine 0.6 mg/ml 1 ml amps.
Sodium Bicarbonate 5% 10 ml amps.
Dobutamine 250 mg dry powder.
Water for injection.

There should be an oxygen supply and facilities for providing artificial ventilation of the patient if necessary. Failing this, an Ambu bag which uses air rather than oxygen and is manually operated, can be used in emergencies, but is unsuitable for long-term ventilation of the lungs.

There should be a **standard resuscitation procedure** (p. 623) for dealing with cardiac arrests, which is known to all nursing staff and displayed where it can be easily seen. An example is given below:

CARDIAC ARREST:
      Call for help
      Note the time
AIRWAY:    Establish clear airway—endotracheal tube
BREATHING:
      Start intermittent positive pressure ventilation (IPPV)—12 per minute with 100% oxygen

CIRCULATION:
      Start external cardiac massage—Sandbag under chest 60 per minute
      Coordinate with IPPV If unsuccessful: Internal cardiac massage
DRUGS:    Establish cause of cardiac arrest
      If available—link up ECG—Asystole or Fibrillation?
      Administer drugs.

### Care and transport of the anaesthetized animal

There are four main aims:
1. To maintain a patent airway.
2. To prevent injury.
3. To protect surgical wounds.
4. To keep the patient warm.

Whenever possible the animal should not be moved from the operating area whilst it has an endotracheal tube in place or until it has a swallowing or cough reflex and can breathe unaided. The animal's body should be stretched out with the head and neck extended and the tongue pulled well forward and out to one side. An anaesthetized animal should remain under constant observation during recovery to ensure that the airway does not become obstructed. It should not be returned to its kennel until it is fully conscious, and even then, constant checks must be made to ensure the wellbeing of the patient. This is particularly important in the brachycephalic breeds and animals which have undergone surgery of the upper respiratory tract.

Vomiting sometimes occurs during recovery from anaesthesia, which may lead to asphyxiation if it is inhaled. To prevent this happening, if retching or vomiting are seen, the animal should be placed in sternal recumbency with the head and neck lowered. The tongue should be pulled forward and the mouth and pharynx wiped out with damp cotton wool, taking care not to get bitten. In cats, it is important to avoid touching the larynx which may lead to laryngeal spasm and subsequent occlusion of the airway. The use of a suction device is very helpful to clear the mouth and pharynx, of vomit, blood and saliva.

When transporting anaesthetized animals it is important to be able to see the colour of the tongue and movement of the chest. For this reason dogs should be carried on a stretcher or trolley—hind-legs first so that the head and chest of the dog can be seen by the person moving forwards. Cats should be transported in a wire mesh cat cage so that they can be seen. Anaesthetized animals should not be carried in the nurse's arms as the head and neck may become kinked and it is difficult to check the breathing and colour of the tongue.

Obviously great care must be taken to prevent the anaesthetized animal being injured during transport or recovery. Two people should always accompany a dog which is being carried on a trolley in case it begins to struggle. Care must be taken when going through doorways and when lifting the animal back into its kennel. Beds, baskets and litter trays should be removed from the kennel and foam beds and blankets used to provide cushioning.

During recovery from anaesthesia, animals may behave unpredictably. The nurse should be aware of this and take precautions to avoid getting bitten or scratched. This is more likely to happen if the animal has an "excitable" recovery, when it will struggle, wander and react violently to stimuli such as noise. Cats should be left in their wire cages and dogs put into kennels if this happens, but they must be watched closely until they are fully conscious. Noise should be kept to a minimum and the kennel or cage darkened if necessary.

It may be necessary to protect surgical wounds with a gauze pad during transport. Bandages are often applied to limbs following orthopaedic operations, but if not, the limb must be protected from injury during transport.

Anaesthetized animals lose their ability to maintain their body temperature and will need to be kept warm. Blankets should be used during transport of patients and during recovery. Heating pads and hot water bottles may be used (if necessary), particularly in small dogs and cats.

## Prevention of interference with dressings and wounds

Although bandages and wounds are usually well tolerated by dogs and cats, they will occasionally scratch or chew them. This usually happens when the dressing is uncomfortable, or the wound is irritant or painful, or through boredom.

There are 4 main ways to prevent interference with dressings and wounds:

1. Elizabethan collars (Fig. 5.3).
2. Bandages.
3. Topical applications.
4. Sedation.

The use of an Elizabethan collar is the most reliable and practical method. This is a cone-shaped collar which is long enough to prevent the animal chewing the wound or bandage. It fits over the head and attaches round the neck using a leather or elasticated collar. The collar must not be fitted so tightly that the animal has difficulty in breathing, or so loosely that it can be removed (or the animal get a paw caught in it). Elizabethan collars are usually made of plastic, making them easy to clean and hard wearing. They can be purchased ready made (Buster collars) or

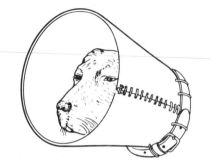

FIG. 5.3.

home-made by cutting the bottom from a plastic bucket or flower pot, and tying it to a collar. Cardboard and x-ray film can also be used but these are less durable. It will usually be necessary to remove Elizabethan collars during feeding and exercise, but the animal must remain under constant observation.

Bandages are sometimes used to protect underlying wounds or to prevent scratching and mutilation of wounds on the body, especially the eyes and ears. In these case, a foot bandage is often applied to the front paw and sometimes the back paw on the affected side.

Proprietary wound dressings are available for topical use e.g. Nobecutane spray, Hibitane spray, or Op-site spray. These taste unpleasant, and so prevent the animal interfering with the wound, but are harmless. They are however generally less reliable than either of the first two methods.

In certain cases the veterinary surgeon may decide to prescribe sedatives for patients who are particularly upset by their wounds and dressings.

### Methods of inducing emesis

It is sometimes necessary to induce vomiting as a first aid measure, following ingestion of certain poisonous substances (p. 547), or occasionally as an emergency measure to empty the stomach prior to anaesthesia.

The most suitable method of inducing emesis is the administration of sodium carbonate (household washing soda)—a piece the size of a walnut for a large dog, or pea sized for a small dog. If this is not available, 20–30 mls of a saturated salt solution (depending on the size of dog), given by mouth will usually make the animal vomit. Alternatively, a teaspoonful of prepared mustard can be used.

### Bandaging

The application of bandages and dressings is a skill in which the nurse should become proficient and be able to carry out without veterinary supervision. A bandage must be comfortable for the patient, serve the purpose for which it is intended and look professional. There are many different types of bandage available and it is impossible to list them all; personal preference will govern the type of materials used in veterinary practices.

### Uses

1. *Protection*—To protect wounds following surgery.
   —To prevent interference with wounds.

2. *Pressure*—As a first aid measure to arrest haemorrhage.

—To prevent swelling following trauma or surgery (especially after using a tourniquet).

3. *Support*—As a first aid measure to prevent a simple fracture becoming compound.

—To immobilize the affected part and thereby alleviate pain following trauma or surgery.

—To rest soft tissues.

4. *To hold wound dressings or intravenous catheters in place.*

5. *Cold Bandaging*—Proprietary bandages are available as cold applications for the treatment of acute sprains and strains.

## Materials

1. *Padding*—Plenty of padding should be used as a first layer for bandages. Particular attention should be paid to ensure that pressure points e.g. the hock and elbow, have extra padding.

Types of padding: cotton wool or orthopaedic wool e.g. Velband, Soffban, Orthoband.

2. *White Open Wove Bandage*—This is a cotton bandage which is applied over the layer of padding. It is fairly strong and gives good support but has been largely superseded by the conforming bandage.

3. *Conforming Bandage*—This can be applied quite firmly over the initial layer of padding and as its name implies, conforms to the area being bandaged. Several layers of conforming bandage may be used, depending on the amount of support required.

Types of conforming bandage: usually cotton based e.g. Crinx, Kling.

4. *Elastoplast*—This is an adhesive stretch bandage. It is usually applied as a protective, external layer and gives additional support to the area. Care must be taken not to apply Elastoplast too tightly. It should not be applied directly to the skin or coat as it will be uncomfortable for the patient and may cause excoriation of the skin.

5. *Zinc Oxide Tape*—This may be used as an alternative to Elastoplast but it does not give so much support or such a professional finish to the bandage. A small piece can be used to secure the free end of the Elastoplast and prevent it from curling back on itself.

6. *Crêpe Bandage*—This is not used routinely in bandaging but it is still useful on occasions. It can be used when support as well as some degree of "give" is required e.g. when bandaging the chest, abdomen and head. These bandages are relatively expensive, but can be washed and re-used a limited number of times.

7. *Stockinette Bandages*—These are elasticated, tubular bandages manufactured for human use but which are quite suitable for veterinary work. They are made of cotton or cotton with nylon, have a net-like appearance and are available in a wide range of sizes. The smaller ones are useful for bandaging legs and tails, and the larger sizes are particularly useful for chest and abdomen. They can be washed and re-used several times and are applied using cylindrical metal applicators.

Types of stockinette bandage: Tubegauz, Frafix, Tubigrip.

## Wound dressings

There are two different types of non-stick dressings which may be applied to wounds prior to bandaging:

(a) Paraffin gauze which is particularly useful for wounds which need to be

Both ears taped above the head

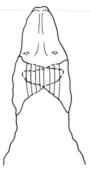

Fig. 5.4.

kept moist e.g. for burns and scalds. It may be impregnated with an antibiotic e.g. Fucidin Tulle.

(b) Absorbent, dry dressings e.g. Melolin, for suppurating lesions.

**Rules for bandaging**

1. Collect all materials including scissors, together before commencing.
2. Only a small amount of bandage should be unwound at a time; this helps to maintain an even tension.
3. The bandage needs to be tight enough to remain in place, but not so tight that the blood supply is impeded.
4. Only in exceptional circumstances should adhesive tape be stuck to the hair or skin.
5. Ends of bandages should be secured using a reef knot or a piece of adhesive tape. Safety pins and elastic bands should not be used.
6. The foot should generally be included when bandaging limbs. Failure to do so invites swelling of the limb distal to the bandage. It is also important in the case of fractured limbs that the joints above and below the fracture are included.

**Practical application of bandages**

The patient should be suitably restrained. This will generally require one person to hold the animal and one person to do the bandaging. Occasionally a sedative may be necessary for uncooperative animals. All the bandaging equipment should be placed on a clean tray and hands washed thoroughly before commencing. When changing dressings, care should be taken to avoid contamination of the wound with the animal's coat. In some instances a protective drape may be required.

*Ears*

Following aural surgery or injury to the ear flaps it may be necessary to bandage the ears to prevent further damage or haemorrhage. There are two common methods for bandaging the ears:

1. The ears are taped above the head using zinc oxide tape.
2. The head is bandaged, including one or both ears in the bandage.

To tape the ears above the head, a dry wound dressing such as Melolin should be placed between the two ears. The ears are then taped together above the head using

One ear enclosed in
a head bandage

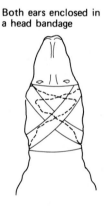

Fɪɢ. 5.5.

Both ears enclosed in
a head bandage

Fɪɢ. 5.6.

2″ wide zinc oxide tape. (Fig. 5.4.) This method is often used following aural resection to allow ventilation of the wounds, or after surgical treatment of an aural haematoma to keep the ear flaps flat and prevent recurrence. It is also occasionally used in the treatment of otitis externa, to allow ventilation of the ear canals.

When both ears are included in a head bandage a thin layer of padding should be applied on the top of the head and between the two ear flaps. Another layer of padding is then applied over the top and under the neck. A conforming bandage is then applied in a figure of eight pattern, see Figs. 5.5 and 5.6. The end is secured with zinc oxide tape and if required a layer of Elastoplast applied, taking care not to apply it tightly as this may interfere with breathing.

**Limbs**

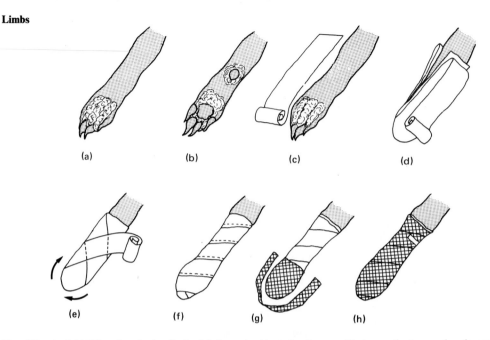

Fig. 5.7. (a & b) When bandaging limbs it is important to put cotton wool between the toes and pads, and under the dew claw, if present, to prevent excoriation due to movement and sweating. (c & d) The leg can be wrapped in either cotton wool or Velband. The latter has the advantage of being easier to apply although it is more expensive. (e & f) The conforming bandage is then applied in the same way and the end secured with zinc oxide tape. (g & h) An external layer of Elastoplast is then applied.

It may be difficult to keep bandages in place on small dogs and cats. In these cases the use of the "stirrup" method can be very useful to help anchor the bandage. See Fig. 5.8. This is one of the few occasions when it is necessary to stick tape to the fur.

As an alternative method, Tubegauz can be used on limbs especially in cats. A layer of cotton wool is used between the toes and the Tubegauz then applied using the metal applicator. This provides a firm, light bandage which is usually well tolerated by the patient. The end may be secured with zinc oxide tape. It is not usually necessary to apply Elastoplast.

*Tail*

It may be necessary to bandage the tail following trauma or surgery. Such ban-

dages may slip due to their weight or due to movement of the tail. The bandage should therefore be kept as light as possible. It is generally sufficient to apply a layer of Kling or Crinx covered with zinc oxide tape (Tubegauz is a useful alternative). (See Fig. 5.9). A plastic syringe case with holes pierced in the bottom to allow ventilation can be usefully applied to protect the end of a dog's tail. This is one of the exceptional circumstances when it will be necessary to secure the syringe case to the coat with zinc oxide tape.

*Chest*

The chest may require bandaging when there are wounds or a chest drain present. The wound or drain should have a protec-

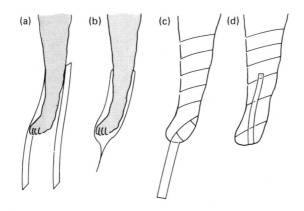

FIG. 5.8. (a) 2 strips of zinc oxide tape are applied: one to the dorsal and one to the plantal or palmar aspect of the paw. (b) The 2 strips are stuck together distal to the foot. (c) The bandage is then applied leaving the strip protruding. (d) The strip is folded back and incorporated in the final layer.

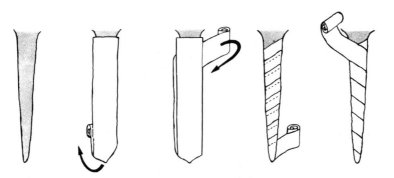

FIG. 5.9. Bandaging the tail.

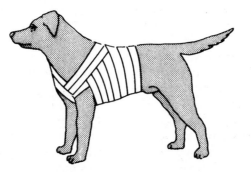

FIG. 5.10. The bandage is applied around the chest wall and then anchored by performing a figure of 8 between the front legs.

tive dressing and a fairly light bandage which will not restrict chest movement. A layer of Velband and conforming bandage is usually sufficient. Alternatively, crêpe or stockinette may be used. (Fig. 5.10).

*Abdomen*

The abdomen is not commonly bandaged, but on occasions it may be necessary to apply pressure to control swelling or haemorrhage. This is a difficult area to bandage successfully because dressings tend to slip and roll up. Wounds, if present, should be dressed and a layer of padding and conforming bandage applied. It is useful to put stockinette on top to help keep the bandage in place.

A body stocking for both chest and abdomen can be made by cutting the legs off two pairs of tights. One pair is put over the front end with an additional hole for the head and the other is put over the hind end with a hole for the tail. The tops of both pairs of tights are then stitched together thus enclosing the whole of the chest and abdomen.

## The Robert Jones bandage

This is particularly useful as a first aid support dressing for fractured limbs and joint injuries. It involves the use of alternate layers of cotton wool and conforming bandage. Any wounds should be dressed, the paws padded and then the leg wrapped tightly in cotton wool. This produces a thick cylindrical layer conforming to the shape of the leg. Alternate layers of conforming bandage and cotton wool are applied until there are at least 3–4 layers of each. About 500 gms of cotton wool will be necessary to bandage a large dog's leg in this way. On completion, a resonant sound should be heard when flicking the bandage with a finger. Although this is a bulky bandage, it acts as a very good splint and is comfortable for the patient. Fig. (5.11).

## Figure of eight bandage

This type of bandage is applied following closed reduction of a dislocated hip. The leg is bandaged in extreme flexion, the foot rotated inwards and the hock rotated outwards. (Fig. 5.12).

## Care of bandages

1. Always protect from dirt and wet when the animal is outside. A sock or polythene bag is useful, but should be removed on return, to prevent sweating.
2. When the patient is discharged, the owner should be asked to report the presence of any sores, unpleasant smells, discharges or discoloration of the bandage, any swelling of the limb or movement of the bandage.
3. The animal must be prevented from interfering with the bandage.
4. The dressing should be changed on Veterinary advice.

## Removal of dressings

Bandages should be removed using round-ended scissors, taking care not to cut the skin or to interfere with a wound. Contaminated dressings should be disposed of, scissors washed and sterilized and hands washed before applying a clean dressing.

## The Administration of Medicines

### Choice of route

It is possible to administer medicines by a number of different routes and in choosing the appropriate route various factors have to be considered.

1. *Compatibility of the drug and route.* It is essential that drugs are only adminis-

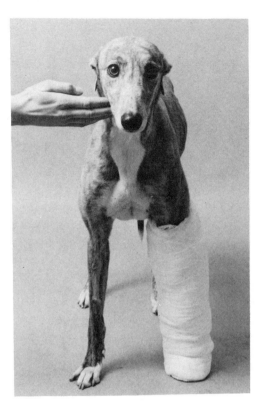

Fig. 5.11.

tered by the manufacturer's recommended routes. Some drugs are ineffective if given by the wrong route e.g. insulin is destroyed by the digestive juices if given orally. Others may be dangerous or have serious side effects if given by the wrong route e.g. thiopentone sodium causes sloughing of the skin if given subcutaneously.

2. *Compatibility of the disease and the route.* It is inadvisable to give oral preparations to a patient with respiratory distress. Some drugs are contraindicated in certain conditions. e.g. acepromazine should not be given to animals with a history of epilepsy.

3. *The speed of onset of the drug.* Parenteral administration generally has a more rapid effect than oral administration of drugs.

4. *The patient's temperament.* A fractious animal may defy attempts to administer drugs topically, orally or intravenously. In each case an alternative method will need to be found. It can be almost impossible to administer tablets to some cats, and a parenteral route may be necessary.

5. *The convenience of clients and veterinary staff.* It is impractical to present an animal at the surgery four times a day for injections if the drug may be given satisfactorily by the oral route at home.

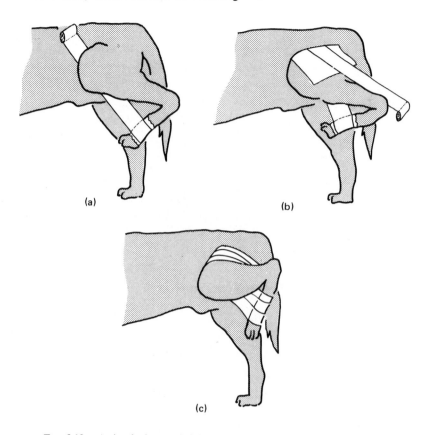

(a)                                    (b)

(c)

FIG. 5.12.  A simple figure of eight bandage for support of the hip joint.
(a) The foot is padded around the metatarsus. The leg is flexed. The bandage applied to the foot is drawn up and over the anterior aspect of the femur from the medial side of the stifle.
(b) Cotton wool or padding is applied over the femur to prevent pressure sores. The bandage is continued by bringing it over the lateral aspect of the thigh, medial to the hock and back to the starting place.
(c) The figure of 8 is continued until the bandage is strong enough to retain the leg in flexion. In some cases it is necessary to bandage the leg to the body. Padding should then be applied to the whole limb and around the abdomen before bandaging the flexed limb to the body. Elastoplast can then be applied as a final covering layer. The bandage, is usually left on for 5–7 days.

## Routes for the administration of drugs

A.  Systemic routes:

> *oral*
> *rectal*
> *parenteral i.e. by injection.*

B.  External routes; by application to:

> *mouth and nose*
> *eyes and ears*
> *mucous membranes*
> *skin*

## Oral administration of medicines

Drugs are administered orally in the form of:

> *tablets*
> *capsules*
> *liquids*
> *semisolids e.g. pastes/gels*
> *powders*

*Advantages*

(a) There is no penetration of mucosa or

epithelium and thus the risk of introducing infection is minimized.

(b) Clients are usually able to administer drugs by the oral route.

(c) Parenteral drugs may become painful if repeated administration is necessary.

*Disadvantages*

(a) Danger of choking especially when administering fluids.

(b) Variable rate of absorption.

(c) It is difficult to ensure that the required dose is administered.

(d) Some animals strongly resent administration by this route.

(e) Some oral preparations may cause irritation of the mucosa resulting in salivation and possibly vomiting in some individuals.

The procedure for administering tablets or capsules to a tractable dog is as follows:

One hand is placed over the top of the upper jaw. The mouth is opened by gentle pressure on the lips behind the canine teeth with the forefinger and thumb and the head is tilted backwards. The lower jaw can then be pressed downwards and the tablet is pushed over the back of the tongue with the forefinger of the other hand. The mouth is closed and if necessary the throat stroked to encourage swallowing. (Fig. 5.13.)

In uncooperative dogs it is more practical to give tablets in food or a titbit such as butter or chocolate. Powders are usually administered in food.

To administer a tablet to a cat, the head should be held firmly and tipped backwards. In most cases, the mouth can then be opened with very little resistance, the tablet pushed over the back of the tongue and swallowing should follow. Occasionally it is necessary to have an assistant to hold the forelegs and prevent the cat moving backwards. (Fig. 5.14.)

Blunt forceps are sometimes used to push tablets over the back of the tongue. However, this method is *not* recommended as it can result in severe injury to the pharynx if the patient moves during the procedure.

The administration of fluid by mouth is most successful using a syringe. The head is tipped back, the syringe inserted behind the canine teeth and the drug instilled on to the back of the tongue in the same way as tablets. It should be introduced slowly to prevent choking. The head is restrained and the throat stroked until swallowing occurs.

**Administration of medicines using the rectal route**

It is possible to administer drugs by the rectal route in the form of enemata or suppositories, although this route is not commonly used in cats and dogs. A suppository is torpedo shaped and made of glycerine or some similar inert soft material into which the drug is incorporated. The patient is restrained and the suppository gently introduced into the rectum. Any difficulty encountered is usually overcome by gentle pressure on the anal ring.

**Administration of medicines by the parenteral route**

Injections made through the thickness of the skin are termed hypodermic.

Common routes for hypodermic injections are:

*subcutaneous*
*intramuscular*
*intravenous*

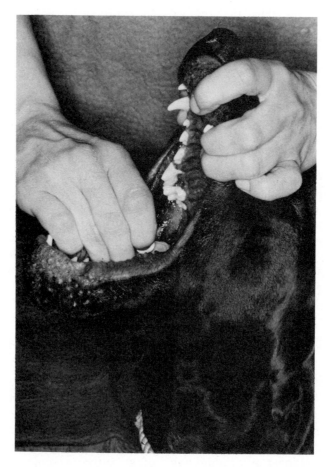

Fig. 5.13.

The following routes are occasionally used:

*intracardiac*
*intraperitoneal*
*intrapleural*
*epidural*
*intra-articular*

The choice of route will depend on various factors:

1. *The drug being administered*—some substances can be given by any route; others require a specific route e.g. tetracycline often produces a local reaction if given subcutaneously, and is therefore usually given by deep intramuscular injection.

2. *The desired speed of effect*—time intervals from administration to effect will vary with the drug, its preparation and the individual animal, but are approximately as follows:

intravenous route   1–2 minutes
intramuscular route   20–30 minutes
subcutaneous route   30–45 minutes

3. *Volume of solution to be administered* —relatively large quantities of solution may be given by the subcutaneous and intravenous routes, but might be very painful if given intramuscularly.

4. *Temperament of the animal*—a fractious or excitable animal may be difficult to restrain for administration of intravenous injections.

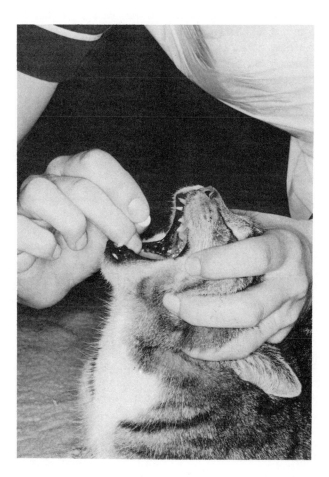

FIG. 5.14.

5. *Assistance available*—subcutaneous injections can usually be administered single handed, but two people are generally required to administer injections by the intravenous and intramuscular routes.

### Preparation and techniques for administration by injection

If the drug is contained in a multidose bottle, the procedure is as follows:

1. The contents are checked, the bottle shaken to resuspend contents if necessary and the dose computed:

If a vial holds 30 ml of solution with a concentration of 10 mg/ml and you wish to administer 20 mg of the drug, the volume to be withdrawn is 2 ml.

2. A sterile needle and syringe of appropriate size are selected.

3. The rubber cap of the bottle is swabbed with alcohol.

4. The plunger of the syringe is withdrawn to the 2 ml mark, the needle inserted through the rubber cap, the bottle inverted and 2 ml of air injected.

5. Two ml of the solution are then drawn up by withdrawing the plunger.

If there are great differences of pressure between the outside and inside of the vial, the contents of the vial may bubble out or air may be sucked in.

When glass ampoules are used, the top is snapped off, preferably using gauze to protect the hands from shattering glass. The ampoule is tipped to the horizontal position and the solution withdrawn into the syringe (there is no need to inject air beforehand). Any air bubbles contained in the syringe should be expelled before the injection is administered.

Most syringes and needles are disposable and after administration of the injections the needle should be disposed of in a "sharps" container and the syringe disposed of in a suitable receptacle after breaking off the nozzle.

### Subcutaneous injections

The most common site for subcutaneous injection in the dog and cat is the back of the neck since it is poorly supplied with nerves and the skin is fairly loose. Other sites often used are the sides of the neck or behind the shoulder.

A fold of skin is raised from a suitable area, the site is swabbed with spirit (except in the case of a site for injection of a vaccine).

The patient is restrained as necessary and the needle inserted into one side of the fold, taking care not to push it through both layers of skin. The plunger is withdrawn to ensure that a blood vessel has not been punctured. The injection is then made and the needle withdrawn. If blood flows back into the syringe when the plunger is withdrawn, the needle is in a vessel and it should be withdrawn and redirected.

### Intramuscular injections

The most common site for intramuscular injections is the quadriceps group of muscles in front of the femur. The muscles of the upper arm behind the scapula and the lumbar muscles can also be used. Injections should not be made in the gluteal region or behind the femur as there is a danger of injury to bone or to the sciatic nerve which runs in this region.

It is usually necessary for one person to restrain the animal and one person to give the injection. The site is selected and swabbed. When using the quadriceps group, one hand is placed on the inside of the leg to immobilize the muscle; the

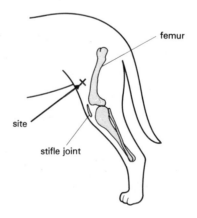

FIG. 5.15.

needle is then inserted at right angles, the plunger withdrawn to ensure that a blood vessel has not been punctured and the injection made.

### Intravenous injections

The common sites for intravenous injection in the dog and cat are the cephalic, saphenous and jugular veins (the sublingual vein is sometimes used in anaesthetized or unconscious animals). To allow visualization of the vein, the site of injection is clipped with scissors or electric clippers and swabbed with spirit. An assistant then holds the animal and "raises" the vein above the clipped area. Slight tension is applied to the skin on either side of the vein to immobilize it. The point of the needle is inserted through the skin and into the vein—the needle is then gently slid further up the vein. The plunger is then withdrawn slightly and blood should flow back into the syringe, ensuring that the needle is still in the vein. The needle is stabilized in the vein by holding the hub and nozzle of the syringe between the thumb and forefinger of the hand supporting the leg. The assistant then releases the pressure on the vein and the injection is made (Fig. 5.16 and 5.17).

The speed of injection will depend on the drug being given. When the needle is withdrawn, a swab is placed over the injection site and firm pressure applied to avoid haemorrhage and the formation of a haematoma. The injection should not be given if there is any doubt as to whether the needle is in the vein, as extravascular injections of some substances can be very irritant and lead to sloughing of the skin. Treatment of accidental extravascular injections of irritant anaesthetic solutions is discussed in the section on anaesthetic accidents and emergencies (p. 626).

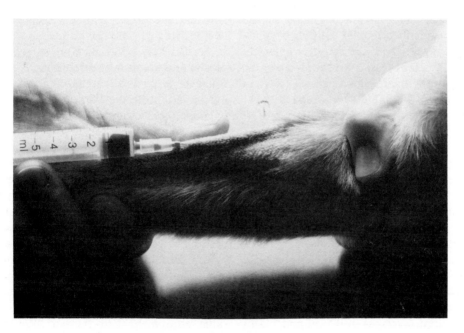

FIG. 5.16.

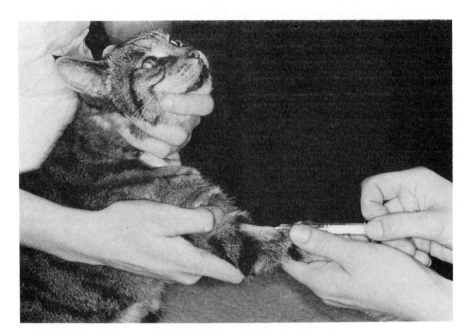

FIG. 5.17.

### Syringes and needles

*Syringes* may be made of glass, glass and metal, nylon, nylon and metal, plastic or occasionally all metal. Disposable plastic syringes are used most commonly nowadays. They are purchased ready for use in individual, sealed packs. A variety of sizes are available with a capacity of: 1 ml, 2 ml, 5 ml, 10 ml, 20 ml, 50 ml and 60 ml. The nozzle may be centrally or eccentrally placed on the barrel—the latter being most suitable for intravenous use.

*Diabetic syringes* are available which have graduations representing International Units of Insulin. This enables very small doses to be given accurately. Until recently, insulin was available in strengths of 40 I.U./ml. of 80 I.U./ml. This has now been changed to a strength of 100 I.U./ml. It is very important that the syringe used corresponds to the strength of insulin being used. Syringes of 0.5 ml and 1.0 ml capacity are available.

*A Waites' dental syringe* is designed for the administration of local anaesthetic. A cartridge containing the local anaesthetic is loaded into its barrel and a special fine needle screwed onto the hub.

*Needles* may be all metal or metal and plastic and are usually disposable. A wide range of sizes and lengths of needle are available. The needle diameter is measured in gauge. The larger the gauge the finer the needle. The choice of needle will depend on personal preference, size of animal and substance to be injected. 25 g and 23 g needles are most suitable for cats and small dogs. 23 g and 21 g needles are most suitable for larger dogs. Needles are usually supplied in different coloured containers according to gauge for easy identification.

The size of needle hub and syringe nozzle must be matched. Most disposable needles, syringes, catheters and cannulae have "Luer" fittings. Formerly, non-disposable equipment had thinner "Record" fittings.

Non-disposable syringes are sterilized by autoclaving, boiling or by using a hot-air oven. Prepacked disposable syringes have usually been sterilized by gamma radiation.

## Topical administration of medicaments

Topical administration means the application to the external surface of the body, including the eyes, ears and nostrils. The presentation of the drugs vary and includes: ointments, creams, lotions, drops, sprays, shampoo and powders.

### The Skin

Skin disorders can be generalized or localized to one or more areas. Treatment may consist of the application of ointments, creams or sprays to individual lesions, or medicated baths, shampoos or powders to the whole body.

Disposable gloves should be worn when treating skin conditions if the disease is transmissible to man or if the medicament is likely to be harmful to human skin. It is important when bathing or shampooing dogs or cats to protect the eyes by the application of an eye ointment beforehand.

### The Eyes

Drops, ointments or lotions may be prescribed in the treatment of eye conditions. Ointment is more commonly used because it persists longer in the eye, but it is more difficult to apply than drops.

Before applying any medication, the animal's eyes should be cleaned with damp cotton wool. If drops are being used the patient should be restrained and the head tilted upwards. The eye should be held open by applying gentle pressure to the skin above and below, and the required number of drops placed in the centre of the eyeball. The animal is then allowed to blink while the head is kept still for a moment.

If ointment is being used the patient is held as before with a hand resting on the animal's head to prevent inadvertent injury. The nozzle of the tube is held flat in relation to the eyeball and a short distance away. The ointment is then squeezed in a line across the inside of the lower lid. Blinking and tear secretion will then disperse it.

If a number of different medicaments are to be applied to the eye, it is very important that they are applied in the correct order and time allowed for absorption. Bottles of drops and tubes of ointments should be used for one particular patient only (and labelled accordingly), to prevent the risk of infection being transferred to other patients.

### The Ears

Drops and lotions are most commonly prescribed for the treatment of ear conditions. The patient is restrained and the head held firmly. The pinna should be held up and any wax, etc., should be cleaned away before applying any medicaments. The nozzle of the container is introduced into the entrance to the external auditory meatus and the lotion or drops applied to the ear canal. The pinna is allowed to return to its normal position and the external auditory meatus massaged, enabling the application to work down the canal. Ater a few moments the patient is released and will often shake his head. It may be advisable to administer topical applications prior to feeding or exercising to divert the animal's attention from licking or scratching. Clients may also find it useful to administer ear medications outdoors to prevent their houses being spattered with eardrops, ointment or ear secretions.

### The recording of medicines administered

Instructions regarding the administration of medicines to in-patients should be recorded on the patient's record card by the veterinary surgeon in charge of the case. The following information should be recorded: date, name of drug (approved or proprietary name), strength, route of administration, dose rate, duration of treatment.

When the treatment has been given, this should also be entered on the record card. Additionally, drugs given during consultations should be recorded on the case notes.

### The Preparation and Administration of Enemata

An enema is a fluid preparation for instilling through the anal sphincter into the rectum and colon.

There are three main reasons for the administration of enemata:

### (1) *To Empty the Rectum*

An evacuant enema may be given to relieve constipation and impaction of the rectum and colon. This can occur for a number of reasons including the presence of bony material, furballs, neoplasia and prostatic enlargement.

An enema may be given to evacuate normal faeces prior to radiography of the pelvis or abdomen or before surgery of the pelvic or anal regions.

*Solutions Used*

Liquid Paraffin
Saline solution—1 dessertspoonful of salt in 1 litre of water.
Mild soap (not carbolic) and water
Glycerine and water
Olive oil and water
Obstetrical lubricant
Proprietary brands e.g. Micralax enema
                              Phosphate enema

### (2) *As a Diagnostic Aid*

A barium sulphate enema may be administered as a diagnostic aid in radiography to outline the rectum and colon. This is useful, for example, in cases of suspected intussusception, neoplasia and ulcerative colitis.

Following evacuation of the barium, air may be introduced to produce a double contrast study which will outline the bowel wall. The quantity of barium sulphate solution to use is 7–14 ml/kg body weight.

### (3) *As a Route for Drugs*

Although this route is not commonly used it is possible to administer some drugs per rectum in the form of an enema.

### Equipment used

There are different types of equipment available for the administration of enemata. Choice will depend on the size of the animal and reasons for administration.

(a) *Higginson's Syringe.* This consists of a short length of soft rubber tubing which incorporates a bulb in the middle. (Fig. 5.18.)

At one end is a nozzle and valve and at the other, a suction cup and valve. Both ends are immersed in the liquid in order to fill it. The valve and suction cap remain in

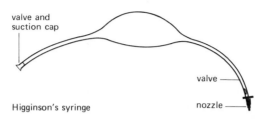

valve and
suction cap

valve

nozzle

Higginson's syringe

Fig. 5.18.

the liquid and the nozzle is inserted into the rectum. The bulb is squeezed to administer the enema.

(b) *An enema can or funnel with a length of rubber tubing* and a clamp can be used. The can is held higher than the patient and the flow of the enema can be altered by opening and closing the clamp.

(c) *An ordinary syringe with a nozzle or length of rubber tubing.*

(d) *Proprietary brands of disposable enema* normally come in a bag or tube with a nozzle attached.

## Administration of enemata

1. All equipment should be prepared and the solution warmed to blood heat.
2. The patient should be restrained in a suitable place i.e. an area that is easily cleaned, preferably outside for dogs.
3. It is advisable to wear a protective apron and disposable gloves.
4. The nozzle and anal ring should be lubricated with vaseline, K.Y. jelly or Xylocaine gel.
5. The nozzle should be introduced into the rectum and held in place.
6. The operator should stand to the side the enema is administered. The rate of administration will vary but care should be taken to prevent overdistension of the bowel.
7. Dogs should then be allowed to exercise to empty the rectal contents and cats provided with a litter tray.

8. It is important to ensure that the animal is cleaned and then dried afterwards.

## Quantities to use

Cats and very small dogs: up to 150 mls.
Medium sized dogs: 500 mls—1 litre.
Large dogs: 1–2 litres.

## Local Applications

This term refers to the application of heat, cold, pressure or medicants to certain areas of the body.

## Hot applications

The application of heat to the skin causes dilation of superficial blood vessels (vasodilation), thus increasing the blood supply to the area. This hastens the removal of fluid from the area e.g. oedema resulting from sprains and strains. It also increases the number of white blood cells available, thus speeding the healing of infected wounds and abscesses.

Heat can be applied locally with cotton wool soaked in hot water, or a warm solution of sodium chloride or magnesium sulphate. This is known as hot fomentation. It should be applied as hot as the patient will tolerate and be repeated 2–3 times daily. An alternative method of applying hot fomentations to the lower parts of limbs or the tail is to immerse the affected part in the solution.

## Cold application

The effect of cold is the opposite to the effect of heat; it causes constriction of blood vessels (vasoconstriction). Cold applications are used on lesions where there is extravasation of fluids into the tissues, the aim being to reduce the passage of fluids. The application of cold also helps to arrest haemorrhage, reduce pain and to lower the body temperature in cases of heatstroke. Cold may be applied in the form of a compress—a swab or cloth soaked in cold water and applied to the affected part, or an extremity may be immersed in a bowl of cold water. Ice cubes may be wrapped in a cloth and applied to the affected area.

## Management of Wounds

Surgical wounds will not usually require much treatment, but they should be examined daily to ensure that satisfactory healing is taking place. Dressings and bandages will need to be changed on veterinary advice.

Infected and granulating wounds should be flushed using a syringe and a mild antiseptic solution such as Savlon diluted 1:200 with water. For wounds near the eyes and mouth a dilute solution of povidone iodine which is non-irritant should be used.

Accidental wounds include road traffic injuries, bite wounds, gunshot wounds, lacerations etc. Such wounds will probably be contaminated by micro-organisms, oil, dirt, etc., and possibly contain foreign bodies e.g. splinters, glass. The best method of cleaning is by flushing with an antiseptic solution and plenty of water. Any foreign bodies should be removed, the wound cleaned and if necessary a dressing and bandage applied.

For suppurating and penetrating wounds a 1:20 dilution of hydrogen peroxide in water can be used. This is non-irritant and will effervesce and allow pus and debris to rise to the surface to be flushed away. This process is usually repeated 2–3 times daily. Drainage tubes are sometimes sutured into the cavity of this type of wound. Certain types of drainage tubes may need regular flushing.

Excoriation of surrounding skin may accompany suppurating wounds. This should be anticipated and prevented wherever possible by the application of vaseline or a cream such as zinc and castor oil, over the areas likely to be affected. Acriflavine lotion is often used in the treatment of granulating wounds, and being oil based, helps to protect the skin.

## (d) Fluid Therapy

## S. B. WATKINS

### The Water Content of the Body and its Distribution

The water content of the body is, on average, 60% by weight, ranging from 50–70% in normal healthy animals. Water content varies with age, young animals containing about 70% whereas older animals contain 50–55% water on a body weight basis. This means it is important to ensure prompt and adequate fluid therapy in neonatal and young animals suffering from excessive fluid loss especially as their kidneys are less efficient at producing concentrated urine. Fatty tissue contains a much smaller amount of water than other organs so overweight animals will have a slightly lower fluid content than that calculated from their total body weight. Fluid therapy in obese animals should be based on the requirement for their ideal body weight to avoid the danger of overhydration.

There is a definite pattern of distribution of water within the body. The two main compartments consist of the intracellular fluid (ICF) and the extracellular fluid (ECF). These two fluids differ in both composition and function. ECF may be further divided into plasma water (PW), i.e. the water within the blood vessels, and the interstitial fluid (ISF) which fills the spaces between the cells. PW and ISF are similar in composition but the ICF is very different. These differences are due to the metabolic processes occurring within the cells. Water can diffuse freely throughout body tissues but the volume of water in each compartment is a direct result of carefully controlled metabolism.

Plasma water contains sodium as the main cation, with smaller amounts of potassium, calcium and magnesium. Chloride and bicarbonate are the main anions with small amounts of phosphate, sulphate, organic acids and protein. The ISF is an ultrafiltrate of plasma and contains everything found in plasma except the proteins.

Intracellular fluid has potassium and magnesium as its main cations and relatively small amounts of sodium. The major anion is phosphate with a significant amount of protein. There is also some bicarbonate and sulphate in ICF.

Sodium may be thought of as the "backbone" of the ECF with chloride and bicarbonate as its neutralizing anions. Potassium is the "backbone" of cell fluid with phosphate and protein as its neutralizing anions.

A **solution** consists of solute dissolved in solvent. e.g. salt (solute) in water (solvent).

An **electrolyte** is a substance which dissociates into its constituent ions when in solution.

Chemists discuss the strength of solutions in terms of grams-percent (gm%) i.e. grams per 100 mls of solution. Biological solutions such as ECF and ICF are better considered in terms of their ionic composition or electrical equivalents as this gives more information about their potential activity. The sum of the concentrations of the anions (negatively charged ions e.g. $Cl^-$, $HCO_3^-$ proteins) equals the sum of the cations (positively charged ions e.g. $Na^+$, $K^+$, $Ca^{++}$). These must balance to ensure electrical neutrality. 1 mEq (milliequivalent) of cation balances 1 mEq of anion.

The concentrations of solutes in biological fluids are expressed in terms of millimoles per litre (mM/L) or milliequivalents per litre (mEq/L).

$$1 \; mole = \text{Molecular weight in grams}$$
$$= 1 \text{ gram molecular weight (relative molecular mass)}$$

$$1 \; millimole = \frac{1}{1000} \times \text{gram molecular weight}$$

$$mEq/L = \frac{mg/L \times \text{valence}}{\text{atomic or radical weight (relative atomic mass RAM)}}$$

Table 5.1 shows the main constituents of venous blood in terms of both mg% and mEq/L. From the figures it can be seen that the anions balance the cations but no useful information is gained from knowing the mg% concentrations of the substances.

**Osmosis** is the movement of pure solvent (water) from a region of low solute concentration to a region of high solute concentration separated by a semipermeable membrane, to equalize, or at least minimize the difference in concentrations.

Semipermeable membranes are very common in the body and many body fluids contain both salts, which can diffuse through these membranes, and non-diffusable substances such as proteins which cannot. The **osmotic pressure** of a solution is proportional to the number of particles in the solution. The particles are ions and undissociated molecules. **Isotonic solutions** exert equal osmotic pressures. A fluid or solution having a higher osmotic pressure than body fluid is described as

TABLE 5.1.    *Canine Venous Blood (from Parker)*

| Cations | mg/100 ml | mEq/L | Anions | mg/100 ml | mEq/L |
|---------|-----------|-------|--------|-----------|-------|
| $Na^+$ | 336 | 146 | $HCO_3^-$ | $\equiv 49$ mls $CO_2$ | 22 |
| $K^+$ | 20 | 5 | $Cl^-$ | 365 | 110 |
| $Ca^{++}$ | 10 | 5 | $HPO^-$ | 5 | 3 |
| $Mg^{++}$ | 3 | 2 | $SO_4^-$ | 1 | 1 |
| | | | Protein | 5090 | 16 |
| | | | Organic acids | | 6 |
| Total | 369 | 158 | | 5461 | 158 |

*Intracellular Fluid*

| Cations | mEq/L | | Anions | mEq/L |
|---------|-------|---|--------|-------|
| $K^+$ | 140 | | Protein | 65 |
| $Mg^{++}$ | 43 | | $SO_4^=$ | 20 |
| $Na^+$ | 5 | | Organic | |
| | | | $HPO_4^-$ | 90 |
| | | | $Cl^-$ | 3 |
| | | | $HCO_3^-$ | 10 |
| Total | 188 | | | 188 |

**hypertonic**; one with a lower osmotic pressure is **hypotonic**.

Protein molecules contribute to the osmotic pressure of body fluids. Since the proteins in plasma are large molecules that cannot diffuse out of the capillaries, but the salts can move freely through the capillary walls, there is a steady osmotic pressure exerted on the plasma side of the capillary due to these proteins. This is the effective osmotic pressure of plasma. The difference between the osmotic pressure of blood plasma and tissue fluid is due to the osmotic pressure of the blood proteins. This is an important factor in maintaining an adequate volume of fluid within the blood vessels. Similarly non-diffusable proteins within the cells contribute to the intracellular osmotic pressure.

Ideally when choosing fluids for parenteral injection isotonic solutions should be used. When we administer fluids, by whatever route, initially the fluids go into the ECF. If hypertonic fluids are added to the ECF water will be drawn out of the cells into the ECF which will result in cellular dehydration. When hypotonic solutions are added to the ECF this may result in cellular overhydration, although if the kidneys are working normally excess water is readily excreted.

**Fluid balance in the body**

Fluid is normally obtained orally both directly as water and indirectly in the food. Water is produced in the body as a product of fat and carbohydrate metabolism.

Water is lost from the upper respiratory tract during breathing, from the surface of the skin by evaporation, in the faeces and in the urine. Respiratory, skin and faecal losses are referred to as insensible losses and cannot be regulated by the animal. The body can control, within certain limits, the amount of water lost in the urine and the urine composition can be altered to compensate for changes in hydration.

*Normal Water Losses per 24 Hours*

|  | DOG | CAT |
|---|---|---|
| Urine | 22 ml/kg | 44 ml/kg |
| Skin, faeces, respiratory tract | 22 ml/kg | 48 ml/kg |

Water balance in the body is the result of matching water intake and water output. If water loss increases then the thirst centre is stimulated to promote thirst, to encourage drinking, and ADH (antidiuretic hormone) is produced to decrease loss of water in the urine. Water balance can be upset by an abnormally increased output or decreased input see Table 5.2.

TABLE 5.2. *Factors affecting overall water balance*

| Increased Output | Decreased Input |
|---|---|
| vomiting | coma |
| diarrhoea | vomiting |
| chronic nephritis | pain around head/neck |
| Diabetes Insipidus | toxicity due to illness |
| Diabetes Mellitus | forgetful owners |
| uterine discharge | |
| wound drainage | |
| haemorrhage | |
| excess panting | |
| accumulation in bowel e.g. due to foreign body obstruction. | |

TABLE 5.3.    *Fluid Therapy Record*

| CASE NO: | | | | DATE: | | | | | |
|---|---|---|---|---|---|---|---|---|---|
| WEIGHT: | | | | | | | | | |

| Existing deficit | = | mls |
|---|---|---|
| Maintenance requirement | = | mls |
| Total requirement | = | mls |

| TIME | FLUID INTAKE | | | | FLUID OUTPUT | | | Balance | Comments |
|---|---|---|---|---|---|---|---|---|---|
| | Type | Route | Amount | Running Total | Type | Amount | Running Total | | |
| | | | | | | | | | |
| | | | | | | | | | |

PCV:
Plasma Proteins:
Specific Gravity Pooled urine:

Recording water input and output is an important part of nursing care in veterinary patients especially those that have been suffering from a water imbalance.

Recording will range from simply monitoring the drinking and urinary habits of elective surgical patients to accurate observations of volumes of fluids given orally and parenterally and the measurement of urine, faecal and abnormal fluid losses. Water balance ideally should be recorded on a chart, with each page representing a 24-hour period. A glance at the chart will then be a useful guide to the animal's needs and indicate how far these requirements have been met. A sample chart is shown in Table 5.3 as a guide, although these charts can be readily made up to suit the conditions in an individual practice.

Fluid loss may be a pure water loss e.g. due to decreased water intake or loss due to panting in which case water is the only requirement. Alternatively there may be loss of both water and electrolytes e.g. due to vomiting, diarrhoea or wound drainage and these losses need to be replaced with suitable electrolyte solutions.

Taking an accurate history of the animal's behaviour plays an essential part in assessing dehydration. It is important to know if the dog has been eating and drinking, about any vomiting or diarrhoea or other abnormal losses noted by the owner.

*Determining Fluid Losses*

Clinical signs of dehydration are not seen until 5% of body weight has been lost.
*Signs of 5% loss* : skin lacks pliability
: mouth is dry
: eye is slightly sunken
6% loss represents an obvious fluid deficit.
*Signs of 6% loss* : skin does not return to normal position after "tenting"
: produces decreased volume concentrated urine
: severely sunken eye.

8% loss represents serious fluid loss.

*Signs of 8% loss* : pulse may be weak
: oliguria
: animal is depressed
: apparent increase in PCV and plasma proteins.

10–12% dehydration is life threatening and the animal shows clinical signs associated with shock.

## Objects of fluid therapy

The purpose of fluid therapy is to replace deficits from previous losses, improve renal function and supply maintenance requirements.

The most important initial treatment is to restore an adequate circulating volume as severely dehydrated animals may present showing signs of shock.

After this, present deficits can be estimated from the clinical appearance and known losses e.g. vomiting, diarrhoea, haemorrhage if a history is available.

e.g. 20 Kg dog 6% dehydrated requires

$$\frac{6}{100} \times 20 \text{ litres} = 1.2 \text{ litres to replace deficit}$$
(1 litre $H_2O$ weighs 1 kg)
$$= 1200 \text{ mls.}$$

After deficits have been calculated it is also necessary to supply the normal daily requirements, approx. 45 mls/kg/24 hrs.
$45 \times 20$ mls = 900 mls.
∴ Total fluid requirement = 1200 + 900 mls
$$= 2100 \text{ mls}$$

Subsequently any continuing losses must be met using fluids matching the composition of the loss e.g. vomiting, diarrhoea, wound drainage.

## Administration of fluids

It is essential to provide fluids both to make up existing deficits and to supply the daily maintenance requirements. The ideal way to provide fluids is to encourage the animal to drink normally. Fluids, electrolytes and calories can be given more cheaply and effectively by mouth than by injection. Unfortunately very often when an animal has become dehydrated it is either unwilling or unable to drink. Other cases may be unable to absorb fluids given by mouth due to gastrointestinal inflammation. When the oral route is impractical several alternative (**parenteral**) routes may be used.

Occasionally fluids may be given directly to the stomach if the animal is unable to drink but is capable of absorbing food and water. A *nasogastric tube*, lubricated with local anaesthetic gel, may be passed via the nostril to the stomach and fluids given directly into the stomach. This tube should not remain in place if the animal is to be left unattended.

If the animal has an operation that means it will be difficult for it to eat for several days afterwards, the vet may choose to place a *pharyngostomy tube*. This is performed under anaesthesia via an incision in the skin of the neck and the tube is introduced via the pharynx into the oesophagus and stomach so that fluids and food can be given during recovery from surgery, by-passing the mouth.

## Parenteral routes of administration

Whenever fluids are given parenterally they should be warmed to body heat before administration. Cold fluids can rapidly result in hypothermia.

### Rectal Administration

The rectal route is probably only appropriate if no other routes are available. It is an easy way of administering fluids and does not require the use of sterile equipment. However absorption from here is often erratic and the route is contraindicated in animals with diarrhoea. It will eventually have an enema-like action in most animals.

### Subcutaneous Injection

The subcutaneous route is suitable for giving isotonic, non-irritant solutions. When large volumes need to be given the total amount should be divided and given at different sites. This increases the area for absorption and is less painful for the patient. The addition of hyaluronidase (2 mg/500 mls solution) aids the spread of fluid subcutaneously and this increases the area for absorption. This route is unsuitable for animals that are collapsed or severely dehydrated as they will have a constricted peripheral circulation and so will be unable to absorb fluids very rapidly from this site.

### Intraperitoneal Injection

This method of introducing fluids directly into the abdominal cavity may be useful for puppies, kittens and small exotic pets in which it is difficult to find a vein and the peripheral circulation is poor. The animal should be held almost vertically and a fine, short needle introduced aseptically just behind the umbilicus in the mid line into the abdomen in a cranial direction. Fairly rapid absorption occurs but only isotonic fluid should be given by this route for fluid therapy. Other solutions are used by this route for peritoneal dialysis. Care should be taken when using this route to avoid puncturing abdominal organs and aseptic technique is essential to minimize the danger of peritonitis.

### Intravenous Infusion

The intravenous route is the **method of choice for effective fluid therapy.**

It ensures that the fluid is delivered directly into the circulation. It is the only suitable route of administration for fluids that are not isotonic with plasma. All infusions should be given through an administration set so that the rate can be controlled and constant supervision is advisable to ensure complications do not arise.

Short-term infusions may be given via a needle inserted in a vein but prolonged infusions should be given via an indwelling catheter which will cause less damage to the blood vessel wall. The largest possible catheter should be used as this will determine the maximum flow rate possible.

Catheters should be placed under strictly aseptic conditions and should be maintained in a sterile manner. Catheters must be adequately secured to the skin to prevent movement at their point of entry. Movement of the catheter predisposes to infection, phlebitis and thrombus formation, and to "kinking" and subsequent blockage of the line. Catheter contamination can be minimized by maintaining a closed system i.e. not frequently disconnecting and reconnecting administration sets. The use of a 3-way tap between the catheter and the administration set is useful as it allows other substances e.g. antibiotics to be injected through the catheter without disconnecting the administration set. Administration sets should be changed daily and the site of entry of the catheter cleaned and maintained under a sterile dressing. If the fluid is to be discontinued the catheter should be flushed with 0.5–1.0 mls heparin saline and should be sealed either with a sterile cap or 3-way tap. Heparin saline (5 I.U. heparin per ml) should always be used to flush the catheter after injection of any agents or if the fluid type is changed to ensure that incompatible substances do not precipitate in the catheter.

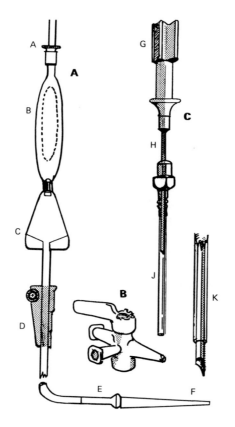

FIG. 5.19.   Apparatus for fluid administration

A: *Fluid Administration set comprises parts*
  A:  point for insertion into fluid bag or bottle.
  B:  filter—essential when giving blood or blood products.
  C:  drip chamber.
  D:  flow controller—enables accurate control in drops/min. and hence mls/minl. to ensure correct administration rate.
  E:  injection port useful for adding drugs.
  F:  adaptor to fit needle, catheter or 3-way tap.
B:  *Three-way tap.*
C:  *Over-the-needle catheter—ideal for peripheral veins.*

G:  bung.
H:  stylet—aids in puncturing vein and inserting catheter.
J:  catheter.
K:  close up to show position of stylet and catheter tip before insertion into vein. The stylet acts as a guide to allow the catheter to slide into the vein, after which the stylet is withdrawn and the catheter attached to an administration set, a 3-way tap or sealed with a sterile cap.

Intravenous infusions should be closely monitored to ensure the infusion rate continues as planned and that the catheter has not been pulled out so the fluid is going outside the vein. It is best to give the bulk of the fluid requirement during the daytime when supervision is available.

If the infusion is to continue for several days the jugular vein is the best route and will allow measurement of the CVP.

### Central venous pressure

Measurement of central venous pressure (CVP) may be a useful guide when monitoring intravenous fluid administration. CVP is a measure of pressure in the right atrium, i.e. the chamber of the heart to which all the venous blood is returned. A long catheter is placed aseptically in a jugular vein and advanced until the tip of the catheter lies within the chest. Ideally it should lie in the right atrium itself but often it is in the cranial vena cava which will reflect changes in atrial pressure. A fluid manometer is set up to measure the CVP. CVP may be easily measured in practice using fluid administration sets, a 3-way tap and a ruler (see Fig. 5.20). The fluid to be administered can be used to fill the manometer line. To measure CVP the 3-way tap is turned so the catheter is connected directly to the manometer and the height of the column of fluid in the tube is read. The zero line of the scale should be level with the right atrium, i.e. at approximately the level of the sternum when the dog is lying on its side. If the tip of the catheter is in the correct place the meniscus in the manometer tube will fall and rise with inspiration and expiration reflecting the changes in intrathoracic pressure that accompany respiration. If this is not seen either the catheter is blocked or the catheter tip is not in the chest.

Blood is returned from the great veins to the right atrium and from there enters the right ventricle which pumps the blood to the lungs. The CVP therefore measures the filling of the great veins which is an indicator of the total circulating fluid volume. The CVP will continue to rise if either too much fluid is being given too fast or if the heart is unable to pump efficiently. The normal CVP in the dog is 0–5 cms water and the level should return to this range within 20–30 minutes of stopping a test infusion. If the CVP continues to rise the fluid administration should be discontinued and the animal should be reassessed by the veterinary surgeon. Provided that the CVP does not rise significantly during fluid administration the infusion may be safely continued at its current rate.

### Solutions commonly used in fluid therapy

*Whole Blood*

Blood is obtained from a donor animal and collected in commercially available collection sets containing an anticoagulant (either ACD acid citrate dextrose or CPD citrate phosphate dextrose) to prevent the blood from clotting. Blood can be taken from cats into a syringe containing ACD or CPD. Before infusion into the recipient animal a cross-matching test should be carried out in the laboratory to ensure the blood is compatible for transfusion. The A antigen is the most important factor in canine blood typing and ideally donor dogs should be A negative. Blood samples can be taken from both donor and recipient animals for cross-matching to ensure compatibility before obtaining a large volume of blood from the donor. Blood in collection bags may be stored for 3 (ACD) or 4 (CPD) weeks in a normal refrigerator after which it is not suitable for transfusion and should be discarded. Blood stored in a refrigerator is useful for replacement of red cells. It should be warmed in a water bath to a temperature not greater than 40°C before infusing. If

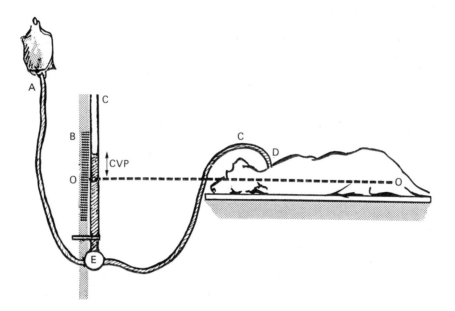

FIG. 5.20. Measurement of Central Venous Pressure. A. Infusion fluid and administration set. B. Centimetre scale. C. Administration extension tube. D. Connection with jugular cathether. E. 3-way tap.

platelets are required for a dog with a clotting abnormality the blood must be given to the recipient immediately it has been collected as refrigerated blood is unsuitable.

Whole blood is useful for treatment of acute and chronic haemorrhage, acute and chronic anaemia and diseases of the blood cells.

### Canine Plasma

If the practice is able to obtain fresh blood from donor dogs plasma may be extracted and stored. To make best use of donor animals, unless the blood is needed at once, the blood should be centrifuged immediately after collection. The plasma is then separated from the red cells and can be deep frozen. It can be stored for 6 months at $-70°C$ and can be thawed and warmed as required. The red cells may be kept refrigerated for 3 weeks and can be given to dogs needing red cell replacement. The red cells may be diluted with any isotonic solution that does not contain calcium e.g. 0.9% $NaCl$, since calcium reacts with the citrate used to prevent clotting.

### Plasma Replacement Fluids

When whole blood or plasma are unavailable commercial plasma replacement fluids can be used. These contain molecules that will remain within the circulation thus increasing the osmotic pressure and allowing for expansion of the plasma volume. These fluids may be used when there has been haemorrhage, although they will not replace red cells, or when the plasma volume is reduced for other reasons e.g. sodium depletion, hypoproteinaemia.

*Gelatin Solutions* e.g.
"Haemaccel"* "Gelofusin"*

These are solutions derived from gelatin which are isotonic with plasma. They are non-antigenic and do not interfere with cross-matching tests if blood is to be given later. The solution remains in the circulation for about 5 hours and most of it has been excreted within 24 hours.

*Dextrans*

There are solutions containing high molecular weight (MW) glucose polymers in either 0.9% NaCl or 5% dextrose. The solutions are classified by the MW of the glucose molecule and remain in the circulation for times ranging from 2–24 hours depending on their MW. Unfortunately these solutions tend to interfere with the red cells, some solutions promoting clumping of cells and others, producing haemolysis. They interfere with the interpretation of cross-matching tests. These solutions are hypertonic so will tend to draw water from the cells into the ECF so crystalloid fluids should be given at the same time.

*Crystalloid Solutions*

These are non-colloidal substances which in solution pass readily through animal membranes. This means that they will not remain in the ECF for very long but will rapidly equilibrate with the ICF and if renal function is normal will be excreted in the urine.

The most useful solutions to keep in general practice are:
*0.9% sodium chloride* (NaCl) commonly referred to as Normal Saline
*5% Dextrose in water*
*Hartman's solution*
*0.18% sodium chloride in 4% dextrose.*

*Trade name.

The main constituents of these fluids are listed in Table 5.4 together with some indications for their use. 5% dextrose and 0.18% NaCl with 4% dextrose are used to replace water alone.

Normal saline and Hartman's solution are useful for replacing water and electrolyte losses. Normal saline is especially useful for vomiting patients and Hartman's is the solution of choice for post-gastric losses e.g. diarrhoea or intestinal foreign body.

Providing the kidney is working normally it will be able to excrete any electrolytes surplus to its needs.

Animals that are unable to eat or drink for prolonged periods not only require fluids but also need calories and proteins to prevent excessive breakdown of body tissues. However caloric balance is difficult to achieve by any route other than by mouth and it is unimportant during short, acute illness since deficits can be corrected during convalescence. In chronic illness fluids containing electrolytes, amino acids and dextrose may be given to attempt correction of deficits. Requirements for replacement and maintenance can be calculated in a similar manner to fluid replacement. Several commercial solutions that contain amino acids and calories are now available. Fat emulsions may also be given intravenously and provide an excellent source of calories in dogs but may be dangerous in cats. Once an appropriate amount has been given to provide the required calories other fluid requirements may be met using conventional crystalloid solutions. The more complex fluids are often irritant and not isotonic and therefore need to be given via a jugular catheter to ensure adequate mixing with blood and minimal damage to the blood vessels. Manufacturers' recommendations about rates of administration should always be followed to avoid side effects associated with over rapid administration.

TABLE 5.4.   *Constituents of useful replacement fluids mmol/L*

| Solution | | Na+ | K+ | Ca++ | Cl⁻ | Others | Indications |
|---|---|---|---|---|---|---|---|
| Haemaccel | Isotonic | 143 | 5 | 6 | 145 | gelatins | ⎫ |
| Dextrans | hypertonic | 150 | — | — | 150 | — | ⎬ to restore |
| | hypertonic | — | — | — | — | 5% dextrose | ⎭ circulating volume |
| 0.9% NaCl | isotonic | 150 | — | — | 150 | — | replacement of ECF especially gastric losses when vomiting |
| Hartman's Solution (Ringer-lactate) | isotonic | 131 | 5 | 2 | 111 | lactate | replacement of ECF especially for diarrhoea or when fluid is lost into gastrointestinal tract distal to stomach |
| 5% Dextrose | isotonic | — | — | — | — | 5% dextrose | water replacement |
| 0.18% NaCl +4% Dextrose | isotonic | 30 | — | — | 30 | 4% dextrose | neonatal ECF replacement |

## Acid-base balance

The acidity of substances is measured on the pH scale, pH being determined from the hydrogen ion concentration of the solution. The pH range is 1–14 with pH 7 being termed "neutral". Solutions which have a pH of less than 7 are acids and those with a pH greater than 7 are alkalis or bases. The normal pH of plasma is 7.35–7.45. It is essential for proper cellular and enzyme function that the pH remains within this narrow range. Large changes in plasma pH result in a sequence of changes in other body compartments which rapidly lead to the animal becoming depressed and may ultimately result in death. When the plasma pH falls, i.e. becomes more acidic the animal is said to be acidotic. Conversely if the plasma pH rises, i.e. becomes more alkaline the animal is said to be alkalotic. In general, acidosis is associated with a net gain of hydrogen ions or loss of bicarbonate, and alkalosis is associated with a net loss of hydrogen ions or gain in bicarbonate. The acid-base balance of an animal may be upset either by pathological changes resulting in excessive production or loss of acid or base, by accidental ingestion of toxic substances or by inappropriate fluid therapy or treatment.

The body maintains its pH within the normal range in 3 general ways.

### (1) *Buffer Systems*

These are chemicals within the body fluids which interact to cushion the effects of extra acid or base. They are able to compensate for small changes in acid-base balance but the other two methods are more important in dealing with major changes.

### (2) *Respiratory System*

The lungs excrete carbon dioxide from the alveoli in normal respiration. Carbonic acid in solution in the body fluids is in equilibrium with carbon dioxide. Therefore increasing respiration tends to remove more carbon dioxide from the body, thus decreasing acidity and a decrease in respiration will cause carbon dioxide to be retained in the body thus increasing acidity.

TABLE 5.5.    *Examples of Acid-Base Imbalance*

*Metabolic Acidosis*
Causes:   diabetic ketoacidosis
          chronic renal failure
          aspirin poisoning
          ethylene glycol poisoning
          severe diarrhoea
Physiological response: hyperventilation.
Treatment: therapy of underlying condition. Sodium bicarbonate (very slowly) may be needed.
*Metabolic Alkalosis*
Causes:   profuse vomiting
          diuretic treatment
          excess alkali administration
Treatment: 0.9% NaCl and may need potassium.
*Respiratory Acidosis*
due to hypoventilation
Causes:   severe lung disease
          CNS disease
          anaesthetic accidents/drug overdosage
          respiratory failure due to nerve or muscle disease.
Treatment: correct problem by improving ventilation.
*Respiratory Alkalosis*
Very rare—usually iatrogenic or compensatory for metabolic acidosis.

### (3) *Metabolic System*

Various metabolic changes, mostly in the kidneys, can result in the excretion of an acid or alkaline urine in an attempt to rid the body fluids of excess acid or base.

Since the respiratory system and other metabolic processes are involved in the maintenance of a normal body pH it is obvious that interference with these functions will itself result in the creation of acidosis or alkalosis. For example, when the cause of acid-base disturbance is due to respiratory malfunction the physiological compensation is renal. When the imbalance results from metabolic disturbances the physiological compensation is respiratory.

Treatment of acid-base disturbances involves correcting the underlying lesion responsible for the imbalance e.g. Respiratory acidosis should be treated by attempting to improve the animal's breathing. Infusion of solutions containing acids or bases may occasionally be useful but will not produce a long term solution if the disturbance is caused by underlying disease. Inappropriate fluid therapy may often make the situation worse and when treating animals with disturbed acid-base balance it is essential to monitor blood pH and electrolytes frequently to assess the effects of the treatment.

Once a good circulating volume has been restored and the kidneys are functioning normally the body is usually able to correct acid-base disturbances by the methods described above, providing adequate fluids are administered.

# CHAPTER 6

# The Theory and Practice of Nursing—II

(a) Catheterization

B. M. BUSH

## Introduction

Catheterization is the insertion of a narrow tube (the **catheter**) into the body, usually to withdraw a body fluid. Catheters can be inserted into the larger blood vessels and heart, the bile duct, the ureters and at other sites, but the catheterization most commonly performed is catheterization of the urethra and urinary bladder (**urinary catheterization**). Catheterization of the larger blood vessels may be carried out in veterinary practice using flexible narrow plastic catheters (e.g. "Braunula") to facilitate either the long-term administration of intravenous fluids or the collection of repeat blood samples. However, the description which follows is of urinary catheterization alone.

## Urinary Catheterization

Urinary catheterization may be undertaken for the following reasons:

(1) To collect a urine sample for examination. Although it is often preferable to collect a mid-stream urine specimen (MSU) which has been passed naturally, this may not be possible where:

(a) the animal is available for only a short period, e.g. during a consultation;

(b) tests are being performed which require samples to be collected at specific times; or

(c) the animal is aggressive or otherwise unco-operative in allowing collection of an MSU.

(2) To drain an abnormally distended bladder, i.e. where there is some obstruction to the passage of urine but it is still possible to pass a catheter. This is often associated with (3) and (4) below.

(3) To check the urethra for abnormalities, e.g. stricture, the position of a calculus, etc.

(4) To help dislodge an obstruction in the urethra or bladder neck.

(5) To check that urine is being formed and passed into the bladder. (This may *not* be occurring in acute renal failure or with ureteral obstruction.)

(6) To drain the bladder prior to an operation upon the bladder.

(7) To drain the bladder after an operation upon the bladder; to prevent undue pressure upon the operation wound.

(8) To introduce contrast media into the bladder or urethra before radiographic examination. The media may be either negative contrast media (air) or positive contrast media (radio-opaque liquids).

(9) To introduce drugs into the bladder.

The main disincentives to catheterization are:

(1) it may cause trauma (including bleeding, which can interfere with urinalysis), and

(2) it may result in a significant bacterial infection of the urine, referred to as a urinary tract infection (UTI). The external portion of the urethra is always colonized by bacteria, some of which will be pushed into the bladder by a catheter, even if the catheter is sterile. Usually these bacteria will be eliminated but they are much more likely to become established in the bladder if,

   (a) trauma is produced during catheterization,
   (b) non-sterile catheters are used,
   (c) an infected discharge is picked up from the prepuce or vagina and introduced by the catheter, or
   (d) an indwelling catheter is used.

**Indwelling catheters** (catheters left in position in the bladder for a long time—sometimes several days) are occasionally employed. They need to be secured in position and carry an increased risk of introducing bacterial infection into the bladder.

## Sizes of Urinary Catheters

Catheter diameters are expressed in the French gauge. Each unit on this gauge (written as F or FG) is one-third of a millimetre and refers to the *external* diameter of the catheter.

## Types of Urinary Catheters

Urinary catheters for small animals have been made from a variety of materials. Nowadays the preferred material for flexible catheters is usually a plastic (in general nylon or polyvinyl chloride (PVC)), but soft latex rubber catheters can be used in the bitch. Rigid metal catheters have also been used in bitches, made from brass plated with silver.

## Plastic (nylon and polyvinyl chloride) catheters

These flexible catheters are recommended for the catheterization of male dogs, and male and female cats (Fig. 6.1). A type which can be used in the bitch is available, though some veterinary surgeons prefer to use a latex rubber (or even a metal) catheter.

As supplied for veterinary use each catheter is individually packed within two transparent packets—an inner and an outer—and sterilized by gamma-irradiation. The nylon catheters for cats and male dogs are enclosed by two polythene packets; the PVC "bitch" catheters have an inner polythene packet and an outer paper and plastic peel pack. Before use the outer packet is removed and the end of the inner packet, nearest to the catheter tip, is cut off. At this stage care must be taken not to damage or even touch the end of the catheter. The catheter can then be inserted directly from the inner packet without the inserted portion being touched by the hands.

As the cost of these catheters inevitably increases there is more incentive for catheters to be cleaned, re-sterilized and re-

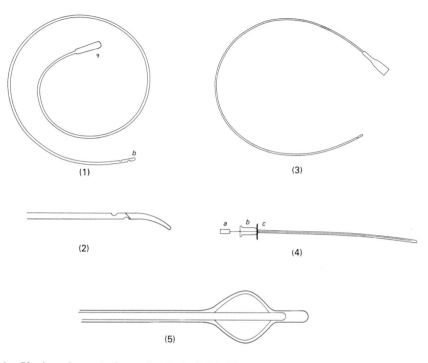

FIG. 6.1. Plastic catheters (nylon and polyvinyl chloride). (1) Male dog catheter, 50 cm or 60 cm long. *a*, Luer mount; *b*, eyes (drainage holes). (2) Tip of Tieman's catheter, suitable for use in the bitch, showing the curved end. (3) Conventional cat catheter, 30 cm long with Luer mount. (4) Jackson cat catheter, 11 cm long, *a*, removable wire stylet; *b*, Luer mount; *c*, nylon flange for suturing to prepuce. (5) Tip of Dowse's catheter, a type of indwelling (self-retaining) catheter, showing the two flexible strips which stand out from the wall. *Note* (1) and (3) are shown curved only for convenience in illustration; as supplied they are completely straight.

used rather than discarded after being used once.

If they are undamaged, nylon and PVC catheters can be individually re-packed and successfully re-sterilized by autoclaving (although they may become slightly more opaque), or failing that ethylene oxide gas (see later). However, re-use of the Jackson cat catheter is *not* recommended, as explained later.

Plastic catheters have the advantages of being relatively smooth, non-irritant and transparent. It is easy to see through the wall both the flow of urine and any debris causing blockage which must be removed before re-use.

The end of the catheter which remains outside is fitted with a **Luer mount** to which, if necessary, a disposable syringe can be securely attached. This is not often needed for drainage but it greatly facilitates introducing liquid or air into the bladder. If a large volume is to be introduced the air or liquid already inserted will flow out again when the syringe is removed to be re-filled *unless* a three-way tap is fitted between the catheter and syringe. Alternatively the catheter can be clamped with artery forceps close to the Luer mount whilst the syringe is removed, but this usually causes irreparable damage and the three-way tap is preferred.

### (a) *Male Dog Catheters*

These are made of nylon and are similar

to but longer than the Nelaton pattern used in man, i.e. they have a rounded **tip** behind which are the two lateral drainage holes, or **eyes**. Three sizes are available; 6FG (length 50 cm), 8FG (length 50 cm) and 10FG (length 60 cm). The size of catheter should be matched to the size of dog. Although it is, of course, possible to pass the smallest size in large as well as small dogs, this is not advisable because:

(a) its length may not be sufficient to reach the bladder;
(b) drainage will be slower;
(c) urine will flow not only along the lumen (i.e. the inside space) but also down the *outside* of the catheter, and thus over the fingers of the person holding the catheter mount.

### (b) *Bitch Catheters*

Some veterinary surgeons find it convenient to catheterize bitches with **Tieman's catheters**, although these are *not* specifically manufactured for veterinary use. These PVC catheters are similar to those used in male dogs but the tip of each is prolonged by a 1–2 cm length of plastic which is tapered and curves slightly to one side. This curve at the tip makes it easier to insert into the urethral opening of the bitch. Catheters are available in diameters from 8FG upwards.

Tieman's catheters are primarily intended for catheterization of the human male, and this means that they are much longer (43 cm) than is necessary for the bitch. The main drawbacks are,

(1) their extreme length,
(2) the absence of catheters less than 8FG in diameter, and
(3) the greater risk of damage to the bladder (and even vaginal) mucosa by the rigid tapered tip.

To minimize trauma some veterinary surgeons prefer to use a Foley catheter for routine catheterization of the bitch (see under **Indwelling Catheters**).

### (c) *Cat Catheters*

These are made of nylon especially for use in cats and are of two types.

### (1) Conventional Cat Catheters

Two sizes are available, 3FG and 4FG (both 30 cm long). These are essentially smaller versions of those intended for the male dog.

### (2) Jackson Cat Catheters

These are also made in sizes 3FG and 4FG. These catheters have a number of special features and are appreciably more expensive. They are designed primarily to treat cases of feline urological syndrome (FUS) in male cats, a condition in which the penile urethra becomes blocked by a plug of material consisting equally of struvite (triple phosphate) crystals and colloid (protein) particles, plus a small quantity of epithelial cells. This plug can often be dislodged by inserting the catheter into the urethra. To make it sufficiently rigid for this purpose the narrow catheter as supplied has a wire stylet (or stilette) inserted along the total length of its lumen (internal space). The stylet is removed once the catheter is in position. If the catheter alone cannot dislodge the plug, it may be removed using a fine metal rod with a rounded end and *then* the catheter inserted.

To dissolve the struvite crystals once the catheter is in place in the bladder Walpole's buffer solution can be introduced from a syringe connected to the Luer mount. Just behind the mount the catheter has a small circular nylon flange, or collar, with tiny holes in it. These allow the flange, if required, to be stitched to the prepuce thereby retaining the catheter in position (i.e. as an indwelling catheter) to facilitate further treatment. The catheter is much shorter than usual (11 cm) so that when the flange is up against the tip of the penis the tip of the catheter is just inside the neck of the bladder. Also the eyes (drainage openings) are much nearer the catheter tip than in other catheters to prevent them becoming blocked by crystals within the urethra (Fig. 6.1(4)).

The re-use of this pattern of catheter is not recommended because it can become damaged in being passed (i.e. scratched by crystals) and subsequently might harm the urethra of another cat.

Although intended for a specific purpose this catheter *can* be used for all other purposes in both male and female cats.

## Metal Catheters

Metal catheters may be used for careful catheterization of the bitch but tend to damage the mucose of the vagina, urethra and bladder (Fig. 6.2). For these reasons they are also not recommended for use in cats. Metal bitch catheters are usually around 20–25 cm long and between 2 and 4 mm in diameter (corresponding to sizes 6FG to 12FG). The 4–5 cm nearest the tip are slightly curved to facilitate introduction. Some are supplied with a wire stylet which is useful in cleaning but is not, of course, required to give added rigidity as with plastic or gum elastic catheters.

These metal catheters do not have mounts for attachment to syringes. However, a syringe can be attached by using a short connecting length of narrow rubber or plastic tube.

## Bitch specula (Fig. 6.2)

Both plastic and metal catheters may be inserted "blind" in bitches which are large enough, sometimes after first feeling inside the vagina with a finger for the small elevation upon which the urethra opens. However, this technique is not easy and the use of a **speculum** (plural—*specula*) is advisable in order to part the vaginal walls allowing the urethral orifice to be seen.

The type of speculum often employed is a *nasal* speculum (Killian pattern) or one of similar design, having two flat blades that can be separated by pressing the handles together. It is also possible to attach a very small light source to one of the blades (connected by cable to a battery or transformer) in order to illuminate the interior of the vagina. A child-sized nasal speculum is unsuitable for all except the smallest bitches because the blades are so short that they will not part the vaginal walls sufficiently far forward for the urethral opening to be seen.

Other types, intended for use as human *rectal* specula (e.g. Brinkerhoff pattern), resemble a conical tube, either with a segment removed from the wall, or a removable sliding panel, which allows the urethral opening to be seen and catheterized.

Also available is a tapered speculum (similar to an ear speculum but with a segment missing from its wall), which attaches to an auriscope, and **it is possible to make a suitable speculum** from the plastic container of a "Monoject" disposable syringe by cutting away part of the wall and sandpapering off the rough edges.

Both catheters and specula must be sterilized before use; if pre-packaged by autoclaving or ethylene oxide gas, *or* alternatively, if made of metal, by dry heat without packaging.

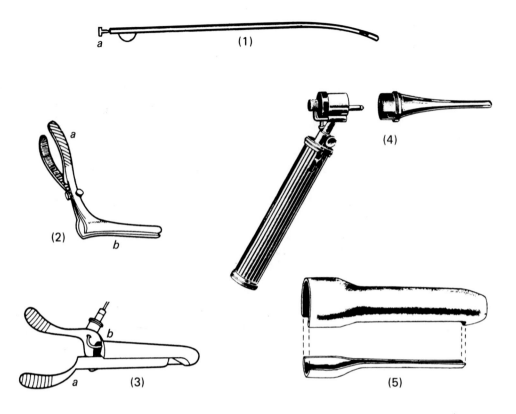

Fɪɢ. 6.2.   Metal bitch catheter and specula. (1) Metal bitch catheter (20–25 cm long) showing the removable wire stylet labelled *a*. (2) Nasal speculum—Killian pattern, suitable for use as a bitch vaginal speculum. Pressing together the handles *a* causes the blades *b* to move apart and open the vagina. (3) Rectal speculum—Brinkerhoff pattern, suitable for use as a bitch vaginal speculum. The lower sliding panel *a* is removed after insertion into the vagina to expose the urethral opening. The lighting attachment *b*, which is connected to a battery, provides a self-contained light source. (4) Catheterization speculum for attachment to an auriscope resembles an ear speculum except that a segment of its wall (positioned on the vaginal floor) is absent. (5) A speculum made from the container of a "Monoject" disposable syringe by cutting away a segment of the plastic.

### Indwelling catheters

The smaller sizes of indwelling (self-retaining) catheters made for human use can also be used in most adult dogs but are too large for small breeds, or puppies or for the cat. Indwelling catheters are employed where, (a) the alternative would be frequent re-catheterization, for example where continuous drainage is necessary because the urethra becomes blocked, or (b) continuous monitoring of urine production is required, to check that urine is being produced and to measure the rate. Less commonly indwelling catheters are used (c) to introduce drugs at frequent intervals (e.g. antibiotics which when given orally or parenterally do not reach sufficiently high concentration in the urine to kill bacteria). Two types are common:

(a) **Foley catheters** (Fig. 6.3) are made of soft latex rubber (with a polystyrene core) and each incorporates an inflatable balloon just behind the eyes (similar to an endotracheal tube). After insertion of the catheter into the bladder the balloon is inflated along an inflation channel built into the wall which terminates in a side arm. This prevents the catheter being removed when in place. Sterile water or saline has conventionally been used for inflation, but air appears to be just as effective. The balloon can be deflated by compressing the external valve on the inflation side-arm. Do not inflate the balloon before it is in its correct position and always deflate the balloon before attempting to remove the catheter. If the balloon is inflated for more than a short time it can become weakened and therefore should not be re-used. If it is re-sterilized ethylene oxide gas is preferable to heat.

Foley catheters can also be used to seal the penile urethra of male dogs before a positive radiographic contrast medium is injected, when some urethral defect is suspected.

Because they cause less trauma than other types of catheter some veterinary surgeons prefer to use Foley catheters routinely for catheterization of bitches. However they lack rigidity and therefore some form of stiffening is usually devised. Some veterinarians strengthen the catheter by placing a wire stylet, having a slight curve to its tip, along the length of the lumen. Others put the end of a straight metal probe in through one of the Foley catheter eyes and push it forwards the little way to the tip, so that just the end of the probe is inside the catheter tip with the remainder of the probe outside and beneath the catheter. (This arrangement can be used to catheterize bitches positioned on their backs.) These "stiffeners" are removed once the catheter is in place.

Neither Foley nor Tieman's catheters have Luer mounts, and if it is required to attach a Luer disposable syringe a plastic (or metal) adapter must first be fitted.

(b) **Dowse's catheter** is made of PVC and has two flexible strips which stand out on either side of the tip. When the catheter is being pushed or pulled through the urethra the strips lie flat against the side of the catheter, but when the tip is in the bladder they spring out stopping the catheter from working free.

Always there is the danger with an indwelling catheter that the animal may interfere with it, either removing it completely or chewing at the protruding end. For this reason the Jackson cat catheter may be sutured in position with stainless steel wire. Animals with an indwelling catheter in place are probably best fitted routinely with an Elizabethan collar or similar device.

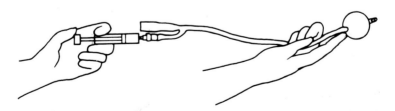

FIG. 6.3. Foley catheter, a type of indwelling catheter made of latex rubber, showing how liquid or air inserted from a syringe through the side-arm inflates the balloon just behind the tip. This is done after the catheter has been inserted. The balloon will not deflate until an external valve in the side-arm is pinched, allowing the liquid or air to escape.

## Care and Sterilization of Catheters

Urinary catheters must be clean and sterile, and therefore those which are to be re-used will require cleaning and re-sterilization.

### (a) Cleaning

As soon as possible after use, the catheter should be washed outside and inside with *cold* water to prevent coagulation of any protein. Water is best flushed through after attaching a syringe; this also confirms that the catheter is patent, i.e. not blocked. Any blockage should be carefully removed by inserting a wire stylet or failing that a length of any wire (e.g. bone wire) of suitable diameter. The wire must not damage the wall or the eyes.

After flushing with cold water the catheter should receive a thorough washing both inside and out with warm detergent solution, followed by the rinsing away of the detergent with warm water. As much water as possible should be drained and shaken from the lumen and the outside carefully dried. If it is intended to use ethylene oxide gas "sterilization", complete drying in a warm room beforehand is recommended.

### (b) Sterilization

For convenience it is advisable for catheters and bitch specula to be prepackaged before sterilization. This allows them to be stored for up to 1 month afterwards.

Autoclaving for a minimum of 10 minutes is the preferred method for nylon, PVC and metal catheters after they have been individually sealed in packets made of autoclavable nylon film. Water-repellent paper can also be used, but it is an advantage to be able to see the contents of the packet.

The use of ethylene oxide gas (e.g. "Anprolene" system) is not as reliable as autoclaving under practice conditions but it is considered acceptable, again after individually sealing the catheters in bags of the appropriate nylon film.

Packets must be long and narrow to conform to the shape of the catheter. If it has been sharply bent, i.e. "kinked", the plastic material does not recover but remains weak at that point and the catheter will easily bend again at the same place. At the "kink" the flattened edges of the catheter protrude laterally and will damage the urethra. To avoid this, plastic catheters should *not* be bent, folded or coiled to fit shorter packets, and any already damaged must *not* be re-used.

Also, since plastic materials soften with heat, when they are packed in the autoclave there must be no heavy weight on them which could produce distortion.

Metal catheters and specula can also be efficiently sterilized by dry heat in an oven. However, this method is less convenient because it cannot be performed more than a short time before the instruments are required.

In all cases where a catheter stylet is supplied it should be re-sterilized *with* the catheter but not actually inside its lumen because this can interfere with sterilization of the internal surface.

Boiling is not recommended—it will not truly sterilize, only disinfect, and in any case plastic catheters tend to float. Furthermore boiling in any water other than distilled or deionized results in the precipitation of calcium salts, and if done repeatedly produces a rough and potentially irritant coating on the outer surface of the catheter.

Liquid chemical disinfectants and paraform tablets (releasing formaldehyde gas within a closed catheter container) are *not* adequate; neither will produce sterile catheters. In addition chemical disinfectants may attack the material of the catheter.

### (c) Care of catheters and specula

Metal catheters, and other catheters that are intended for re-use, must be checked for any damage, i.e. splits or protruding fragments that could damage the urethra or bladder. Forcing catheters into the urethra will not only damage the urethra but may also weaken the catheter. Plastic catheters may "kink"—the most common site being at the eyes. Brass bitch-catheters are also easily bent if mishandled.

Damaged catheters should either be discarded or, in the case of metal catheters, repaired if that is possible. If a catheter is passed with a stylet in place the latter must not protrude through a catheter eye, otherwise serious damage to the urethra will be caused.

Plastic or rubber catheters, new or resterilized, should be stored flat and straight inside their individual packets in a dry, cool place out of direct sunlight, and with no heavy load on top of them. Stainless steel specula stored for a long period can be lightly oiled to prevent rusting, but this oil has to be removed before sterilization and re-use. An occasional spot of light (sewing machine) oil at the fulcrum of a nasal speculum ensures that it opens and closes smoothly.

### Methods of Male and Female Catheterization in the Dog and Cat

Attention should be paid to a number of general points.

1. **Dogs and cats need to be effectively restrained** on a table about 85–90 cm high. Dogs of both sexes can be catheterized when standing. Also the lateral position can be used for male dogs, and bitches can be placed in sternal recumbency or on their backs. Difficult animals should be tape-muzzled.

Cats are best restrained in lateral recumbency, and it may sometimes help to tape their forelegs together and their hindlegs together.

2. The application of a local analgesic spray, or in the case of the bitch a local analgesic gel, will desensitize the penis or vagina after a few minutes, so that nervous animals will more readily accept catheterization. However, this is seldom necessary with male dogs.

Animals which prove very difficult to handle (particularly cats) are best given a tranquillizer or even a general anaesthetic—though if this is necessary it clearly limits the number of times it can be done, i.e. it is no longer a simple procedure.

3. A good source of light is important especially with bitch catheterization. It may be possible to incorporate the light source in the speculum, although this may not be as useful as a good movable auxiliary light correctly positioned.

4. Disposable gloves should be worn when inserting the catheter, both to minimize contamination of the catheter and to protect the hands from urine.

5. The catheter must not be placed on any unsterile surface or allowed to touch an unsterile object, i.e. the animal's hair, the table, unsterile clothing or dishes, etc. Ideally it should be fed out of the packet in which it has been sterilized (i.e. the *inner* packet for *new* plastic catheters).

6. Any discharge on the penis or in the vagina which could be picked up by and inserted with the catheter should be wiped away with a dampened sterile gauze swab or medical wipe (e.g. "Clinipad"), or if profuse washed away with a mild detergent solution, e.g. "Savlon". However, any antiseptic solution should be well rinsed

away with tepid water if it is intended to collect urine for culture.

7. The use of a lubricant on the catheter is best avoided. Often lubricants are not sterile, those containing antibacterial substances may affect bacterial culture of urine and greasy lubricants will give rise to oil droplets in the urinary sediment. Although they can serve to reduce trauma in the vast majority of cases the catheter can be passed just as easily without them.

8. A vessel in which to collect any urine that is passed (e.g. a kidney dish) should be handy, and if a urine sample is required for testing, a sterile Universal bottle should also be available. If the urine sample is to be examined, the *middle* part of each flow of urine is required, i.e. the first and last portions of the flow should pass into the kidney dish.

9. Great care should be taken to avoid trauma to the urethra and catheter. Force must not be used to insert the catheter, and it is much better to use one that is too small than one which is slightly too large. Any attempt at catheterization should be stopped if blood appears.

10. A surplus length of catheter should not be placed in the bladder; as soon as urine appears no further length should be inserted. Whilst the catheter is still inside its protective packet the approximate length to insert can be judged by placing the tip of the catheter on the flank of the animal in the region of the bladder neck, and then using the catheter to trace the route of the urethra back to the opening of the penis or vagina.

An excessive length of catheter will follow the curve of the bladder wall and may pass completely around to re-enter the urethra or even, on rare occasions, tie a knot in itself (which has to be surgically removed).

11. Once the catheter is in the bladder a poor urine flow can be increased by *gentle* pressure on the bladder through the abdominal wall (though excessive pressure can cause bleeding and produce other changes in the urine), or if urine is required for testing a sample can be withdrawn into a sterile disposable syringe attached to the catheter.

12. Although not essential instilling an antibacterial into the bladder after catheterization will decrease the likelihood of a UTI developing. Alternatively an antibacterial injection may be given as a routine precaution.

### The male dog

If the operator performing catheterization is right handed he/she should stand on the right-hand side of the animal which is restrained, on the table in the standing position, by an assistant positioned on the animal's left side. The assistant's left arm should be around the animal's neck and the right hand beneath the abdomen to prevent the animal from sitting.

After cutting off the end of the packet next to the catheter tip, about 8–10 cm of catheter should be fed out. The catheter should then be held by the assistant (clasping the part still within the packet) while the prepuce is reflected by the operator.

The left hand is placed between the animal's hindlegs and the root of the penis grasped. The prepuce is then taken between the thumb and fingers of the right hand and pushed back towards the left hand exposing the tip of the penis. The fingers of the left hand can then be used to hold the prepuce and prevent it coming forwards again. At this stage any discharge is removed.

Holding the catheter about 15 cm from its tip in his/her right hand, the operator inserts the catheter tip into the urethral opening and carefully introduces it along the urethra. The catheter needs to be held more or less parallel to the surface of the table. As the catheter is inserted the polythene covering can be gradually pulled back and further lengths of catheter introduced. In this way the catheter is gradually "fed" into the urethra without being directly handled.

If there is any difficulty in insertion it usually occurs when the catheter encounters the narrow groove through the os penis. If it cannot be passed beyond this point it should be removed and a smaller size inserted, gradually rotating the catheter whilst it is being passed. Sometimes when the catheter reaches the part of the urethra which curves around the ischial arch some difficulty in advancing it may be experienced.

When urine begins to flow the end of the catheter should still be held, otherwise the tip may move out of the neck of the bladder causing the urine flow to cease.

If considerable struggling is experienced the dog may be better restrained on its side with the assistant holding the lower foreleg above the carpus and lower hindleg above the hock (with both legs pointing away from him/her). Pressure is then exerted by the assistant's elbows on the neck and in front of the hip joint (Fig. 3.4).

### The bitch

The bitch should stand near to the end of the table and be restrained by an assistant standing on one side with one arm under the bitch's neck or if she attempts to sit down under her abdomen and the other holding the tail. If the operator is right-handed the assistant should stand on the right-hand side of the bitch and the operator, standing behind and slightly to the left of the bitch, can insert the speculum with his/her left hand. The speculum should first be inserted

vertically upwards between the lips of the vulva and then turned to run horizontally into the vagina. If a nasal speculum is employed it is most convenient to have the handles uppermost, and by gentle pressure on them the blades will open, parting the walls of the vagina.

With a good source of light, either attached to the speculum or directed at the vulval opening, the opening of the urethra can usually be seen. With the right hand the operator can pass the tip of the catheter into the urethral opening, (taking care not to confuse it with the nearer, and blind-ended, clitoral fossa) and onwards into the bladder. The opening of the urethra is located on a small elevation on the vaginal floor, and in a medium-sized bitch is approximately 4 cm from the exterior.

An alternative is to have the bitch **restrained on her back by two assistants** (holding the fore and hindquarters respectively). If the hind legs are drawn forwards and a speculum put in place the opening of the urethra becomes visible and the tip of a catheter can be inserted. Then the hind legs are drawn backwards and the catheter moved further in until it enters the bladder.

In either position if difficulty is encountered, force should not be employed but an attempt made to re-introduce the catheter at a slightly different angle. Particular difficulty is encountered with the narrow urethral opening of very young, very small, or spayed bitches, and in obese bitches and bitches in heat the extensive mucosal folds tend to obscure the urethral orifice.

### The male cat

With the animal restrained on its right side the assistant should draw the hindlegs forwards. If the operator is right-handed the prepuce should be retracted with the left hand and drawn slightly towards the anus. The tip of the catheter can then be introduced and the catheter "fed", with slight rotation, along the urethra from its packet (in the same way as described for the male dog) more or less parallel to the vertebral column.

### The female cat

Again the cat should be restrained on its right side with the hindlegs drawn slightly forwards. The operator should then clean the lips of the vulva with a medical wipe and pull them slightly up towards the anus with the left hand. The right hand can then insert the tip of the catheter along the vaginal floor and guide it into the opening of the urethra.

If the above procedures present difficulty in conscious cats, more success may be obtained if, a few minutes before inserting the catheter, the penis or vaginal entrance are sprayed with a local analgesic spray.

In all the above descriptions if the operator is left-handed the directions "right" and "left" should be exchanged.

### Alternatives to Catheterization

The other ways in which urine samples can be obtained are as follows.

### 1. *Natural Urination*

This has the advantages that samples can be collected by owners and without any risk, of trauma or infection, to the patient. Unfortunately animals do not urinate to order and, in cats particularly, collection during urination may prove impossible. Because samples are readily

contaminated by bacteria from the urethra and (especially in long-haired bitches) from the coat when it is disturbed, they are less suitable for culture than catheterized samples. Ideally a midstream urine (MSU) should be collected, avoiding the first and last portions of the flow, into a metal or ceramic dish (previously sterilized in an oven or by boiling without subsequent wiping) and transferred to a Universal container. Collection directly into a Universal container is possible but a rubber glove should be worn as almost inevitably some urine will pass on to the hand.

Although collection from the surroundings is generally unsuitable, at times a satisfactory sample from a cat can be collected in a litter tray (empty of litter, newspaper, etc.) previously scalded with boiling water.

### 2. *Manual Compression of the Bladder*

Provided it is reasonably full, gently squeezing the bladder of an animal in the standing or lying position may provoke a flow of urine which can be collected. The introduction of infection is avoided. Although there will be no trauma due to a catheter, squeezing the bladder may itself cause damage, including haemorrhage. Pressure should be steadily and slowly applied to the bladder from either side and directed backwards, i.e. towards the urethra. Sudden violent compression could result in rupture of an overdistended bladder, especially if the urethra was obstructed.

### 3. *Cystocentesis*

This term refers to urine collection via a needle inserted through the abdominal and bladder walls. The bladder needs to be reasonably full. Usually general anaesthesia, or even local analgesia of the skin site, is unnecessary but the procedure should not be attempted in conscious animals that are inclined to struggle.

After clipping, cleaning and disinfecting the skin, a 22 gauge needle of appropriate length, with syringe attached, is inserted through the ventral abdominal wall at a 45° angle backwards entering the bladder near its junction with the urethra. During this procedure the animal is restrained on its back or side, and the bladder is immobilized through the abdominal wall by the fingers, but is not squeezed.

The procedure is surprisingly well tolerated, and if the urethra is blocked may be the only way to achieve emergency drainage of the bladder. In general infection is much less likely than with catheterization, but poor sterility could give rise to UTI or even peritonitis. It may also give rise to trauma and haemorrhage, both to internal organs (e.g. the intestines) and the abdominal wall, and after removal of the needle may allow leakage of urine from the bladder.

(b) Geriatric Nursing

B. M. BUSH

## Introduction

**Geriatrics** is a branch of medical science dealing with old age and its diseases. The word **geriatric** is also used (both as a noun and an adjective) to refer to the elderly and matters affecting them, particularly illnesses.

All living things grow older and eventually die, and, of course, pet animals are no exception. Extreme old age may be referred to as **senility**. Old age itself should not be regarded as a disease but as a state in which there are decreased powers of survival and adjustment to change. Two main factors are responsible.

## 1. Ageing

As all animals grow older there occur generalized structural and functional changes, which are natural and irreversible and which lead to a loss of normal function.

(a) There is a gradual reduction in the *number* of cells in each organ. This is because as the older cells "wear out" naturally not *all* of them are replaced. This leads to there being progressively fewer neurons in the brain with increasing age, and the weight and volume of the kidneys can fall by a quarter.

(b) There is a gradual reduction in the *efficiency* of the surviving cells in performing their function. One reason is a decrease in the amount of enzymes in the cells, (e.g. in the liver). Also cell mutations occur at the approximate rate of one per million cell divisions, and these mutant cells subsequently multiply in the tissues. Most mutant cells are simply non-functional (or at least less functional), but occasionally neoplastic cells appear.

These age changes are most pronounced in nervous tissue, which has very limited powers of regeneration. They are also more marked in muscle and connective tissue than in epithelial tissue (e.g. liver and intestinal epithelium) which has the greatest ability to regenerate.

Although these retrogressive changes go on continuously, dogs and cats are generally considered to be entering old age when they have lived for about 8 years. Ageing occurs more rapidly in the larger breeds of dog (e.g. Great Dane) than in the smaller breeds (e.g. small terriers), so that the normal life-span of the larger breeds is correspondingly shorter. The average life-span for all dogs is about 13 years; for the domestic cat slightly longer at 14 years. Exceptionally an individual animal may live for 20–25, or even up to 35, years but this should *not* be regarded as normal.

There is also *individual* variation in the rate at which ageing takes place. This is due both to the genetic constitution and to the amount of stress to which animals are subject. Animals which enjoy good nutrition and are well cared for, live longer.

## 2. Accumulated injury

In addition to the normal ageing process which affects all animals, some will have sustained during their lifetime illnesses or accidents which have resulted in permanent damage to one or more organs. The older the animal the greater is likely to be the accumulated injury.

The changes due to both *ageing* and *previous injury* produce a loss of **functional reserve**; this means that the maximum amount of work of which an organ is capable is less in old age. However, since normal healthy organs are capable of much more work than is usually required (e.g. the kidneys can function efficiently with less than 40% of their total number of nephrons), there has to be a very considerable loss of function before an organ fails.

Failure of an organ is most likely to become apparent in a stress situation when increased work is demanded. For example, in severe exercise the heart is required to pump more blood at a faster rate to keep the voluntary muscle tissue supplied with oxygen; if it is unable to perform this extra work the animal will collapse.

Stress may be imposed on the body in a number of ways both physical and mental. These include increased activity (exercise and excitement), inadequate nutrition, dehydration, illness, accident, anaesthesia, surgery, changes in routine (e.g. changes in housing and food) and changes in environmental temperature. If an acute illness is superimposed on functional changes then a crisis will occur. Consequently as far as possible stress situations should be avoided.

### Special Factors and Problems Involved in the Care of Aged Animals

#### Physical and mental changes

Both physically and mentally the aged animal is less active and less adaptable than formerly.

#### (a) *Physical Changes*

An early sign of advancing age is greying of the coat, especially around the muzzle. The skin becomes thickened and pigmented and the haircoat thinner and harsher.

The mass of the skeletal musculature is reduced, particularly in the thighs and the upper part of the forelimbs, so that the animal has less physical strength and stamina. It moves more slowly and is more restricted in its movements, i.e. is less agile. It is unable to exercise as strenuously or for as long a period. Immobile animals, particularly of the larger breeds, are prone to develop pressure sores on the bony prominences—hocks and elbows.

There is also a decreased mass of bone, due chiefly to resorption (osteoporosis).

The body is less able to adapt to physiological changes. As stated in the introduction, there is less ability to withstand stress. Fluid loss takes much longer to correct than in the younger animal, so that old animals are especially prone to dehydration. Temperature regulation is often impaired, and exposure to cold can easily result in hypothermia.

Reduced powers of regeneration result in any damage to tissues taking longer to repair, and the decreasing efficiency of the immune responses produces reduced resistance to infection and to cancer. (At the same time there is an increase in the frequency of auto-immune diseases.)

The special senses, (smell, taste, sight and hearing), are all impaired to some degree. Deafness and failing eyesight are common.

#### (b) *Mental Changes*

Elderly dogs and cats show less response to stimuli; they are less interested in what is happening and often prefer to remain inactive for lengthy periods. Their sensitivity to pain appears to be reduced so that minor injuries, or the attentions of ectoparasites, cause little discomfort. However, they tend to resent any interference and become irritable; i.e. more inclined to growl, scratch or snap. They may forget previous training and fail to obey commands.

Mentally they are less adaptable, and changes in their environment, food and daily routine can produce confusion and resentment. Therefore such changes should be avoided if possible.

### Diseases of old age

Certain disorders are especially common in the geriatric dog and cat. The incidence of almost all neoplasms increases with age, and **cancer is the largest single cause of death**. Particularly common are small tumours of the skin and, in the bitch, malignant tumours of the mammary glands. The old male dog is especially prone to neoplasms of the circumanal glands and to enlargements of the prostate gland. Chronic renal disease is very common in both species and chronic heart disease (mitral valve incompetence) occurs frequently in dogs, especially the small and miniature breeds. Acquired heart disease (cardiomyopathy) also occurs more frequently as cats get older. Chronic obstructive lung disease, degenerative nervous diseases, urinary tract infections and diabetes mellitus are also more common with increasing age.

Osteo-arthritis and cataract (opacity of the lens of the eye) occur frequently in aged dogs. In both dogs and cats dental disease is common in old age, with the accumulation of tartar on the teeth, inflammation of the gums and infection of the tooth sockets causing the loosening and loss of teeth (periodontal disease).

Chronic ear conditions are also frequently encountered in both species.

A less active life style, combined with a 20% fall in the metabolic rate (i.e. the rate at which foodstuffs are utilized by the body) means that if the previous daily intake of calories is not reduced obesity will result. On the other hand undernutrition may occur especially if the appetite is impaired.

Constipation in the older dog is due in large part to insufficient exercise, whereas in the older cat there may be an absence of tone in the large intestine and abolition of the normal defaecation reflex. Inability to control the sphincters of the bladder and/or anus can result in urinary and faecal incontinence.

### The Care of Aged Animals

When caring for aged animals, either in the home or in hospital, it is necessary to take into account the particular problems described in the previous section. The existence of a disease condition may also require special nursing techniques which are described later in Chapter 8 on Medical Nursing.

The doses of drugs (including anaesthetic agents) require careful calculation to avoid overdosage which can arise if the metabolism and/or excretion of drugs is impaired.

### Feeding

As well as providing all the essential nutrients the diet of elderly animals should be easily digestible. This is to compensate for diminished tone in the gastrointestinal tract and a reduced output of digestive juices. Canned foods are usually perfectly adequate. However, any drastic change from the existing familiar diet may not be accepted, or it may cause a digestive upset such as diarrhoea. Consequently any modification of the diet should take place gradually. Where there are deficiencies they are best corrected by adding the necessary nutrients to the existing, readily accepted, diet.

The frequency of feeding need not be altered but the total quantity of food should be regulated to prevent the onset of obesity. In the absence of special problems, such as chronic renal failure, the reduction in the daily ration should be chiefly in the amount of energy foods, especially carbohydrates. Dietary protein should be of good quality (high biological value) to aid tissue repair. Obesity is particularly harmful to animals suffering from cardiac disease or osteoarthritis, and can facilitate the development of many other disorders. The life expectancy of obese animals is markedly reduced.

## Water

Provided drinking is not followed by vomiting there should be no restriction of the amount of water that is drunk. All of the diseases which cause dogs and cats to drink increased amounts of water are (with only one rare exception) due to a failure of the kidney to retain water. The most common cause in aged animals is chronic renal failure, due principally to chronic nephritis. If an animal with this type of illness is not allowed to drink as much as it wants it will be unable to replace all of the water lost through the kidneys, resulting eventually in dehydration and stress.

## Exercise

Strenuous exercise and excessively long periods of exercise are inadvisable for old animals because they may result in cardiac failure (i.e. a "heart attack") particu-larly in animals known to suffer from cardiac disease. Old dogs should not be encouraged to race about (e.g. chasing after sticks or balls) and should not be placed in exciting or stressful situations which may stimulate or demand vigorous exertion.

A number of short periods of exercise on a lead is preferable to one long or strenuous period. The complete absence of exercise, however, is undesirable. A regular routine of short walks is beneficial both in stimulating interest and facilitating urination and defaecation.

## Defaecation and urination

Regular bowel habits and urination should be encouraged in the dog principally by providing regular mild exercise.

## Grooming

Regular grooming is important since the animal may make little effort to keep itself clean. Food and excreta should be removed from the coat, by regular bathing if necessary, especially in the summer, because blowflies can be attracted to lay their eggs on the skin.

## Bedding

A warm soft bed, out of draughts, is recommended. For example, a foam mattress will reduce the likelihood of pressure sores occurring. Dogs should be discouraged from lying directly on hard surfaces, e.g. tiles, concrete, paving slabs. A waterproof covering to the mattress covered with a disposable material such as newspaper is advisable for regularly incontinent animals.

## Vaccination

With decreasing efficiency of the immune responses aged animals may be unable to maintain adequate immunity against infectious diseases for long periods so that revaccination at least annually is advisable.

### Stress

Stress should be avoided wherever possible. Factors which are commonly responsible have been mentioned previously, but in particular excessive exercise and excitement should be avoided, as should extremes of temperature (chilling can occur if wet animals are not quickly dried). Changes in routine and environment (as will happen with hospitalization) should be avoided if at all possible. Younger dogs, especially puppies, may irritate aged animals provoking displays of bad temper.

The avoidance of stress is particularly important in animals that have managed to compensate for such diseases as chronic renal failure or heart disease because stress may cause this compensation to break down.

### Parts of the Body Requiring Regular Attention

The coat should be kept clean and any ectoparasites eliminated. Incontinent animals should have urine and/or faeces washed from the skin at least once daily to avoid scalding. Clipping away continually soaked hair (especially in the long-haired breeds) will simplify regular cleaning. The application of a waterproof lubricant such as petroleum jelly (e.g. "Vaseline") will provide a barrier to protect the skin from the urine or faeces. Paraplegic animals will also require assistance to move.

Attention should be paid to the hock and elbows in particular to check for the development of pressure sores or lacerations. Any known skin tumours or wounds should be checked for signs of haemorrhage or infection. The nails become brittle and easily split, and in some dogs receive so little wear that they can interfere with walking and even grow into the pads. Such excessive overgrowth is particularly likely in the case of the dew-claws. Regular clipping and trimming will keep their growth under control.

The pads of the feet can also become overgrown—thickened and cracked—as can the nose. The application of petroleum jelly may help to smooth and soften these areas and prevent further cracking. Any nasal discharge should be removed.

The ears, both the ear canal and pockets in the flaps, should be examined frequently and wax and other debris cleaned out. If necessary a wax-softener (e.g. "Cerumol") can be used. Some improvement in hearing may result.

The eyes should be kept clean, i.e. free from discharges and crusts. If necessary they can be bathed with warm water or a warm boric (boracic) acid solution. The teeth and gums should be checked regularly for evidence of pain and inflammation. Any thick saliva in or around the mouth should be wiped away, and it can be beneficial to wipe the gums and the inside of the lips with a gauze swab soaked in normal saline or a solution of glycerine and thymol (at blood heat). The lip folds should be kept dry, and free from food, especially in the Cocker Spaniel.

Other body orifices where excreta or discharges may collect (anus, prepuce, vulva) should be examined and cleaned regularly. The creases around the vulva, particularly in obese bitches, should be kept clean and dry. Again warm water or if necessary a mild antiseptic detergent solution (e.g. "Savlon") can be employed.

In cleaning, cotton wool-tipped cleaning sticks (e.g. "Cotton Buds", "Q-Tips") are useful, and it is advisable to wear disposable gloves.

## Points for Discussion with the Owners of Aged Animals

Advice on the management of geriatric dogs and cats should be given along the lines indicated in the previous sections, and any problems relating to a specific animal can be discussed in detail. For example, precise recommendations can be made about the animal's diet having regard to its body weight and preferences for particular foods.

When the animal has to be hospitalized the owner can provide much useful information as to the animal's command words, its likes and dislikes in respect of food, its bowel habits and, as is often the case, whether it prefers being handled by a man or a woman. If the animal is receiving medication routinely it is important to learn and record the type of drug(s), the dose and when the animal last received it. If the owner can provide a favourite blanket or toy it may ease the stress of being away from familiar surroundings.

It is important that the owner should appreciate that the degenerative ageing process cannot be reversed and that chronic progressive diseases, such as affect the kidneys and the heart, cannot be "cured". It should be explained that medical treatment is designed to allow the animal to live with (and despite) its disabilities by improving its clinical condition, alleviating pain and generally making the animal more comfortable.

The value of regular check-ups should be mentioned together with the importance of an early consultation if signs of deterioration appear. Excessive medication, particularly with home remedies or patent medicines, should be discouraged.

In discussion with the client the significance to them of the geriatric pet should be appreciated. In many cases it represents a link within the family between parents and children who have grown up and moved away from home. Often it reminds the owner of people and events long past and is therefore particularly well regarded. Also some discretion should be exercised in discussing a geriatric animal with an elderly client: statements about old age can be equally applicable to both client and patient and, indeed, both may suffer from the same disorder.

## (c) Elementary Bacteriology

B. M. BUSH

### Introduction

Bacteria and viruses are members of the group of very small organisms known as micro-organisms; a group which also includes yeasts, moulds, algae and protozoa.

Bacteria and viruses exist throughout the environment of man and animals and are normally present on and within the body. They are present in the air which is inhaled, the food which is eaten and on the surfaces which are touched. They are normal inhabitants of the skin, the alimentary tract and the outermost parts of the respiratory and urinary tracts. **Infection** is the process by which micro-organisms become established in the host.

Essentially micro-organisms may be divided into:

(1) **saprophytes** (saprophytic micro-organisms) which live on dead organic matter; and

(2) **parasites** (parasitic micro-organisms).

In veterinary practice when we speak of "parasites" we are usually referring to those larger organisms which live on or in the body, such as the skin mites or intestinal worms. However, many micro-organisms can also properly be described as parasites. Bacteria may either be saprophytic or parasitic, and there are some (*e.g. Pseudomonas*) which can, depending on circumstances, adopt either mode of living. However, viruses are always parasitic because they cannot multiply unless they are within a living cell.

**Parasitism** is an association between two different living organisms in which the smaller one (the parasite) lives upon or within the larger one (the host) and receives food and/or shelter. The parasite's food may be either part of the host's own food supply or it may be the host's cells or body fluids. In the past a parasite was strictly defined as being an organism which always harmed the host. However, it is now appreciated that the most successful parasites cause little or no damage to the host since if they are to survive the host must survive also.

This has led to parasitic micro-organisms being sub-classified into three main categories.

1. **Pathogenic** (i.e. disease-producing) **micro-organisms**. The diseases such pathogenic micro-organisms (*pathogens*) cause are termed infectious diseases.

2. **Mutualistic micro-organisms**. These are ones which are of benefit to the host (e.g. those in the rumen of cattle which break down cellulose into substances which nourish the host). Therefore in *mutualism* both parasite and host derive an advantage from their association. (Mutualism used to be called symbiosis, but this latter term is now usually given a wider meaning to include all associations, harmful and beneficial, between the host and parasite.)

3. **Commensal micro-organisms. Commensalism** (or neutralism) refers to an arrangement in which the para-

site does no damage to the host but is of no advantage to it either. Many of the bacteria usually found in or on the body are often placed in this category. However, it is difficult to be confident about this description since many so-called "commensals" may be found to be either of some benefit to the host in that they provide natural competition for pathogenic micro-organisms and limit their multiplication, or to be pathogenic if they are allowed the opportunity. If the natural body defence mechanisms are weakened or fully occupied dealing with a pre-existing serious infectious disease, they may be unable to control the growth and spread of such "commensal" micro-organisms, usually bacteria, which are therefore referred to as opportunists, secondary invaders or potential pathogens.

Bacteria are named by the binomial system universally employed in biology. Using this an organism has a first name (given a capital first letter) indicating its **genus**—that is the small group of similar organisms to which it belongs—and an individual second name, the **species** name (given a small initial letter).* The generic name is often abbreviated to one or two letters, e.g. *Escherichia coli* may be abbreviated to *E. coli*. However, viruses are not named on this system and the important viral pathogens are usually referred to by the name of the disease which they produce, e.g. distemper virus and feline leukaemia virus. Viruses are classified into groups according to common features they possess such as their shape and symmetry and the type of nucleic acid they contain (either RNA or DNA).

*The plural of genus is genera; the plural of species is also species.

## Basic Structure and Mode of Reproduction of Bacteria

Bacteria (singular = bacterium) are minute single-celled organisms most of which are large enough to be visible under a normal microscope (light microscope) but not with the naked eye. Their size is measured in micrometres, written as $\mu$m. $1 \mu m = \frac{1}{1000}$th (one thousandth) part of a millimetre (mm). In general they do not exceed 5 $\mu$m in either length or diameter although there are important exceptions. One square inch of surface could accommodate about 9 trillion bacteria.

Bacteria may be classified by their shape, and those of importance in the dog and cat may be:

(1) Spherical, termed **cocci**, e.g. streptococci, which occur in chains and staphylococci which occur in clusters.
(2) Relatively straight rods of varying length and thickness termed **bacilli**, e.g. *Escherichia coli*.
(3) Definitely curved rods, belonging to the group *Campylobacter*.
(4) Thin spiral filaments known as **spirochaetes**, e.g. *Leptospira* (Fig. 6.4).

They are also classified by their reaction to Gram's method of staining; those which stain violet are termed Gram-positive and those which stain red are termed Gram-negative.

### Structure

Despite differences in shape each bacterium, which is an individual cell, shows certain basic features (Fig. 6.5).

1. There is a strong and rigid **cell wall** to provide support and to protect the contents in most bacteria. The properties of the cell wall are different in Gram-positive and Gram-negative bacteria, and this causes the difference in staining.

2. The part inside the cell wall (called

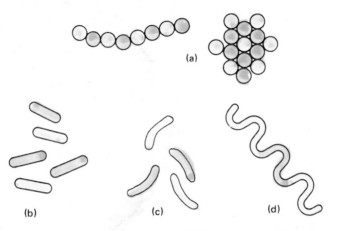

FIG. 6.4.   Classification of bacteria by shape. (a) Cocci: spherical bacteria which may occur in chains (e.g. streptococci) or in clusters (e.g. staphylococci): (b) Bacilli; i.e. straight rod-shaped bacteria. There is considerable variation in length and width. Some species are only slightly longer than they are wide, others are long and thin. (c) Campylobacters; i.e. curved rod-shaped bacteria. (d) Spirochaete, a long, spiral filament.

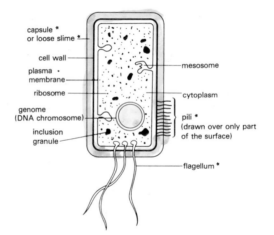

FIG. 6.5.   The structures of a bacterial cell. The structures marked with an asterisk (*) do not necessarily occur in every bacterial cell but are included for the sake of completeness. All the structures within the cell wall are known collectively as the protoplast.

the **protoplast**) consists of **cytoplasm** containing several small structures.

3. The outer flexible layer of the cytoplasm just inside the cell wall is the **plasma membrane** (or cytoplasmic membrane) which controls the passage of materials into and out of the cell. Intrusions, or extensions of the plasma membrane into the cytoplasm (*mesosomes*) are involved in (a) the formation of a dividing septum when the cell reproduces, discussed in more detail later, and (b) other vital processes including, it is believed, cell respiration.

4. There is no nucleus such as occurs in mammalian cells. In mammalian cells the

genes which determine the genetic characteristics of the individual lie along separate strands of DNA called chromosomes which are gathered together in the nucleus and separated from the rest of the cell by a nuclear membrane. In a bacterium the genes all lie on a continuous ring of DNA which can be regarded as a single chromosome or **genome**. It is not separated from the rest of the cell contents. The genome divides just before the cell does, and therefore at times it is possible to see two, or with rapid growth even four, genomes in a bacterium. (The genome has also been referred to as the chromatin body or nucleoid.)

5. The cytoplasm also contains: (a) numerous minute granules, **ribosomes**, containing ribonucleic acid (RNA), which are responsible for protein synthesis, and (b) various larger structures, **inclusion granules**, most of which represent food reserves (lipids or polysaccharides).

Other features shown by *some* bacteria include:

1. Another protective layer outside the cell wall, designated a **capsule** or **loose slime**, depending on its properties. This layer protects against drying and against phagocytosis by white blood cells.

2. One or more long whip-like structures protruding through the cell wall called **flagella** (singular = flagellum), which enable bacteria to swim about. Bacteria exhibiting motility are referred to as **motile bacteria**. Flagella develop from granules within the cytoplasm.

3. Numerous fine filaments, protruding from the surface, called **pili** or fimbriae. They can have a number of functions, including attachment of the bacterium to host cells. A special sex pilus may be formed to transfer genetic material between two bacteria—a process called "bacterial mating" or **conjugation** (see later).

4. A spherical or eliptical structure within the bacterium called an endospore, or more simply a **spore** (see Fig. 6.8). It has a very thick protective wall and is very resistant to heat, to drying (desiccation) and to the action of chemicals, e.g. disinfectants. Since only one is formed in each cell it is not considered as a means of reproduction but simply as a means of survival in adverse circumstances. Only two groups of bacteria form such spores —members of the genera *Bacillus* and *Clostridium*.

Spores are formed when the supply of nutrients is inadequate (the process is described later) and they can survive without food or water in an inactive (dormant) state for long periods, certainly for many years. In the presence of water and nutrients at a suitable temperature, and probably triggered off by other factors, a spore is transformed back through a number of stages to the normal, so-called "vegetative", bacterial cell.

Whole bacteria with their capsules and endospores may be distinguishable using an ordinary microscope, particularly after special staining of the bacteria, but the other small structures described, such as flagella and pili, require much greater magnification before they can be seen.

## Reproduction

With an adequate supply of nutrients and under suitable conditions (temperature, pH, oxygen level, etc.) bacteria can reproduce very rapidly.

Most bacteria will grow in the presence of free oxygen; these are called aerobes or **aerobic bacteria**. (Those which will not grow unless free oxygen is available are called obligatory aerobes, and those which are able to grow whether free oxygen is present or not are called facultative anaerobes.) Bacteria which will only grow if free oxygen is absent are called obligatory anaerobes or **anaerobic bacteria**. Microaerophilic bacteria grow best in the presence of minute quantities of free oxygen.

Those bacteria which prefer to live in or on the animal body usually grow, i.e. reproduce, most rapidly at normal body temperature. This is the optimum temperature for their growth. Other bacteria may have a lower or higher optimum temperature for growth.

### Binary fission

Bacterial cells *usually* reproduce by **simple binary fission** in which a pre-existing cell divides into two. Each of these new cells later divides into two and so on. This is an example of asexual reproduction, otherwise called vegetative reproduction. If adequate nutrients are available they are taken into the cell and converted into nucleic acids and protein thereby increasing the size of the cell. The cell elongates and the genome divides. Half-way along the cell the plasma membrane grows inwards to form a **septum**, or cross-plate, which separates the genomes and also the cytoplasm. Then a cell wall develops in this septum and the final stage is a splitting of the new transverse cell wall (Fig. 6.6). However, not all bacteria separate immediately, and some characteristically appear still joined together in chains or clusters when viewed under the microscope (e.g. streptococci and staphylococci).

The multiplication of parasitic bacteria usually takes place *outside* the host's cells, which is the opposite of what occurs with viruses.

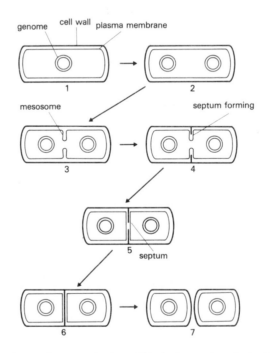

Fig. 6.6. Binary fission (vegetative reproduction). This is the usual method of bacterial reproduction in which one bacterial cell divides into two cells. The genome first divides, then a mesosome grows inwards from the plasma membrane to form a septum. The cell wall grows into this septum and finally the new transverse cell wall divides.

The time interval required between successive bacterial cell divisions is called the **generation time** and, even under optimum conditions, it varies for different bacterial species. For *E. coli* it is about 15 minutes and therefore one *E. coli* cell can give rise to well over a million within 5 hours.

Two non-reproductive processes which occur in bacteria might conveniently be described at this point:

## 1. Conjugation or "Bacterial Mating"

This process is sometimes referred to as sexual reproduction but such an expression is misleading since, unlike sexual reproduction in mammals or other animals, conjugation between bacteria does *not* lead to the production of another individual.

The term conjugation refers to the passage of genetic material from one bacterium (the donor) to another (the recipient). DNA passes through a short tube, the **"sex pilus"**, formed by the donor and which connects the two cells (Fig. 6.7).

Conjugation rarely occurs, only involving approximately one bacterial cell in a million and probably only Gram-negative bacteria. It is, however, of importance since extra genes can be transferred by conjugation to another bacterium. Bacteria having extra genes are created as a result of mutations which occur fairly frequently in organisms able to reproduce so rapidly. The extra genes are called *plasmids* and are separate structures from the genome. One of the plasmids can be the so-called antibiotic resistance factor, or R-factor, which confers resistance to antibiotics. Often antibiotic-resistant bac-

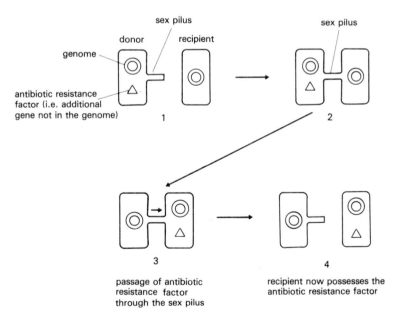

FIG. 6.7. Conjugation, or "bacterial mating". After the formation of a sex pilus by the donor bacterial cell and connection with the recipient, the antibiotic resistance factor passes from one to the other. All the offspring of the recipient (produced by binary fission) would also possess the factor, i.e. would have the same antibiotic resistance as the original donor cell.

teria (i.e. bacteria possessing an antibiotic resistance factor) are relatively harmless bacteria which normally inhabit the body, e.g. the intestine. However, if an important disease-producing bacterium at some time gains entry to the intestine, the antibiotic resistance factor may be passed to it from one of the normal inhabitants via the process of conjugation. Now the previously antibiotic-sensitive pathogen suddenly becomes resistant, possibly to a whole range of antibiotics all at the same time, and treatment of the disease caused by the pathogen can become very difficult or even impossible. It should be emphasized that *all* types of bacteria may possess an antibiotic resistance factor (e.g. staphylococci resistant to penicillin possess one). However, the transfer of an antibiotic resistance factor by conjugation appears to be confined to Gram-negative bacteria, and the intestine is a particularly suitable area for conjugation to take place.

## 2. Spore Formation

When an endospore is formed the sequence begins in the same way as in binary fission but a septum forms nearer one end of the bacterium and grows to completely surround one genome, including the cytoplasm. This "coat" around the genome separates from the plasma membrane and other coats form in succession around it giving rise to the thick wall of the spore. Finally, the cell wall of the original cell lyses (i.e. is broken down by cell enzymes) to release the spore (Fig. 6.8). It should be emphasized that this is not a method of reproduction but a means of survival.

## Major Differences between Bacteria and Viruses (Table 6.1)

Individual viruses are much smaller than bacteria and cannot be seen using the normal light microscope. They are visible using the much greater magnification of the electron microscope. Their size is measured in nanometres (nm); a nanometre is one-millionth part of a millimetre. In certain diseases such as canine distemper small patches called inclusion bodies can be seen in virus-infected cells using a light microscope. These represent a *large number* of growing viruses clustered together. There is discussion as to whether viruses should be considered as living organisms since they are not able to move and cannot grow or reproduce unless they are within a living host cell.

TABLE 6.1.    *Major differences between bacteria and viruses*

| Bacteria | Viruses |
|---|---|
| 1.  Larger | Smaller |
| 2.  Have a cell wall which contains muramic acid | Lack both a cell wall and muramic acid |
| 3.  Carry out chemical changes necessary for metabolism and reproduction using their own enzymes | Depend essentially for growth and reproduction on the enzymes of the host cells |
| 4.  Usually reproduce by binary fission | Do not replicate by binary fission |
| 5.  Contain both DNA and RNA | Contain either DNA or RNA but not both |
| 6.  All can, and most usually do, multiply outside cells: some also live in cells | Can only multiply inside living cells |
| 7.  Can be grown on non-living media | Will not grow on non-living media |
| 8.  Some may form toxins | None form toxins |
| 9.  Some are motile (able to move) | None are motile |
| 10.  Can be saprophytic or parasitic | Always parasitic |

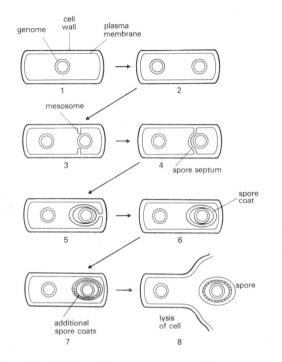

FIG. 6.8.   Spore formation. After division of the genome a septum forms near one end of the bacterial cell. This septum surrounds one of the genomes and other protective coats develop around it. Finally the original bacterial cell wall lyses to release the spore.

Viruses are always parasitic and reproduce by **replication**, a process which takes place after the viral nucleic acid has entered the host cell. The viral nucleic acid either enters the cell within the intact virus (i.e. the virus enters the cell) or it is injected by the virus from outside. The viral nucleic acid (which may be either DNA or RNA but never both) then takes over control of the cell metabolism and "directs" it to manufacture more virus particles. Usually 100 to 300 are manufactured and released by rupture (lysis) of the host cell's wall.

Most viruses are very host specific and will grow only in one, or very few, host species. All the diseases that dogs and cats are routinely vaccinated against, with the exception of the leptospiral diseases (which are bacterial diseases) are caused by viruses. Viruses also infect plants and some infect bacteria; these latter are called bacteriophages. However, very commonly, as with bacteria, the effects of viruses are hardly noticeable, i.e. they cause an inapparent infection. If such a virus is transferred from its natural host to another host it may in some instances produce violent changes and a serious disease.

## Media Suitable for Bacterial Growth and Multiplication

The term *media* (or culture media) denotes nutrient substances upon which micro-organisms are cultivated in the laboratory. To isolate and identify different bacteria they are grown in or on an artificial non-living culture medium which must contain the essential growth requirements of moisture, carbon and nitrogen. However, viruses will not grow on non-living media as they demand living cells for growth. This discussion of media is limited to those employed for bacterial culture.

In consistency bacterial culture media may be either liquid or solid. Although liquid media are most useful where there are only a few organisms to culture, they have the disadvantages that bacterial growths within them have no characteristic appearance and it is virtually impossible to separate two or more organisms growing in the same liquid medium. On solid media the differences in the size, shape and colour of bacterial colonies can be used to identify the organisms and they can be separated if more than one is present. The basis of solid media is the jelly-like substance called agar.

Both liquid and solid media may be classified into the following categories:

1. *Simple media* containing the basic growth factors for most bacteria, and also providing the basis for more complex media. Examples: liquid—nutrient broth; solid—nutrient agar.

2. *Enriched media.* The addition of blood or serum to the simple media enhances the growth of fastidious organisms. Blood agar, containing 10% animal blood, is widely employed and is also used to distinguish certain pathogenic species which produce haemolysis. Chocolate agar is another example; the blood in this medium has been heated beforehand to rupture the red blood cells and release their nutrients. Because of this chocolate agar is more nutritious than blood agar.

3. *Selective media.* These are media on which only certain bacteria will grow and consequently are used for their isolation and identification. Selenite broth (a liquid medium) is used to enhance the growth of

*Salmonella* organisms and inhibit the growth of others. Of the solid media, McConkey agar, which distinguishes organisms able to ferment lactose, and desoxycholate citrate agar (DCA), which is able to distinguish salmonellae, are two widely employed examples.

4. *Biochemical, or characterization, media.* These are used to identify bacteria by their particular biochemical reactions with the media. Separate 1% solutions of a number of different sugars (e.g. dextrose, sucrose, fructose) in peptone water are widely used as liquid media because each of the sugars can be fermented only by certain bacteria. The fermentation produces acid which is detected by an indicator in the solution, and some bacteria also produce gas. A commonly employed solid medium is one containing urea which can only be broken down by bacteria that produce the enzyme urease. The ammonia which results from urea breakdown affects an indicator in the medium producing a colour change.

The majority of bacteria routinely isolated from the dog and the cat will grow satisfactorily upon blood agar, although specialized media may be required to distinguish particular bacterial species.

### Pathogenic and Saprophytic Bacteria

As mentioned earlier, pathogenic bacteria are those which cause disease; usually, but not always, they are parasitic. Some will almost always cause disease, i.e. are invariably pathogenic, and others only become pathogenic when the body defence mechanisms are less efficient. The capacity of a particular strain of a bacterial species to produce disease is termed its **virulence**. Virulence depends upon invasiveness (the ability to become established and multiply within the host) and toxigenicity (the ability to produce toxins).

Saphrophytic bacteria live upon dead organic material. Their enzymes pass through the cell wall to digest this non-living material outside the cell and the digested nutrients are then absorbed back into the cytoplasm. A very few bacteria can be classed as both pathogenic and saprophytic; for example *Clostridium tetani*. This organism lives on dead tissue in the wound of an animal but produces a powerful exotoxin that causes the disease tetanus.

### Significance of Toxin Production

Some bacteria can produce poisonous substances known as toxins. They are of two types: **endotoxins**, produced within each bacterium and only liberated when it dies, and **exotoxins**, secreted by the living bacterial cells.

**Endotoxins** are part of the cell wall structure of certain types of Gram-negative bacteria which are released by autolysis (digestion of the cell by its own enzymes when the cell dies). They are normally of low toxicity but will withstand heat, e.g. autoclaving at 120°C. Endotoxins produce signs of generalized shock and fever.

**Exotoxins** are soluble protein poisons secreted by the living cells of certain bacteria (Gram-positive organisms). They may be formed within the body or, in food poisoning, they may be formed outside the body and then ingested. Many of them are extremely powerful poisons and even a small quantity may prove lethal. Each toxin produces a very specific type of damage to certain body cells. However, exotoxins are readily killed by heating to boiling point.

**Exotoxins produced within the body** may act only locally or throughout the body, i.e. systematically. Classed as **locally acting exotoxins** are various enzymes produced by bacteria to aid their spread through the host's tissues. They include hyaluronidase (which breaks down the intercellular cement holding the cells together) and leucocidin (which kills phagocytes).

*Clostridium tetani* is a bacterium which produces a **systemically acting exotoxin.** The endospores of *C. tetani,* which occur frequently in soil, may enter a skin wound, often a very small wound. In the wound they are transformed to the vegetative (growing) form of the bacterium. The bacteria require a low level of oxygen and dead tissue to live on (i.e. are anaerobic and saprophytic), both of which conditions exist in the wound, and they produce a potent exotoxin. The organisms remain at the wound site but the exotoxin diffuses up the peripheral nerves to the central nervous system and is also carried by the blood to peripheral nerves in other parts of the body. It is a neurotoxin and produces the muscle spasms and paralysis of the disease tetanus.

**Exotoxins produced outside the body**. Some strains of *Staphylococcus aureus* growing in contaminated food produce an exotoxin known as an enterotoxin (acting on the bowel) which causes vomiting and diarrhoea when the food is eaten, i.e. **food poisoning**. *Clostridium botulinum*, a saprophyte which does not infect animals, produces in contaminated food (often incorrectly preserved meat) a neurotoxin which when consumed acts throughout the nervous system causing paralysis. It is one of the most poisonous substances known and is frequently lethal.

These examples serve to show that some bacterial toxins can affect body cells which are at a considerable distance from the site in the body of the bacteria which produce them, and in some cases where the bacteria have never even entered the body.

In the body of an animal an exotoxin stimulates the production of an antibody called an antitoxin. If at a later date the same exotoxin reappears in the body the antitoxin will react with it and neutralize it. This is an example of immunity. In the laboratory, animals deliberately infected with small non-lethal doses of exotoxin will produce antitoxin in this way. The antitoxin can then be separated from their blood and stored and later given as part of treatment to any "non-immune" animal in which the toxin is present.

Also in the laboratory exotoxin can be treated with chemicals (e.g. formalin) to produce a non-poisonous substance called a **toxoid** which when injected into the body will still stimulate it to produce antitoxin. In this way tetanus toxoid is used to immunize animals, i.e. provide immunity against tetanus. It is essential for those working with animals to be immunized against tetanus because *C. tetani* spores are widespread in the environment and wounds, e.g. scratches and bites, can readily be infected.

Endotoxins will not form toxoids and they cannot readily be neutralized with antitoxins.

### Bacteria and Disease

In the previous section mention was made of a few bacteria that can cause disease by means of toxins that are formed outside the host or in the alimentary tract and then absorbed through the gut. However, in general bacteria must first enter the tissues of the host in order to produce disease. They may then either remain at their site of entry or spread further within the body. To prevent this invasion the body has developed a number of defence mechanisms which the bacteria must overcome if they are to survive (Fig. 6.9). In broad terms these defence mechanisms may be said to constitute the animal's resistance, or immunity to disease, although the term **immunity** is usually given a more restricted meaning (see Principles of Immunity p. 356) and is used only for specific acquired immunity.

Bacteria may enter the tissues through the skin, conjunctiva or the mucosal lining of the alimentary, respiratory or urinogenital tracts. Various **external defence mechanisms** (mechanical and chemical barriers) exist to prevent them doing this. Although bacteria are normally present in the alimentary tract, particularly the intestines and in the outer part of the respiratory and urinogenital tracts, this is not the same as being *within* the tissues of the body. The external defence mecha-

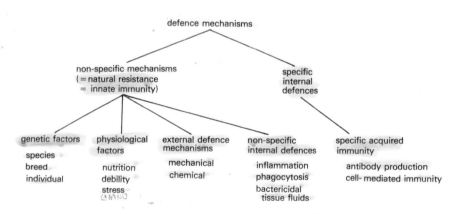

Fig. 6.9. Defence mechanisms of the host animal. Although classified above as internal defences the mechanisms of inflammation and phagocytosis can also occur at the surface of the skin and mucous membranes.

nisms prevent these bacteria progressing further.

The dry horny outer layer of the skin is impermeable, so that breaks in the surface are required for entry, either due to wounds or burns, including insect or animal bites and injection sites, or natural openings like hair follicles. The conjunctiva is washed by tears and the mucous membranes of the body tracts produce mucus to which organisms stick. In the respiratory tract cilia "sweep" mucus and bacteria towards the exterior, and natural functions such as coughing, sneezing, sweating, salivating and urinating help to flush bacteria from the body. Many body secretions contain substances which inhibit or destroy bacteria e.g. the enzyme lysozyme which can rupture ("lyse") Gram-positive bacteria. The stomach contains a high concentration of acid which kills many ingested organisms.

If the bacteria penetrate these defences they may multiply in the epithelial surfaces and remain relatively confined there, as with staphylococci causing skin pustules and streptococci in the throat. Others may penetrate into the sub-epithelial tissues around the point of entry (called **local spread**), and some types of bacteria regularly overcome the local defences and spread throughout the body (called **systemic spread**). Systemic spread occurs through the lymphatic circulation and/or the blood circulation; sometimes the bacteria are carried in the liquid portion of the lymph or blood, whereas other bacteria are transported in or on the red blood cells or white blood cells.

Although bacteria spreading systemically may cause damage in a number of tissues throughout the body, many prefer to settle in one particular part, i.e. to localize, and multiply there, e.g. lung or heart. (This affinity for one particular kind of tissue is particularly strong with viruses.)

Inside the body bacteria have to overcome a whole variety of **internal defence mechanisms** which may be non-specific or specific. **Specific acquired immunity**, however, is dealt with separately in the next sub-section.

The **non-specific internal defence mechanisms** consist of inflammation, phagocytosis and the presence of bactericidal (bacteria-killing) substances in the tissue fluids.

1. **Inflammation**. When bacteria grow in tissues, substances appear, both produced by bacterial metabolism and also released from the cells they damage, which cause an inflammatory response (acute inflammation). These substances cause the capillary blood and lymphatic vessels to dilate and become more permeable to fluid, and they also attract phagocytes. This allows cells and protective substances such as antibodies to pass easily from the blood to the infected area. Initially the phagocytes are chiefly neutrophils, but after one or two days large numbers of macrophages start to appear. Inflammation of tissues is characterized by the well-known signs of redness, heat, swelling, and pain. Inevitably there is a loss of normal function.

2. **Phagocytosis**. The two main types of phagocytes (eating cells) in the body are the **neutrophils**, often called polymorphs, which circulate in the blood and **macrophages**, which are both in the blood and scattered throughout the body in the tissues. The macrophages of the blood are called monocytes.

Neutrophils are most active in the phagocytosis (= eating) of bacteria which occurs in two stages; (i) attachment of the bacteria to the phagocyte, and (ii) ingestion (Fig. 6.10).

(i) **Attachment**. If the bacterium has a large capsule it is difficult for it to adhere to the phagocyte. Attach-

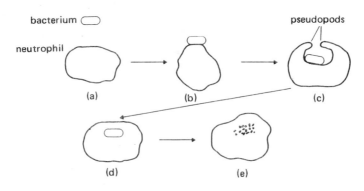

FIG. 6.10.   Phagocytosis by a neutrophil. The first stage is attachment of the bacterium to the neutrophil ((b) above). This is followed by ingestion (c) and (d) in which pseudopods flow around the bacterium to enclose it. Finally (e) the bacterium is killed and broken down by enzymes produced by the neutrophil.

ment is made easier if the bacterium is first coated in antibody.

(ii) **Ingestion**. Pseudopods flow from the neutrophil around the bacterium. Once enclosed the bacterium is killed and broken down by various substances, including enzymes produced by the neutrophil.

Some species of bacteria are very resistant to being ingested and others when ingested may kill the phagocyte leading to the production of large numbers of dead neutrophils which form pus. There are even bacteria, e.g. *Mycobacterium tuberculosis,* which after ingestion are not killed but actually multiply inside the phagocyte.

The macrophages, which appear in greater numbers later, phagocytose dead neutrophils and tissue debris.

Bacteria passing through the lymphatic system will encounter macrophages in each lymph node. If large numbers of organisms reach a node it may become inflamed, and if it is unable to arrest or destroy all of them some organisms will pass on. However, provided the node is not the last before the lymph enters the blood there will be further nodes on the course of the lymphatic vessel where arrest may occur.

3. **Bactericidal substances in tissue fluids**. The chief one of these is **complement**. Complement is a complex system of proteins, normally present in serum, which assist (i.e. are complementary to) antibodies in destroying bacteria. The attachment of antibody to the bacterium enables the complement to recognize its target. It also sets in motion (or activates) a progressive increase in the number of attacking molecules of complement, a process called amplification. The complement molecules produce an enzyme to lyse the bacterial cell. Both inflammation and phagocytosis (by neutrophils and macrophages) are also increased by the action of complement.

(Although not involved in bacterial infections it might be valuable just to mention **interferon**, which is a substance synthesized by body cells infected by a virus. It stimulates uninfected cells to produce another protein which protects them from viral attack.)

Bacteria produce disease by:

(1) direct damage to body cells (including phagocytes);

(2) the action of toxins which cause cell lysis or interfere with their normal function;

(3) provoking    inflammation,    which

causes many of the signs of disease; and

(4) initiating reactions between bacterial antigen and antibody formed by the host, which can lead to severe cell damage or an allergic reaction.

There are a very limited number of bacterial species known to produce a specific named disease in the dog and cat in the United Kingdom (Table 6.2). A further small number of other bacteria are responsible for producing disease at a variety of sites in the body (Table 6.3). Many of these are regarded as normal harmless inhabitants of the body (known as **commensals**) which only cause disease when the body defences are weakened allowing them to gain access to a part of the body from which they are normally excluded (**opportunistic invaders**).

An **endemic disease** is one which is normally present in a particular area; e.g. rabies is endemic in most countries of Asia and northern Europe. An **epidemic** is the sudden widespread occurrence of a large number of cases of an infectious disease in an area, such as the sudden appearance of a large number of cases of influenza in the human population. Strictly speaking, where animals are affected the correct terms to use are respectively **enzootic** and **epizootic**, rather than endemic or epidemic.

### Principles of Immunity

**Non-susceptibility** refers to the protection from certain diseases possessed by some species because of their genetic constitution. For example, the dog does not contract foot-and-mouth disease or the cow get canine distemper. To a lesser extent certain breeds or strains of species, and even particular individuals, may be more immune because of their genetic characteristics.

Certain **physiological factors** may make the host more susceptible to an infectious disease. For example, if an animal is poorly nourished, debilitated due to other diseases, or suffering from stress in the form of shock, fatigue or a lowered body temperature, the phagocytes are not as active as normally and phagocytosis of pathogens is less efficient.

**Specific acquired immunity** is so-called because it is specific for a particular disease-producing organism and is acquired by an animal during its life (after exposure to the organism). It consists of two different defence mechanisms; the production of antibodies and of cell-mediated immunity.

### 1. Antibody production

**Antibodies** are proteins formed by cells of the lymphoid system, known as **plasma cells** (which are derived from B lymphocytes). In the blood most antibodies are found in that group of plasma proteins called the gamma-globulins. The formation of an antibody occurs in response to the presence in the body of a foreign substance, which must be either a protein or linked to a protein. By foreign is meant that the substance is not a normal constituent of the body. Such a substance, which causes the production of an antibody, is called an **antigen**.

The formation of an antibody is a specific response to a particular antigen. Any other antigen would result in the production of some other specific antibody.

All living organisms, including bacteria and viruses, are composed of several antigenic materials. Bacterial exotoxins are also antigens. Consequently the presence of a particular micro-organism or toxin in the body causes the production of one or more antibodies against it. If the

TABLE 6.2.   *To show the limited number of infectious diseases of the dog and cat in the United Kingdom that are caused by specific bacteria.*

| Disease | Bacteria responsible |
|---|---|
| **DOG and CAT** | |
| Tetanus | *Clostridium tetani* |
| Tuberculosis | *Mycobacterium tuberculosis;* |
| | *Mycobacterium bovis* |
| *"Trench mouth" | *Fusobacterium fusiforme* + |
| | *Borrelia vincentii* **together** |
| Nocardiosis | *Nocardia* species |
| Actinomycosis | *Actinomyces* species |
| Listeriosis | *Listeria monocytogenes* |
| Salmonellosis | *Salmonella* species |
| Campylobacter infection | *Campylobacter coli;* |
| | *Campylobacter jejuni* |
| | |
| **DOG ONLY** | |
| Brucellosis (abortion) | *Brucella canis* |
| *Leptospirosis | *Leptospira canicola; Leptospira* |
| | *icterohaemorrhagiae* |
| Actinobacillosis | *Actinobacillus* species |
| Tularaemia | *Francisella tularensis* |
| *Canine respiratory disease (kennel cough) | { *Bordetella bronchiseptica* |
| | { *Mycoplasma* species |
| | |
| **CAT ONLY** | |
| Pseudotuberculosis | *Yersinia pseudotuberculosis* |
| Feline leprosy | *Mycobacterium lepraemurium* |
| *Feline respiratory disease (cat 'flu) | |
| { Feline pneumonitis | *Chlamydia psittaci* |
| { Mycoplasm infection | *Mycoplasma* species |
| *Haemobartonellosis | *Haemobartonella felis* |
| (feline infectious anaemia) | |

* = Most common; the others are rare.

*Note.* Viruses are commonly the cause of canine or feline respiratory disease but the bacteria listed above can also be responsible.

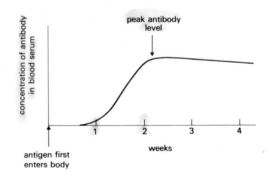

FIG. 6.11.   Antibody production when the body first encounters a particular antigen. After approximately a week's delay antibody is produced and reaches its peak level one week later.

TABLE 6.3. To show that most bacterial conditions in the dog and cat are due to a very limited range of bacteria which are normal inhabitants of the skin and mucous membranes. Also *Moraxella lacunatus* can cause conjunctivitis and rhinitis in the cat.

| Part of body | Disease | Bacteria most often responsible | | | | | |
|---|---|---|---|---|---|---|---|
| | | Staphylococci (chiefly aureus) | Streptococci (chiefly haemolytic) | Escherichia coli | Pseudomonas aeruginosa | Pasteurella multocida | Proteus species |
| Skin | Pyoderma (skin infections with pus) | + + | + | | | | |
| Ear | Otitis externa | + | + | | | + | |
| Eye | Keratitis/conjunctivitis | + + | + | | + | | |
| Joints | Arthritis | + | + | | | | |
| Bone | Osteomyelitis | + + | | | | | |
| Upper Respiratory Tract | Rhinitis | | | | | | |
| | Pharyngitis | + | + | | + | + | |
| | Laryngitis | | | | | | |
| Lower Respiratory Tract | Bronchitis and pneumonia | + | + + | + + | | + | + |
| Uterus | Pyometra | + + | + + | + + | | | |
| | Metritis/vaginitis | + | + + | + + | | | + |
| Prostate Gland | Prostatitis | + | + + | + + | | | |
| Urinary Tract | Urinary infection | + | + + | + + | | | + + |
| Alimentary Tract | Gastritis and enteritis | + + | + + | + + | | | |
| Heart | Endocarditis | + | + + | + + | + | | |
| Mammary Gland | Mastitis | + + | | | + | | + |
| Neonatal septicaemia | | + | + + | + + | | | |

+ + = most important.

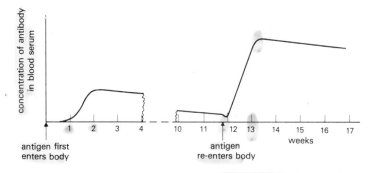

FIG. 6.12.    Subsequent antibody production. When the body re-encounters the same antigen the antibody
against it is more rapidly produced and reaches a much higher peak level.

body has not encountered the antigen
before it normally takes about 1 week
before producing detectable amounts of
the antibody and 2 weeks before the
maximum level of antibody is reached
(Fig. 6.11).

The formed antibody combines with the
antigen. Where the antigen is part of a
micro-organism or its toxin, this antigen–
antibody combination is beneficial to the
host because:

(a) it makes phagocytosis easier;
(b) it stops viruses entering more cells;
(c) it prevents bacteria from attaching
    to mucosal surfaces;
(d) it neutralizes toxins; and
(e) it activates complement which stim-
    ulates inflammation and increases
    the supply of phagocytes.

When the antigen has been successfully
eliminated the level of antibody in the
body gradually falls but the plasma cells
"remember" the antigen and if it reappears in the body the specific antibody
against it is very quickly formed again
(Fig. 6.12).

When the antibody has been made by
the immune animal itself the immunity is
called **active**. The antibody may be
formed either because the animal has
contracted the disease, which is a natural
process, or because it has been vaccinated,
or injected with toxoid, which are artificial

processes i.e. do not occur in nature. The
injection of a vaccine or toxoid introduces
the antigen(s) into the body so that
antibody will be formed against them, but
the antigen is in a form which will not
produce the disease. For example, in a
vaccine the micro-organisms are either
killed or specially altered (attenuated) to
reduce their virulence. If the animal later
encounters the natural disease, antibody
can be rapidly formed. Re-vaccination
at varying intervals of time is often
advised to maintain high antibody levels
(p. 361).

It is also possible for an animal to
receive antibodies against particular diseases which have been made by another
animal and not itself. These will give the
animal protection for a short time. The
immunity conferred in this way is called
**passive**. It can occur naturally in the dog
and cat when antibodies are passed from
the blood of the mother into that of the
new-born animal via ingestion of the
colostrum (i.e. the first milk). These antibodies are not digested but are absorbed
from the young animal's gut into the
blood stream for the first 1–2 days. (Very
little antibody passes to the foetus through
the placenta in the dog and cat, about 5%
of the total, although this is the only route
used by man.) The transferred maternal
antibodies provide some protection for the

young animal whilst its own active immunity is developing.

Also passive immunity can be artificial, i.e. if antibody formed in one animal is injected into another the latter becomes immune as a result. Commercially antibodies against certain diseases are produced in animals, usually horses, by vaccinating them with the particular antigen. The antibodies are then separated, purified and bottled. Such a product is usually called an **antiserum** or a **hyperimmune serum**, e.g. distemper antiserum. The use of antisera is valuable whenever instantaneous protection against the disease in question is required; for example:

(a) when the animal is due to contact other possibly infected animals as when entering a boarding kennels or cattery, or attending a dog or cat show; and

(b) when other in-contact animals have the disease but the animal in question is not yet showing signs of disease.

In the case of tetanus, an antiserum (called in this case an antitoxin) is also used if the animal sustains a wound which could permit the causal bacteria to enter or if the animal shows signs of the disease process. In viral diseases if clinical signs are evident it is probably too late for antisera to stop viral replication in the cells, i.e. to be of much value in treatment.

Immunization therefore may be either active or passive and each may be either natural or artificial (Table 6.4). The main points of difference between active and passive immunity are set out in Table 6.5.

## 2. Cell mediated immunity

In some infectious diseases as well as, or instead of, the production of antibodies another acquired immune response called

TABLE 6.4. *Examples of active/passive and natural/artificial immunization*

| | Active | Passive |
|---|---|---|
| N a t u r a l | Natural infection (not necessarily giving signs of disease) | Maternal antibodies are transferred (mainly in colostrum in dog and cat) |
| A r t i f i c i a l | Vaccination or injection of toxoid | Injection of antibody (in antiserum) |

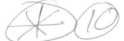

cell mediated immunity (CMI) operates, as follows. There are some lymphocytes in the body derived from the thymus gland called T lymphocytes or **T-cells**, and each type of T-cell is able to react with a particular type of antigen. If an infectious organism enters the body the antigen of which it is composed will eventually encounter the specific T-cells for that type of antigen. When this happens the T-cells respond in a number of ways, including;

(1) releasing substances called **lymphokines** which initiate an inflammatory response and attract phagocytes; and

(2) reacting with antigen on the surface of the micro-organism, to produce holes in its cell wall through which the cell contents leak. This causes the death of the micro-organism.

In diseases such as tuberculosis, in which the micro-organism is able to multiply inside cells, CMI is believed to be of supreme importance in killing the micro-organism and bringing about the recovery of the host.

TABLE 6.5.   *Main differences between active and passive immunity due to antibodies. In addition cell-mediated immunity is a form of active immunity; it cannot be transferred*

| Active | Passive |
| --- | --- |
| 1. The immune animal has produced the antibodies | The immune animal has **NOT** produced the antibodies |
| 2. Antibodies take at least 1 week to form after the first contact with the micro-organism or toxin, i.e. protection is not immediate | As soon as antibodies are transferred there is immunity, i.e. it is immediate |
| 3. Antibody level only gradually falls after antigen disappears | Antibodies stay in the body a much shorter time, e.g. maternal antibodies 8–20 weeks, injected antisera 2–4 weeks |

### Vaccines

As mentioned previously, a vaccine contains antigen from a micro-organism (or other parasite) which can be used for the artificial immunization of an animal. Ideally the vaccine should be effective, safe, stable (i.e. not easily broken down) and reasonably cheap. Two main types of vaccine are employed;

(1) **killed vaccine** (dead or inactivated vaccine) where the antigenic material is from dead micro-organisms;

(2) **live vaccine** where the antigen is in the form of living organisms which have been weakened in some way (i.e. attenuated) so that they will not cause the disease.

The amount of antibody produced by an animal is much greater when it encounters an antigen for the second time and further doses give further but lesser increases (Fig. 6.13).

Therefore, with dead vaccines, where the antigen is quickly removed, e.g. by phagocytosis, it is customary to give two doses of vaccine 2 or 3 weeks apart to boost the antibody level, e.g. with leptospiral vaccines. Often the first dose will merely sensitize the immune system.

However, the live micro-organisms in live vaccines (e.g. canine distemper vaccines) multiply in the host for a time after being administered, in fact until the antibody levels produced are high enough to destroy them. Therefore there is a con-

siderable increase in the amount of antigen which persists for long enough to produce very effective boosting of the antibody level. Consequently only one dose of live vaccine is required. There is, however, always the risk (though usually very slight) that the weakening of the live bacteria may not have been as effective as intended and therefore that it *might* cause disease.

In recent years the potency of some dead vaccines has been increased by adding **adjuvants** (adjuvenated vaccines) which slow down the rate of release of the antigen from the vaccination site. By extending the period of antigenic stimulation in this way antibody production is enhanced and the vaccine manufacturer may advise that a *single* injection of such a vaccine (e.g. against canine parvovirus) will confer adequate immunity.

With either type of vaccine the following statements apply:

(1) The vaccinated animal should as far as possible be kept away from other animals of the same species and places which they might regularly visit (streets, parks, etc.) to avoid becoming infected with the micro-organism before peak antibody levels have been produced. This usually takes at least 2 weeks.

(2) In general, vaccination should not be practised before 8 weeks of age and, ideally, not until 12 weeks of

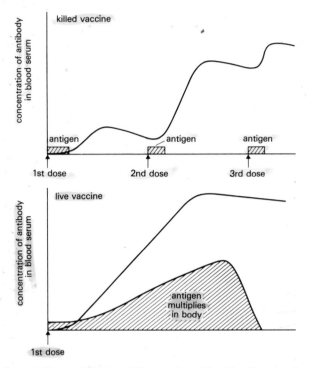

FIG. 6.13.   Comparison of effects of killed and live vaccines. The "dead" antigenic material of the *killed vaccine* lasts only a short time in the body. Each successive administration of the killed vaccine "boosts" the antibody level but this effect gets progressively less after the second dose. The amount of antigen from the live organisms in the *live vaccine* increases as the organisms multiply in the body. Only when high antibody levels have been produced is the antigen eliminated.

age, to avoid the antigen of the vaccine reacting with, and being neutralized by, the residual maternal antibodies. If this happened it would leave the animal with no protection.

In cases where particularly vulnerable animals need to be vaccinated before 12 weeks of age they are usually re-vaccinated at 12 weeks old to ensure antibody development.

(3) Vaccination should not occur if there is evidence of a disease being present (high temperature etc.) because the antibody-producing cells may already be fully occupied reacting to the antigens of the present disease.

(4) Further "booster" injections of vac-cine are usually advisable at yearly intervals (or longer with some diseases) to boost the antibody level which, in the absence of natural contact with antigen, will gradually decline.

Certain respiratory pathogens such as *Bordetella bronchiseptica* only inhabit the surface mucous membrane and never enter the bloodstream. Consequently antibodies in the blood provide little protection against these infections. The best defences are **local antibody production** and **local cell-mediated immunity**. Therefore if the vaccine can be administered locally, e.g. intranasally (e.g. *B. bronchiseptica* vaccine), the local antigenic stimulation is likely to be greater and to result in greater protection.

## (d) Elementary parasitology

B. M. BUSH

### Introduction

Parasitology is the study of parasites. As was mentioned in the previous section on Elementary Bacteriology, the term parasite is commonly used in veterinary practice to refer to the larger parasitic organisms found in or on animals. Customarily the term excludes the smaller micro-organisms, the bacteria and viruses (even though their way of life is parasitic), but includes the larger micro-organisms found both in and on the body, i.e. the protozoa (e.g. coccidia) and the fungi (e.g. ringworm). Consequently parasitic organisms found in animals can be broadly classified into bacteria, viruses and parasites, the last category including everything which is *not* a bacterium or virus.

Parasites can be divided into those which live on the outside of the body (in or on the skin), called **external parasites** or **ectoparasites**, and those which live somewhere inside the body (frequently in the intestines), called the **internal parasites** or **endoparasites**.

The majority of parasites are members of the animal kingdom, the one important exception being the fungi which belong to the vegetable kingdom.

The presence of any micro-organisms (bacteria, viruses, protozoa or fungi) in or on the body is termed an **infection** and any disease which they may cause is called an **infectious disease**. (All other diseases are non-infectious diseases.) In practice the term infection is often stretched to include the presence of *any* parasitic organism. Formerly the term **infestation** was used to describe the presence of parasites, but nowadays this term is usually only used in connection with ectoparasites.

The ability of parasites to produce disease in the host varies considerably: some cause little or no signs of illness, others are consistently pathogenic. In general the disease is likely to be more severe if the host is young, has poor health or immunity or is poorly nourished, or if a large number of parasites are involved (i.e. with a heavy infection).

Some parasites spend all their life in or on the host (e.g. lice), whereas others spend only part of their time there (e.g. fleas). Again some of the intestinal parasites require a second host (the intermediate host) of a different animals species in which to carry out the early stages of development before being transferred to the final host. The **final host** (or **definitive host**) is the animal in which the adult, or reproductive stage, of the parasite occurs. An **intermediate host** is one in which part of the immature phase of the parasite's life-cycle is spent. An essential feature is that some development of the parasite occurs in the intermediate host, i.e. its life-cycle cannot be completed without a period in the intermediate host.

A **transport host** and a **paratenic host** both resemble an intermediate host in that they are animals in which part of the parasite's immature phase is spent but *no* development occurs in these hosts. The

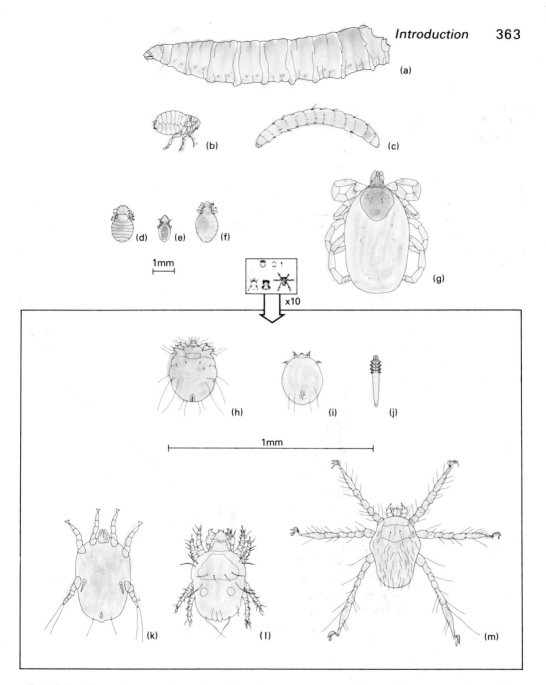

Fig. 6.14.   Common external parasites of the dog and cat in the United Kingdom (excluding fungal parasites). The parasites in the upper part of the drawing are five times life size and those in the lower panel have been enlarged a further ten times, i.e. they are fifty times life size. (The small panel in the centre indicates the size that the lower panel would be if drawn to the same scale as the parasites in the upper part.) (a) blow-fly larva; (b) cat flea (*Ctenocephalides felis*); (c) flea larva; (d), (e), (f) are lice: (d) *Trichodectes canis,* (e) *Felicola subrostratus,* (f) *Linognathus setosus*; (g) hedgehog tick (*Ixodes hexagonus*); (h), (i), (j) are subsurface mites: (h) *Sarcoptes scabiei* (variety *canis*), (i) *Notoedres cati,* (j) *Demodex canis* or *Demodex cati*; (k) ear mite (*Otodectes cynotis*); (l) fur mite (*Cheyletiella yasguri*); (m) harvest mite (*Trombicula autumnalis* larva). Although only marginally larger than *Otodectes* the harvest mite is usually regarded as being a macroscopic parasite.

immature phase of the parasite may be shed from a transport host at any time. In contrast, a paratenic host cannot get rid of the immature phase of the parasite from its tissues. Further development of the parasite only occurs if the paratenic host is ingested by the final host. In some cases the effect of the parasite on the intermediate host or paratenic host is far more damaging than its effect on the final host.

As with bacteria, a binomial system of naming parasites is employed, e.g. *Toxocara canis*. The first name is that of the genus—the smallest sub-group to which the parasite belongs and given a capital letter, and the second name is the individual name of the species and is given a small letter. Frequently where there is only one important species in a genus the first name is used alone, e.g. *Otodectes*. Where different strains of a parasite exist each can be described as a variety, e.g. *Sarcoptes scabiei* (variety *canis*).

### Common External Parasites found on Small Animals

In Table 6.6 are listed the common external parasites (ectoparasites) found on the dog and cat in the United Kingdom. They are divided into microscopic and macroscopic parasites. Macroscopic parasites can be readily seen with the naked eye, but microscopic parasites are not visible and are best detected and examined using a microscope. However, the surface mites (*Otodectes* and *Cheyletiella*) may be just discernible to the naked eye, especially if a hand lens or otoscope lens is used. These ectoparasites are shown in Fig. 6.14.

Conventionally the term ectoparasite includes only those parasites which are animals and not the fungal parasites (the ringworms and yeasts). However, for the purposes of this section these have been

TABLE 6.6. *External parasites of the dog and cat in the United Kingdom*

| External Parasite | Found in Dog | Cat |
|---|---|---|
| **Microscopic parasites** | | |
| Subsurface mites | | |
| *Sarcoptes scabiei* (variety *canis*) | + | |
| *Notoedres cati* | | ± |
| *Demodex canis* | + | |
| *Demodex cati* | | + |
| Surface mites | | |
| Ear mite | | |
| *Otodectes cynotis* | + | + + |
| Fur mite | | |
| *Cheyletiella yasguri* | + | |
| *Cheyletiella blakei* | | + |
| Fungal parasites | | |
| Ringworm (dermatophytes) | | |
| *Microsporum canis* | + | + |
| Other *Microsporum* species | + | |
| *Trichophyton mentagrophytes* | + | |
| Yeasts | | |
| *Candida albicans* | + | |
| **Macroscopic parasites** | | |
| Fleas | | |
| *Ctenocephalides felis* | + + | + + |
| *Ctenocephalides canis* | + | |
| Lice | | |
| Biting lice | | |
| *Trichodectes canis* | + | |
| *Felicola subrostratus* | | + |
| Sucking lice | | |
| *Linognathus setosus* | + | |
| Harvest mite | | |
| *Trombicula autumnalis* (larva) | + | + |
| Ticks | | |
| *Ixodes hexagonus* | + | |
| *Ixodes ricinus* | + | |
| *Ixodes canisuga* | + | |
| Maggots | | |
| Blow-fly larvae | + | + |

+ = occurs
+ + = very commonly occurs
± = extremely rare

included in Table 6.6 under the heading of microscopic parasites since they require microscopic examination to distinguish their features.

Other ectoparasites, not listed in Table 6.6, may be found on quarantined dogs and cats, especially when they have come from tropical climates. Pet animals other than dogs and cats may be infested with parasites similar to those described in Table 6.6, although usually different species are involved and they are mentioned only briefly.

Ectoparasites live in, or on, the skin for part, or all, of their lives. They may feed on dead and flaking skin scales at the surface of the skin, e.g. biting lice, or they may suck blood or lymph, e.g. fleas and ticks. Ectoparasites, particularly in large numbers, may damage the skin, and/or provoke an allergic reaction, both of which can result in inflammation and severe irritation ( = **pruritus**). This in turn leads to biting and scratching of the skin, and an affected animal can severely damage itself ( = **self-trauma**).

## Mites

The mites commonly found on dogs and cats with the exception of *Trombicula autumnalis,* are permanent parasites and spend their entire life on the host. In all cases where the life-cycle is known it lasts for a period of approximately 3 weeks, (i.e. 3 weeks is the length of time taken for a newly passed egg to develop through the larval and nymphal stages into an adult mite).

### Sub-surface Mites

Two of these are round-bodied mites with short stubby legs which burrow through the skin: *Sarcoptes scabiei* (variety *canis*) and *Notoedres cati. Sarcoptes* is fairly common and affects dogs, whereas *Notoedres* is very rare and infests cats. They cause respectively **sarcoptic** and **notoedric mange**. There is intense pruritus and alopecia ( = hair loss) initially affecting the ears and elbows but later spreading in the case of *Sarcoptes* ulti-

mately to affect the entire body. *Sarcoptes* mites found on the dog are contagious to man, and produce a transient skin disorder. A similar mite, *S. scabiei* (variety *hominis*) affects man, producing the disease called *scabies*.

Their presence is diagnosed positively by finding them in skin scrapings, although neither mite can be seen unless a microscope is used. Although they can be distinguished by anatomical features, in practice there is little point in doing this since both mites can be killed by the same drugs. The mites cannot live longer than a few days off a host. Male and female mites mate and eggs are laid in the skin tunnels. The eggs hatch after about 1 week, producing larvae which in turn become nymphs and then adults. Some of the larvae, nymphs and adults wander on the skin surface, and transmission to a new host requires them to transfer during direct skin to skin contact.

The other sub-surface mites are from the genus *Demodex,* the so-called follicular mites. *Demodex canis* occurs in very small numbers in the hair follicles of almost all dogs but only in certain animals does it produce disease, i.e. **demodectic mange** or **demodicosis**. Most animals develop an immunity to the mites which restricts their spread. In animals which do not develop an adequate immunity, or where the immunity is later suppressed (e.g. by cancer), the mites proliferate and generalized skin disease results. In the past it has occurred mainly, but not solely, in the short-haired breeds of dog.

Demodectic mange, in which the skin becomes reddened and itches and hair is shed, has two main forms:

(1) a **localized** form (otherwise called the **squamous** or **dry** form) where lesions are usually confined to the head and forelegs and heal spontaneously, i.e. without treatment. In some large breeds of dog only the feet may be affected.

(2) a **generalized** form, most common in dogs under one year old. Instead of improving the lesions spread across the body and the infected follicles become secondarily infected with bacteria, usually staphyloccoci, producing small abscesses (=pustules). For this reason it is also known as the **pustular** form.

All the life-cycle of *Demodex* is spent on the host, with eggs laid by adult females developing through larval and nymphal stages to new adults. The transmission of mites is from nursing bitches to their puppies by direct contact during the first 2–3 days of life. Larvae, nymphs and adult mites are all cigar-shaped with stubby legs, and this quite distinctive appearance provides easy identification. Again, their presence is confirmed by the microscopic examination of skin scrapings

*Demodex cati* is a similar mite to *D. canis* occurring in the hair follicles of some cats. Rarely it causes demodectic mange (demodicosis) which is almost always localized to the head, and only in exceptional cases becomes generalized.

*Sarcoptes* also occurs in primates, rabbits and hamsters, and *Notoedres* occurs in rats, rabbits and hamsters. A similar round-bodied mite, *Trixacarus,* can give rise to severe irritation in guinea-pigs, and another, *Cnemidocoptes pilae,* infests cage birds, producing the diseases **scaly beak** (most commonly in the budgerigar) and **scaly leg** (most commonly in the canary). Some *Demodex* species probably occur in all hamsters and gerbils but only cause significant skin disease in debilitated animals.

*Surface Mites*

The most common surface mite is the ear mite *Otodectes cynotis.* It is found in the ear canals of both dogs and cats,

particularly the latter, causing inflammation (=**otitis**). However, mites do sometimes occur on other parts of the body, especially the tail. The life-cycle takes about 3 weeks, in which the eggs hatch into larvae and progress through nymphal stages to the adult mite. This is a round-bodied mite but much larger than *Sarcoptes* or *Notoedres,* and its legs are long and not stunted. Moving mites are just visible using the naked eye and are easily seen with a hand lens.

Another surface mite of similar size is *Cheyletiella,* the **fur mite.** *Cheyletiella yasguri* is most important in the dog and *C. blakei* in the cat. These mites produce "dandruff", i.e. excessive shedding of the superficial skin scales, and mild irritation along the body from head to rump, although cats may show little pruritus. The mites spread by direct contact and are very contagious for man.

Characteristic features of the adult mite are the combs on the ends of its legs in place of claws and the hooks on its accessory mouth-parts. It is readily found in brushings or shallow scrapings from the coat of infected animals.

Of the "fur mites" *Cheyletiella parasitivorax* can infect rabbits and is usually non-pathogenic, but large numbers may result in considerable pruritus. The mite *Listrophorus gibbus* is a non-pathogenic fur mite of rabbits, easily seen on albino animals.

*Chirodiscoides* on the guinea-pig seldom gives ill-effects. On hamsters the mite *Ornithonyssus* may occur, and rats and mice are subject to several other fur mites (the most important being *Myobia* and *Mycoptes*).

*Otodectes* occurs in the ears of ferrets and primates and a similar mite is found in the ear canal of rabbits. This mite is *Psoroptes,* and infestations produce irritation with crusts and a cheesy exudate in the canal.

## The Harvest Mite, *Trombicula autumnalis*

This differs from the other mites in that only the larvae are parasitic. The adult mites live in the soil and are non-parasitic. In late summer and early autumn the larvae attach themselves to the skin of animals, including dog and man. In the dog the limbs (especially the skin between the digits) and the ears are favourite sites. The mites cause intense pruritus and can be seen with the naked eye as pin-head-sized red spots.

## The Red Mite, *Dermanyssus gallinae*

This mite feeds on cage birds such as budgerigars during the night and retreats to crevices during the day. A heavy infestation can give rise to anaemia.

(At times this mite has migrated into a house from abandoned birds' nests under the eaves and fed from humans, causing skin reactions.)

## Fleas

Few dogs and cats pass through life without at least a temporary infestation with these small, brown wingless insects. In England the most common flea on dogs, as well as cats, is the cat flea *Ctenocephalides felis* except in the case of racing greyhounds where the dog flea *C. canis* predominates. Rabbit fleas, hedgehog fleas and human fleas may also occur on pet dogs and cats.

The bodies of fleas are flattened from side to side and powerful legs enable them to jump to a considerable height, by which means they can transfer from host to host.

Adult fleas suck the blood of the host and their bites can cause extreme irritation. Some animals also become allergic to flea saliva which is injected into the skin when the animal bites (so-called **flea-allergy dermatitis**) and such animals can react to even a single flea bite. Fleas are also the intermediate host of the tapeworm *Dipylidium caninum* and are responsible for carrying this parasite to its final host in which it will develop to an adult tapeworm (see later). Fleas are important carriers ( = **vectors**) of the bacteria pasteurellae, and also *Haemobartonella felis*, and the virus of feline panleukopenia.

Fleas are easily seen with the naked eye moving swiftly over the skin surface and are usually particularly numerous at the base of the tail and behind the ears. Flea dirts, looking like specks of dark grit, may also be found on the skin. These consist mainly of dried blood and can be distinguished from grit by being placed on a piece of damp cotton wool or filter paper. If they are flea-dirts a red–brown stain spreads out from them over the dampened surface.

After mating, the female flea lays its eggs in cracks and crevices in the environment of its host, e.g. behind the skirting-boards, between floor-boards, tiles and sections of lino, in the pile of fitted carpets and in pet baskets and bedding (including chairs and beds if the pet is allowed on them). If they are laid on the host, the eggs soon drop off because they are not sticky. Several hundred eggs may be laid by each female during her 6 months of life.

After about 1 week each egg hatches into a yellowish-coloured larva which feeds on flea-dirts (which are the faeces of adult fleas). At approximately weekly intervals there occur two moults—the first to a red-brown larva and the second to a white larva. These larval stages resemble short worms with bristles and are usually found in the surroundings and not on the host. After a further week the third (white) larva spins a cocoon and becomes a pupa. Depending on such conditions as temperature and humidity the pupa may remain for a period of between 1 week and 1 year before the adult flea hatches out. Low temperature prolongs the pupal stage.

Adult fleas spend only short periods of time on their hosts, just sufficient to obtain a meal of blood, and therefore may not be found when looked for on the coat. They are most numerous in the host's environment. Also they are not confined to using one species of animal as a host and will readily feed from man as well as the dog and cat. Infestation of a new host is by direct contact (e.g. with an already infested animal) or indirect contact, i.e. acquiring fleas from infested surroundings. The latter is the most common. This fact is important in treating flea infestations since all the surroundings must be treated with insecticide at the same time as all the pets in the household (see Table 6.10).

On soft furnishings the application of gamma-BHC powder (vacuumed off after half-an-hour), or fly spray, or "Nuvan Staykil", is particularly useful. If a fly spray is used the animal is best kept off the area for several days afterwards. Old bedding and baskets, etc., are best burned. Dichlorvos is used to impregnate some brands of "flea-collars" and is released slowly as a vapour which kills fleas. Since many dogs are allergic to contact with these collars the use of dichlorvos fly strips above the beds of dogs and cats may be preferable.

The wild rabbit flea *Spilopsyllus cuniculi* rarely affects domesticated rabbits (most commonly on the inner surface of the ear).

### Lice

These are dorso-ventrally flattened wingless insects which are host-specific (i.e. will not develop on other host species) and spend *all* their life on the host. They spread by direct or indirect contact; that is to say either directly from infected animals or by contact with contaminated brushes and combs used in grooming.

Lice are divided into **biting lice** and **sucking lice**; both types occur in the dog. The sucking louse is *Linognathus setosus*—the most common dog louse, and the biting louse is *Trichodectes canis*. In the cat only a biting louse, *Felicola subrostratus,* is usual. (Some parasitologists use the term "chewing lice" in preference to "biting lice" because it more accurately describes their method of feeding.)

Lice are often most numerous around the ears, especially in long-coated dogs such as Cocker Spaniels. *Trichodectes canis* can act, like the flea, as an intermediate host of the tapeworm *Dipylidium caninum.*

Sucking lice have mouth-parts adapted for sucking blood, whilst biting lice feed chiefly on dead epithelial cells and, being more mobile than sucking lice, result in irritation to the host.

After mating, the female louse lays her eggs (called nits) and these are cemented to the hair. This cement makes it extremely difficult to remove nits from the hair. They cannot be combed out (except laboriously with a special metal comb which consists essentially of a series of slits in a metal plate—a "Derbac" comb) nor soaked off with water or most solvents. Clipping off infested hair is the best way of removing lice.

The egg hatches to release a nymph which resembles the adult in appearance but is smaller. This first nymph moults to produce a second nymph, which then moults to a third nymph, and this in turn moults to the adult. All stages occur on the host, and because of this control is made easier. The life-cycle (egg-laying to adult) occupies around 2–3 weeks.

*Polyplax* species of sucking lice occur on rats and mice and can be vectors carrying bacteria. Biting lice can occur in guinea-pigs (*Gliricola* and *Gyropus*) and may be transferred to new individuals in hay and straw. Rabbits (most commonly wild rabbits) may be infested with the sucking louse *Haemodipsus,* which is a vector for the bacterium *Francisella tularensis,* the cause of tularaemia. Primates are affected with the sucking louse *Pediculus longicepus.*

## Ticks

The ticks found on dogs and cats in the United Kingdom are ixodid ticks (hard ticks). They are almost always acquired from either farm livestock or wild animals. The most common is the hedgehog tick *Ixodes hexagonus.* The true dog tick. *I. canisuga* is much less common, being found most frequently in kennels (e.g. of greyhounds), particularly in northern areas of Britain. The sheep tick *I. ricinus* frequently occurs on dogs in rural areas where sheep farming predominates.

Ixodid ticks have a life-cycle which usually lasts several months and each stage can be considerably prolonged at lower temperatures, e.g. in Britain that of *I. ricinus* usually takes 3 years. Eggs, laid on the ground by the female tick, hatch to produce a larva or "seed" tick which becomes attached to and feeds from a host (i.e. sucks blood and/or lymph). The larva then drops off the host and after a rest moults to become a nymph. This in turn attaches to a host and sucks blood, then drops off, rests and finally moults to an adult tick. Adult males and females again attach to a host and suck blood, and usually mate whilst on the host. The female then drops off to lay her eggs.

Each stage (larva, nymph and adult) may prefer to feed from a different species of host to each other, and usually only the adults are found on the dog or cat. However, in the case of *I. canisuga* all three stages will feed from the dog and may be found on it. Adults are most commonly found on the legs, flanks, head and neck of dogs and may become engorged up to 1 cm or more in diameter. They appear greyish when unfed but are dark-brown black when distended with blood and may be confused with small pigmented tumours. Their **mouth-parts are deeply embedded in the skin** and may be left behind (possibly resulting in the formation of an abscess) if the tick is merely pulled off. It is therefore advisable to cause the tick to first slacken its grip, either by anaesthetizing it with a swab of ether or chloroform or spraying it with an insecticidal aerosol spray, before removing it carefully with forceps. Large numbers of ticks are best removed by bathing or spraying with a suitable insecticide. The removed ticks are best burnt. Outbreaks of infestation in kennels necessitate treatment of the surroundings to kill the resting stages which hide in cracks and crevices.

Tortoises can be imported bearing more exotic ixodid ticks (*Hyalomma* species) which can inflict unpleasant bites on humans. Exotic ticks (*Rhipicephalus* species) can also occur on dogs in quarantine kennels.

## Maggots

These are the larvae of calliphorid flies (**blow-flies**), which are otherwise called blue-bottles and green-bottles. In the summer these flies may lay their eggs in open wounds or in the dirty coats of neglected and debilitated animals. The larvae which hatch from the eggs feed from the living animal just as they would on non-living animal tissue, e.g. a carcass or piece of meat. The secrete enzymes which digest proteins in the tissues producing craters in the skin and can cause considerable damage.

### Fungal parasites

Mention should be made of two microscopic fungal parasites:

(1) **The ringworm fungi** or **dermatophytes**. Much the most important of these in the dog and cat is *Microsporum canis*. Of lesser importance are *Trichophyton mentagrophytes* and occasionally other ringworm species. These fungi grow on keratin in the cornified parts of the skin and its appendages, e.g. the outer horny layer of skin, the hair and the nails. With *M. canis* there may be the formation of skin crusts, breaking of affected hairs and actual hair loss. However cats, especially long-haired breeds, often show *no* obvious lesions. *Trichophyton* infestation can result in an inflammatory skin reaction.

(2) **The yeast**, *Candida albicans*. This organism is considered to be a saprophyte in the intestine but when the host's resistance is lowered it can spread to other parts of the body, including the skin, and become a parasitic pathogen. However, it rarely causes skin lesions in the dog or the cat.

Mice, rats, rabbits, hamsters and guinea-pigs can all be affected with *Microsporum* or *Trichophyton* species of ringworm. *Microsporum* is the more common in rats and mice; *Trichophyton* in the others.

### Common Internal Parasites found in Small Animals

The parasites listed in Table 6.7 are those encountered in the dog and cat in the United Kingdom, some of which are much more common than others. Other parasitic species such as the heartworm and giant kidney worm may be found in imported animals, e.g. those in quarantine kennels. All of the worms of the dog and cat in their adult stage (together with the coccidia) are found in the small intestine with the exception of the whipworm (found in the caecum), tongue worm (nasal cavities), bladder worm (bladder), tracheal worm (trachea) and lungworms (lungs and bronchi).

The most common internal parasites throughout the dog and cat population in the United Kingdom are the ascarid worms *Toxocara* and *Toxascaris*, the tapeworms *Dipylidium caninum, Taenia hydatigena* and *Taenia taeniaeformis,* the cat lungworm *Aelurostrongylus abstrusus* and the coccidian organism *Toxoplasma gondii.* The hookworm, whipworm, the dog lungworm (*Filaroides osleri*), bladder worm and coccidia other than *Toxoplasma* and *Sarcocystis* are most frequently found in animals bred or housed in large kennels or catteries. Having a large number of animals gathered together makes transmission of these parasites much easier. Other parasites (chiefly other tapeworms) are not commonly encountered, being most frequent in rural areas.

It is important to realize that many of these internal parasites do not produce obvious diseases in the affected dog or cat and usually there are no clinical signs to suggest that the host is infected. The effects of infection are greatest where there are a large number of parasites within the host and where the host is a debilitated or young animal; particularly the latter since young animals will not yet have developed immunity to parasites.

In the life-cycle of some of the parasites an intermediate host or paratenic host of another species is necessary. At times this

TABLE 6.7. *Internal parasites of the dog and cat in the United Kingdom*

| Internal Parasite | Found in Dog | Cat |
|---|---|---|
| Nematode worms | | |
| Ascarids (roundworms) | | |
| *Toxocara canis* | + + | |
| *Toxocara cati* | | + + |
| *Toxascaris leonina* | + + | + + |
| Hookworm | | |
| *Uncinaria stenocephala* | + | + |
| Whipworm | | |
| *Trichuris vulpis* | + | |
| Lungworms | | |
| *Filaroides osleri* | + | |
| *Angiostrongylus vasorum* | + | |
| *Aelurostrongylus abstrusus* | | + + |
| Tracheal worm | | |
| *Capillaria aerophila* | + | + |
| Bladder worm | | |
| *Capillaria plica* | + | |
| | | |
| Cestode worms (tapeworms) | | |
| *Dipylidium caninum* | + + | + + |
| *Taenia pisiformis* | + | |
| *Taenia ovis* | + | |
| *Taenia hydatigena* | + | |
| *Taenia taeniaeformis* | | + |
| *Taenia multiceps* | + | |
| *Taenia serialis* | + | |
| *Echinococcus granulosus* | + | ± |
| | | |
| Tongue worm | | |
| *Linguatula serrata* | + | |
| | | |
| Protozoa | | |
| Coccidia | | |
| *Toxoplasma gondii*[a] | + | + + |
| *Hammondia* species | + | + |
| *Sarcocystis* species | + | + |
| *Isospora* species | + | + |

+ = occurs
+ + = very commonly occurs
± = extremely rare
[a] Cat is final host, dog is intermediate host.

intermediate host can be man, and therefore parasites which invade man in this way have an added importance because of their potentially harmful effect on human health. The internal parasites have been divided up into the major groups of nematode worms, cestode worms (tapeworms), tongue worm and the protozoan parasites (coccidia).

## Nematode worms

This group includes the ascarids, hookworm, whipworm, lungworms, tracheal worm and bladder worm (Fig. 6.15). Ascarids are commonly referred to as **roundworms**, although this term should properly include all worms of this group. All are cylindrical (i.e. round in cross-section), slender worms, tapering at the ends, and there are separate male and female individuals. Their length varies up to 10 cm or more for the ascarids, around 4–6 cm for the whipworm and bladder worm, 2–3 cm for the tracheal worm and 1–2 cm for the hookworm and lungworms. The eggs passed out by these worms produce larvae, which may in some circumstances remain within the egg-shell for a period of time before hatching out. The larvae then go through a series of moults, sometimes outside, and sometimes inside, a host animal, before becoming adult worms. The successive larval stages between the egg and the adult stage are known as $L_1$, $L_2$, $L_3$, etc. **Only larvae at a certain stage of development** (e.g. $L_2$ stage) **are capable of infecting a new host.** This is spoken of as being the **infective stage**.

### (a) Ascarids

#### 1. *Toxocara canis*

Adult female worms in the small intestine of the dog pass out eggs which leave the dog in its faeces. These eggs lie on the ground, and by the action of wind and rain and the movement of pedestrians and vehicles, can become distributed over a wide area, e.g. in parks. Inside the egg-shell the egg develops first into an $L_1$ (first-stage larvae) and then into an $L_2$ (second-stage larvae). The $L_2$ is the infective stage, **and for it to develop may take only 2–3 weeks** in the summer but several months in the winter, i.e. development depends on

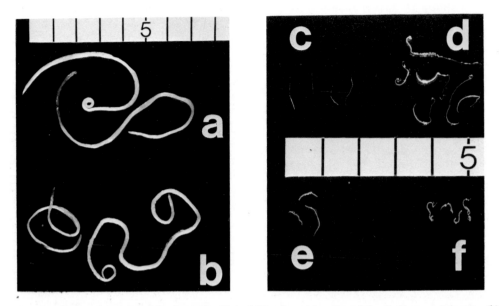

FIG. 6.15.    Nematode worms of the dog in the United Kingdom. (a) male and female *Toxascaris leonina*; (b) male (immature) and female *Toxocara canis*; (c) bladder worm (*Capillaria plica*); (d) whipworm (*Trichuris vulpis*); (e) hookworm (*Uncinaria stenocephala*); (f) lungworm (*Filaroides osleri*). The scale in both parts of the figure is 1 cm wide and marked off at intervals of 1 cm.

temperature. Each $L_2$, still within the eggshell, may then be ingested by a dog, usually because it sticks to the feet or coat and is then licked off. If eggs are eaten *before* $L_2$ are produced, **no further development takes place, i.e. they pass straight through the intestines and out in the faeces.** Some eggs containing $L_2$ are still capable of infecting a dog after 2 years or longer in the ground. (Occasionally an $L_2$ will hatch out *before* it is ingested. Although still infective if eaten, such a larva does not now have the protection of the shell and cannot survive very long.)

In the intestine of the dog the $L_2$ hatch from the egg. The $L_2$ now burrow through the intestinal wall and are carried by the blood stream, first to the liver, then to the right side of the heart and, finally, to the lungs. What happens next depends on the age and sex of the dog. There are two possibilities.

1. In young dogs (particularly those under 5 weeks of age) the following sequence occurs. In the lungs the $L_2$ moult to $L_3$ (third-stage larvae) which then wriggle up the trachea, are coughed up into the pharynx and are re-swallowed. In the stomach the $L_3$ moult to $L_4$. Finally, in the duodenum the $L_4$ moult to produce adult male and female worms, which are then able to mate. From ingestion of $L_2$ to the production of adult worms takes 3–4 weeks. The female adults are producing eggs after a further week.

2. In older dogs (over 5 weeks of age) a protective immunity develops and an increasing proportion of all the $L_2$ in the lungs follow another route, until in those dogs 10 weeks of age and older *almost* all the $L_2$ follow this other route, which is as follows. The $L_2$ leave the lungs in the blood stream and go to the left side of the heart and are then distributed to the

tissues throughout the body; muscles, liver, lungs, etc. This is called a **somatic migration**. In these tissues they remain as $L_2$ without developing further, i.e. they are dormant.

If at some later date, perhaps many years later, the bitch becomes pregnant the $L_2$ are reactivated (in fact at the start of the sixth week of pregnancy), and these $L_2$ larvae, plus any from newly ingested eggs, pass in the blood stream to the placenta. This occurs because during late pregnancy and lactation the bitch's normal protective immunity is suppressed. The larvae cross the placenta and enter the foetus, lodging in the foetal liver and lungs.

When the puppies are born, the $L_2$ in each puppy's liver and lungs moult to $L_3$. One week after birth of the puppy the larvae then follow the route described previously, i.e. from the lungs up the trachea, to be coughed up and swallowed, finally producing adult worms in the small intestine. These **adult worms can commence passing out eggs when the puppy is only 2–3 weeks old.**

The eggs passed out by the adult worms in the puppy contaminate the surroundings, so that later the puppy may reinfect itself and other animals, and in particular they stick to the puppy's coat. Eggs which stick to the coat are likely to be ingested by the nursing bitch as she licks the puppy to clean it in the early weeks of life. If any of these have developed to the $L_2$ stage, i.e. if the egg is infective, the $L_2$ will infect the bitch.

Most of these $L_2$ larvae entering the bitch pass from the intestine to the liver and the heart, and then undergo the somatic migration described previously to again give rise to dormant $L_2$ larvae in tissues throughout the body; these will be reactivated at the *next* pregnancy. Also, because the lactating bitch's immunity is suppressed, some of these $L_2$ larvae undergo migration through the lungs and

trachea to become adult worms in the intestine. However, *some* of the eggs ingested by a lactating bitch will pass straight through her intestines without any further development taking place and these appear unchanged in her faeces (for clarity this feature has been omitted from Fig. 6.16).

An additional complication is that in the puppy *some* of the $L_3$ which are coughed up and swallowed, and some of the $L_4$ pass straight through the alimentary tract without developing further, and appear in the faeces. These larvae can be ingested by the bitch as she licks the coat and cleans faeces from the young puppy, and in the bitch they develop into adult worms which pass out eggs to further contaminate the environment.

Consequently the lactating bitch can be a major source of contamination of the environment with *T. canis* eggs. These eggs come both from adult worms in her intestines (mainly the result of ingesting $L_3$ and $L_4$ larvae) and from the faeces of the puppies (i.e. those which pass straight through her intestine).

Seven to ten days after the end of lactation the bitch regains her immunity and most of the adult worms are spontaneously eliminated from her intestine. (An adult dog's immunity to ascarids can also be suppressed by high doses of corticosteroids, similarly permitting adult worms to develop in the alimentary tract.)

Two additional sources of infection should also be mentioned:

(a) Some of the $L_2$ larvae which are reactivated in the pregnant bitch may migrate to the mammary gland and pass out with the colostrum and milk ingested by the puppies.

(b) Some of the infective eggs (i.e. containing $L_2$) or hatched $L_2$ larvae, which lie on the ground, may be

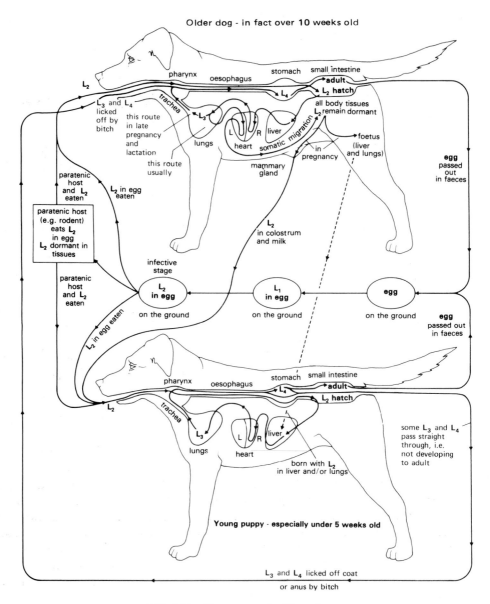

FIG. 6.16.    *Toxocara canis*—life-cycle.

eaten by other species such as rodents, earthworms, and house-flies. They do not develop in these species but lie dormant in their tissues and are carried by them; such hosts are transport or para-tenic hosts. If any of these hosts are subsequently eaten by a dog, the $L_2$ in their tissues will infect the dog in just the same way as if an infective egg had been eaten.

If man consumes an infective egg he will also act as a transport host and the $L_2$

will migrate into the tissues (presumably to await subsequent consumption by a dog). These migrating larvae in man can produce damage to the eye (**ocular larva migrans, OLM**) or to the liver, brain or other tissues (**visceral larva migrans, VLM**). The risk of this occurring is higher in children because they often put unwashed fingers, which can carry infective eggs, into their mouths.

It is clear that the environment of puppies is particularly likely to become heavily contaminated with infective eggs. In addition, about 10% of adult dogs are infected with egg-laying *Toxocara* at any one time.

To control the spread of *T. canis* in both the dog and man, the following recommendations are made:

1. *The pregnant bitch should be routinely wormed* before parturition to remove any adult worms.

   Effective drug treatment to kill dormant *Toxocara* larvae in the bitch are being developed. One is commercially available now, fenbendazole (Panacur), and others are expected in the near future.

2. *Puppies should be routinely wormed at intervals of about 2–3 weeks* from 2–3 weeks of age until weaning, and then again at 3 months of age and 6 months of age. Subsequent worming at 12 month intervals (e.g. at the time of booster vaccination), or preferably every 6 months, is probably adequate. Newly acquired dogs should always be wormed.

3. *Ideally at intervals throughout life, and especially after worming, faecal examinations should be performed.*

4. *In kennels, gardens, etc., all faeces should be regularly removed and burned to destroy any eggs.* Eggs will withstand all disinfectants, long-term freezing and even short periods in boiling water. Only the use of horticultural flame-guns on concrete runs effectively destroys the eggs.

5. *Faeces containing eggs, and hair and dust to which eggs readily stick, can be removed by scrubbing surfaces in kennels,* etc., with hot detergent solution and then hosing them down. However, this will not *kill* the eggs.

6. *Dogs should be encouraged to defaecate in especially reserved* (ideally concreted) *areas* in streets and parks from which the faeces are regularly and efficiently removed, or alternatively over drains.

7. *Young children should be discouraged, even prevented, from handling young puppies or sharing the same environment.* The sticky eggs are easily transferred to hands which frequently enter the mouth.

8. *Personal hygiene is most important.* All those who handle dogs should wash their hands afterwards.

*Toxocara canis* infection produces noisy breathing and coughing (especially during suckling) in puppies under 2 weeks old. In older puppies, up to 3 months of age, there is persistent diarrhoea often with vomiting, whining and a pot-bellied appearance. Adult worms may be vomited up, and infected animals have poor growth rates. In older animals clinical signs of *Toxocara* infection are virtually non-existent.

### 2. *Toxocara cati*

This ascarid is common in the small intestine of cats. It has a similar life-cycle to *T. canis* with some important differences.

SIMILARITIES

(1) Infective $L_2$, which cause *T. cati* infections may be ingested by cats who:

    (a) eat infective eggs;

(b) eat paratenic hosts, e.g. rodents, earthworms, birds, etc., which have previously eaten infective eggs and which carry the $L_2$ in their tissues;

(c) suckle (in the case of kittens) milk from an infected lactating queen.

(2) When infective eggs are eaten the larvae undergo an identical liver-lung migration before returning to the intestine to grow into adults. From eggs being ingested to adult females passing eggs takes approximately 2 months.

(3) $L_2$ can infect man, who becomes a paratenic host, i.e. *T. cati* **can be a cause of ocular or visceral larva migrans in humans.**

DIFFERENCES

(1) When an infected transport host is eaten the $L_2$ do not migrate through the liver and lung but develop through their larval stages to adults entirely within the stomach and intestines.

(2) There is no pre-natal infection of kittens, i.e. there is no migration of larvae to the foetus. However, some $L_2$ can remain dormant in the female cat's tissues and at parturition pass to the mammary gland and out in the milk to be consumed by kittens. Only *some* of these larvae then undergo the liver–lung migration in the kitten; the rest grow to adulthood entirely within the gut.

Clinical signs due to *T. cati* infection appear to be even less common in kittens than those due to *T. canis* infection are in puppies.

### 3. *Toxascaris leonina*

This ascarid is common in both dogs and cats. Its life-cycle is, however, simpler than either *Toxocara canis* or *T. cati*. First the infective larvae are eaten. These may be *either*:

(a) still within the eggs which have been passed out in the faeces of an already infected cat or dog (these are $L_2$); *or*

(b) within the tissues of an intermediate host, e.g. mouse or rabbit.

$L_2$ develop to $L_3$ within the intermediate host but these are still infective.

After ingestion by the dog or cat **the larvae develop to adult worms in the intestine without any migration** through liver and lungs. Eggs are passed out in the faeces of the host—in the dog about 2 months after egg ingestion, in the cat after $10\frac{1}{2}$ weeks. There is *no* transplacental migration and *no* infection via the mother's milk.

This worm can infect man, but has not been shown to cause disease and is *not* considered to be a public health risk. Like the *Toxocara* species, it seldom appears to cause illness in infected dogs and cats.

Note on roundworms: 1, the major route by which cats become infected with both *T. cati* and *T. leonina* appears to be ingestion of transport hosts; 2, the same methods, i.e. hygiene and worming, are used to control infections with *Toxocara cati* and *Toxascaris leonina* as are recommended in the case of *Toxocara canis*. The same anthelmintic drugs are also used to remove the adult stage of all three ascarids from the intestines of dogs and cats.

### (b) Hookworm

The hookworm is so-called because of its hook-shaped anterior end.

*Uncinaria stenocephala* is the only hookworm commonly found in the United Kingdom and it can infect both dogs and cats. It is most common in sheepdogs and also in kennels or wherever several dogs are exercised on grass runs (e.g. greyhound or hunt kennels). Infections in pet or show-dogs are rare (p. 528).

*Uncinaria* does not suck blood, unlike tropical hookworms, so that anaemia does not occur unless a large number of worms have produced extensive damage to the intestine. A large number of the worms in the intestine is more likely to produce diarrhoea and/or poor growth and loss of condition. However, most hookworm infections produce *no* detectable signs.

Eggs are produced by adult female worms and pass out in the infected animal's faeces. The $L_1$ develops within the egg, and after hatching moults twice to become the $L_3$. The $L_3$ are the infective stage. $L_3$ larvae which are swallowed pass to the stomach, where they moult to $L_4$, and then to the intestine, where they moult to adult worms.

The $L_3$ larvae of *Uncinaria* can also enter the body by burrowing through the skin, particularly of the feet, *but* they do not go any further, whereas when tropical hookworm larvae enter the skin they then undergo a migration through the body. **Large numbers of larvae entering the feet may produce dermatitis** (skin inflammation) on the paws; less often the abdomen is affected.

Control of the worm is based on regular worming, hygiene (including regular removal of faeces) and in kennels avoiding the regular use of grass runs. These measures prevent the accumulation of large numbers of eggs and larvae.

### (c) Whipworm

The whipworm is so-called because the posterior part is clearly thicker than the slender anterior part, as in a whip.

This worm, *Trichuris vulpis,* occurs in the dog, especially kennelled dogs, but seldom in the cat. Most dogs show no clinical signs of infection although some have intermittent diarrhoea.

The worms inhabit the caecum, and eggs are passed out in the host's faeces. The infective first-stage larva ($L_1$) develops within the egg-shell (a process which takes weeks or months in the United Kingdom) and remains there until it is eaten. Unless killed by desiccation (rare in the United Kingdom) the $L_1$ within the egg can remain infective for 5 years or more. After being eaten the $L_1$ hatch out in the small intestine, and after a short period there pass to the caecum. Here they moult through the succeeding larval stages to the adult male and female worms.

The same control measures are employed as for hookworms.

### (d) Lungworms

1. *Canine Lungworms*
A. *Filaroides osleri*

Although this parasite can occur in dogs kept singly, **transmission is from the dam to suckling puppy in breeding kennels.** It can cause serious respiratory disease in infected animals which are usually puppies 4–6 months of age but sometimes young adults.

The small adult worms are found in raised nodules in the trachea, especially at the point where it divides, and in the bronchi. The nodules can be up to 2 cm across (i.e. like a finger-tip pushing out from the wall). The partial blockage of the air passages causes a dry cough, particularly noticeable after exercise, and eventually results in wasting of the dog. The tail of the female worm projects out of the nodule so that it can lay its eggs into the air passages. The eggs hatch almost immediately to larvae ($L_1$) which are coughed up in sputum. They are then either passed out of the mouth in sputum or swallowed to appear later in the faeces. Ingestion of these infective first-stage larvae by puppies results in them moulting to the $L_2$ stage. The $L_2$ pass through the intestinal wall and are carried in the blood to the lungs where they undergo further moults to become adult worms. These migrate up the airways to the tracheal bifurcation where they enter the tracheal wall, causing development of the raised nodules around them.

Drug treatment for a month or more can kill many of the worms and leads to their nodules gradually becoming smaller. However, it is important to be able to pick out affected animals, some of which do not show marked signs, and to isolate them from young puppies before the latter become infected. Recognition of affected animals is best achieved by endoscopic examination of the trachea and bronchi.

### B. Angiostrongylus vasorum

This lungworm occurs only sporadically in most of the U.K. but is known to be endemic (i.e. established) in Cornwall. It inhabits the pulmonary artery (or rarely the right ventricle of the heart) and its eggs are carried in the blood until they block the lung capillaries. Here they hatch to $L_1$ larvae which enter the albeoli and pass up the trachea. The larvae are swallowed when they reach the pharynx and pass through the alimentary tract and out in the faeces. Infected dogs can excrete the $L_1$ larvae continuously for up to 5 years.

The $L_1$ larvae then need to be eaten by certain slugs or snails which act as intermediate hosts and in which they develop into $L_2$ and then $L_3$ larvae.

The dog can be infected by ingesting slugs or snails containing $L_3$ larvae which pass to the lymph nodes adjacent to the intestine. Here they undergo a further 2 moults before migrating via the liver to the heart and pulmonary artery where they develop into adult worms.

Damage to the heart and lungs can result in difficulty in breathing and even death. A feature of chronic infection is interference with blood clotting which leads to anaemia and the development of subcutaneous swellings.

### 2. Feline Lungworm— Aelurostrongylus abstrusus

This worm appears to affect up to a quarter of all cats, and not only those housed together in catteries. It does not affect dogs. Adult worms appearing like short pieces of black thread occur within the lung air passages from the bronchioles to the alveoli. Eggs laid in the alveoli hatch to $L_1$, which then pass up the trachea. In the pharynx they are swallowed and pass through the alimentary tract and out in the host's faeces. If these **$L_1$ are eaten by certain slugs or snails**, which act as intermediate hosts, the larvae moult first to $L_2$ and then to $L_3$. The slugs and snails may be eaten by a cat but are more likely to be eaten by birds, rodents, frogs or snakes, which are then in turn eaten by a cat.

In the cat the $L_3$ burrow out of the intestine and are carried by the blood to the lungs. Here they moult to adult worms.

Most damage is due to inhalation of the eggs and an infected animal may show persistent coughing and lose condition. However, most affected animals do not show clinical signs, probably because immunity to the parasite is gradually acquired so that the number of worms decreases.

## (e) *Tracheal Worm—*
## *Capillaria aerophila*

In the United Kingdom this worm occurs occasionally in kennelled dogs and probably in cats. Adult worms live mainly in the trachea as white coiled masses surrounded by eggs, embedded in the mucous membrane. Eggs from the adult females are coughed up, swallowed and passed out in the faeces. The infective $L_1$ stage develops in the egg.

If the infective egg is eaten by a host the $L_1$ hatches out in the intestine, passes through the bowel wall and is carried by the circulation to the lungs. Here it passes into the air passages and up them to the trachea, where it moults to become the adult worm.

Mild infections produce no clinical signs; severe infections produce inflammation (tracheo-bronchitis) with a cough and wheezing respiration.

## (f) *Bladder Worm—*
## *Capillaria plica*

The adult worms, which occur in the bladder of dogs, are most frequently found in kennelled animals, e.g. packs of hounds. Eggs laid by female worms pass out in the urine and $L_1$ develop inside the eggs. These constitute infective eggs, and when eaten by the intermediate host, the earthworm, the larvae hatch out. If a dog eats an infected earthworm the $L_1$ moults to $L_2$ and then enters the intestinal wall and moults to $L_3$. (There is also the possibility that if a dog eats an infective egg directly from the ground a similar sequence of moults occurs.)

$L_3$ pass into the blood stream, eventually reaching the kidneys, and then pass through the glomeruli and tubules and down the ureters to the bladder. Here they moult to the $L_4$ stage and then to adult worms. Perhaps, surprisingly, *Capillaria*

*plica* seldom causes any disorder and treatment is not usually required.

## Nematodes in other species

The pinworm *Syphacia obvelata* occurs in the small intestines of hamsters and, together with *Aspiculuris*, in rats and mice. The most common parasite of the rabbit *Passalurus ambiguus* occurs in the caecum and colon, and also an inhabitant of the caecum is *Paraspidodera* in the guinea-pig. Only rarely do any of these worms produce disease.

In the rabbit the lungworm *Prostrongylus* usually causes no clinical signs unless there is secondary bacterial infection. In primates, infections include the hookworm, threadworm and pinworm of children. Nematode worms may occasionally be present in large numbers in tortoises.

## Cestode worms (tapeworms)

These worms are not round in section like the nematodes but flattened and appear like a length of tape or ribbon (Fig. 6.17).

Each worm consists of a **head** (or **scolex**) and a body consisting of a number of segments (or **proglottids**). The head bears a number of hooks and suckers by means of which the worm attaches itself to the small intestinal lining of the final host. The segments grow successively from the lower part of the head to produce a worm which in some instances may eventually be of considerable length. Consequently the segments furthest from the head are the oldest and the most mature. If an anthelmintic drug cannot successfully eliminate the head of the tapeworm, even although all of the segments are shed and removed, a complete new worm will regrow.

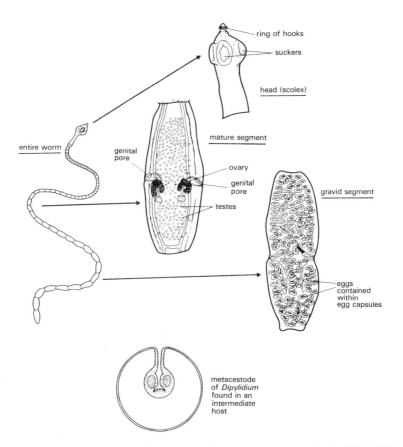

FIG. 6.17.   *Dipylidium caninum,* the commonest tapeworm of the dog and cat in the United Kingdom. A full-grown worm may reach 0.5–0.75 m in length.

Each segment contains both male and female sexual organs, and fertilization may occur either within the individual segment or between segments. The terminal segments are filled with eggs ( = **gravid segments**). Eggs are eliminated from the final host by the terminal segments becoming successively shed from the end of the worm and passed out in the host's faeces, or segments may even pass through the anus independently. A released segment possesses powers of muscular contraction and may at times be seen moving over the animal's coat near the anal region or over the floor covering. Segments seldom burst releasing their eggs, but eggs can pass out of a segment through the genital pore. Inside each egg is an embryo, but for further development ingestion of the eggs (usually still contained within the segment) by a particular intermediate host is required (see Table 6.8).

If it is successful in being eaten by the intermediate host the embryo is released in the host's intestine and passes through the intestinal wall. It passes either to particular body tissues (in the case of mammalian intermediate hosts) or to a body cavity (in invertebrate intermediate hosts). It then develops into a **metacestode**, a bladder-like larval structure containing a head which will develop into an

TABLE 6.8. *Tapeworms and their hosts*

| Tapeworm | Final host | Intermediate host |
|---|---|---|
| *Dipylidium caninum* | Dog or cat | Flea or louse |
| *Taenia pisiformis* | Dog | Rabbit |
| *Taenia ovis* | Dog | Sheep |
| *Taenia hydatigena* | Dog | Sheep, cattle, pig |
| *Taenia multiceps* | Dog | Sheep |
| *Taenia serialis* | Dog | Rabbit |
| *Taenia taeniaeformis* | Cat | Mouse or rat |
| *Echinococcus granulosus* | Dog or cat* | Sheep, cattle, pig, man and horse |

\* *Echinococcus granulosus* in the cat does not produce eggs.

adult tapeworm when eaten by the final host. The metacestodes of different tapeworms vary in their size and structure. Those of *Taenia multiceps* and *T. serialis* contain several heads, each capable of giving rise to a tapeworm. The metacestode of *Echnococcus* is a large cyst (a **hydatid cyst**), inside which float many free heads and bunches of heads. Clearly a hydatid cyst can produce a very large number of tapeworms.

After consumption of the larval structure by the final host each head attaches to the intestinal wall (having in some cases turned itself inside out to expose the hooks and suckers), the rest of the structure is digested off and the head begins to produce segments.

Tapeworms vary in length; *Dipylidium*, *T. serialis* and *T. taeniaeformis* reach about 0.5–0.75 m, *T. ovis* and *T. multiceps* may reach 1 m and *T. hydatigena* and *T. pisiformis* can reach 2–3 m or more. *Echinococcus* however, seldom exceeds about half a centimetre in length and consequently individual segments are very small and difficult to detect with the naked eye.

greyhounds), but is rather less common in cats. It is certainly the commonest tapeworm of both dogs and cats. It is not usually pathogenic, causing mainly loss of condition and anal irritation as segments migrate through the anus to the exterior. The segments resemble grains of rice (or cucumber seeds) and as they move about they shed eggs (contained within egg capsules). If an egg is eaten by a larva of the cat or dog flea, the egg develops into the metacestode when the flea becomes an adult. However, if the egg is eaten by a biting louse (*Trichodectes canis*) the metacestode develops straight away. The cat or dog becomes infected by eating a flea or louse carrying the metacestode, which is then released, in the intestine, and develops to an adult tapeworm in 3–4 weeks.

If an infected flea or louse is eaten by a child the same development of an adult tapeworm in the intestine will take place.

Undoubtedly it is because fleas are so common in the dog that *Dipylidium* is so common, particularly in urban dogs.

### 1. *Dipylidium caninum*

This tapeworm probably occurs in about a third of all dogs (though up to 75% of

### 2. *Taenia species*

The *Taenia* species found in the dog all produce larval stages in meat animals including the rabbit and hare. Meat so affected is condemned at the abattoir, not because of the hazard to human health so much as because it is aesthetically unacceptable, and this represents an economic loss. In the case of *T. multiceps* the cystic metacestode occurring in the central nervous system can produce marked brain damage with staggering and blindness.

Dogs become infected by being fed uncooked, or imperfectly cooked, meat or offal containing metacestodes which develop in the intestine to adult tapeworms. Dogs in rural areas or kennels are most likely to be fed uncooked carcasses. The eggs produced by the adult worm can be spread by the dog over a large area of grassland, so infecting many intermediate hosts. Though the effect of the adult worms on the dog is very slight (as with *Dipylidium*) *T. hydatigena* can infect up to 50% of dogs in farming areas or kennels. *T. pisiformis, T. serialis* and *T. multiceps* infect between 5 and 10%, and *T. ovis* even less.

*Taenia taeniaeformis* probably infects about 10–15% of cats. Its metacestode stage occurs principally in the rat and mouse (but also other rodents) which the cat catches and eats, thus becoming infected. The adult worm produces little ill-effect in the cat. The eggs it sheds, when eaten by a rodent, produce the larval stages. Since it is difficult to control mouse-catching, worming is the principal way of reducing the number of infected cats.

3. *Echinococcus granulosus* appears to occur in two main strains. One strain prefers the sheep as an intermediate host, and is particularly common in farm dogs in areas where sheep are grazed extensively, such as South and Mid Wales and some of the Scottish Isles. Dogs take in the metaces-tode (larval stage) by scavenging carcasses of dead sheep (e.g. in the hills) or being fed uncooked offal. This strain will also readily infect man as an alternative intermediate host.

The other strain prefers the horse as an intermediate host, and dogs (e.g. those in hunt kennels) become infected by being fed raw horse meat or offal. This strain seems to infect man rarely.

In all cases the intermediate hosts are infected by consuming the eggs. In the case of both sheep and horses they ingest the eggs when grazing pasture on which an infected dog has defaecated.

The adult worm causes no disease in the dog but in the intermediate host the larval stage **the hydatid cyst can grow in the liver or lung** (occasionally other organs) to 10 cm or more in size and interfere with the organ's function. In man the disease which is produced is called **hydatidosis**. Rupture of the hydatid cyst may result in the heads it contains being distributed all over the intermediate host's body—each one of which can then give rise to a further hydatid cyst.

In the cat adult *E. granulosus* worms occur but they die before reaching sexual maturity so that they are not infective, i.e. are not transmitted to intermediate hosts.

### Tapeworms in other species

The metacestode (larval stage) of *Taenia taeniaeformis* can occur in the tissues of rats, mice and gerbils, which act as intermediate hosts. Similarly, the metacestode stages of *T. pisiformis* and *T. serialis* are found in the tissues of rabbits acting as intermediate hosts.

Tapeworms of the genus *Hymenolepis* (especially *H. nana* and *H. diminuta*, which can also infect man) occur in rats, mice, hamsters and gerbils.

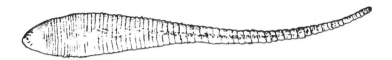

FIG. 6.18. *Linguatula serrata,* the tongue worm (ventral view).

**The tongue worm** (*Linguatula serrata*)

The parasite is not in fact a worm but a variety of mite which has no legs. In shape it is long and flattened, i.e. like a tongue (Fig. 6.18). There are separate male and female "worms"; the latter are much longer and can grow to 12 cm.

The "worms" attach themselves high up in the nasal chambers of the dog and the irritation they cause results in sneezing, coughing and difficulty in breathing. Eggs are passed out by the female "worms" and eaten by an intermediate host, which can be horse, sheep, cattle or rabbit. In the intestine of the intermediate host each egg hatches to produce a larva which then passes to the mesenteric lymph nodes. There it develops to the nymphal stage which can infect the dog. Dogs fed on uncooked rabbit, or on the infected glands or larger meat animals, take in the nymphal stage which then migrates to the nasal chamber and becomes an adult "worm".

**Parasitic protozoa—coccidia**

Protozoa are micro-organisms (i.e. microscopic unicellular organisms) and there are some parasitic members of the group which cause diseases in man and animals. The parasitic protozoa of importance in the dog and cat in the United Kingdom belong to those called the **coccidia**, and all of them live in the small intestine of the final host. They include *Toxoplasma gondii* and species belonging to the genera *Hammondia, Sarcocystis* and *Isospora.*

The basic life-cycle of all coccidia consists of stages inside the host and stages outside the host.*

However, it is now known that all the coccidia of the dog and cat in the United Kingdom can also infect various intermediate hosts. Indeed, with some of these coccidia infection of an intermediate host is *essential* for the parasite to complete its life-cycle.

The member of the coccidia that has received most attention because of its public health importance is *Toxoplasma gondii.*

1. *Toxoplasma gondii*

The final host for this parasite is the cat. The life-cycle of *T. gondii* differs from the general life-cycle of coccidia shown in Fig. 6.19 in the following respects.

1. In a cat (final host) which consumes a sporulated oocyst (Fig. 6.20), the sporozoites released from the oocyst do not immediately pass to the intestine and

*This is summarized in Fig. 6.19. Provided conditions (temperature, moisture, etc.) are suitable an oocyst shed by an animal undergoes **sporulation**, resulting in the formation of sporocysts containing sporozoites. This makes the oocyst infective to the next host. After ingestion the sporozoites are released and pass into epithelial cells, there to undergo two or more asexual reproductive cycles followed by a sexual reproductive cycle. The union of a microgamete and a macrogamete produces a zygote and this becomes surrounded by a wall forming an oocyst which is shed in the faeces.

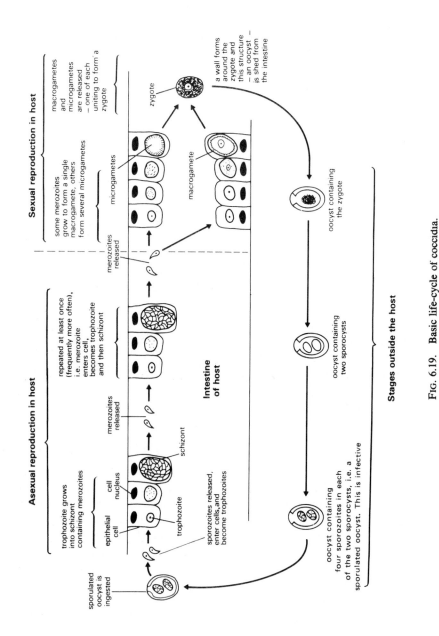

FIG. 6.19.   Basic life-cycle of coccidia.

undergo the cycles of asexual and sexual reproduction as in Fig. 6.19. Instead sporozoites are carried in the circulation to other parts of the body where they become trophozoites and undergo repeated asexual reproduction. After about 3 weeks some pass back to the intestine to start sexual reproduction with the production of oocysts. Some, however, remain in the tissues.

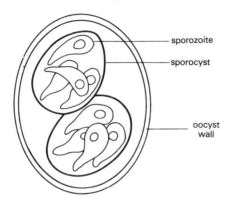

FIG. 6.20. Sporulated oocyst. The coccidian species which infect dogs and cats in the United Kingdom have two sporocysts, each containing four sporozoites, within each sporulated oocyst.

2. Oocysts may be swallowed not only by the final host but by intermediate hosts (e.g. man, dog, cattle, sheep, pig, rodents and birds). This occurs when cat faeces contaminate their food (e.g. pasture or via human hands). Some animals may even consume invertebrates (earthworms, flies) which have previously eaten, and are therefore carrying, the oocysts. In the intermediate hosts the sporozoites are released and go to *all* parts of the body, there to undergo repeated asexual reproduction producing more and more trophozoites. This is similar to the process which occurs in the cat *except* that it is not followed by sexual reproduction in the intestine and oocyst formation.

3. Trophozoites in the tissues of an intermediate host may be ingested, *either* by the final host (i.e. the cat) *or* by another intermediate host. For example, cats and dogs may be fed raw meat (e.g. from cattle or sheep) containing trophozoites, and, similarly, man may eat infected raw meat products or undercooked meat. Also cats, and certain birds, and even dogs, can catch and eat infected mice.

(a) In *the cat* the trophozoites released from the tissues of the intermediate host which has been eaten behave like those trophozoites which develop from the sporozoites released from ingested oocysts. That is to say they undergo asexual reproduction in the tissues, which may be followed by sexual reproduction in the intestine, and the shedding of oocysts. However, if the ingested trophozoites are contained in a cyst in the tissues of the intermediate host, some of them pass directly into the intestinal epithelial cells and undergo there the stages of asexual and sexual reproduction—as in the typical coccidian life-cycle.

(b) If *another intermediate host* eats the tissues of a previously infected intermediate host the same process occurs as before, i.e. there is asexual reproduction of trophozoites in the tissues.

By the repeated ingestion of one animal by another *Toxoplasma* can pass along a food chain. Eventually some *Toxoplasma* organisms may return to the final host—a cat.

4. In both the intermediate host and the cat the tissues in which the trophozoites survive and multiply are most often the brain, eye, skeletal muscle and cardiac muscle.

If the host has very little immunity, multiplication occurs rapidly producing an acute phase (**acute toxoplasmosis**). However, after a period of time the host develops a specific immunity and the rate of multiplication slows down (chronic phase). At this time the trophozoites are stored in minute **cysts** in the tissue cells. Such intact cysts may last throughout the life of the host and cause no harm. But as the immunity gradually declines these cysts can break down releasing the trophozoites to result in another acute phase, i.e. a relapse. (This is especially likely to occur after a cat receives corticosteroid therapy.)

5. Congenital infection, i.e. infection of the foetus through the placenta, can take place in **a female intermediate host**, such as a woman or a bitch, if the female becomes infected during pregnancy. However, congenital infection does not occur in the final host—the cat (Fig. 6.21).

It would appear that in the main cats become infected by ingesting trophozoites (i.e. by being fed infected meat or catching infected mice or birds), rather than by ingesting oocysts. In summary, therefore:

(a) Cats—the final host—are usually infected by eating already infected tissues, *either* as small animals which they catch *or* as food (i.e. infected meat) from a meat-producing animal.

(b) Intermediate hosts are usually infected by eating already infected meat (containing trophozoites) or food contaminated with cat faeces (containing sporulated oocysts).

By checking for antibodies against *Toxoplasma* in the blood it has been found that at least one-third of cats in the United Kingdom have been infected with toxoplasmosis and therefore have been excreting oocysts at some time. Also about one-third of the dogs in the United Kingdom have been infected. Approximately half a billion humans around the world have been infected with *T. gondii,* and in some areas, such as central France, 90% of adults have been infected.

Rarely does *Toxoplasma* produce clinical signs in either the final or the intermediate hosts. However, a host may die or suffer severe injury with acute toxoplasmosis because the organisms can cause the death of a large number of cells in vital organs such as the eye or heart. If the host develops immunity (i.e. produces antibodies) cysts form in the heart and CNS, but the existence of immunity does not eradicate infection and the *Toxoplasma* may stay in the cyst for several years and later reactivate to again produce cell damage.

In man congenital infections can result in ocular lesions and brain damage, whereas infection acquired after birth most often causes lymph node enlargement (though occasionally there is damage to the CNS, heart or lungs). In sheep abortion is a serious problem due to toxoplasmosis. In dogs, adults appear to be resistant to *Toxoplasma,* and the disease is most severe in puppies producing respiratory distress, pneumonia and diarrhoea. It can also complicate cases of canine distemper.

The final host—the cat—may also suffer from toxoplasmosis, the most important feature being pneumonia.

After an infection cats only shed oocysts for about 2 weeks (so that it is very difficult to find the parasite in cat faeces), but several million may be shed during this time. Oocysts can survive in moist conditions for at least a year, and may be spread by flies and earthworms. There is still some doubt as to whether chronically infected cats continue to shed oocysts later; possibly they do. Stray cats are a major problem in the spread of toxoplasmosis.

Although the oocysts are resistant, the

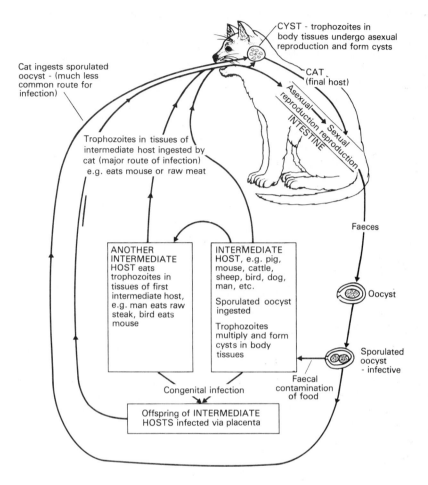

FIG. 6.21.    Life-cycle of *Toxoplasma gondii*.

trophozoites which occur in meat (especially pork or mutton) are easily destroyed by heat or even by water. So washing the hands after handling meat is a useful hygienic precaution. To minimize *Toxoplasma* infection it is recommended that one should:

(a) *Heat meat to 68°C throughout before eating.*

(b) *Wash hands with soap and water after handling meat.*

(c) *Never feed raw meat to cats; feed only dry or canned food or cooked meat.*

(d) *Keep cats indoors, thus necessitating the use of litter boxes.*

(e) *Change litter boxes daily and flush cat faeces down the toilet or burn them; this is to dispose of cat faeces before the oocysts can sporulate, i.e. become infective. Sterilize litter boxes daily by immersing them in boiling water—chemical disinfectants are not able to kill the oocysts.*

(f) *Use gloves while working in the garden to avoid faecal contamination.*

(g) *Cover children's sand pits when not in use.*

## 2. *Hammondia species*

One species occurs in the cat and one in the dog. In both cases the parasite undergoes asexual and sexual phases of reproduction in the intestine and passes out oocysts in the faeces. When sporulated, i.e. infective, these have to be eaten by an intermediate host to complete their life-cycle. In the case of the cat the natural intermediate host is probably rodents and in the case of the dog probably cattle, although this is still not certain.

In the intermediate host a cyst is formed in the muscles and this has later to be ingested by the final host for completion of the life-cycle. Unlike *Toxoplasma* there appears to be no infection of further intermediate hosts or any congenital infection. The parasites appear not to cause illness in dogs or cats.

## 3. *Sarcocystis*

There appear to be at least half a dozen species in both the dog and the cat whose life-cycle is superficially similar to that of the *Hammondia* species. The intermediate host, which is essential to the life-cycle, varies in each case but is usually a particular species of herbivore, e.g. cattle, sheep, deer, rabbit. However, the mouse, the pig and man are the intermediate hosts for some of these coccidia. Cysts form in the skeletal muscles of the intermediate host. The dog and cat appear to show no signs of illness, and only particular species of *Sarcocystis* cause disease in the intermediate host. *Sarcocystis* species are believed to occur in between a quarter to a third of farm and kennel dogs in the United Kingdom.

## 4. *Isospora*

Two species of these coccidia have the dog as final host, and a further two species occur in the cat. Unlike the other coccidia considered here, intermediate hosts are *not* essential in the life-cycle, although rodents and chickens *may* act as intermediate hosts. It appears that the final host can become infected by eating *either* sporulated oocysts *or* cysts from the tissues of an intermediate host that has itself eaten sporulated oocysts. *Isospora* seem not to produce disease in either the final or intermediate hosts.

## Coccidia in other species

Coccidia belonging to the genus *Eimeria* can cause disease in rabbits, rats, mice and guinea-pigs. Intestinal coccidiosis of rabbits is a major, though self-limiting disease. There are also coccidian species which cause disease in caged birds. As previously mentioned, *Toxoplasma gondii* and *Sarcocystis* can occur in tissues of rabbits, rats and mice which act as intermediate hosts.

## Parasites as Disease Vectors

A **disease vector** is an animal (very often an insect) that transmits a disease-producing organism to a new host. A distinction is made between a biological vector and a mechanical vector. A **biological vector** is one in which the infecting organism must pass part of its life-cycle, i.e. one which acts as an intermediate host. A **mechanical vector**, on the other hand, is one which merely carries the organism mechanically and is not in any way affected by it.

Of the important canine and feline parasites described very few act as disease vectors.

## Biological vectors

The flea and louse act as biological vectors in transmitting *Dipylidium caninum* to the dog or cat. An essential stage in the life-cycle of this tapeworm is development of the metacestode stage within the body of the flea or louse. (Similarly, the mosquito acts as a biological vector in the transmission of the malarial and yellow fever parasites to man.)

## Mechanical vectors

The flea acts as a mechanical vector in carrying bacteria of the genus *Pasteurella* from one dog or cat to another as it sucks blood. Also the flea in sucking blood from successive hosts may transfer the virus of feline panleukopenia (= feline infectious enteritis). It can be taken in by the flea from a cat which is in the viraemic stage (i.e. has the virus circulating in its bloodstream) and be transmitted to the next cat bitten by the flea. Ticks may implant bacteria in their bite wounds, and on other pet animals lice are also mechanical vectors carrying bacteria, e.g. transferring *Rickettsia* organisms to rats and mice and *Francisella tularensis* to rabbits. (The flea is well known as a mechanical vector for its transference of the plague organism *Yersinia pestis* from the rat to man).

(e) Prevention of Spread of Infection

B. M. BUSH

## Introduction

In the previous two sections various aspects of the diseases caused by pathogenic micro-organisms and larger parasites have been considered. This section explains how diseases are transmitted from one animal to another and how this information can be used to control the spread of disease.

There are three stages in the transmission of a disease-producing organism (i.e. pathogen) to a new host:

(1)  the organism leaves the first host;
(2)  the organism passes from the first to the second host;
(3)  the organism enters (or stays on the surface of) the second host.

In some instances the three stages follow one another very rapidly as when lice crawl from the hair of one dog to that of another, which is in direct contact, or when one cat bites another and *Pasteurella* organisms pass from the mouth into the wound. In other cases there may be a long interval of time between the organism leaving the first host and entering the second, e.g. *Toxocara canis* eggs passed out in a dog's faeces may require several months just to become infective, and even then it may be several months more before they are ingested by another dog.

## Infectious and Contagious Diseases

An **infectious disease** is a disease produced by micro-organisms, i.e. viruses, bacteria, fungi or protozoa. It may or may not also be contagious.

**A contagious disease** is a disease which is transmitted by direct or indirect contact. The term includes not only infectious diseases but also diseases due to external parasites transmitted by direct or indirect contact.

**Direct contact** denotes that part of the body of one animal meets part of the body of another, e.g. when skin surfaces come into contact or when one animal licks another's skin, nose or anus. Venereal transmission of disease, involving direct contact between the reproductive organs, occurs in the dog and cat but is not of great importance.

**Indirect contact** refers to two or more animals coming into contact, usually within a short period of time, with the same inanimate object, e.g. with bedding material or a feeding bowl. (However, with some micro-organisms this period can be up to 1 year, e.g. the viruses of feline infectious enteritis and canine parvovirus infection.) A pathogenic organism can be transferred to the inanimate object by one animal, and subsequently the organism may be transmitted to a second animal when it in turn contacts this object. Inanimate objects contaminated in this way are known as **fomites**, and therefore indirect contact can also be referred to as **contact via fomites**.

### Routes of Transmission

In most cases pathogenic micro-organisms are acquired from animals which at some stage show clinical signs of disease (i.e. are obviously infected). Sometimes they are obtained from carrier animals (see below), and occasionally from the environment *without* having first been shed by another animal (e.g. the spores of *Clostridium tetani,* which is a saprophytic organism often present in soil).

A **carrier** of an infectious disease is an individual who does not show clinical signs of the disease but whose body harbours the disease-producing organism and may continue to pass it out (i.e. to excrete it). Carriers may be of two types:

(a) Individuals who have had the disease, with the usual clinical signs, but who do not rid themselves of the organism completely, either for a long time, or, in some cases, ever. These are called **convalescent carriers**. For example, dogs recovered from leptospirosis can excrete the bacteria for 3 months or more, and following recovery from infectious canine hepatitis (ICH) may excrete the virus in their urine for up to 6 months afterwards. Approximately 80% of cats that recover from feline viral rhinotracheitis (a form of "feline influenza") become carriers.

(b) Individuals who never show clinical signs of the disease. These are so-called **healthy carriers** (immune carriers) who possess an innate immunity to the organism, as, for

example, with some *Salmonella* infections and ringworm infestations in cats. Some dogs are believed to be healthy carriers of canine herpesvirus.

Carriers of either type (i.e. convalescent or healthy) which shed the pathogenic organism can be termed **open carriers** e.g. healthy dogs excreting ICH virus), and carriers which do *not* shed the organism can be termed **closed carriers** (e.g. many cases of tuberculosis). Open carriers are an important, and often unsuspected, source of infection.

Clinical cases (i.e. animals showing clinical signs of disease) can also be classed as open or closed, again depending on whether they are or are not shedding the pathogen (e.g. open and closed cases of pyometra).

### A. The routes by which pathogenic organisms leave an animal

The common routes are as follows:

(1) **From the nose, mouth and eyes**. The organism may be contained in a secretion such as:

(a) saliva, e.g. rabies virus;

(b) nasal or ocular secretions, e.g. the viruses of canine and feline respiratory diseases (including canine distemper virus and the "feline influenza" viruses—herpesvirus and calcivirus) and the eggs of the tongue worm *Linguatula serrata*;

(c) sputum, e.g. the tuberculosis bacterium *Mycobacterium tuberculosis* and the larvae of the canine lungworm *Filaroides osleri.*

Nasal secretion is spread particularly by sneezing, which causes the secretion to break up into millions of droplets, and saliva and sputum are particularly spread by coughing.

In addition, the normal expiration of air will take organisms (principally staphylococci) from the nose out into the surrounding air, and biting other animals will cause organisms in the mouth to be implanted in the wound—particularly pasteurellae.

(2) **In urine**. The leptospiral bacteria, many viruses (particularly those causing feline infectious enteritis (FIE) and infectious canine hepatitis) and also the eggs of the bladder worm *Capillaria plica* are passed in the urine.

(3) **In faeces**. This is the route by which most internal parasites leave the host, e.g. the larvae of lungworms, the oocysts of coccidia, the segments of tapeworms and the eggs of other intestinal worms. It is also a route for the excretion of the viruses of canine distemper, infectious canine hepatitis, canine parvovirus infection and feline infectious enteritis.

(4) **From the skin**. This is most important in the spread of external parasites, including ringworm. However, bacteria (chiefly staphylococci) can also be shed from the skin surface as the superficial skin scales flake off.

Less common routes by which pathogens leave the body are:

(5) **In vomit**. For example this occurs in the diseases canine parvovirus infection and infectious feline enteritis.

(6) **In blood** taken as food by blood-sucking parasites, e.g. fleas can transmit the virus of feline panleukopenia ( = feline infectious enteritis or FIE) and *Haemobartonella felis* the bacterium responsible for feline infectious anaemia.

(7) **In semen**. (8) **In discharges after parturition**. (9) **Venereal contact**, i.e. between genitalia. The organism *Brucella canis,* responsible for canine brucellosis (and capable of producing abortion) is probably the only organism commonly spread by these routes, although leptospirae are occasionally spread venereally.

(10) **In milk**. *Toxocara* larvae and possibly some viruses are spread by this route.

(11) **From dead bodies**. Although important as the means by which anthrax organisms are released into the environment from farm animals, anthrax is a rare disease in small animals, and consequently this route is of little significance in dogs and cats.

## B. The transfer of organisms from one host to another

This may occur by the following routes:

(1) **By direct contact**, i.e. between parts of the body of two animals.

(2) **By indirect contact** i.e. the organism is present upon and may be carried from one site to another on fomites such as bedding (e.g. in the case of fleas) and feeding bowls (in the case of many viruses).

(3) **Through the air**, usually by the **aerosol route**, i.e. by infected droplets, resulting from sneezing or coughing, passing through the air. Ringworm spores from skin and staphylococci from the nose can also pass through the air using air currents. (Some authors include this route as a direct contact method.)

(4) **In contaminated food**, e.g. *Toxoplasma* trophozoites, **and in contaminated water**, e.g. leptospirae.

(5) **From the environment**, e.g. floors, walls, soil, runs. This may simply be a variant of indirect contact but also includes the ground in parks contaminated with infective *Toxocara* eggs and runs infected with hookworm larvae.

(6) **By a vector**, i.e. by another host which carries the organism and in which, in some cases, the organism undergoes development. These are subdivided into:

(a) **Biological vectors**—those in which the organism undergoes part of its life-cycle. These are the intermediate hosts of the internal parasites, particularly the tapeworms and cocidia.

(b) **Mechanical vectors**, which are those which merely carry the organisms and in which *no* development takes place. These can be further subdivided into:

  (i) **transport hosts**, which can shed the organism at any time (e.g. the flea carrying feline panleukopenia virus);

  (ii) **paratenic hosts**, which cannot shed the organism and which need to be eaten by the final host if the organism is to complete its life-cycle; e.g. the mouse-carrying *Toxocara canis* $L_2$ larvae.

## C. The routes by which organisms gain entry onto or into a host

These are as follows:

(1) **Via the mouth**, i.e. by ingestion. This includes: eating infected food or drinking infected water; eating faeces, either deliberately or because it contaminates food, etc.; eating vectors, both intermediate hosts (for instance of tapeworms, e.g. the flea carrying the metacestode stage of *Dipylidium caninum*) and paratenic hosts (such as the mouse infected with the larval stage of *Toxocara cati*); licking at infected urine (e.g. containing viruses such as those of ICH and feline infectious peritonitis), licking an infected animal (direct contact); and licking or chewing at infected fomites, e.g. bowls or blankets (indirect contact).

(2) **By inhalation**, i.e. through the respiratory tract. This includes inhaling infectious organisms in droplets (aerosol transmission) or in dust.

(3) **Through the skin surface**. This can be the result of:

(a) the skin having *already* been broken, e.g. following wounds or burns (this will allow easy entry of micro-organisms, especially bacteria, including leptospirae, and also can attract blowflies to lay eggs which develop into maggots);

(b) implantation beneath the skin when *being* bitten or scratched by another animal (usually it is bacteria which are transmitted in this way, but it is also the route of entry for the rabies virus);

(c) implantation with an insect bite, e.g. flea bites can implant *Pasteurella, Haemobartonella felis* and the virus of FIE;

(d) actual penetration by a complete parasite; as with hookworm larvae (internal parasite) and *Sarcoptes* (external parasite);

(e) penetration by infected hypodermic needles or surgical instruments which implant bacteria, viruses, etc.

(4) **Through other mucous membranes**, including the conjunctiva, especially following previous damage, e.g. leptospirae can enter through the mucosal surfaces of the eye, nose and mouth.

(5) **On to the skin surface**. This is the route used by the surface ectoparasites, including ringworm spores. Fleas and lice are attracted by body heat and blowflies are attracted by faecal contamination.

One route of transmission not listed above and which takes place entirely within the body of pregnant females is the **congenital route**. Organisms may pass to a foetus either through the placenta or the wall of the uterus. This route is important in the transmission of:

(a) *Toxocara canis*, from bitch to puppy foetus;

(b) *Toxoplasma gondii*, from a pregnant intermediate host to its foetus;

(c) canine parvovirus, causing damage to the heart muscle (myocarditis);

(d) the virus of FIE producing cerebellar hypoplasia in kittens resulting in juvenile feline ataxia;

(e) *Brucella canis*;

(f) canine herpesvirus;

(g) feline leukaemia virus (FeLV).

The last four micro-organisms cause resorption of the foetus or abortion (occurring in early and late pregnancy respectively) or stillbirths or the birth of weak, sickly animals which die soon afterwards ("fading puppies" and "fading kittens"). Abortion can also follow infection with the virus of feline viral rhinotracheitis, and fading puppies may result from transplacental infection with the viruses responsible for canine distemper and ICH (i.e. canine adenovirus-1).

Congenital transmission may also be possible at times with other organisms such as leptospirae. Also organisms may be acquired from the birth canal at the time of birth ( = parturition).

### Methods by which Groups of Organisms are Commonly Spread

#### (a) Virus infection

In general viruses leave an infected host in its secretions and excretions (saliva, nasal and other discharges, urine and faeces) and are spread by direct or indirect contact or by the aerosol route. The last method is very important in diseases which produce signs of respiratory damage. They enter the body of the new host usually by ingestion or inhalation. However, rabies virus is an important exception in that it usually enters via wounds, frequently bite wounds inflicted by an infected animal.

#### (b) Bacterial infection

Bacteria can enter and leave the body by any of the routes previously described, although some are more commonly used by particular organisms. For example, leptospirae are frequently shed in the urine and ingested by a new host and *Pasteurella* is commonly passed from animal to animal in bite wounds.

It is important to remember that the bacteria responsible for many of the common diseases of the dog and cat are normal inhabitants of the body (Table 5.3). Such "commensal" bacteria are potential pathogens (opportunists) and they can cause disease either when introduced into a part of the body where they do not normally occur or when the body defence mechanisms are weakened.

Other bacteria such as *Pseudomonas* and *Clostridium tetani,* both of which can live saprophytically, may not be transferred from other hosts but simply acquired from the environment, e.g. the soil.

Bacteria can also be transmitted from man; tuberculosis in the dog is usually due to airborne infection transmitted from the owner.

#### (c) Ectoparasite infestation

Ectoparasites are almost always transmitted from host to host by direct or indirect contact. Where only one stage in the life-cycle of an animal is parasitic the parasite need not be acquired from another host, e.g. the larvae of *Trombicula autumnalis* (harvest mite) in pasture, or the maggots derived from eggs laid by blowflies.

#### (d) Endoparasite infection

Endoparasites, in the form of eggs, larvae, segments (tapeworms) and oocysts (of coccidia), almost always leave the host (final host) in the faeces. (However, canine lungworm larvae may be coughed out, and the eggs of the tongue worm and the bladder worm are expelled from the nasal chambers and bladder respectively.)

The endoparasite usually enters a new final host by ingestion. With some parasites the eggs or oocysts need to be infective to this new final host when eaten; they pass from one host to the other by direct or indirect contact. In some parasitic life-cycles a vector is involved which may be a transport host, paratenic host or intermediate host, as explained previously. The use of a vector may be an essential part of the parasitic life-cycle (as with the flea carrying *Dipylidium*) or it may simply be another method whereby the parasite can gain entry into the final host (as with the mouse carrying *Toxocara canis*).

In some cases a pet animal may itself act as a vector, e.g. the dog can act as an intermediate host for *Toxoplasma gondii*, whose final host is the cat.

### Elementary Methods of Disease Control

With knowledge of how diseases are normally transmitted their spread can be checked or minimized in a number of ways. Education, not only of veterinary surgeons and animal nurses but of owners and handlers of animals, is very important in ensuring the prompt control of disease. Important methods of controlling disease are as follows.

### 1. Quarantine and isolation

This refers to the separation and segregation of infected, or potentially infective, animals from those known, or presumed, not to be infected. The term quarantine is usually used in connection with the isolation of animals (particularly cats and dogs) entering the United Kingdom from abroad, for a period of 6 months because of the possibility that they might be infected with rabies virus. It is believed that almost all quarantined animals would begin to show clinical signs of rabies within the 6 month period if they harboured the virus, thereby enabling the infected animals to be recognized and destroyed.

Whenever animals are gathered together, particularly in large numbers, e.g. in kennels, catteries, animal hospitals, centres for stray animals, etc., the transfer of disease is made much easier and therefore more likely. It is particularly likely to occur by direct and indirect contact and the aerosol route. Consequently animals showing signs of infectious disease *and* those known to be carriers of an infectious disease or of parasites, although not showing signs of disease, should be kept separate from apparently healthy animals.

If the animal is in a kennel or cattery of a hospital the ideal is to transfer it to a separate building or room where it can be treated in isolation or, alternatively, to send it home again to be nursed by the owner. Since few of the infectious diseases of cats (and none of the viral diseases with the exception of rabies) are transmissible to dogs, and vice versa, in an emergency an infected cat can be placed temporarily in a room housing only dogs, or conversely an infected dog can be placed in isolation with cats.

Animals in isolation should have their own feeding bowls and bedding if non-disposable materials are used, which are washed separately. Ideally these animals should be attended by different staff to those dealing with other animals to prevent infectious organisms being transferred on clothing and shoes, etc.

Ideally animals which are known to have been in contact with an infected animal for some time before clinical signs were noted should themselves be isolated in this way and treated.

It is wise *not* to house animals in *large numbers* in a building because all are likely to be affected if one of the number develops an infectious disease.

Other points are:

(a) New animals entering an existing colony (e.g. breeding colony) of animals should be kept separate for at least 3–4 weeks in case they are carrying an infectious disease. In this time vaccination may be carried out (see later).

(b) Young animals usually have no, or poor, immunity to many of the larger parasites, whereas older animals usually have immunity and may carry and transmit the parasites without showing disease signs. Therefore young animals are best isolated from kennels, and particularly runs, used for older animals in which there can be a gradual accumulation of the infective stages of parasites which have been passed out in faeces.

## 2. Immunization

This is a way of limiting the spread of an infectious disease by providing some degree of protection against it. For example, if the virus of canine distemper enters the body of a dog which is immune to this disease the virus will probably be destroyed. In a non-immune animal the virus may multiply within the body tissues and then be excreted in large numbers in discharges, urine, etc., to infect other dogs in turn.

Immunity may be provided either by vaccination or by the administration of a hyperimmune serum (containing ready-made antibodies). The latter is comparatively short-acting (3 weeks) and is administered chiefly to unvaccinated (and presumed non-immune) animals when *immediate* immunity is required, e.g.:

(a) *after* they have been exposed to an infectious disease but *before* clinical signs of disease appear;

(b) before contacting other, possibly infected, animals, e.g. at cat shows or in kennels at holiday times.

## 3. Hygiene

In reducing the transmission of pathogenic organisms hygiene is extremely important.

(a) The thorough cleansing of all surfaces will remove many of the viruses, bacteria and parasitic eggs and oocysts which may be present. This applies to feeding vessels, non-disposable bedding, all surfaces in kennels and catteries, cat trays, concrete and asphalt runs, and paths. If the number of infective organisms can be greatly reduced in this way, the small number which remain to infect the animal are more likely to be successfully destroyed should they enter the body.

The efficient cleaning of surfaces with soap or detergent plus water (preferably hot), or even plenty of water alone, is much more effective than using disinfectants to try to kill organisms. Mechanical cleaning in this way actually *removes* organisms so that they are no longer present to produce infection. Disinfectants are frequently ineffective; many kill few infectious organisms and none will reliably kill bacterial spores or *Toxocara* eggs. Even the best are likely to be rendered much less effective by the presence of dirt, blood, pus or faeces. It is extremely unwise to rely on disinfectants alone and to assume that they will destroy all infectious agents because this they cannot do.

Regular cleaning of the animal's own haircoat (i.e. bathing) will help to reduce the population of infectious organisms that accumulate there.

If it is feasible, heat sterilization of feeding bowls and cat trays is even more efficient in reducing the burden of organisms. The use of flame-throwers on concrete runs may be the only way to destroy *Toxocara* eggs, but regular scrubbing and washing will loosen and flush away a high proportion.

(b) There should be regular and efficient removal of soiled bedding, which should preferably be burned, as should faeces from runs. Certainly, soiled bedding should be placed in areas where animals will *not* have access to it.

(c) To avoid contaminated food being fed, *either* all food must be cooked *or, alternatively,* dried or canned foods from a manufacturer should be used. This is particularly important in preventing the transmission of tapeworms and *Toxoplasma* to dogs and cats. Cooked meat must not be replaced on surfaces used for the preparation of *uncooked* meat because it can be recontaminated with the organisms which the cooking is intended to kill.

(d) Cats and dogs should be discouraged from catching rodents, birds and even slugs and earthworms as far as is possible, since it is by ingesting them that they acquire many internal parasites, including *Toxocara, Toxoplasma,* certain tapeworms and the feline lungworm. Of course a cat may be kept expressly to catch rodents; in that situation it will obviously be more likely to acquire and transmit these parasites.

(e) Vermin, such as rodents, and flies should be controlled since these act as vectors for infection, e.g. keep lids on dustbins, remove faeces and uneaten food, use fly-sprays, vapour strips or electric fly-catchers in kennels.

## 4. Treatment of infected animals

All infected animals (including healthy carrier animals if it is possible to identify them) should be treated to remove and kill the pathogenic organisms, not only to benefit the infected individual but to prevent the organism being transmitted to more and more animals.

At the present time there is no generally available drug which will effectively kill viruses. Antibiotic treatment is used in viral diseases solely to limit the effect of the "opportunist" bacteria, which, because of the animal's weakened body defences, are better able to attack its body tissues—a phenomenon known as **secondary bacterial infection**.

Antibacterial drugs consist of the antibiotics (which can be produced from living micro-organisms) and some other substances which can only be produced synthetically, e.g. the sulphonamides and nitrofurans.

The drugs used to kill all parasites can properly be called *parasiticides,* though in practice this term is usually reserved for those used against *external parasites alone.* Drugs used against the worm parasites (helminths) are referred to as antihelmintics, or more usually **anthelmintics**. The parasiticides and anthelmintics in common use at the time of writing are listed in Tables 6.9 and 6.10. Regrettably the drug amitraz which is particularly effective against Demodex is currently not available in the UK. It is not yet possible to destroy the metacestode stage of the tapeworms, or the cysts of *Toxoplasma* within the tissues of the final or intermediate host.

However the transmission of *Toxocara canis* larvae from the tissues of a pregnant

TABLE 6.9.  *Anthelmintics in common use in dogs and cats in the United Kingdom*

| Name of drug | Trade name | Size of tablet(s) | Dose rate (drug/body wt.) | Notes |
|---|---|---|---|---|
| **Anthelmintics against ascarids** | | | | |
| *Piperazine citrate* | "Citrazine" | 500 mg | | |
| *Piperazine adipate* | "Coopane" | 450 mg | | |
| | "Verocid" | 500 mg | Dog and cat: one tablet (416—500 mg)/5 kg | Piperazine also has low activity against hookworms. Dose for hookworm treatment = 1½–3 tablets/5 kg |
| *Piperazine phosphate* | "Canovel" | 416 mg | | |
| | "Catovel" | 416 mg | | |
| | "Endorid" | 416 mg | | |
| Also fenbendazole, mebendazole and nitroscanate (see below) | | | | |
| **Anthelmintics against hookworms** | | | | |
| Use piperazine, fenbendazole, mebendazole or nitroscanate (see below) | | | | |
| **Anthelmintics against whipworms** | | | | |
| Use fenbendazole or mebendazole (see below) | | | | |
| **Anthelmintics against tapeworms** | | | | |
| Bunamidine* | "Scolaban" | 100 mg and 200 mg | Dog: 100 mg/5 kg maximum dose—600 mg Cat: 100 mg only (unless under 2 kg) | *Contraindicated* in unweaned animals. For *Echinococcus* repeat after 2 days and after 4–6 weeks. Fast and dose 3 hours before feeding. Do not break tablet. |
| Niclosamide* | "Yomesan" | 500 mg | Dog: 500 mg/4 kg Cat: up to 2 kg:250 mg above 2 kg:500 mg | Fast 12 hours before dosing. *Contraindicated* in animals with acute diarrhoea or intestinal atony. |
| Praziquantel* | "Droncit" "Droncit injectable" | 50 mg Solution 56.8 mg/ml | Dog and cat: 5 mg/kg Dog and cat: 0.1 ml/kg | No fasting required. S/C or I/M injection. (S/C injection may give brief period of pain; therefore maximum 3 ml at any one site.) |
| Also fenbendazole, mebendazole and nitroscanate (see below) | | | | |

TABLE 6.9. *continued*

| Name of drug | Trade name | Size of tablet(s) | Dose rate (drug/body wt.) | Notes |
|---|---|---|---|---|
| **Broad spectrum anthelmintics** | | | | |
| Fenbendazole (effective against ascarids, hookworms, whipworms and *Taenia* spp. of tapeworms—including pre-natal ascarid infection) | "Panacur" | Suspensions (2.5% and 10%), powder (4%) and granules (22%) | Dog and cat: 100 mg/kg once or *better* 20 mg/kg daily for 5 consecutive days. Pregnant bitches: 50 mg/kg daily from 45th day of pregnancy to 18 days after whelping. | No fasting required |
| Mebendazole (effective against ascarids, hookworms, whipworms and tapeworms except *Dipylidium*) | "Telmin KH" | 100 mg | Dog and cat with ascarids only, dose twice daily for 2 consecutive days; under 2 kg : 50 mg, otherwise 100 mg. Dog and cat with mixed infection dose twice daily for 5 consecutive days; same doses, though dogs above 30 kg : 200 mg. | No fasting required |
| Nitroscanate (effective against ascarids, hookworms and tapeworms—though limited effectiveness against *Echinococcus*) | "Lopatol" | 100 mg and 500 mg | Dog: 50 mg/kg | *Contraindicated* in cat. Do not break tablets |

*Worms usually disintegrate in the intestine and whole tapeworms are seldom passed in the faeces.

The above notes are not necessarily complete and reference should be made to the manufacturers' data sheets before using these drugs.

TABLE 6.10.  *Parasiticides in common use on dogs and cats in the United Kingdom (Trade names within inverted commas)*

SULPHUR PREPARATIONS
(a) *Inorganic substances*
  Powdered sulphur
    "Skin dressing No. 3" (Dales)
    "Skin dressing Sulphur 22%" (Vet. Drug)
  Selenium sulphide
    "Seleen"
(b) *Organic compounds*
  Monosulfiram
    "Tetmosol"
    "Oterna"
  Mesulphen *plus* γ-BHC and benzyl benzoate
    "Temadex"

PLANT DERIVATIVES
Derris
  "Skin dressing No. 1" (Dales)
Rotenone
  "Demodectic mange dressing (concentrate)"
Permethrin*
  "Wellcare insecticidal spray"
  "Wellcare insecticidal powder"
  "Wellcare insecticidal dog shampoo"
Pyrethrins *plus* piperonyl butoxide
  "Pybuthrin dusting powder"

ORGANOCHLORINE COMPOUNDS
Gamma-benzene hexachloride (γ-BHC) = lindane
  "Skin dressing No. 3" (Cooper)
  "Skin dressing No. 2" (Dales)
  "Gammexane skin dressing"
  "Framomycin ear drops/skin lotion"
  "Lorexane No. 3"
  "Lorexane cream 1%"
  "Parasitic dusting powder" (Dales)
  "Quellada veterinary shampoo"
  "Auroid ear drops"
  "GAC ear drops"
  "Clendrol ear drops"

"Otoryl ear drops"
Also the active ingredient in many "flea collars"
γ-BHC *plus* mesulphen and benzyl benzoate
  "Temadex"
Bromocyclen
  "Alugan"

ORGANOPHOSPHORUS COMPOUNDS
Fenchlorphos ( = ronnel)
  "Ectoral"
Cythioate
  "Cyflee tablets"
Iodofenphos
  "Nuvanol Vet"
Diazinon
  "Canovel insecticidal collar"
  "Catovel elasticated insecticidal collar"
Fenitrothion *plus* dichlorvos
  "Nuvan Top"
  "Zeprox"
Dichlorvos
  Active ingredient in many "flea collars" e.g. "Vivopets"
  Also combined with iodofenphos in "Nuvan Staykill" for the control of insects in the environment

OTHER ORGANIC SUBSTANCES
Piperonyl butoxide
  "PB Dressing"
Piperonyl butoxide *plus* pyrethrins
  "Pybuthrin dusting powder"
Carbaryl
  "Derasect"
Propoxur
  "Bolfo"
Thiabendazole
  "Auroto ear drops"
Benzyl benzoate *plus* γ-BHC and mesulphen
  "Temadex"

*Actually manufactured synthetically.

bitch to her puppies whilst they are in the uterus can now be controlled by the drug fenbendazole.

Coccidial infections in small animals have been routinely treated with sulphonamides, which appear to be more effective when combined with pyrimethamine. However, clindamycin is reported to be most effective in treating cats with toxoplasmosis.

Although certain topical treatments are still employed the most effective drug against ringworm infestations of small animals is the anti-fungal antibiotic, griseofulvin, which is administered orally.

In all cases it is wise to refer to the drug manufacturer's recommendations concerning dose rates (which may be modified in the light of experience), the time of dosing in relation to feeding, the need for repeat dosage and any special precautions.

It should be borne in mind that most

drugs are toxic, some more so than others, and that indiscriminate use may impair rather than improve the animal's condition. Debilitated animals are more likely to develop toxic signs than healthy animals. Owners should always be given clear instructions about a drug's use and a warning about problems which may occur.

Having regard to cost effectiveness and availability, the most commonly used anthelmintics at the present time are: for ascarids—piperazine; for tapeworms—bunamidine (though to control Echinococcus infection regular dosing with praziquantel is most effective); and for hookworms or whipworms—one of the broad spectrum drugs.

### Zoonoses

Zoonoses are diseases that are transmitted from animals to man. There are in fact very few that are spread by the dog and cat in the United Kingdom although some of these are extremely important. (Diseases transmitted from man to animals are *not* zoonoses.)

External parasites transmitted to man are *Sarcoptes, Cheyletiella,* ringworm fungi and fleas, and the internal parasites are *Toxocara, Echinococcus* and *Toxoplasma.* The transmission of rabies virus to humans by cats and dogs is, of course, extremely important, although fortunately not yet recorded in the United Kingdom. It is also believed that there is a virus which, although causing no ill effects in cats, can be transmitted by cat scratches producing a fever in man (cat-scratch fever virus). The leptospiral bacteria are known to be the cause of the human diseases **Weil's disease** (in the case of *L. icterohaemorrhagiae*) and **Canicola fever** (in the case of *L. canicola*). Other bacteria may also be transmitted to humans of which *Pasteurella* from bite wounds is probably the most important, but also at times salmonellosis, tuberculosis and Campylobacter infection can be transmitted.

Because of the lack of immunity in young animals, such conditions are usually more serious in children.

To control the spread of such diseases to man it is important not only to treat the infected animals (e.g. routine worming to remove possible *Toxocara* infection) but also to observe hygienic precautions in addition to those already mentioned. They include the following recommendations:

(1) **Wash the hands thoroughly** after handling animals and before putting the hands on the face, particularly in the mouth, i.e. before eating, smoking, etc. Also wash the hands after handling raw meat.

(2) Do not allow animals to lick the face, or the plates and utensils, etc., used for human food.

(3) Wash animal feeding bowls quite separately from crockery and utensils used for human food.

(4) Keep young children (babies and toddlers especially) away from the environment of young puppies and cats.

(5) **Keep children's sand pits covered** when not in use and ensure animal faeces are cleared from play areas, e.g. gardens, patios, etc.

(6) Wear gloves when gardening, particularly if pregnant, to avoid possible contact with *Toxoplasma.*

(7) **If pregnant avoid being involved in looking after a cat.**

(8) Feed cats and dogs only dried, canned or cooked meat. *Toxoplasma* and *Echcinococcus* in particular are spread via raw meat and offal.

## (f) Antiseptics and Disinfectants

B. M. BUSH

### Introduction

It is important as a first step to understand the meaning of the various terms used in connection with the destruction of micro-organisms.

**Sterilization** is the removal or destruction of *all* living micro-organisms including bacterial spores. It can be achieved by moist heat at raised pressure (autoclaving), dry heat at normal atmospheric pressure, ionizing radiations and filtration. A few chemicals, ethylene oxide (gas), formaldehyde (gas) and glutaraldehyde (solution), *used under carefully controlled conditions* are able to kill bacterial spores, i.e. *can* produce sterilization. However, these ideal conditions are difficult to achieve in practice, and where other methods are available these chemicals should *not be relied upon* to produce sterilization.

**Disinfection** is the removal or destruction of pathogenic micro-organisms, though not necessarily of bacterial spores. The number of "vegetative" micro-organisms is thereby reduced to a level which is not harmful to health. Chemical solutions which destroy micro-organisms are described as **chemical disinfectants** or disinfectant solutions.

However, using a disinfectant solution is not the only way of achieving disinfection; it can also be obtained using heat (e.g. boiling, or the technique of pasteurization) or by cleaning (physically removing the micro-organisms). These methods are usually cheaper and more effective than using chemical solutions.

**Antisepsis** is the destruction of micro-organisms, but not bacterial spores, on living tissue. The term was used originally to denote the prevention of sepsis, or decay, by either killing or inhibiting the growth of micro-organisms. Chemical solutions which produced antisepsis are described as **chemical antiseptics** or antiseptic solutions. Antiseptics may be applied to tissues, usually the skin, not only as solutions but also as components of creams, ointments and aerosol sprays, e.g. those designed for the treatment of wounds.

**Antiseptics** are therefore essentially disinfectants which do not damage the patient's cells and can therefore safely be used on living tissue. Nowadays the term **skin disinfection** is often used instead of antisepsis, and consequently antiseptics are referred to as **skin disinfectants**.

Not all disinfectants are safe to use on living tissues. Some are so damaging to cells that they should only be used to disinfect inanimate objects—a process called **environmental disinfection**. Others can be used both as environmental disinfectants and also, though often at a lower concentration (i.e. when more diluted), as skin disinfectants (antiseptics). Some chemicals are either so expensive or so easily inactivated by dirty surroundings that they are usually *only* employed as skin disinfectants.

It must be appreciated that disinfection is quite different from sterilization since disinfectants *cannot* be relied upon to kill bacterial spores. Consequently disinfection is not able to produce sterile conditions. Terms such as "cold sterilization" or "emergency sterilization" when referring to soaking in a disinfectant solution are incorrect and misleading. Similarly, reference to disinfectant solutions as "sterilizing solutions" or "sterilants" implies that the solution is able to achieve more than in fact it can (with the possible exception of glutaraldehyde solution).

Again a clear distinction should be made between chemical disinfectants, cleaning agents and deodorants. Chemical disinfectants will *not* facilitate the removal of dirt. If mixed with the wrong type of detergent the efficiency of both the detergent and the disinfectant may be severely reduced. Chemical disinfectants should not be used to mask bad smells. These are usually associated with the accumulation of grease which harbours micro-organisms, and this is best removed from sinks, drains, etc., using scouring powder and/or washing soda as a strong solution in hot water. If necessary, deodorizers can be obtained to scent the air, as blocks, gels or aerosol sprays—the latter in cans or electrically dispelled. However, deodorizers do nothing to remove the micro-organisms which may be the underlying cause of unpleasant odours.

Chemical disinfection *after thorough cleaning* is recommended for operating theatres, food preparation areas and where walls and floors, etc., are contaminated by excretions (faeces, urine) and secretions (nasal discharge, sputum).

## Common Antiseptics and Disinfectants

The large and rather bewildering array of disinfectants which are commonly used can be conveniently classified into the twelve chemical groups listed in Table 6.11. To simplify description both antiseptics and environmental disinfectants are referred to as disinfectants.

Other substances which have some slight antibacterial activity may also be used but principally for other properties which they possess, e.g. hydrogen peroxide is used in veterinary practice chiefly as a wound cleanser.

The **choice of disinfectant** for a particular purpose must take into account the properties of disinfectants and the factors which affect their action, and these are described below.

### Activity against micro-organisms

The activity of disinfectants is measured in terms of their ability to destroy bacteria. The earliest tests devised (Rideal–Walker test and Chick–Martin test) only give accurate results for phenolic disinfectants. However, the more recent Kelsey–Sykes test is suitable for the assessment of all disinfectant solutions.

Of the **bacteria**, Gram-positive organisms are the group most easily destroyed by disinfectants; Gram-negative bacteria are generally more resistant; the tuberculosis (acid-fast) group of bacteria are even more resistant; and bacterial spores are the most resistant of all to disinfectant action. In Table 6.11 disinfectants have been graded 1–5 according to their ability to destroy a lesser or greater part of this range of bacteria. The disinfectants which are most effective against bacterial spores are the aldehydes, ethylene oxide and, to a lesser extent, the halogens. Some disinfectants do actually destroy the organisms ( =**bactericidal**); others do not kill but merely stop bacterial growth ( =**bacteriostatic**). Bactericidal chemicals are always preferable because following the dilution

TABLE 6.11. *Common antiseptics and disinfectants*

| | Disinfectant | Examples of brand names | Use | Antibacterial activity | Resistance to inactivation |
|---|---|---|---|---|---|
| 1. | Alcohols (ethyl, isopropyl) | | Ⓔ Ⓢ | 5 | 5 |
| 2. | Aldehydes* | | | | |
| | (a) Formaldehyde | | E | 5 | 5 |
| | (b) Glutaraldehyde | "Cidex" | E | 5 | 5 |
| 3. | Ampholytic surfactants | "Tego" | E | 2 | 1 |
| 4. | Chlorhexidine | "Hibitane", "Hibiscrub", "Dispray" | Ⓢ | 2 | 1 |
| 5. | Dyes Acriflavine, Proflavine, Gentian violet | | S | 1 | 4 |
| 6. | Ethylene oxide* | "Anprolene" | E | 5 | 4 |
| 7. | Halogens | | | | |
| | (a) Hypochlorites** (bleaches) | "Chloros", "Domestos", "Milton" | Ⓔ | 5 | 3 |
| | (b) Chloramine** | "Halamid" | Ⓔ | 5 | 3 |
| | (c) Iodine | | Ⓢ | 5 | 3 |
| | (d) Iodophors | "Pevidine", "Wescodyne" | Ⓢ | 5 | 3 |
| 8. | Organic mercurials*** Thiomersal | "Merthiolate" | S | 2 | 3 |
| 9. | Phenol compounds | | | | |
| | (a) Black fluids | "Jeyes' fluid" | E | 4 | 4 |
| | (b) White fluids | "Izal" | Ⓔ | 4 | 4 |
| | (c) Clear soluble | "Stericol", "Hycolin", "Clearsol" | Ⓔ | 4 | 4 |
| | (d) Chlorinated phenols | | | | |
| | Chloroxylenol | "Dettol", "Ibcol", "Rycovet antiseptic" | E   S | 2 | 2 |
| | Hexachlorophane | "Mastisept", "Phisohex", "Disfex" | S | 2 | 2 |
| | Triclosan | "Irgasan", "Zalclense" | S | 2 | 2 |
| 10. | Pine oil fluids | Many household and commercial brands | E | 1 | 2 |

TABLE 6.11. *continued.*

| Disinfectant | Examples of brand names | Use | Antibacterial activity | Resistance to inactivation |
|---|---|---|---|---|
| 11. Quaternary ammonium compounds | | | | |
| (a) Cetrimide | "Cetavlon" | E S | 2 | 1 |
| (b) Benzalkonium chloride | "Roccal", "Marinol", "Agriclens" | E S | 2 | 1 |
| 12. Quaternary ammonium compound plus a diguanide (i.e. in combination) | | | | |
| (a) Cetrimide plus chlorhexidine | "Savlon" | Ⓢ | 3 | 1 |
| (b) Benzalkonium chloride plus picloxydine | "Residuard" | Ⓔ | 3 | 1 |

*Key:* *Use:* E = Environmental disinfectant.
S = Skin disinfectant (i.e. antiseptic).
◯ = Suitable for routine use because of their antibacterial efficiency or special properties (see text).

*Antibacterial activity and resistance to inactivation:* the higher the number the better, although this should only be considered as a guide. The antibacterial activity of the hypochlorites is graded higher than that of phenol compounds only because of their greater ability to destroy bacterial spores. Although the aldehydes are given a high grading their antibacterial action is slow.

*The aldehydes and ethylene oxide are specialized disinfectants, i.e. employed in specialized ways and not used for routine purposes.

**Another similar chlorine-releasing solution is "Eusol". This solution should be freshly prepared from a mixture of chlorinated lime (bleaching powder) and boric acid and remains effective for up to 2 weeks.

***Other organic mercurials, especially mercurochrome, are less effective against bacteria than thiomersal.

Ampholytic surfactants and quaternary ammonium compounds possess detergent as well as disinfectant properties so that it is unnecessary to add a detergent to them for cleaning purposes.

of a bacteriostatic disinfectant bacterial growth may begin again. The ampholytic surfactants and quaternary ammonium compounds are essentially bacteriostatic, and consequently less desirable.

**For destroying viruses** the hypochlorite disinfectants (i.e. bleaches), which release chlorine, are particularly effective.

Equally valuable against viruses is chloramine, the active component of sodium tosylchloramide ("Halamid", available as a powder). Chloramine also releases chlorine, and "Halamid" used as a 2.5% solution is believed to kill most viruses. However, available information relates chiefly to farm animals and in the absence of severe organic contamination a 0.5% solution would be expected to inactivate all feline and canine viruses. Glutaraldehyde ("Cidex") 2% is also very effective against viruses but slow acting and too expensive to use for the cleaning of floors, walls, etc. However, it is suitable for bowls and instruments. Ampholytic surfactants (e.g. "Tego") can kill some, but not all, viruses, though they have the advantage of being odourless and non-toxic.

Although not mentioned in Table 6.11 a 0.5% solution of sodium carbonate (washing soda) has proved very effective in inactivating the virus of ICH.

**Fungal spores** are less resistant than bacterial spores, and all the disinfectants listed in Table 6.11 have good activity against fungal spores, with the exception of the dyes, pine oil fluids and quaternary ammonium compounds.

### Efficiency

*Thorough physical cleaning* before, or as part of, the disinfection process is *important* for the following reasons.

(1) The smaller the number of bacteria (or any type of micro-organisms) which are present in a particular area the higher the proportion which will be killed by the disinfectant.

(2) If the bacteria are protected by covering layers of dirt or grease the disinfectant cannot readily come into contact with them.

(3) Disinfectants are *inactivated* (some more than others—see later) by the presence of large amounts of organic material, e.g. pus, blood, faeces, food, etc.

Washing away the dirt, grease, organic material and also many of the bacteria themselves, increases the efficiency of the disinfectant in killing those bacteria which remain. Simply pouring a disinfectant solution on to dirt containing bacteria is unlikely to be an effective method of removing them.

Disinfectants are also more effective under the following circumstances:

(1) When used at higher temperatures, i.e. in hot rather than cold water.

(2) The longer the disinfectant is in contact with the micro-organisms, up to a maximum of 24 hours (alcohol and hypochlorites act most rapidly).

(3) When a large, rather than a small, volume of prepared disinfectant solution is used, as this reduces inactivation by organic matter.

(4) When the disinfectant is used in a higher concentration within the recommended range. In general higher concentrations of disinfectants are more effective (though the difference may be slight) but phenol compounds and alcohol are *less* effective in very high concentrations (e.g. 70% ethyl or isopropyl alcohol is the *most* effective concentration). Because costs rise when more disinfectant is used it is gener-

ally wasteful to exceed the recommended concentration. However, to go *below* the recommended concentration is even more wasteful as total failure of the disinfectant is likely.

(5) When freshly prepared. With age disinfectant solutions deteriorate (i.e. become less effective), and even worse any bacteria which survive in them (e.g. in solutions retained in mop buckets) may multiply. When the solution is used again these bacteria will be spread around. *Where possible diluted solutions should not be kept longer than 24 hours.* Containers of diluted disinfectant solution should never be "topped up" with more of the diluted disinfectant solution as the level falls, because of the danger of resistant bacteria surviving and multiplying in the solution. Even worse is the practice of "topping up" by simply adding more water; here the reduction in concentration which is produced makes it much easier for the bacteria to multiply in the solution.

## Inactivation of disinfectants

All disinfectants are inactivated to a greater or lesser extent by a variety of materials with which they may come into contact.

The ampholytic surfactants, chlorhexidine and pine oil disinfectants are seriously inactivated by hard water and by such organic materials as pus, blood, faeces, vomit and foodstuffs. These same disinfectant groups are also inactivated by such natural materials as cork, rubber, wood and cotton, and by the many types of plastic. This is significant because **plastic bowls and buckets**, plastic squeezee

bottles and plastic-sponge mopheads are frequently used with disinfectants.

The halogen disinfectants (including the hypochlorite bleaches) are also seriously inactivated by organic materials, but only slightly by the other substances mentioned above. Phenolic and mercurial compounds are inactivated by rubber, and phenolic compounds may also be inactivated to some extent by certain plastics (although plastic buckets appear to produce little inactivation).

Care is needed when combining disinfectants with soap or detergents for cleaning purposes. Soap interferes with the action of chlorhexidine and the quaternary ammonium compounds. Detergents are classified as cationic, non-ionic or anionic according to their properties. Cationic detergents (including the quaternary ammonium compounds which have detergent as well as disinfectant properties) inactivate phenolic and hypochlorite disinfectants. Therefore phenols and hypochlorites should only be used with soap or with anionic or non-ionic detergents such as "Teepol", "Decon 90" or household washing-up liquids; they should not be mixed with such preparations as "Cetavlon" or "Roccal".

These facts form the basis of the assessment of the resistance to inactivation appearing in Table 6.11. Reputable disinfectant manufacturers provide information about substances which are not compatible with their products.

## Types of chemical disinfectants

(1) *Alcohol.* Seventy per cent ethyl alcohol (ethanol) or 70% isopropyl alcohol (isopropranol) is an effective environmental disinfectant (for thermometers and trolley tops) and skin disinfectant. Markedly weaker or stronger alcoholic concentrations are *less* effective. Its high cost limits its use as an environmental disinfectant.

Although not inactivated by organic materials, alcohol cannot easily penetrate them and therefore surfaces (both of the skin and of objects) should be cleansed before its application. Chlorhexidine or iodine may be added to alcohol for an increased effect.

2. *Aldehydes.* Formaldehyde is used either as a gas (chiefly for fumigation of infected buildings) or as a solution of dissolved gas (=formalin). Although effective it is extremely irritant to the eyes and skin. Glutaraldehyde used as an alkaline 2% solution can kill bacterial spores following their prolonged immersion, but it is expensive, penetrates poorly, is slightly irritant, and stable for only a maximum of 2 weeks after preparation. Neither aldehyde is suitable as a routine environmental disinfectant for hospital use.

3. *Ampholytic surfactants.* These have detergent as well as disinfectant properties but are inactivated by many materials and are expensive. They are unsuitable for routine hospital use.

4. *Chlorhexidine.* Although expensive and inactivated by many materials, including soap, this disinfectant is useful for skin disinfection especially in alcoholic solution. It is also available combined with a detergent (e.g. "Hibiscrub").

5. *Dyes.* These are feeble disinfectants whose use has largely been replaced by other antiseptics and by sulphonamides and antibiotics.

6. *Ethylene oxide.* Used *under carefully controlled conditions* this gas can produce sterilization of fabrics and instruments, etc., but the process is less reliable than autoclaving. Ethylene oxide mixtures with air are explosive and its vapours are irritant. Because it is an uncontrolled system the "Anprolene" method of using ethylene oxide is not recommended for sterilization by the Department of Health and Social Security.

7. *Halogens.*

(a) *Hypochlorites.* Popularly known as "bleaches" these are **cheap and effective environmental disinfectants.** As well as having good activity against bacteria and fungi they are very effective against viruses and very suitable for use in food preparation areas. A concentration of 0.175% sodium hypochlorite is able to inactivate feline viruses, including FIE virus which most disinfectants are unable to inactivate.

At the time of writing the concentration of sodium hypochlorite in commercial bleaches (when manufactured) is: "Domestos" 8.8% (dilute 1 part in 50), "Chlorox" (USA) 5.6% (dilute 1 part in 32), "Brobat" 3.5% (dilute 1 part in 20) and "Milton" 1% (dilute 1 part in 6). All bleaches lose potency with age (especially if exposed to sunlight) and 1 year after manufacture these recommended dilutions should be halved. Also, because hypochlorite can be seriously inactivated by organic material, it is advisable for the concentration to be doubled or trebled (i.e. a half or a third the normal volume of water added) where there is contamination with blood, faeces etc. Preferably the surfaces should first be prepared by thorough cleaning.

Most hypochlorite solutions are strongly alkaline and undiluted are corrosive, i.e. will damage fabrics, plastics, enamelled ware and metals (aluminium and stainless steel). Even diluted they are irritant to the skin. However "Milton" is stabilized with sodium chloride and diluted solutions are less irritant.

They do not wet surfaces well and therefore are best used with a compatible (anionic) detergent, e.g. "Teepol" or a household washing-up liquid.

Some scouring powders contain hypochlorites.

(b) *Chloramine.* Solutions can be prepared from a powder. The higher concentrations (2½–5%) used against some viruses should be rinsed off plastic, rubber and metal-work after use, but the lower concentration (0.5%) routinely used against bacteria and other viruses is non-corrosive and non-irritant to the hands or animal skin. Chlorine is released slightly more slowly than from the hypochlorites.

(c) *Iodine.* One per cent iodine in 70% alcohol is an effective pre-operative skin disinfectant, though it may produce a skin reaction.

(d) *Iodophors.* These have the advantages over iodine of being less irritant and non-staining and the colour of iodophor solutions can be used as an indicator of potency; once the colour has disappeared the solution will usually be ineffective. They are used similarly for skin disinfection, mainly of the hands, in the form of "surgical scrubs", e.g. povidone–iodine and detergent mixtures ("Pevidine", "Wesco-dyne"), but also (in alcoholic solution) of operation sites.

8. *Organic mercurials.* These comparatively feeble disinfectants have largely been replaced by other compounds.

9. *Phenol compounds.*

(a) *Black fluids.*

(b) *White fluids.*

(c) *Clear soluble phenolics.*

All three are irritant to varying degrees and cannot be used on the skin. They are also, because of their toxicity and their strong residual odour and flavour, unsuitable for food preparation surfaces. However, because they are cheap and not inactivated by organic material they are valuable for cleaning purposes.

Black fluids leave dark sticky residues in buckets and consequently white fluids are preferred; both have strong, possibly, objectionable smells. As effective as both of these but less pungent are the clear soluble phenolics, (e.g. "Hycolin") which are often combined with a detergent (e.g. "Stericol", "Clearsol").

(d) *Chlorinated phenols.* Chloroxylenol is non-irritant but inactivated by hard water and organic material. Hexachlorophane has been widely used in soap and detergent preparations for skin disinfection, e.g. of the hands ("Phisohex"), but it is slow-acting. Reports of its cumulative toxicity have resulted in its use being restricted and the less effective substance triclosan has been used as an alternative.

10. *Pine oil fluids.* These pleasant-smelling liquids sold for household use have minimal disinfectant effect and should not be seriously considered for hospital use.

11. *Quaternary ammonium compounds.* These are non-toxic with good detergent properties which makes them suitable for cleaning wounds (e.g. 1% cetrimide solution), but as disinfectants they are only bacteriostatic and are inactivated by many materials. (Cetrimide ("Cetavlon") is in fact an important ingredient of the culture medium used to *grow* the pathogenic bacterium *Pseudomonas* in the laboratory.) Apart from use in food preparation areas, these disinfectants have few other uses.

12. *Quaternary ammonium compound plus a diguanide.* The addition of a diguan-

ide to a quaternary ammonium compound makes the combination more effective against bacteria. Cetrimide plus chlorhexidine ("Savlon") is useful for skin disinfection as a 5% solution, or for cleaning wounds as a 1% solution. Benzalkonium chloride plus picloxydine ("Resiguard") is employed for the cleaning of areas where phenolics are undesirable, e.g. food preparation areas.

## Choosing Disinfectants and Antiseptics

**A. For environmental disinfection** (that is of surroundings, instruments, equipment, etc.).

Chemical disinfectant solutions should only be used where sterility is not required, where disinfection by cleaning is inadequate or where disinfection by heat (e.g. boiling) is not possible.

Where sterility is essential *either* autoclaving (or some other sterilizing procedure) must be undertaken, *or* alternatively pre-sterilized disposable equipment must be used. **Disinfectants cannot be relied upon to produce sterility**.

No more than *two* types of disinfectant solutions are required for routine use in any one premises. The two generally recommended (after considering efficacy, toxicity, cost and acceptability, e.g. odour) are a clear soluble phenolic compound (preferably with detergent already added) and a hypochlorite.

The *clear soluble phenolic plus detergent* is used (generally as a 1–2% solution depending on the manufacturer's instructions) for such routine purposes as:

(1) Disinfecting contaminated instruments for 30 minutes *before* cleaning with detergent and then autoclaving (the same procedure, but without autoclaving, is suitable for rectal thermometers).

(2) Cleaning operating theatres and their equipment.

(3) Cleaning floors, walls, examination tables and other equipment contaminated with organic material (excreta, vomit, etc.). Where floors, etc., are *not* contaminated using disinfectant has *no* advantage over cleaning with water and detergent alone. With heavy contamination the concentration of phenolic disinfectant should be doubled.

The *hypochlorite* is used, following thorough cleansing with an anionic detergent such as "Teepol" in the concentrations recommended previously.

The hypochlorites, and *not* the phenolic solution, should be used on rubber articles.

Other points to note about environmental disinfectants are:

(1) There are no advantages in using disinfectant solutions for damp dusting or for cleaning drains.

(2) Floor mops and buckets should be thoroughly washed with clean water after use and the mops then placed in a clean 1% hypochlorite solution for an hour followed by drying upside down (i.e. with mophead uppermost). To avoid them becoming breeding grounds for bacteria both mops and buckets not in use must be stored *dry*.

(3) Great care should be taken to *measure out* the amounts of disinfectant and water to *ensure* that the recommended dilution is always used.

## B. For skin disinfection

In veterinary practice antiseptics are used for two main purposes:

(1) disinfection of the hands, usually

prior to operating but occasionally after handling contaminated material;

(2) disinfection of the patient's skin, again usually prior to operation.

*(1) Disinfection of the Hands*

An initial washing in running water with soap or detergent, particularly if a brush is used, will remove the dead skin scales plus those bacteria which are on them. The resident bacteria can then be removed by applying either:

(a) a chlorhexidine plus detergent solution (e.g. "Hibiscrub"); or

(b) a povidone–iodine (= an iodophor) plus detergent solution (e.g. "Pevidine surgical scrub").

An alternative to using one of these solutions prior to surgery is to rub on, *without added water,* two successive 5 ml applications of a preparation containing chlorhexidine, isopropyl alcohol and emollients (e.g. "Hibisol hand rub"). Other than prior to surgery, *one* application is generally sufficient.

The use of any of these three preparations is superior to a single application of preparations containing either hexachlorophane plus detergent ("Phisohex") or triclosan plus detergent ("Zalclense").

**Frequent washing of the hands without disinfection** will do much to minimize the spread of infection, particularly before giving injections, collecting blood samples or applying dressings and also after handling infected material. Hands should *always* be washed before consuming food or drink.

*(2) Disinfection of Operation Sites*

First the skin should have been cleansed with soap and water and dried with a sterile towel or sterile swabs. Then a quick-acting antiseptic is required, and 70% ethyl alcohol containing 0.5% chlorhexidine ("Dispray No. 1", or "Dispray No. 3", which also contains a red dye) has been found to be the most effective. (1% iodine in 70% alcohol is equally effective but may cause skin reactions). The alcoholic solution is applied on a sterile gauze swab using friction.

Sites ingrained with dirt which may contain a large number of bacterial spores should have a compress soaked in povidone–iodine applied for 30 minutes *after* cleansing and *before* applying the alcoholic antiseptic.

(g) Pharmacy and Dispensing

B. M. BUSH

## Introduction

**Materia medica** is an out-dated term which refers to the study and knowledge of all matters relating to drugs, including their sources, preparation, effects and usage. Nowadays, if a similar broad term is required, the word **pharmacology** (science of drugs) may be employed. However, pharmacology is often used in a more restricted way to refer primarily to knowledge about the actions of drugs and their fate in the body.

**Therapeutics** is concerned with the use of drugs in the prevention and treatment of disease, and **pharmacy** with the preparation and dispensing of drugs.

**Dispensing** refers to the "giving out" of drugs. In veterinary practice the dispensing of drugs often takes place on the practice premises but, as is more usual in human medicine, it may be performed by a pharmacist upon receipt of a prescription, that is a written instruction from the veterinary surgeon or physician to dispense a particular drug preparation.

## Definitions

The most useful way in which to classify drugs is by their effect in or on the body, which determines the purposes for which the drugs can be employed. Drugs are therefore grouped together because of some similarity of action, and the group is given a name descriptive of the effect they produce (e.g. analgesics—pain-relievers)

or the use to which they are put (e.g. antidiarrhoeals—drugs to control diarrhoea). Much less frequently a group of drugs may be named according to a similarity of source (e.g. hormones—produced by endocrine glands) or of chemical structure (e.g. sulphonamides—which all possess the same chemical nucleus).

It should be appreciated that some drugs have more than one major effect and therefore can belong to more than one group, e.g. aspirin may be described as an antipyretic drug, an analgesic drug and an anti-inflammatory drug. It should also be noted that all drugs produce effects in addition to those for which they are principally employed and which are called **side-effects**. These are sometimes of little consequence but they are often harmful and are then described as **toxic actions**.

On the pages which follow there are definitions of the names used to describe the different types of drugs. Some of these classes of drugs are much more important in human medicine or large animal practice than in small animal practice and are marked with an asterisk.

After each definition one or two examples of the particular type of drug are given; in each case these examples are given their **approved** (or official) **name** rather than any **proprietary** (or brand) **name**. In each case the definition can be made more complete by inserting the words "is a drug which" after the descriptive name; these words have been omitted to avoid repetition.

**Adsorbent**—adsorbs on to its surface bacterial toxins and other substances, usually from the intestines. Examples: kaolin, magnesium trisilicate.

**Anabolic**—promotes anabolism, i.e. the conversion of food into body tissues. Anabolic drugs with a steroid structure are termed anabolic steroids. Examples: boldenone, nandrolone.

**Anaesthetic**—produces a reversible (i.e. temporary) loss of sensation, especially pain, in the body. It may affect only a limited area, when it is described as a local analgesic or local anaesthetic, or it may produce a complete loss of sensation accompanied by unconsciousness, when it is described as a general anaesthetic. Examples of these two types of anaesthetics are given under the respective headings.

**Analeptic**—stimulates the cerebral and medullary centres of the brain. This type of drug is used mainly as a respiratory stimulant; given to conscious animals convulsions can be produced. Examples: nikethamide, bemegride.

**Analgesic**—relieves pain (without producing general anaesthesia). Examples: pethidine, paracetamol.

**Androgen**—possesses masculinizing properties. Examples: testosterone (natural), methyltestosterone (synthetic).

**Antacid**—neutralizes the hydrochloric acid in the stomach. Examples: sodium bicarbonate, bismuth glycinate.

**Antagonist**—reverses, completely or partially, the effect of another drug. This is not a single drug group but some drugs are spoken of as being antagonists to others, e.g. bemegride is a barbiturate antagonist and nalorphine is a morphine-group antagonist.

**Antemetic (or anti-emetic)**—suppresses vomiting (emesis). Examples: chlorpromazine, chlorbutol.

**Anthelmintic**—kills parasitic worms and/or removes them from the host's body. Examples: piperazine, bunamidine.

**Antibacterial**—acts against bacteria, either killing them or stopping their growth. Drugs capable of *killing* bacteria are described as **bactericidal** (examples: penicillin, streptomycin) whereas those capable only of inhibiting the *multiplication* of bacteria are termed **bacteriostatic** (examples: oxytetracycline, chloramphenicol, sulphonamides).

**Antibiotic**—is produced by a micro-organism and is antagonistic to the growth or life of other micro-organisms (usually bacteria but occasionally fungi) at low concentration. Examples: penicillin, oxytetracycline. As well as being either bactericidal or bacteriostatic antibiotics can also be classified as either narrow spectrum or broad spectrum.

**Narrow spectrum** antibiotics are effective against a relatively narrow range of bacteria, usually either Gram positive (e.g. penicillin) or Gram negative (e.g. streptomycin), whereas **broad spectrum** antibiotics are effective against a wide variety of bacteria (e.g. ampicillin, oxytetracycline).

**\*Anticoagulant**—prevents blood clotting. Examples: heparin, sodium citrate.

**Anticoccidial**—kills or prevents the multiplication of coccidia in the host (alternatively known as a coccidiostat). Examples: sulphadiazine, clindamycin.

**Anticonvulsant**—suppresses convulsions. Examples: primidone, phenytoin.

**Antidiarrhoeal**—decreases diarrhoea, usually by coating and protecting the intestinal mucosa (alternatively known as an antidiarrhoeic). Examples: kaolin, attapulgite.

**Antidiuretic**—decreases the production of urine. Example: desmopressin.

**Antifungal = antimycotic**—kills or stops the growth of fungi. Examples: griseofulvin, nystatin.

**Antihistaminic**—antagonizes the effects of histamine (other than its effect on gastric acid secretion). Examples: diphenydramine hydrochloride, mepyramine maleate.

**\*Antihypertensive**—reduces blood pressure when it is continuously raised (alternatively known as a hypotensive). Examples: methyldopa, propranolol.

**Anti-inflammatory drug**—reduces inflammation in the tissues. Examples: phenylbutazone, prednisolone (and other corticosteroids).

**Antipruritic**—reduces itching (pruritus). Examples: antihistaminics, local analgesics (for specific examples see under those headings).

**Antipyretic**—lowers an abnormally high body temperature (e.g. in fever) but not when caused by a high environmental temperature (e.g. heatstroke). Examples: aspirin, phenacetin.

**Antiseptic**—removes or destroys pathogenic micro-organisms (though not necessarily bacterial spores) and does not damage living tissue (alternatively referred to as a skin disinfectant). Examples: ethyl alcohol, chlorhexidine.

**Antiserum**—contains a high concentration of antibodies against a disease-producing agent, usually a micro-organism or its toxin (alternatively referred to as hyperimmune serum, or, in the case of an antiserum against a toxin, an antitoxin). Examples: antisera against canine distemper and feline infectious enteritis.

**Antisialogogue**—reduces the flow of saliva and increases its viscosity (i.e. "thickness"). Alternatively known as an antisialic. Examples: atropine, hyoscine.

**Antispasmodic**—relaxes all smooth muscle and reduces intestinal motility, i.e. diminishes gut contractions (alternatively known as a spasmolytic). Examples: atropine, diphenoxylate.

**Antitoxin**—contains a high concentration of antibodies against a specific toxin. Example: tetanus antitoxin.

**Astringent**—precipitates protein when applied to the skin or a mucous membrane. Only the surface proteins are precipitated to produce a protective coating; the underlying cells are not killed. Examples: silver nitrate (skin astringent), tannic acid (intestinal astringent).

**Ataractic**—reduces anxiety without producing excessive drowsiness or otherwise impairing consciousness (otherwise referred to as a tranquillizer). Examples: acetylpromazine, trimeprazine.

**Blood-volume expander** (otherwise known as a **plasma expander** or **plasma substitute**)—produces and maintains an increase in the volume of circulating blood. Examples: dextran, gelatin.

**\*Carminative**—causes the expulsion of gas from the stomach. Example: peppermint.

**Chemotherapeutic drug**—has an adverse effect on pathogenic organisms in or on the host's body. Examples: antibiotics and anthelmintics (for specific examples see under those headings).

**Coagulant**—acting internally arrests minor haemorrhages by promoting the coagulation of blood. Sometimes used as synonymous with haemostatic, although the latter term is most commonly applied to drugs which stop haemorrhage by acting locally, i.e. on the surface of the body. Example: a mixture of malonic and oxalic acids.

**Coccidiostat**—prevents the multiplication of coccidia in the host and may kill them. Examples: sulphadiazine, clindamycin.

**Corticosteroid** (or corticoid)—is either naturally produced by the cortex of the adrenal gland or is a synthetic equivalent. The effects of corticosteroids in the body are of two types: glucocorticoid and mineralocorticoid. Because one type of effect usually predominates corticosteroids are often classified into glucocorticoids (e.g. cortisol) and mineralocorticoids (e.g. aldosterone). The synthetic corticosteroids are usually glucocorticoids (e.g. betamethasone, triamcinolone).

**Cough suppressent (antitussive)**—reduces coughing, usually by depression of the cough centre in the brain. Examples: codeine, pholcodine.

**Cytotoxic drug ( = antimitotic)**—is toxic to cells and used in the treatment of cancer. Examples: chlorambucil, cyclophosphamide.

**Demulcent**—lubricates, soothes and protects the mucous membrane of the mouth, pharynx, oesophagus or stomach. Examples: dextrose ( = glucose), glycerol ( = glycerine).

**Disinfectant** (chemical disinfectant)—destroys pathogenic micro-organisms, though not necessarily bacterial spores. Examples: hypochlorite bleaches, phenol compounds.

**Diuretic**—increases the volume of urine produced, usually by increasing the excretion of sodium and therefore water. Examples: hydrochlorothiazide, frusemide.

**Ecbolic**—causes contraction of the uterus (alternatively known as an oxytocic). Example: oxytocin.

**Emetic**—causes vomiting (emesis). Examples: washing soda (orally), apomorphine (by injection).

**Emollient**—softens, soothes, lubricates and protects a skin surface. Examples: lanolin, petroleum jelly.

**Expectorant**—decreases the viscosity (i.e. "thickness") and increases the volume of respiratory secretions. Helps to "loosen" mucus (phlegm) in the respiratory tract. Examples: ammonium chloride, ipecacuanha.

**Fungicide**—kills fungi. Examples: griseofulvin, nystatin.

**General anaesthetic**—produces, in a controlled way, unconsciousness, muscle relaxation and a reduction in the sensitivity to stimuli and the motor response to them. Examples: thiopentone, halothane.

**Haemostatic**—arrests minor haemorrhages at the surface of the body. Sometimes used as being synonymous with coagulant, although the latter is more commonly applied to drugs administered *internally* to control haemorrhages. Examples: Strong solution of ferric chloride, fibrin foam.

**Heart stimulant ( = cardiac stimulant)**—increases the heart rate and/or the output of the heart. Examples: digoxin, etamiphyllin camsylate.

**Hormone**—is produced in the body by an endocrine gland (although some can now be produced synthetically) and is transported by the circulation before influencing the metabolism of cells in other tissues. Examples: insulin, thyroxine.

**Hypnotic**—produces moderate sedation (depression of the central nervous system) resulting in sleep from which the patient can easily be roused. Example: sub-anaesthetic doses of barbiturates.

**\*Hypoglycaemic**—produces a marked fall in the blood glucose level. Examples: chlorpropamide, insulin.

**Inhalant**—acts as a local expectorant when vaporized—usually with hot water, i.e. increases the volume and decreases the viscosity ("thickness") of respiratory secretions. Examples: Friars' balsam, eucalyptus oil.

**Insecticide**—kills insects. Examples: gamma-benzene hexachloride, fenchlorphos.

**Laxative**—results in defaecation due to a slight increase in intestinal movements, i.e. a mild purgative. Example: liquid paraffin.

**Local anaesthetic or local analgesic**—temporarily prevents the conduction of impulses when applied to nerve terminals or nerve fibres. Analgesia results from the lack of sensory stimuli. It also blocks motor fibres producing paralysis. Examples: lignocaine, procaine.

**Miotic**—causes constriction of the pupil

of the eye. Examples: physostigmine, pilocarpine.

**Muscle relaxant**—excluding general anaesthetics and local analgesics, produces generalized skeletal muscle relaxation (i.e. muscle paralysis). Usually this is because it prevents the transmission of impulses from the end of motor nerves to the muscle fibres, i.e. at the neuromuscular junction. Examples: gallamine triethiodide, pancuronium bromide.

**Mydriatic**—causes dilation of the pupil of the eye. Examples: atropine, ephedrine.

**Narcotic**—produces heavy sedation (i.e. depression of the central nervous system) resulting in stupor and insensibility to pain. Example: morphine.

**Oestrogen**—produces feminizing characteristics including oestrus. Naturally is formed in the ovary but synthetic equivalents are available. Examples: oestradiol (natural), stilboestrol (synthetic).

**Oestrus suppressant**—prevents or postpones oestrus. Examples: megestrol acetate, medroxyprogesterone acetate.

**Oxytocic**—causes contraction of the uterus. Example: oxytocin.

**Parasiticide**—kills parasites; commonly applied only to those drugs effective against external parasites excluding fungi. Examples: gamma benzene hexachloride, fenitrothion.

**Progestagen (progestin)**—possesses the properties of progesterone, e.g. inhibits ovulation. Naturally produced in the body by the corpus luteum of the ovary but synthetic equivalents are available. Examples: progesterone (natural), megestrol acetate (synthetic).

**Purgative**—markedly increases intestinal peristaltic movements resulting in defaecation. Examples: danthron, phenolphthalein.

**Respiratory stimulant**—stimulates respiration usually by stimulating the respiratory centre in the medulla. Examples: nikethamide, bemegride.

**\*Rubefacient**—causes mild inflammation of the skin producing redness. Examples: kaolin poultice, turpentine liniment.

**Sedative**—produces mild depression of the central nervous system so that the subject is calm and possibly drowsy. Example: barbiturates in low doses.

**Spasmolytic (antispasmodic)**—relaxes all smooth muscle and reduces intestinal motility, i.e. diminishes intestinal contractions. Examples: atropine, diphenoxylate.

**Sulphonamide**—has a characteristic chemical nucleus responsible for its antibacterial activity. All members of the sulphonamide group are synthetically produced. Examples: sulphadiazine, sulphacetamide.

**Toxoid**—can stimulate the formation of antibodies against a toxin without producing disease. It is prepared by chemical treatment of a toxin. Example: tetanus toxoid.

**Tranquillizer (ataractic)** reduces anxiety without producing excessive drowsiness or otherwise impairing consciousness. Examples: acetylpromazine, trimeprazine.

**Urinary acidifier**—makes the urine acid. Examples: ammonium chloride, sodium acid phosphate.

**Urinary alkalizer**—makes the urine alkaline. Examples: sodium bicarbonate, potassium citrate.

**Urinary antiseptic**—produces an antibacterial effect, usually only slight, in the urine. The term is not applied to antibiotics or other antibacterial drugs able to act at other sites in the body. Examples: hexamine, mandelic acid.

**Vaccine**—contains antigen from a micro-organism (or other parasite) which can be used for the artificial immunization of an animal. Examples: infectious canine hepatitis vaccine, leptospirosis vaccine. (**Autogenous vaccine** is a vaccine for administration to an *individual* animal and prepared from material (usually bacteria) taken from that individual.)

**Vasoconstrictor**—produces vasoconstriction, i.e. constriction of blood vessels. Examples: adrenalin (in the blood vessels of the skin), angiotensin.

*****Vasodilator**—produces vasodilation, i.e. dilation of blood vessels. Examples: isoxuprine, isoprenaline.

**Vitamin**—is an organic compound essential to normal tissue metabolism in a very small quantity. Examples: cyanocobalamin (vitamin $B_{12}$), cholecalciferol (vitamin $D_3$).

### Types of Preparation

Drugs can be introduced into or applied on to the body in a variety of forms. The choice of preparation depends not only on the properties of the drug concerned, including any harmful effects it may have, but also where it is required to act, the speed of action desired, and the convenience of administration.

A drug can be applied directly to the affected part of the body if this is at the surface or communicates with the surface. This is described as **local** or **topical** administration, e.g. application to the skin, eye, ear canal, rectum, vagina or mammary gland.

When a drug is required to act on an internal organ or throughout the entire body (i.e. systemically), **systemic** administration is required. This is achieved by giving the drug either **orally**, i.e. by mouth, or **parenterally**, i.e. by injection—usually intravenous, intramuscular or subcutaneous injection, occasionally intraperitoneal injection. Injections are very rarely given into *other* parts of the body and usually only when it is difficult to achieve a high concentration of drug in that particular area, e.g. intra-articular injection (into a joint cavity) and intrathecal injection (into the cerebrospinal fluid). (Parenteral administration means by any route *other than* the oral route, but in practice this invariably means by injection.)

Oral administration is invariably chosen for the treatment of disorders of the alimentary tract. Where systemic treatment is required the drug has first to pass from the site of administration (either the alimentary tract or the site of an injection) into the blood which will then carry it to the part of the body where it is required. This passage from the site of administration is called absorption. It is, of course, immediate with an intravenous injection. In general absorption is faster after intramuscular injection than subcutaneous injection and slowest of all after oral administration (Fig. 6.22). However, if absorption is slower it often means that there will be an effective concentration in the blood for a longer period. Higher doses are commonly required if the oral route is used because following absorption the drug passes first to the liver where some of it may be inactivated.

### A. Oral preparations

#### 1. Tablets

A tablet is a circular, flattened, compressed or moulded mass of a drug or drugs. Some tablets contain other non-active (inert) ingredients to increase the bulk, e.g. lactose. Tablets are the most common form in which drugs are administered orally to small animals.

Some tablets are coated; this is done for one or more of the following reasons:

(1) To improve their appearance and/ or give a characteristic recognizable colour, e.g. the orange or yellow colour of oxytetracycline tablets.

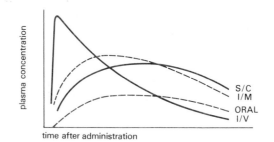

FIG. 6.22.   Plasma levels of a typical drug following its administration by different routes. I/M = intramuscular injection; I/V = intravenous injection; S/C = subcutaneous injection.

(2) To protect them from the atmosphere, particularly from moisture.

(3) To hide an unpleasant taste. For example uncoated "Tribrissen 80" tablets will cause cats, though not dogs, to salivate profusely giving frothing at the mouth. Accordingly the coated "Tribrissen 20" tablets are used for the cat. In some tablets the bitter drug forms a distinct inner core to the tablet because an inert material is compressed all around it, e.g. "Scolaban".

(4) To protect the drug from hydrochloric acid in the stomach which could inactivate it. This type of coating is designed to come off in the alkaline environment of the small intestine. Such tablets are called **enteric-coated**, e.g. "Panteric" tablets.

Consequently tablets which have been coated for reason (3) or (4) above should *not* be crushed or even broken before administration; in one case the animal is most unlikely to consume the drug because of its taste and in the other the drug's activity will be reduced. Such coated tablets should not even be vigorously shaken together because in so doing the tablet coating can crack thereby removing its effectiveness.

## 2. Capsules

A capsule (strictly a hard capsule) consists of two cylindrical halves, or shells, made of gelatin (each with a sealed, hemispherical end) fitted together to enclose the drug which is in powder or granular form. The outer half has to be of a slightly larger diameter to fit over the inner half of the capsule.

They are usually used to disguise the bitter taste of drugs, e.g. chloramphenicol. However, with one product ("Tryplase") the capsules are not swallowed but the two halves are pulled apart so that the granules they contain can be sprinkled onto the food.

(Soft or flexible capsules of soft gelatin containing liquids, e.g. halibut-liver oil capsules, are not often used in veterinary practice.)

## 3. Powders, Granules and Flakes, etc.

Certain drugs may be prepared in bulk in the form of a powder or as granules or flakes, etc., for addition to an animal's food, or in the case of dispersible (i.e. soluble) powders to its drinking water. These preparations are particularly suitable:

(a) where the drug affects digestion or faecal consistency and therefore is best given with food (e.g. pancreatin, sterculia), and

(b) for the treatment of very young animals (puppies, kittens) or very small species (budgerigars, hamsters, etc.); e.g. oxytetracycline is available as a soluble powder which can be dissolved in cage birds' drinking water.

It is important that these preparations do not have an unattractive taste.

At one time individual doses of powder were separately wrapped and were referred to as "powders". Although these still persist as human remedies (e.g. "Beecham's Powders") they have disappeared from small animal therapy.

### 4. *Mixtures*

A mixture is a liquid medicine intended to be divided into a number of doses for administration to the patient.

(a) Some drugs are completely soluble in water. Such **solutions** can in some cases be added in small quantity to the drinking water of the smaller species (e.g. cage birds).

(b) Other drugs are insoluble and are dispensed as **suspensions** (e.g. of kaolin in water) which require to be thoroughly shaken in the container before administration.

(c) A syrupy liquid should strictly be referred to as a **syrup** or a **linctus** (e.g. codeine linctus), although the term mixture is also used, e.g. cough mixture.

(d) An **emulsion** is a suspension of oils (or fats) and water stabilized with an emulsifying agent so that the components do not readily separate out again. Although available (e.g.

liquid paraffin emulsion) they are seldom used to treat small animals.

### 5. *Oral Creams*

Occasionally a drug is mixed with other ingredients to form a semisolid mass known as an oral paste or cream. This is most conveniently administered from a plastic "doser" (resembling a disposable syringe) directly into the animal's mouth, e.g. "Penbritin Oral Doser" for the administration of ampicillin to dogs and cats.

### 6. *Other Oral Preparations*

Other oral preparations are seldom used. *Pills,* which consist of drugs and other ingredients made into a spherical or ovoid shape and often coated, have been replaced by tablets. *Cachets* (receptacles made of rice paper containing powdered drug), *pastilles* (soft masses with a basis of gelatin and glycerin plug the drug) and *lozenges* (hard, flat, sugar-based shapes incorporating the drug) are not convenient for administration to small animals.

### B. Parenteral preparations—injections

Drugs for injection are usually prepared ready for use either as a **solution** or if the drug is insoluble as fine particles suspended in the liquid, i.e. as a **suspension**. They are packed in single-dose vials or more usually multi-dose bottles with rubber closures. The preparations must be sterile.

*Solutions* consist of the drug—the solute —dissolved in the liquid—the solvent. If the solvent is water the solution is called an **aqueous solution** (e.g. streptomycin solution), and this usually can be given by any injection route. Highly irritant solutions are preferably given intravenously.

Some drug solutions are only stable for a short period, i.e. the drug changes into an inactive form fairly quickly. Such drugs (e.g. sodium benzylpenicillin) are supplied as a powder in a vial to which sterile water is added to prepare the solution for use. Solutions of such drugs retain their activity for a few days longer if they are stored in the cool compartment of a refrigerator (4°C) after being prepared. Solutions can also be prepared by dissolving soluble tablets of a drug in sterile water.

If a solvent other than water is used it may be dangerous to inject the solution directly into the blood stream; it may be recommended by the manufacturer that an intravenous injection is either not given or that it is given very slowly. Injection by routes other than the intramuscular or subcutaneous is usually not recommended.

*Suspensions* (e.g. of procaine benzylpenicillin) should be well shaken before any liquid is withdrawn to ensure that all the drug is evenly suspended. Suspensions are usually only injected intramuscularly or subcutaneously. Intravenous injection is particularly dangerous because the drug particles can block small capillaries, e.g. in the brain.

## C. Topical preparations

*Applied to external surfaces and organs in close communication with the exterior.*

### 1. Creams

A cream is a semi-solid emulsion of oil, or fat, and water which usually incorporates drugs. It is applied externally without friction, and spreads easily. When made with an animal fat such as lanolin (wool fat) it rapidly penetrates into the skin. Water-soluble drugs are more active in creams than in ointments, and nowadays creams are more commonly used than ointments.

### 2. Ointments

An ointment is a semi-solid substance consisting of a drug or drugs in a base of wax or fat applied externally without friction. Usually soft paraffin (petroleum jelly) is used as the base which produces a non-penetrating ointment acting at the surface only.

(a) **Eye ointments** (ophthalmic ointments) are similar but more liquid, having a base of soft paraffin and lanolin, and possibly also liquid paraffin. They must be sterile when applied.

(b) **Intramammary ointments** (intramammary injections) contain the drug(s), usually antibiotics, in an oily base, either vegetable or mineral oil. Again they should be sterile. These preparations are intended principally for insertion into the udder of cows via the teat canal. However, their semi-fluid consistency and the narrow nozzle of the tubes in which they are presented makes it convenient to insert them into puncture wounds such as those caused by cat bites, which are very common in small animal practice. (Antibiotic intramammary ointments have also been inserted into the abdominal cavity of small animals, but this practice is not recommended as a routine since some animals have died from the toxic effects of streptomycin.) Intramammary preparations should not be used as eye ointments because they have an irritant effect on the cornea.

### 3. Dusting Powders

A finely divided powder intended for application to the skin is referred to as a dusting-powder. In small animal practice they are mainly used:

(1) Containing parasiticides to kill the larger external parasites, e.g. "Pybuthrin Dusting Powder" dusting-powder containing pyrethrins and piperonyl butoxide. The parasiticides employed vary in their toxicity but in general dusting-powders are best (a) *not* applied to breaks in the skin and open wounds, and (b) not licked off and consumed in large amounts by the animal. This is most easily avoided by brushing out the residue of powder half-an-hour or so after application, preventing the animal licking in the meantime.

(2) As an antibacterial dressing on open wounds and eczematous areas, e.g. sulphanilamide powder (a sulphonamide). Such antibacterial powders must be sterile.

**Wettable powders** (e.g. "Cooper's Skin Dressing No. 3") are applied to the skin as a suspension after mixing with a large quantity of water. A treated animal's coat is dried by warmth, rather than rubbing with a towel, so that the powder remains on the coat.

### 4. *Liquid Applications*

(a) **Lotions** are liquid preparations intended for application to the skin without friction. They usually consist of solutions or suspensions of the drug(s) in water, e.g. calamine lotion, and are applied by swabbing.

(b) **Eye lotions** (ophthalmic lotions) are solutions, usually aqueous, of drugs for bathing the eyes to remove infection or foreign bodies, e.g. boric acid eye lotions. They are often prepared more concentrated than required so that they can be diluted with warm water and thereby used as warm solutions.

(c) **Applications** are referred to as semi-liquid preparations, i.e. they are less fluid than lotions, but intended to be used in the same manner; e.g. benzyl benzoate emulsion.

(d) Eye and ear drops. *Eye drops* (opthalmic drops) are sterile aqueous or oily solutions or suspensions of drugs for instillation into the eye. They are used for a variety of purposes including diagnosis of ophthalmic disorders.

*Ear drops* are most commonly used in small animal practice to treat infections of the ear with ear mites (*Otodectes cynotis*) or bacteria. They frequently have an oily base, and may be "thicker" than eye drops, though at least one manufacturer produces drops suitable for application to both ear and eye ("Betsolan Eye and Ear Drops").

(e) **Sprays.** Aerosol sprays are liquid solutions or suspensions of drugs packed under pressure, with a propellant gas, in a metal container. Pressure on the nozzle button causes the contents to be emitted as a fine spray, or aerosol, which is directed on to the affected part of the skin. Aerosol sprays are convenient for the application of antibacterial drugs (particularly to raw areas such as burns) and parasiticides (e.g. dichlorvos and fenitrothion together—"Nuvan Top"). Care should be taken not to spray directly into the eyes.

(f) **Medicated shampoos** are aqueous solutions or suspensions of drugs which have a detergent base. They are usually used for the application of parasiticides (e.g. selenium sulphide and gamma-benzene hexachloride), and the presence of the detergent gives thorough penetration of the coat. After remaining in contact with the skin for the recommended period of time the shampoo should be thoroughly rinsed away.

(g) **Liniments** are liquid or semi-liquid preparations intended for application to the skin with friction, and are commonly referred to as "rubbing oils". They often have a spirit or oily base and are applied with a piece of flannel or lint. Liniments should not be used on broken skin. Generally they have some rubefacient action (e.g. White Liniment) and are used to treat sprains and strains, most commonly in hunting and racing dogs.

(h) **Irrigations** are solutions, usually of antiseptic or other antibacterial drugs, which are diluted with warm water and used to flush out wounds or body cavities.

### 5. Poultices

A poultice is a semi-solid mixture of drugs which is applied externally, as hot as can be borne, sandwiched between two layers of gauze or lint and usually bandaged in place. It is a means of applying heat to a site (usually of bacterial infection or of a sprain). Some types, e.g. kaolin poultice, also exert a considerable osmotic pressure producing a "drawing" effect which is valuable in removing toxic products. A poultice requires to be renewed at least once daily. In small animal practice hot fomentations are often used instead of poulticing (p. 311).

### 6. Suppositories and Pessaries

**Suppositories** are elongated cone-shaped or torpedo-shaped masses containing drugs intended for introduction into an organ.

The name suppository alone, i.e. without the name of the organ into which it is to be inserted, refers to a **rectal suppository**, and in common usage suppositories are names for the masses introduced into the rectum.

**Pessary** is an alternative, and more commonly used, name for a vaginal or uterine suppository.

Both types have an oily (e.g. cocoa butter) or glyco-gelatin base which softens

at body temperature so that the suppository melts releasing the drug. Rectal suppositories have been used in small animals as an alternative to enemas for promoting defaecation, but the latter are usually preferred because they are more often efficacious. Pessaries containing antibacterial drugs are employed in large animals to combat or prevent infection, especially after parturition, but are seldom used in small animals.

### 7. Enemas

These are fluids which are infused into the rectum to soften faecal masses and distend the bowel, thereby stimulating the expulsion of faeces. They are commonly solutions of soap (e.g. soap flakes or soft soap) or may incorporate glycerine, and are used warm.

### 8. Other External Preparations

There is little use in small animal practice of other external applications which are employed in human medicine, e.g. **gargles**, **nasal drops** and **mouth washes**, and large animal medicine, e.g. **paints** (liquid preparations, usually of dyes, for application to the skin or mucous membranes) and **pastes** (solid preparations usually applied on a piece of lint).

## D. Preparations administered by other routes

### 1. Inhalations

An inhalation is a liquid preparation composed of, or containing volatile ingredients which when vaporized (usually by hot water) and inhaled are intended to penetrate as far as the lining of the respiratory tract. (The active ingredients can also be termed inhalations.) Examples are Friar's Balsam and "Vick Vapour Rub". Although of more limited use in small animals than in humans, they can be of benefit to animals with respiratory infections by helping to "loosen" and remove mucus.

## 2. *Implants*

An implant is a small disc or cylinder of relatively insoluble drugs usually including a hormone, e.g. implants of testosterone or of progesterone. The implant is usually inserted beneath the skin, i.e. subcutaneously implanted, in a sterile manner using a special trocar, canula and expeller. The implant dissolves only slowly so that the hormone is slowly released over a period of weeks or months, thus avoiding the need for repeated administration by some other route.

## Legal Aspects of Pharmacy

At the present time the use of medicinal products by veterinary surgeons in the United Kingdom is governed by two Acts of Parliament; these are the **Medicines Act 1968** and the **Misuse of Drugs Act 1971**. The Medicines Act 1968 controls the manufacture and distribution of all medicinal products. The Misuse of Drugs Act 1971 imposes additional, more stringent, controls on the distribution and possession of certain drugs which are subject to abuse (drugs of addiction) and which are termed **controlled drugs**.

The following descriptions of these Acts should not be regarded as comprehensive or authoritative statements of the law. It is intended mainly to draw attention to those parts of the Acts relating to the work of veterinary surgeons in *small animal practice* particularly those that may concern animal veterinary nurses.

## Medicines Act 1968

This legislation controls the manufacture, sale and supply (including importation and exportation) of all medicinal products, including those intended for the diagnosis, treatment or prevention of disease, including anaesthesia and preventing, or interfering with, a normal physiological function (such as oestrus). Medicinal products intended for administration to animals are classed as **veterinary drugs**, even though the same basic product may be used also for the treatment of humans. It should be appreciated that the description refers not only to products supplied to veterinary surgeons by pharmaceutical companies but also includes a large number of patent medicines sold for animal use in such places as pet-shops.

## 1. *Quality, Safety and Efficacy*

The safety, efficacy and quality of medicinal products is controlled by a system of licences and certificates issued by the Secretary of State for Health and in the case of veterinary drugs the Secretary of State for Agriculture.

(a) To ensure that a particular product is safe, efficacious, and of sufficient quality, the person who devises its composition (or imports it from elsewhere) has to supply proof of its quality, safety and efficacy (e.g. from tests); he will then be issued with a **product licence**. Until a product licence is issued, no-one may manufacture or sell the product.

(b) A *manufacturer's licence* is required before anyone can manufacture any medicinal product or assemble it (which means package and label it).

(c) A *wholesale dealer's licence* is required by anyone conducting wholesale trade in medicinal products.

(d) Before a new product can be tested, (i) on humans *a clinical trial certificate* is required, (ii) on animals an *animal test certificate* is required.

However, **a veterinary surgeon does not require a licence to specially prepare a product himself**, or to have it specially prepared for him by someone else (e.g. a pharmacist or another veterinary surgeon), provided it is intended for administration to an animal under his care. Likewise the person who specially prepares the product at the veterinary surgeon's request does not need a licence.

Nevertheless, a licence *is* required by the veterinary surgeon if:

(a) he proposes to keep in stock more than 5 litres (liquid) or 2.5 kg (solid) of the product prepared; *or*

(b) a vaccine (other than a mammalian autogenous vaccine) is to be prepared.

A medicinal product must not be advertised to a veterinary surgeon either by word of mouth (e.g. by a sales representative) or by sending him an advertisement, unless at the same time he receives a **data sheet** (giving essential information on the product relating to its uses, administration, toxicity, dosage, etc.) or has received one in the previous 15 months. False or misleading statements are an offence.

## 2. Sale and Supply

It is considered that in general medicinal products should be sold to the public only by a qualified pharmacist, i.e. a Member of the Pharmaceutical Society (MPS). However, it is recognized that there are some medicinal products (e.g. patent medicines for both human and animal use) which it would be both safe and convenient for members of the public to be able to obtain from a variety of outlets (e.g. grocers, supermarkets, pet shops) and not only from a registered pharmacy.

On the other hand, it is considered that the consequences of misusing certain drugs are so serious that these drugs should only be supplied to a member of the public by a pharmacist if the pharmacist receives written instructions from a doctor, dentist or veterinary surgeon, i.e. upon receipt of a prescription.

Accordingly medicinal products are classified into three main categories, (a), (b) and (c) below.

### (a) General Sale List Products

These are the products which can be sold or supplied to the public by many different types of traders, i.e. without the supervision of a pharmacist. Almost 700 veterinary drugs are on the general sale list but the supply of many of them is restricted in some way. For example there may be a limit on the maximum strength of drug that can be supplied or on the total quantity per package, and some can only be supplied for external use or for administration by a specified route.

Examples of the types of veterinary products on the general sale list are:

(i) certain anthelmintics, namely dichlorophen, diethylcarbamazine citrate and piperazine;

(ii) certain shampoos and parasiticides, including flea collars;

(iii) herbal remedies;

(iv) castor oil.

The types of veterinary products which do *not* appear on the general sale list are those:

(i) for use as anthelmintics (*excepting* those mentioned in the previous paragraph);

(ii) for parenteral injection;

(iii) for use as eye drops or eye ointments;

(iv) for the internal treatment of ringworm.

### (b) Prescription Only Medicines (**POM**)

These are medicinal products which in general may be supplied by a pharmacist upon receipt of a prescription provided by a doctor, dentist or veterinary surgeon.

There is a list of such products which includes:

(i) all controlled drugs (i.e. controlled by the Misuse of Drugs Act 1971);
(ii) antibiotics and sulphonamides;
(iii) corticosteroids and many hormone preparation (though not insulin);
(iv) barbiturates and tranquillizers;
(v) vaccines and antisera,
and many other drugs.

### (c) Pharmacy Medicines

These are medicinal products which in general can only be purchased by the public from a registered pharmacy, but which *do not* require to be prescribed by a doctor, dentist or veterinary surgeon. When supplied by retail (or wholesale) trading pharmacy medicines must be labelled with the symbol,

$$\boxed{\text{P}}$$

There is no list of pharmacy medicines but they include *all* products not specifically listed as either (a) general sale list products, or (b) prescription only medicines.

*Sale and supply by veterinary surgeons.*

Despite the general rules stated above, a veterinary surgeon is able to sell or supply directly to his client *any* product in *any* of the three categories listed (with a few important exceptions) *provided* it is for the treatment of an animal under the veterinary surgeon's care.

Those drugs which a veterinary surgeon cannot supply are:

(a) controlled drugs contained in Schedule 4 of the Misuse of Drugs Act 1971,
(b) phenacetin
(c) stilbenes, e.g. stilboestrol (though not oestradiol), and
(d) thyrostatic drugs, i.e. anti-thyroid drugs, used to increase an animals' body weight (really only applicable to large animal practice).

*Use by veterinary surgeons and others.* Those veterinary drugs which are classified as prescription only medicines, including all parenteral (chiefly injectable) preparations, may only be administered by a veterinary surgeon or *a person following his instructions,* which would include RANAs.

*Prescribing by veterinary surgeons.*

(a) A prescription provided by a veterinary surgeon for a *prescription only medicine* (for a client to obtain it from a pharmacy) must be written in indelible ink (so that it cannot be altered) and must contain:

(i) his usual signature;
(ii) his address;
(iii) an indication that he is a veterinary surgeon (i.e. his qualifications);
(iv) the date on which he signed the prescription;
(v) the name and address of the person to be supplied with the medicine (i.e. the client);
(vi) the declaration "This prescription is issued in respect of animals under my care", or words with a similar meaning.

It is also advisable, though not legally required, for the prescription to state the total amount to be supplied and the dose.

The drug will not be dispensed more than 6 months later *or* more than once on the same prescription (i.e. the prescription will not be repeated) *unless* the prescription states that dispensing *may* be repeated. If the prescription states that it may be repeated but does not specify the total number of times, the drug will be dispensed only twice.

(b) Although there is *no legal requirement* for a veterinary surgeon to provide a prescription in order for his client to be able to purchase a *pharmacy medicine* (or for that matter a general sale list product) from a pharmacy, there is also nothing to prevent him from doing so, e.g. if he feels that his client may not remember what product to ask for. However, a note of the name of the product, rather than a full prescription, would probably be adequate in this situation. Only a prescription only medicine *must* be prescribed before it can be purchased from a pharmacy.

*3. Labelling*

Manufacturers and wholesalers of medicinal products must label each container with certain particulars about the product relating to its composition, use and storage, including any warning or special precautions to be taken.

Of more immediate concern to the veterinary surgeon is the labelling of products he supplies (i.e. dispenses) to his clients.

The container of a medicinal product (i.e. the bottle, box, packet or other receptacle, that immediately encloses the product) dispensed by a veterinary surgeon must be clearly and legibly labelled with the following particulars:

(a) The name of the person who has possession or control of the animal and the address where the animal is kept.

(b) The name and address of the veterinary surgeon.

(c) The date of dispensing.

(d) The words "For animal treatment only" unless the container is too small for it to be reasonably practicable to include them.

(e) The words "Keep out of the reach of children", or words with a similar meaning.

(f) The words "For external use only" in a separate rectangle *if* the product is a liniment, lotion, antiseptic or other *liquid* for external use only. If such liquids contain certain substances they should also be dispensed in fluted bottles, i.e. having vertical ridges, so that they can be readily recognized by touch.

The container need *not* be labelled *provided* that it is enclosed in a package (i.e. another box or packet) which *is* labelled. This is useful where the container (e.g. of eye ointment) is too small to label easily.

It is also valuable, but not a legal requirement, to include on the label:

(i) the name of the product and its strength;

(ii) directions for use;

(iii) precautions concerning its use;

(iv) the name of the animal, especially if there is more than one in the household.

There is no legal requirement for a veterinary surgeon to keep a record of the drugs he supplies (other than controlled drugs), although this is often a wise precaution.

## Misuse of Drugs Act 1971

This legislation controls the possession and use of those drugs likely to be misused, i.e. drugs of addiction, and which are referred to as **controlled drugs**. These used to be termed dangerous drugs.

## 1. Classification

Controlled drugs are classified in one of four schedules according to their harmfulness if misused.

*Schedule 1* contains the least harmful preparations, including products containing:

(a) a very low level of cocaine, morphine or opium which cannot be readily extracted and concentrated, (e.g. Kaolin and Morphine Mixture);

(b) Codeine or pholcodine (e.g. cough mixtures).

Only the manufacture and supply of these products is controlled and they are *not* subject to *any* of the regulations described later (e.g. storage, record keeping, etc.).

*Schedule 2* contains some of the most harmful drugs including those most likely to be of use to veterinary surgeons, e.g. pethidine, etorphine (in "Immobilon"), fentanyl in "Hypnorm" and also morphine, cocaine and the amphetamines. They are subject to *all* the regulations described later (purchase, storage, records, special prescription requirements and destruction).

*Schedule 3* contains drugs less harmful than in Schedules 2 and 4, (e.g. minor stimulants, such as benzphetamine) but these are unlikely to be used in veterinary practice. They are subject to all the regulations described later except those concerning records and destruction.

*Schedule 4* contains drugs which normally have no use in medical or veterinary practice (e.g. cannabis, LSD and mescaline) and consequently veterinary surgeons and others are *not* allowed to possess or use them (unless they have a special licence).

## 2. Regulations

Veterinary surgeons and certain other "authorized persons" are allowed to possess, prescribe, administer and supply all of the drugs in Schedules 1, 2 and 3 (but *not* Schedule 4) provided they are all for professional use. Even so, special regulations apply and these are described in (a) to (e) below.

### (a) Purchase

Schedule 2 and 3 drugs may only be obtained (from a pharmacist, wholesaler or manufacturer) by a veterinary surgeon if he supplies a written requisition (i.e. a written order) which must contain:

(i) his signature;
(ii) his name, address and profession;
(iii) the purpose for which the drug is required;
(iv) the total quantity of drug required.

If a messenger is sent to collect the drug the veterinary surgeon must also supply, as well as the requisition, a signed letter which authorizes the messenger to receive the drug on the veterinary surgeon's behalf.

### (b) Storage

Schedule 2 and 3 drugs must be kept in a locked receptacle (e.g. an immovable cupboard) which can be opened only by the veterinary surgeon or a person authorized by him.

### (c) Records

For Schedule 2 drugs records must be kept in a bound (not a loose-leaf) book, called a *register*, of (i) all drug purchases, and (ii) all drugs administered (to animals) and supplied (to clients for them to administer to their animals). The register must not be used for any other purpose.

Particular requirements are:

(i) A *separate* register is required for each premises where controlled drugs are kept (i.e. for each branch surgery). However, only *one* register must be kept for *each* premises.

(ii) A *separate* part of the register must be used for each drug, e.g. pethidine in one part, etorphine in another etc. The drug to which the entries on a page refer must be written at the *top* of the page. In addition, separate pages are needed for (i) purchase, and (ii) administration and supply.

(iii) Each entry must be made within 24 hours of the actual receipt, administration or supply of the drug.

(iv) Entries on a page must be made in chronological order.

(v) Entries must be indelible and must not be cancelled, obliterated or altered. If any corrections are necessary they must be made by means of a note in the margin or at the foot of the page, which must state the date on which the correction was made.

(vi) The register must be kept for at least 2 years after the date of the last entry.

---

For **purchases** of the drug the following information must be recorded in the following form:

| Date on which supply received | NAME and ADDRESS of person or firm from whom obtained | Amount obtained | Form in which obtained |
|---|---|---|---|
| 14–7–84 | F. Jones Ltd., 4 Market Street, Greenston | 20 × 50 mg | Pethidine tablets |

For the **administration or supply** of a drug the following information must be recorded in the following form:

| Date on which the transaction was effected | NAME and ADDRESS of person or firm supplied | Particulars as to licence or authority of person or firm supplied to be in possession | Amount supplied | Form in which supplied |
|---|---|---|---|---|
| 17–8–84 | W. Smith, 5 Station Rd., Greenston | Dispensed | 6 × 50 mg | Pethidine tablets |
| 18–8–84 | D. Brown's dog, 8 Vale Road, Greenston | Direct administration | 25 mg | Pethidine injection 1 ml |

It is not necessary for a veterinary surgeon to enter in the register drugs supplied *on prescription* and dispensed by a pharmacist.

---

(d) Special Prescription Requirements

A prescription supplied by a veterinary surgeon to a client to permit the client to purchase a Schedule 2 or 3 drug from a pharmacist must be indelible, usually by being written in ink.

It must contain all the information which is normally required on a prescription for a prescription only medicine (the name, address, qualifications and signature of the veterinary surgeon and a statement that the drug is for an animal under his care, plus the name and address of the client and the date of the prescription). But in addition it *must* state:

(i) the dose of the drug:
(ii) the total quantity of the drug (in both words and figures), plus the form and strength of the preparation (i.e. 50 mg pethidine tablets);
(iii) the words "For animal treatment only".

As well as his signature the veterinary surgeon himself must write, i.e. in his *own* handwriting, the client's name and address, the dose and total quantity, form and strength of the drug.

A prescription for a controlled drug will not be dispensed if it is presented more than 13 weeks after the date of issue.

(e) Destruction of Drugs

Schedule 2 and 3 drugs which are no longer required can *only* be disposed of by being destroyed in the presence of an authorized person (e.g. drug squad officers and Home Office inspectors) and following their instructions. An appropriate entry relating to the destruction must be made in the veterinary surgeon's register and witnessed by the authorized person.

## Care and Labelling of Drugs

The *expiry date* on a product should be noted and stocks of that drug arranged so that they are used in rotation, i.e. so that the older ones are used or supplied first. (An expiry date is not required by law if the product will retain its potency for more than 3 years, but rotation should still be practised.)

As has been mentioned previously there are legal requirements for controlled drugs to be stored at all times in a locked receptacle. For other drugs any special recommendations made by the manufacturer should be followed. Drugs which might be stolen and mis-used should be stored in areas not accessible to the public. There are certain preparations which should be kept in the cool compartment (4°C) of a refrigerator, e.g. vaccines, antisera and certain injectable hormone preparations (e.g. insulin). In general all other drugs should be stored in cool, dry conditions away from strong sunlight. Many preparations are adversely affected by heat; drugs may be inactivated and some preparations such as creams and ointments may separate out. On the other hand, damp causes powders to clog and sugar coatings on tablets to become sticky.

For the storage of drugs it is better to use cupboards and shelves rather than to stack a number of boxes of medicinal products one upon the other. The weight can crush and spoil containers at the bottom and may even cause bottles to crack. To reduce breakages and prevent accidents to staff, shelves should not be overstocked and heavy bottles and large containers should be stored near floor level. If boxes are in contact with the floor, care is needed when the floor is washed to ensure that these are not soaked in water. It is preferable not to use shelves above head height, but if this is necessary secure ladders or stools should be provided to reach them safely.

Preparations for dispensing should be neatly arranged alphabetically according to proprietary names. (Alternatively drugs can be arranged so that those with a similar purpose are in a similar location e.g. all anthelminthics together, all eye preparations together, etc.) This will save considerable time in finding the drug in dispensing and in checking stock-lists for re-ordering.

It is advisable to open only one pack of a particular preparation at one time and always to keep the lids on containers. This is particularly important with liquids, especially those containing spirit, because evaporation will take place if the container is not sealed causing concentration of the other ingredients. If a number of tablet preparations have been dispensed at the same time, care should be taken to ensure that any surplus tablets are replaced in the correct containers. Drug preparations should always be handled with clean hands (to avoid contaminating tablets, etc.) and the hands should be washed again after handling toxic drugs, in the meantime taking care not to smoke, eat etc., or even rub the eyes.

Coated tablets should be handled carefully; unnecessary shaking of the container may result in the coating being cracked. Any spillages of powders, liquids, etc. produced in dispensing should be wiped up straight away.

## Methods of Dispensing and Correct Labelling

In former times dispensing in a veterinary practice involved making up products from their basic ingredients, but nowadays (as in most pharmacies) it is chiefly concerned with packaging and labelling ready-manufactured products for supply to clients. Consequently it would be unrealistic to describe how to make ointments, emulsions, powders and other types of preparations. Similarly, describing the dispensing of a prescription

(as occurs in a pharmacy) would be of little value since it is highly improbable that this occurs within any small animal practice.

A knowledge of the use of a **dispensing (pharmaceutical) balance** (Fig. 6.23) was important for dispensing but it is now unusual for any drug to be weighed. Although powders and ointments are solid preparations that can be purchased in bulk and then supplied to clients in smaller quantities the amount being supplied is seldom weighed out in a veterinary practice. Instead the preparation is supplied by volume, i.e. the amount that will fill a certain size of container. If this is the case it would be advisable to weigh a few containers before and after filling with the preparation to know the approximate weight of preparation that is being supplied, particularly for costing purposes.

To do this either a dispensing balance, or a more accurate analytical (laboratory) balance, can be used. With an analytical balance the weights are placed on the right-hand scale pan and the object or material being weighed on the left-hand pan, but with a dispensing balance the opposite is true. With a dispensing balance the right-hand pan is removable and almost always made of glass; preparations can be placed directly upon it (a practice which is not recommended with the fixed stainless steel pan of a laboratory balance). Washing the glass scale pan after use is necessary but easily done.

When using either balance the pointer should rest on the zero mark of the scale when the beam is raised, both:

(i) before use; and
(ii) when the weights and the material being weighed, i.e. in opposite pans, are exactly balanced.

When the beam of a *dispensing balance* is raised during weighing:

(i) if the pointer swings to the left side of the scale it indicates that the

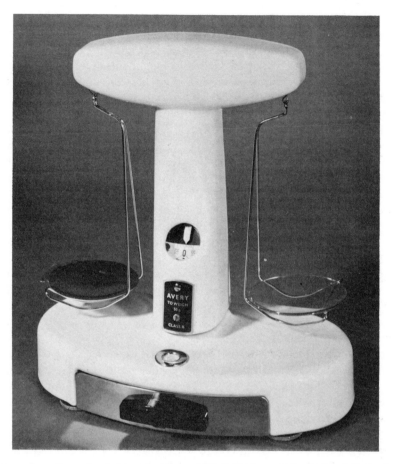

FIG. 6.23.   A modern dispensing balance (courtesy of W. & T. Avery Ltd., Smethwick). In the base is a drawer containing weights and above it is a spirit-level for accurate positioning. This type has no lever to raise the beam and therefore the pans remain permanently in the weighing position. Weights are placed in the left-hand pan and the material being weighed in the right-hand (glass) pan. The pointer and zero mark can be seen contained within the central pillar.

material being weighed is heavier; and

(ii) if the pointer swings to the right side of the scale it indicates that the weights are heavier.

**Use of a dispensing balance**

Always check that a full set of metric weights is available.

(a) **To weigh out a predetermined amount of material** (e.g. to weigh out a certain number of grams of powder).

Place individual weights up to the total weight required in the left-hand pan and add material to the right-hand pan (and later, if necessary, remove some), until the pointer, when the beam is raised, comes to rest on the zero mark of the scale.

(b) **To weigh an object** (e.g. an empty or filled container). Place in the left-hand pan a weight slightly greater than the estimated weight of the object. Thereafter

(i) if raising the beam shows the *total weights* are *heavier* remove the last weight that was added and replace it with the next lightest weight in the set; (ii) if raising the beam shows that the *object* is *heavier* add to the weights the next heaviest weight in the set. Continue in this manner until the pointer comes to rest on the zero mark of the scale. (For the use of an analytical balance refer to *Veterinary Laboratory Manual*, B. M. Bush, Heinemann Medical Books, London, 1975 pp. 75–80).

In general supplying drug preparations to clients in a small animal practice will involve at the time of supply *either,* (a) labelling commercially packed containers, e.g. of eye-drops, creams, cough mixtures, dusting powders, etc., *or* (b) labelling containers which have been filled beforehand (i.e. packaged) in the practice with preparations ordered in bulk, e.g. ointments, powders, liquids, etc.

Usually only tablets or capsules will need to be packed as well as labelled *at the time they are supplied*; this is because the number supplied will depend on the size of the animal and the length of treatment required.

Therefore, with the exception of tablets and capsules all the packaging of preparations which may be required in a small animal practice can be carried out beforehand. This prepackaging of items (usually a dozen or more at a time) is generally carried out at regular intervals as the need arises.

## Packaging

The packaging of medicines should ideally be carried out on a generous area of a working surface which can be easily cleaned. Eating, drinking or smoking at the same time should not be permitted.

### (a) *Powders*

Parasiticide or antibacterial dusting powders, or soluble powders for addition to food or drinking water, purchased in bulk are usually dispensed in cardboard or plastic containers with push-on or screw-top lids. Parasiticides are best supplied with perforated lids on the container to simplify their application. The perforations are usually covered at the time of supply by a removable disc of card or paper.

Containers are most easily filled using a teaspoon which should be reserved solely for this function. Care should be taken not to disturb the powder more than is necessary because powder in the air can be inhaled, and with toxic drugs this is undesirable. For complete filling the container should be tapped gently a few times to remove air mixed with the powder, i.e. to shake it down. Surplus powder on the outside of the container should be wiped away.

### (b) *Ointments*

These can be packaged in ointment boxes (usually of the "seamless" type, stamped out of card), or plastic containers, or proper glass ointment jars with screw-on lids which are, however, relatively expensive. Cardboard ointment boxes are often adequate, but if filled some time beforehand, the greasy base can penetrate the cardboard giving an unpleasant appearance and making it difficult to attach a label.

The containers are best filled using a **palette knife** (referred to as a **spatula**) whose width is less than the internal diameter of the container. The ointment should be taken from the bulk supply on one side of the end of the spatula and deposited in the container by drawing the end of the spatula across the container's edge. This is repeated, taking care not to trap air in the container, until it is full. Finally, the surface is smoothed off, any surplus ointment on the container is wiped away and the container lid applied.

### (c) *Liquids*

Those for internal use are usually dispensed in flattish glass or rigid plastic bottles with smooth sides (medical flats) most commonly holding 50 ml, 100 ml or 150 ml, and fitted with plastic screw-caps with waterproofed cardboard liners.

Liquids for external use only should be supplied in **fluted bottles**, i.e. having vertical ridges.

It is usually difficult to fill the bottles directly from a larger, heavy bottle without spilling the liquid or knocking the bottles over, and therefore it is best to pour a quantity into some other vessel from which the bottles can be filled. If the liquid is a suspension it should be well shaken (i.e. in the container in which it is supplied and with the cap firmly in place) and the container inverted before any is poured out to check that no sediment remains at the bottom.

Any jug or beaker with a lip which allows easy pouring would be suitable from which to fill the bottles. However, if some dilution of the manufactured preparation is required, it is simpler to use a proper pharmaceutical **measuring cylinder** which has volume graduations on its side and a suitable lip for pouring.

If the preparation being diluted is one which readily forms a froth or lather (e.g. "Savlon"), the water should be added slowly, and without force, to minimize its production.

Bottles should usually be filled to the junction of the shoulders and the neck, any spillage being wiped away and the screw-cap then applied. Filling is simplified if a funnel is used.

### (d) *Tablets and Capsules*

These can be carefully shaken out onto a clean and dry surface, e.g. the lid from the bulk container (glass jar or plastic box) or a piece of clean paper. They can then be counted into the container in which they are to be supplied, provided the hands are clean.

An alternative is to use a triangular metal or plastic **tablet counter** which simplifies the counting of large numbers of tablets. This triangle is provided with shallow sides except for one corner, from which the tablets, after being counted, can be poured into the container. If tablets with flattish sides are arranged one layer deep on the tablet counter and the counter slightly tilted towards one of the two enclosed corners, the tablets will be found to arrange themselves in rows; the first containing only one tablet, the second two, the third three, and so on. Simple arithmetic will show that two complete rows contain 3 tablets, three rows will contain 6, four rows 10, five rows 15, six rows 21, and so on. By arranging the tablets in rows and then adding or subtracting individual tablets any desired number can readily be counted. Because of their shape it is not possible to use this device with capsules, and it may not work efficiently with tablets having more rounded edges because these tend to overlap each other and not form distinct rows.

If the tablets are ready-packaged in metal foil strips, sufficient should be torn off, taking care not to tear into a section containing a tablet.

Rigid plastic containers with lids or self-sealing plastic packets are preferable as containers to small cardboard boxes or paper envelopes. Plastic (or paper) packets can be ready-printed with such information as the name and address of the veterinary surgeon and the words "For animal treatment only" and "Keep out of the reach of children", and space left for such other details as the client's name and address and the dose. Any label printed *on* the container should have these other details added *or alternatively* a separate label, again with these details already filled in should be attached to the container, *before* the tablets or capsules are inserted. The container should then be securely sealed.

There is apparently no legal requirement for a veterinary practice to dispense drugs in childproof containers.

## Labelling

The legal requirements for the labelling of medicinal products supplied by a veterinary surgeon have been stated earlier under the heading of the Medicines Act 1968. These requirements are the same for preparations containing controlled drugs.

Gummed-paper labels do not always adhere effectively to plastic surfaces (often peeling off as the gum dries). Increasingly widely used are self-adhesive paper labels which can be peeled from a backing sheet before application to the container; these will adhere to any dry surface. Either type can be ready-printed with the name and address of the veterinary surgeon, the words "For animal treatment only" and the words "Keep out of the reach of children", leaving space for the other necessary information.

A separate label bearing the words "For external use only" within a rectangle can be affixed to bottles containing liquid intended for external use only.

The handwritten part of the label must be clear and legible and it is prudent to write all instructions in full without abbreviation to avoid any misinterpretation. A ballpoint pen or fine fibre-tipped pen is preferable; fountain pen ink will run if the label becomes wet.

Always write the label before attaching it to the container. Usually the label is attached after filling the container, but in the case of labels to be affixed to tablet envelopes or packets they should be completed *and* attached before the tablets or capsules are placed inside. If two or more preparations are being dispensed at the same time particular care must be taken to avoid attaching them to the wrong package.

When attaching self-adhesive labels to bottles, make sure that the bottle is dry. The label should be stuck on straight in the centre of one of the flat sides.

Because the labels needed to contain all the required information are relatively large it may not be possible to attach them to small containers, e.g. tubes of cream or bottles of eye drops, or to the packets within which the manufacturers supply them. In such cases it is permissible to attach the label to another larger package (e.g. a larger paper envelope or plastic packet) into which the drug container is then placed for supply to the client.

Under no circumstances must a veterinary nurse supply a medicinal preparation (possibly at the direct request of the owner) *without* the authority of a veterinary surgeon.

## Weights and Measures

### The metric system

In science and in pharmacy all measurements of weight and volume are made using the **metric system**. All measurements are expressed in multiples of 10, the standards being the **kilogram** (kg) for weight and the **litre** for volume.

However, in pharmacy the smaller units are more commonly employed. The units of weight are the gram (now written as g in both pharmacy and science), the milligram (mg) and occasionally the microgram which should **not** be abbreviated (though previously it was written as mcg in pharmacy). These are related as follows:

1 kilogram (kg) = 1000 grams

1 gram (g) = 1000 milligrams

1 milligram (mg) = 1000 micrograms

The common unit of volume is the millilitre (ml), and 1000 ml = 1 litre.

Formerly, instead of millilitre (ml) the term cubic centimetre (cc) was used, and more recently in science the term cubic centimetre has returned again (though abbreviated now to $cm^3$). Although the units cc, $cm^3$ and ml are not *exactly* identical, the differences between them are so minute that for all practical purposes they can be considered to be the same. In modern pharmacy the abbreviation ml is used exclusively; the only reason for mentioning the other abbreviations is that it may be noticed that some volumetric (i.e. measuring) glassware is calibrated using those units.

In the grocery and wine trades and recently in science the units centilitre (cl) equivalent to 10 ml, and decilitre (dl), equivalent to 100 ml, are often used, these are related as follows:

1 litre = 1000 ml

= 100 cl

= 10 dl

Note that the letter *s* is *not* placed after abbreviations, i.e. 15 millilitres is written as 15 ml *not* 15 mls, and similarly 30 milligrams is written as 30 mg *not* as 30 mgs.

Care must be taken to clearly indicate the position of the decimal point if fractions of a unit are being shown. If the total number is less than one, a 0 should be placed before the decimal point, i.e. half a millilitre is written as 0.5 ml **not** as .5 ml. Less than one gram should be written in milligrams (e.g. 500 mg rather than 0.5 g) and similarly less than one milligram should be written in micrograms.

Apart from all units being in multiples of 10, the other great advantage of the metric system is that there is a direct connection between the units of weight and volume. **1 ml of water weighs 1 gram**.

Strictly speaking this is only completely accurate at a temperature of 4°C. However, the error is so slight and unimportant for pharmaceutical purposes that it can be considered to apply at all normal temperatures (avoiding extremes of hot and cold). This greatly simplifies the calculation of percentage solutions and of doses of drugs.

In pharmacy the metric system has totally replaced the two **Imperial systems** of weights and measures (**Avoirdupois** and the **Apothecaries**), both of which used the units grain, ounce and pound. Unfortunately, confusion was possible because although the grain was of the same weight in both systems there were a different number of grains in an ounce and therefore in a pound. The **American system** also used the same unit names as the Imperial systems but assigned different values to some of them. No such confusion should arise with the metric system, which is used internationally, provided that the user is able to perform simple arithmetical calculations using decimals.

**Percentage solutions**

The fundamental fact in the calculation of percentage solutions is that a **1% solution** is produced by *either*:

(a) *1 gram* of a solid in a total volume of *100 ml* (this applies to a solid dissolved in a liquid and is called a weight/volume solution (wt/vol solution)), *or*

(b) *1 ml* of a liquid in a total volume of *100 ml* (this applies to a liquid dissolved in another liquid, and is called a volume/volume solution (vol/vol solution)).

Weight/volume solutions are more common. It can be readily seen, then, that doubling the weight of solid, or alternatively halving the total volume of the solution, will double the concentration of the solution. From the definition of a 1% wt/vol solution it can be deduced that:

% solution =

$$\frac{\text{weight (in g)} \times 100}{\text{volume of solution (in ml)}}$$

volume of solution (in ml) =

$$\frac{\text{weight (in g)} \times 100}{\% \text{ solution}}$$

*and*

weight (in g) =

$$\frac{\text{volume of solution (in ml)} \times \% \text{ solution}}{100}$$

If it is a volume/volume solution, with a liquid A dissolved in another liquid B, the above formulae can be applied by *substituting* the *volume of liquid A* (in ml) for the *weight* (in g).

*Example 1*

*Q.* How much dextrose is required to prepare 250 ml of a 5% dextrose solution?

*A.* Weight of dextrose (in g).

$$= \frac{\text{volume of solution (in ml)} \times \% \text{ solution}}{100}$$

$$= \frac{250 \times 5}{100} = \frac{1250}{100} = 12.5$$

The answer is **12.5 grams**.

*Example 2*

*Q.* What is the least volume of solution that can be prepared by dissolving 500 mg of a drug in water if the concentration does not exceed 2.5%?

*A.* The first step is always to convert any weight in milligrams (or micrograms) into grams. Therefore we should state that 500 mg = 0.5 g.

volume of solution (in ml)
= Weight (in g) × 100

$$\frac{}{\% \text{ solution}}$$

$$= \frac{0.5 \times 100}{2.5} = \frac{50}{2.5} = 20$$

The answer is **20 ml**. If the volume of the solution was reduced below this its concentration would be increased. (If you are not convinced of this fact try a calculation to prove it for yourself.)

**Calculation of doses**

The information from the previous section may be needed in the calculation of doses. Three other items of information are often involved:

(a) The weight of the animal concerned. Body weights are best measured in kilograms (kg) since most dose rates are expressed in terms of so many millilitres of drug solution, or milligrams of drug, per kilogram body weight. However, if the body weight is expressed in pounds it can be converted to kilograms by the knowledge that 1 kg = 2.2 lb (and conversely 1 lb = 0.45 kg).

(b) A calculated total *daily* dose may need to be split into 2, 3 or more, equal parts for administration throughout the day.

(c) With tablets and capsules only certain sizes are available.

*Example 1*

*Q.* A 33 lb dog needs to be injected with a certain drug every 8 hours. The dose rate of the drug is 20 mg/kg body weight/day and it is produced for injection as a 4% solution. What volume of solution should be injected each time?

*A.* The first step is to convert the milligrams to grams and the pounds to kilograms.

20 mg = 0.02 g (i.e.  $\frac{20}{1000}$)

$$33 \text{ lb} = \frac{33}{2.2} \text{ kg} = 15 \text{ kg}$$

The next step is to discover the total amount of drug required per day.

If a 1 kg dog requires 0.02 g of drug per day a 15 kg dog will require $15 \times 0.02 = 0.3$ g/day.

Now the total amount of solution required per day can be calculated from the formula.

volume of solution (in ml)

$$= \frac{\text{weight (in g)} \times 100}{\% \text{ solution}}$$

$$= \frac{0.3 \times 100}{4} = \frac{30}{4} = 7.5$$

If this total volume per day is given every 8 hours (i.e. three times per day) the volume (in ml) to be injected on each occasion $= \frac{7.5}{3} = 2.5$.

Therefore **the answer is 2.5 ml**.


*Example 2*

*Q.* A cat weighing 4 kg requires to be given oxytetracycline by mouth as tablets for 5 days. The recommended dose is 25 mg per kg body weight per day and should be split into two, or preferably three, equal doses throughout the day. Oxytetracycline tablets are available containing 50 mg, 100 mg and 250 mg per tablet. How many tablets, and of what strength should be supplied?

*A.* Since we do not need to use percentage solution formulae we can calculate the weight of drug throughout in milligrams.

If a 1 kg cat requires 25 mg/day, a 4 kg cat requires $4 \times 25 = 100$ mg/day.

This could only be met by giving the smallest size tablet (50 mg) twice daily i.e. $2 \times 50$ mg = 100 mg.

Since two 50 mg tablets are required per day, for 5 days, $5 \times 2$ tablets = 10 tablets are needed.

Therefore the answer is **10 tablets each of 50 mg**.

In a practical situation, if an animal nurse is expected to calculate and administer a dose of drug, but has doubts about having the ability to do so, the advice of someone else, preferably the veterinary surgeon in charge, should always be sought. However, with experience the approximate dose of common drugs for administration to animals with varying body sizes becomes known, and this serves as a useful guide when checking the accuracy of one's calculations.


### Abbreviations used in Pharmacy

Nowadays very few abbreviations are used in pharmacy—almost all of them in the writing of prescriptions.

Wt/vol (or w/v) and vol/vol (or v/v) have already been mentioned as the abbreviations for weight/volume and volume/volume solutions, respectively. Similarly, the weight abbreviations mg, g and kg for milligram, gram and kilogram and the volume abbreviation ml for millilitre have been noted. Litre can be written as l but to avoid confusion with *one* is best written in full.

In writing a prescription the symbol $P_x$ was employed as a direction that the following "ingredients" listed were to be used to make the product. Nowadays the symbol is usually followed by the name of a commercially manufactured product that is to be dispensed.

The Latin words and abbreviations, Mitte *or* Mitt meaning *Send* (followed by the quantity of the preparation to be dispensed) and Sig. meaning *Label* (followed by the instructions to appear on the label), are still written on prescriptions although increasingly they are being replaced by the English equivalents (i.e. *Send* and *Label*).

The abbreviations BP, BPC, BVetC and BNF following the name of a preparation indicate that its composition is precisely stated in the *British Pharmacopoeia, British Pharmaceutical Codex, British Veterinary Codex*, or the *British National Formulary,* respectively.

The other abbreviations on prescriptions are abbreviations of Latin words, usually the meaning of which the prescriber intends should appear in English in

TABLE 6.12.   *Abbreviations used in prescription writing.*

| Abbreviation | Latin meaning | English meaning |
|---|---|---|
| a.c. | *ante cibum* | before food |
| altern. d. | *alterno die* | every other day |
| b.d.s. | *bis in die sumendus* | to be taken twice daily |
| b.i.d. (b.d.) | *bis in die* | twice daily |
| dies | *dies* | daily* |
| m.d.u. | *more dictu utendus* | use as directed |
| NP | *nomina propria* | proper name—used when the prescriber wants the name of the preparation to appear on the label |
| o.d. | *omnes dies* | every day* |
| o.m. | *omni mane* | every morning |
| o.n. | *omni nocte* | every night |
| p.c. | *post cibum* | after food |
| p.r.n. | *pro re nata* | occasionally (repeat as required) |
| q.d.s. | *quater in die sumendus* | to be taken 4 times a day |
| q.h. | *quatis horis* | every 4 hours |
| q.i.d. (q.d.) | *quater in die* | 4 times a day |
| Qq. hor. | *quaque hora* | every hour |
| QR | *quantum rectum* | correct quantity—to confirm that a dose which may appear unusual is in fact intended |
| quotid. | *quotidie* | daily* |
| repet. (rep.) | *repetatur* | repeat |
| s.o.s. | *si opus sit* | if necessary |
| t.d.s. | *ter in die sumendus* | to be taken 3 times a day |
| t.i.d. (t.d.) | *ter in die* | 3 times a day |
| ut dict. | *ut dictum* | as directed |

*Used to mean "once daily".

the instructions on the label. These abbreviations usually relate to the frequency, and time, of administration. Although long lists of such abbreviations have been compiled, in practice very few are commonly used on veterinary prescriptions. Some of them (e.g. ad lib. meaning "as much as desired" and N.B. meaning "note well") have passed into general usage. Those likely to be of use are given above. (The Latin words are only provided to explain the abbreviations; it is not important to know these.)

# Further Reading

BERESFORD-JONES, W. P. and JACOBS, D. E. (1984) Endoparasites. In *Canine Medicine and Therapeutics* 2nd edn. (Ed: Chandler, E. A. and others) pp 463–481, Blackwell Scientific Publications, Oxford.

BRACE, J. J. (ed.) (1981) Internal Medicine and the Geriatric Patient. Veterinary Clinics of North America, Small Animal Practice, **11** (4), 641–838.

BRANDER, G. C. and PUGH, D. M. (1977) *Veterinary Applied Pharmacology and Therapeutics,* 3rd edn., Ballière Tindall, London.

BUSH, B. M. (1975) *Veterinary Laboratory Manual,* Heinemann Medical Books, London.

DAYKIN, P. W. (1960) *Veterinary Applied Pharmacology and Therapeutics,* 1st edn., Ballière, Tindall & Cox, London.

HALL L. W. and CLARK K. W. (1983) *Veterinary Anaesthesia* 8th. edn. Ballière Tindall, London.

JACOBS, D. E. (1979) In *Parasites and Western Man,* (Ed: Donaldson, R. J.) pp 171–200. MTP Press, Lancaster.

KIRK, R. W. and BISTNER, S. I. (1981) *Handbook of Veterinary Procedures and Emergency Treatment,* 3rd edn., Saunders, Philadelphia.

KNIFTON, A. and EDWARDS, B. R. (1981) In *Legislation Affecting the Veterinary Profession in Great Britain,* 3rd edn., pp 33–55, Royal College of Veterinary Surgeons, London.

LAPAGE, G. (1956) *Mönnig's Veterinary Helminthology and Entomology,* 4th edn., Baillière, Tindall & Cox, London.

LOWBURY, E. J. I., AYLIFFE, G. A. J., GEDDES, A. M. and WILLIAMS, J. D. (1975) *Control of Hospital Infection,* Chapman & Hall, London.

MATHER, G. W. (1971) Geriatrics. In *Current Veterinary Therapy, Small Animal Practice,* **IV,** (Ed: Kirk, R. W.) Saunders, Philadelphia. 33–36.

MAURER, I. M. (1974) *Hospital Hygiene,* Edward Arnold, London.

MIMS, C. A. (1977) *The Pathogenesis of Disease.* Academic Press, London.

MULLER, G. H., KIRK, R. W. and SCOTT, D. W. (1983) *Small Animal Dermatology,* 3rd edn., Saunders, Philadelphia.

OLSEN, O. W. (1974) *Animal Parasites,* 3rd edn., University Park Press, Baltimore.

OSBORNE, C. A., LOW, D. G. and FINCO, D. R. (1972) *Canine and Feline Urology,* Saunders, Philadelphia.

OSBORNE, C. A. and STEVENS, J. B. (1981) *Handbook of Canine and Feline Urinalysis.* Ralston Purina Co., Saint Louis.

REYNOLDS J. E. F. (1982) *Martindale, The Extra Pharmacopoeia,* 28th edn., Pharmaceutical Press, London.

CHAPTER 7

# Diagnostic Aids and Laboratory Tests

J. S. WILKINSON

## Introduction

In this chapter are explained the principles behind the satisfactory maintenance of a diagnostic service that can reasonably be carried out in practice. All the methods described may be used routinely and most are relatively simple. The function of such a service is to examine accurately and quickly various materials from patients with a view to assisting the clinician to make a diagnosis and to assess the severity of the condition and the patient's response to treatment. The tests by themselves are of limited value and the results can only be interpreted in the light of the clinical findings. However, occasionally the results may suggest the presence of a condition not previously suspected; in these circumstances it is wise to repeat the estimation if there is sufficient material left or to obtain a further sample.

It is impossible to include in a book of this scope all the information that may prove of value, and a list of books which give more detailed information is included at the end of the chapter.

The value of a diagnostic laboratory depends largely upon the equipment available. However, while first-class, expensive equipment will not necessarily give first-class results, good results cannot be obtained with second-rate equipment.

The following items of equipment are essential if the laboratory is to fulfil its purpose adequately.

A *microscope* with ×4, ×10, ×40 and ×100 (oil immersion) objective lenses and ×10 eyepiece lens. It should have a cover and a suitable light source.

A *centrifuge*: the separation of precipitates in the chemical tests can be achieved by filtration but this is less satisfactory than centrifugation.

A *rough balance* for the balancing of centrifuge tubes for spinning.

An *accurate balance* for the preparation of solutions is desirable but the local chemist (druggist) will no doubt help if a suitable balance is not available. Most methods are now available in kit form and preparing reagent solutions is less important than it used to be.

*A supply of water, gas and/or electricity.*

Adequate glassware:

*Storage bottles* (screw-capped for solids and glass- or plastic-stoppered for liquid reagents).

*Test tubes* (150×16 mm and 100×7.5 mm tubes of pyrex glass will withstand heat and centrifugation).

*Measuring cylinders* (50 ml, 100 ml and 250 ml).

*Filter funnels* with papers to fit (Whatman No. 1 are satisfactory).

*Glass rod.*

*Slides and coverslips.*

*Sample bottles* (screw-capped McCartney bottles holding about 7 ml, ("bijou" size) 15 ml and 30 ml and Universal bottles holding about 30 ml, are suitable sizes). Camlab* produce sterile, chemically clean, disposable tubes for collecting blood samples. They are relatively cheap, can be spun in the standard centrifuge bucket to give maximum yield of serum and discarded after use. (Tubes containing anticoagulants suitable for the various tests are also available). "Vacuum" tubes containing different anticoagulants are also available; these have the advantage that they require no syringe and therefore reduce the likelihood of contamination or haemolysis as the blood is transferred to another container.

*A bunsen burner or similar gas flame heater.*

*Adequate storage space.*

A *working surface* that can be cleaned easily; wood with a wax polish or Formica are suitable.

*Records books.*

*Wax (Chinagraph) pencils or felt tip pens* (waterproof).

While the following are not essential they are of value in the maintenance of a good service.

A *refrigerator* for the storage of specimens and unstable solutions and an *oven* for drying and sterilizing glassware.

In addition to these general items special investigations require their own equipment.

For **blood investigations** described later the following are necessary:

> *Wintrobe tubes* or capillary tubes for the microhaematocrit.
>
> *Haemoglobinometer.*
>
> *Haemacytometer.*

For the **urine analyses**:

*Urinometer,* the smaller the better, or refractometer.

*Reagent strip tests.* *

*Tubes of suitable size* for the use with the "Clinitest" tablets. (The makers of the tablets, Ames Co.,* will supply suitable tubes and droppers in a rack.)

> *"Sedistain",* which is used to stain the urinary sediment, after centrifugation, for microscopic examination.

For **bacteriology**:

*Bacteriological loop.*

A *37°C incubator.* (This is also useful for the reticulocyte count and the estimation of trypsin faeces. A satisfactory incubator heated by a 60-watt electric light bulb can be built for a few pounds. The most expensive item is the thermostat.)

For **blood chemistry**:

A *boiling-water bath* (a small saucepan or beaker is adequate) or a heat block.

A *colorimeter,* or spectrophotometer, is necessary if more accurate results than can be obtained by unaided visual methods are desired.

For **faecal investigation**:

*A pair of dissecting forceps.*

*A pair of mounted needles are useful.*

For **parasitology**:

Examination of faeces for the presence of worm ova needs no extra equipment unless the more accurate quantitative method is to be used. A concentrated solution of sugar is used to bring the eggs to the surface when centrifuging.

Commercial equipment and kit test methods.

Mallinkrodt    Serometer,    Bidynamics

---

*Camlab (Medical Laboratories) Ltd., Milton Road Cambridge

*Ames Co. Ltd., Stoke Court, Stoke Poges, Buckinghamshire.

Unimeter and Ames BMI Analyzer are instruments specifically designed for **clinical chemistry**. Not all are available in the United Kingdom. They provide a colorimeter and heating block(s) and reagents for the tests. The equipment and reagents vary in price and in ease of manipulation, and the decision as to which should be bought should only be made when their individual merits have been assessed.

Boehringer, Sigma and other firms also provide reagents in kit form, but a spectrophotometer and incubator are not supplied and must be obtained elsewhere.

### Running a Laboratory

### General rules

The following rules should always be observed:
(1) Keep the laboratory clean; unsatisfactory results may arise from contamination of glassware.
(2) *Keep it tidy; many breakages occur through untidiness.*
(3) Carry out all tests as soon as possible and dispose of all samples as soon as they have been fully examined.
(4) Label all reagent bottles, samples and test-tubes used in tests clearly.
(5) Keep all poisonous reagents under lock and key.
(6) Keep clear records and keep records away from the sink and work bench where they may get splashed.

### Labelling and recording

This is probably the most important part of laboratory practice.

There is no value in taking a sample, testing it and recording the results if there is no certainty from which animal it came, and there is no point in knowing from which animal it came if the results are not correctly recorded.

If one sample only is being tested it is wise, but not absolutely necessary, to label any test tubes in use. If two or more samples are being tested it is essential, and for this a chinagraph pencil or a felt tip pen can be used. If several dilutions of the sample are being used each tube should be labelled. Chinagraph wax and felt tip marker ink can be readily removed with a little ether.

Similar rules, of course, apply to any slides that are made. Special ink is available for labelling glassware permanently or a diamond "pencil" can be used. On slides with frosted ends a pencil will do.

Accurate recording of results is essential for the satisfactory running of any laboratory. A small duplicate booklet for each type of sample examined or sent away is satisfactory; one for urine, one for blood, one for faeces. Even if no blood examinations are carried out in the laboratory, it is worth making a note of the date on which they were sent; this will serve as a check in case the laboratory reports are held up and inquiries have to be made.

Records should show:
(1) The date of the sampling and how the sample was obtained.
(2) The date of testing.
(3) The reference; possibly the surgery number, the owner's name, the dog's age, breed and sex, and, if known, the dog's name.
(4) The results of all the tests.
(5) The date the results were entered in the surgery books. Entering the results in case records will, of course, depend on the methods employed in the practice. They should be written down and put where the clinician in charge of the case will see them before or at the same time as he next sees the case.

There is little point in doing the tests if the results are not available when needed.

## Use, preparation and care of glassware and laboratory equipment

New *glassware* should always be carefully washed before it is used.

It should be scrubbed with a good detergent ("Teepol") and rinsed two or three times in really hot running water. It should finally be rinsed well in distilled water. It is advisable to dry it in an oven as this sterilizes it as well; stoppers should be put on as soon as the bottles are cool enough to handle.

Used glassware should be rinsed very well in cold water (if infected, stand in 2% lysol for 24 hours) immediately after use; serum, urine and faeces are frequently very difficult to remove once they have dried. It should then be washed in detergent, rinsed and dried in an oven. Glassware should not be left lying about in the laboratory; as soon as it is cool it should be stored carefully in a cupboard, which should be kept tidy. If precleaned slides are not available, slides should be scrubbed with a nailbrush in hot soapy water, rinsed very well with hot running water and dried with a cloth which does not leave fluff. Coverslips, which are very fragile, should not be washed but cleaned with a tissue ("Kleenex", "Scottie" or "Kimwipe") immediately before use. Once clean, slides can be stored in absolute alcohol and dried carefully immediately before use. Precleaned slides are available.

## The preparation of blood bottles

Where *sample bottles* or tubes are not available commercially they can be prepared quite simply. The containers should be washed and dried as previously described. The choice of anticoagulant is shown in Table 7.1.

Nowadays few tests are run on whole blood; plasma or serum is usually used. **When whole blood is allowed to clot and the clot to retract, serum is produced.** If the clotting process is prevented the sample remains fluid and the cells and plasma can be separated by centrifugation. The **plasma contains fibrinogen and other clotting factors** which are used up when no anticoagulant is used. The clotting process can be speeded up by incubating the sample at 37°C for 30 minutes and then cooling in a refrigerator for 30 minutes before spinning. Plasma can, in contrast, be harvested within minutes and the tests started that much earlier. If serum is required, blood should be allowed to clot in a glass container. The clot attaches itself very firmly to plastic tubes and cannot usually be processed without haemolysis.

For haematology, potassium versenate is added at the rate of 1 mg for each 1 ml of blood. This is not absolutely critical but too much will cause the red cells to shrink and too little will not prevent clotting. Prepare a solution of versenate (5 g per 100 ml) and dispense 0.2 ml into tubes for 10 ml. This amount of fluid will make only a little difference to the blood tests, but if desired the tubes can be put back into the oven and dried out. They should then be closed securely.

A similar method can be used to prepared tubes containing anticoagulant for glucose testing (sodium fluoride and potassium oxalate 2 mg per ml of both per ml of blood). The oven should not be hotter than 150°C or the oxalate will decompose.

Heparin, which is not very soluble, can be used in solution, either actually in the syringe into which the sample is being

TABLE 7.1. *Anticoagulants and their uses*

| | |
|---|---|
| Di-potassium EDTA (potassium versenate) | Haematology BUN |
| Lithium | Haemoglobin, Sodium/potassium |
| | Calcium/magnesium, Enzymes, BUN |
| Fluoride and oxalate | Blood/plasma glucose, BUN |

drawn or in the tube in the usual manner; 200 units will prevent clotting in 10 ml of blood.

To ensure that the anticoagulant dissolves rapidly in the blood, the tube should be inverted 5–10 times but it should not be shaken as this will cause the erythrocytes to rupture (haemolysis).

### The laboratory centrifuge

The *centrifuge* is the backbone of many tests (Fig. 7.1). Basically it consists of a number of "buckets" which hold test-tubes which may contain up to 15 ml (much larger buckets are available but are not needed for clinical chemistry). The buckets are rotated very rapidly with consequent settling of heavier particles to the bottom of the tube and lighter ones to the top. The centrifuge is used for separation of blood cells from plasma or serum for many chemical tests and for sedimenting any precipitate which may develop in the chemical reactions. It is also used to concentrate at the bottom of the tube the solid constituents of urine. In parasitology a very concentrated solution is used and centrifugation of a suspension of faeces in this solution causes the ova to rise to the surface. This flotation and sedimentation, as they are called, occur naturally; centrifugation only decreases the time which it takes.

The most important manoeuvre in using the centrifuge is to ensure that it is balanced, that is to say that the diametrically opposite buckets must contain tubes of the same weight. Some instruments are tolerant enough to allow a "by eye" match, in other words a tube containing 10 ml urine, though heavier, will be balanced by 10 ml water in a matched tube. However, the highly concentrated solutions used for parasitology could not be balanced with water and another tube with the concentrated solution should be used. Some instruments, however, are less tolerant and require that the buckets be matched on a beam balance.

The controls on the simplest centrifuges are an on/off switch and a speed control. Some have a timer built into the on/off switch and the bigger ones have rev/min counters and brakes.

When the buckets have been loaded into the machine the speed control is set at zero, the switch turned on (and timer set if present), and the speed control is slowly turned up to the desired setting. If the buckets are **not balanced** the instrument will "judder" violently and must be turned off immediately. If the switch is turned on with the speed control at maximum the instrument may be damaged. More expensive machines are built so that they will not start except with the speed control at zero. Centrifuges require little mechanical attention beyond cleaning out when a tube breaks and replacement of the brushes. If the instrument is difficult to start, produces a lot of sparks or runs unevenly, the brushes, which carry the electric current into the armature, are probably worn and should be checked. Access to the brush housing depends on the type of machine and if necessary the advice of an expert should be sought.

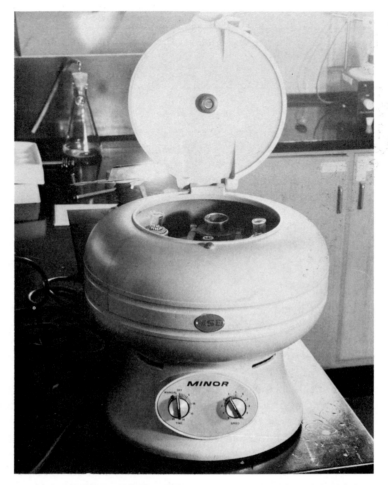

FIG. 7.1.    MSE centrifuge with timer and speed controls and buckets.

*Do not meddle with the "works" until the machine has been disconnected from the mains.*

While the standard laboratory centrifuge, which gives about 4000 rev/min, is adequate for measuring the packed cell volume and all the other needs of the diagnostic lab (see later) there is no doubt that the use of a microhaematocrit is preferable. This latter method uses less blood and is much less time-consuming requiring 5 minutes rather than 30–45 minutes. It also gives a more accurate result. Unfortunately the microhaemocrit

centrifuge cannot be used for anything else and may not represent a reasonable investment.

Occasionally tubes will break while being spun; the bucket must then be thoroughly cleaned, and if necessary disinfected, and the centrifuge bowl cleaned of any broken glass.

## The microscope (Fig. 7.2)

*The microscope* is used for examination of material which cannot be seen adequately by the unaided eye. The main function is to examine stained films of blood for evidence of abnormality in the cells and for doing the cell counts. It is also used for examination of material for the presence of bacteria and for the examination of urine and faeces for evidence of maldigestion or worms. The degree of magnification is determined by the lens in use (this should be noted on the lens itself). The highest power lens ($\times 100$) is usually oil immersed.

Microscopes are often supplied with a built-in light source, but for those that are not a suitable lamp is necessary. The illumination provided should be checked before the microscope is bought; in some makes the bulb does not give sufficient light for the oil-immersion lens.

The microscope must be treated with respect and must be kept as clean as any good glassware. The **stage**, the part on which the slide rests sometimes gets contaminated with material that is being examined and should be cleaned regularly. If the material is infected, it should be swabbed off with a piece of cotton wool just moistened with methylated spirit.

To function properly the lens must be clean and free from scratches. Never use a harsh cloth on microscope lenses; soft paper tissues ("Kimwipes") are most satisfactory. The "oil-immersion" lens should be wiped free of oil as soon as it has been used. The mirror should be kept clean, and occasionally it may be necessary to put a drop of oil on the focusing devices. The microscope should never be left uncovered. It should either be kept in its box or in a safe place under a polythene bag. **Never try to take a microscope lens apart** to clean the inside. This is an expert's job and, if necessary, the lens should be taken out and given to such an expert for cleaning.

A mechanical stage which makes movement of the slide much easier is an optional extra but would be economic in the time saved. Setting the microscope up for use can be time consuming but it is time well spent. Regardless of whether the light source is built-in or is outside the frame and a mirror used to direct the light through the optics, the first step is ensuring that the illumination is optional.

Choose a well-stained film of blood and put it on to the stage. Select the $\times 4$ objective and $\times 10$ oculars and switch on the lamp. Move the condenser lens up until it is 1–2 mm below the slide and close the iris diaphragm until about half the field is illuminated. Now lower the objective lens (or raise the stage) until the lens is 4–5 mm above the slide and adjust the light until the field is evenly lit. This is done by tilting the mirror or by using the adjustment screws in the lamp housing. (Some microscopes are made so that there is no need for this adjustment.) The lens is now racked up from the slide (with the coarse adjustment knob) until the cells are nearly in focus and then finally focused with the fine focus knob. Any unevenness of illumination is now once more corrected.

Remove the eyepiece lens and look down the draw tube. The illumination should be even; if it is not carry out final adjustments as below. The iris diaphragm in the condenser should be sharply visible and should be in the middle of the field. If it is not it can be adjusted in most microscopes with a pair of knurled knobs. The condenser should now be focused to a joint just in front of the lamp. Hold a pencil point (or something similar) just in front of the lamp and adjust the condenser so that it is focused thereon.

Changing the objective lens requires some care. When the slide has been scanned with the low-power lens, more detailed study can be made by switching to an objective of greater magnification. In most microscopes of the sort needed for clinical laboratory use, the lenses are

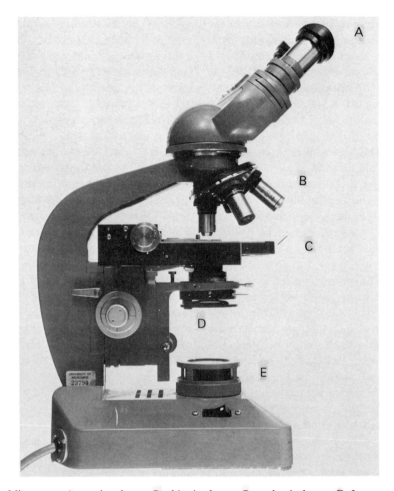

Fig. 7.2.    Microscope. A, eyepiece lenses; B, objective lenses; C, mechanical stage; D, focus controls; E, lamp housing.

arranged so that, when one of greater magnification is swung into place, the lens is nearly in focus. Some older makes may not be constructed this way and damage to both lens and object may result unless the lens is racked up 5–10 mm. The new lens is then lowered until it is just clear of the slide and then racked up until the object is in focus. When the oil-immersion lens is to be used a drop of immersion oil is placed on the slide, the lens lowered until just clear of the slide and again racked up slowly until correctly focused.

The higher the magnification the greater the illumination required. This may be regulated by opening the iris diaphragm on the condenser, increasing output from the light source or in some microscopes by putting another lens into the system.

## The use and care of other laboratory equipment

The **colorimeter** (Fig. 7.3) is an instrument designed to measure the intensity of colour in a solution.

It consists of a light source, a device for

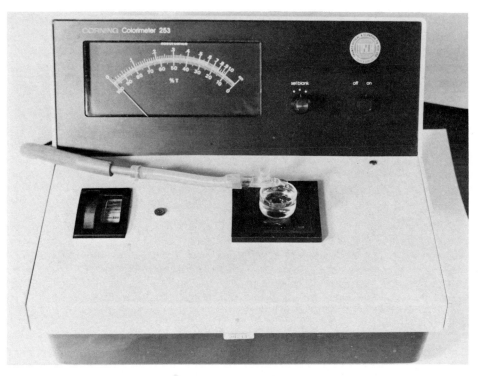

FIG. 7.3. EEL Corning Colorimeter with wavelength, blank controls and "flow through" cuvette.

selecting the right wavelength for the test, a cuvette, which holds the solution being measured, and a barrier layer cell, which measures the amount of light falling upon it and finally a galvanometer with a numbered scale.

There are three controls; the on/off switch, the "Set Blank" and the wavelength control.

Colorimetric methods are based on the fact that when a reaction occurs between two substances the intensity of colour produced is proportional to the ratio of the two reagents. When the amount of one reagent is held constant the intensity of colour is proportional to the amount of the second reagent used.

Tubes are prepared thus; the **reagent blank**, that is the test reagents without the substance being measured, the **standards** which contain known concentrations of the substance under test and the **unknown samples**. All these are treated in exactly the same way; they are heated or they are allowed to stand at room temperature, in the light or in the dark or whatever the test required. In this way the colour developed in the standards and the unknowns are directly comparable. The reagent blank is included in case the procedure produces a colour change in the reagents, even in the absence of the substance under test, and also in the tests in which the initial reagents are coloured and the test is measuring a change in the intensity of the initial colour.

*Use of the colorimeter.* The "Serometer" (Fig. 7.4), "Unimeter" and similar units have their own particular methods and there is no need to discuss these here, but the basic principles for any colorimetric test are the same.

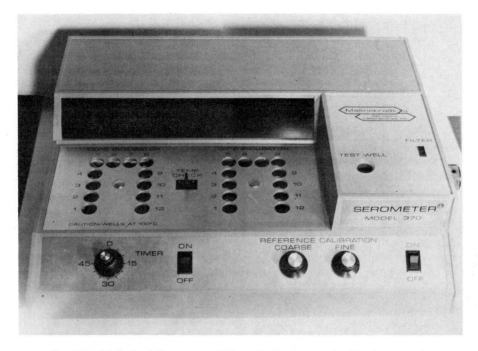

Fig. 7.4.    Mallinkrodt Serometer with heat blocks, timer and calibration controls.

When the test is complete the wavelength or colour filter necessary for that test is chosen and a cuvette, a thin-walled glass tube designed for the instrument, filled with the reagent blank is placed in the colorimeter and the machine set to zero with the "Set Zero" knob. The blank is then discarded, another cuvette is filled from the standard tube and the reading noted. This is then repeated with the remaining tubes.

If more than one standard is used a calibration curve is constructed (a plot of standard concentration against colorimeter reading) and the unknowns read from this. If only one standard is used the concentration of the unknowns is derived arithmetically.

The cuvettes are fragile and should be washed carefully immediately after use. (A "flow through" cuvette which is not removed from the machine, while initially expensive, saves time and the expense of replacing cuvettes.)

Any spills should be mopped immediately. It is necessary occasionally to replace the globe; this is relatively easy in most instruments but care should be taken to avoid handling it by the glass unless a glove is worn.

A **haemoglobinometer** (a photometer specifically designed to measure haemoglobin) is not essential if a colorimeter is to be used for clinical chemistry.

A **spectrophotometer or colorimeter** is essential for reading the end result of the colorimetric tests. The latter uses glass or gelatin filters of known wavelengths while a spectrophotometer uses a prism or a diffraction grating. The former are more expensive and probably unnecessary for most practice laboratories.

A **water bath** is necessary for several reactions which require temperature above normal to go to completion. The two most commonly used temperatures are 37°C and 100°C. These temperatures can be achieved with a thermostatically controlled water bath (one for each temperature) or a heating block, again one for each temperature. Heating blocks can be manufactured for specific requirements; they are, in some ways, more convenient than water-filled baths, which need topping up at regular intervals.

An **electronic particle counter** for red and white cell counts is expensive and can really only be justified if it is intended to count many samples each day. If not a haemacytometer will suffice.

A **urinometer** or **refractometer** is needed for the measurement of concentration of urine. The former has been used largely in the past and measures the weight of the urine as compared to the weight of the same volume of water. The refractometer measures the change in refractive index due to the dissolved solids. The urinometer is cheaper but is relatively fragile and requires at least 30 ml of urine. The refractometer is sturdier and more expensive but requires only 1 drop of urine. It can also be used to measure the protein concentration of plasma. Since the kidney concentrates the urine by osmosis the best measurement of concentration is to measure osmotic pressure (osmolality), but this requires a much more expensive piece of equipment.

All electrical apparatus should be kept clean, and for safety ensure that it is adequately earthed and that it is far enough away from the sink not to get splashed. If there is any doubt about the serviceability of any equipment it should be checked; if it is not functioning properly it will probably stop working when it is needed most.

## The Collection of Material for Examination

Several points have to be borne in mind when dealing with samples for analysis.

The most important of these is absolute cleanliness both from the infection and chemical aspects. There is no point in putting a sample into a dirty bottle and there is no excuse for hazarding a patient's health by using dirty techniques. It is, therefore, essential to use clean sterile bottles and catheters, syringes and needles, preferably disposable.

Samples should be tested as soon after collection as possible since delay frequently results in deterioration.

### Collection of blood samples

This requires skill and practice. Both needle and syringe must be clean and dry; if disposable needle and syringe are used this presents no problems.

Since frequent boiling soon takes the edge off a needle it is best to dry sterilize it. After washing and shaking dry, the needle is put into a small glass tube with cotton wool in the top. This is then "cooked" in an oven Regulo 1 or similar setting for 3 hours.

Blood is usually taken from the cephalic vein of the foreleg vein, the one used for giving intravenous injections, or the jugular vein. The technique for taking blood is very similar to that for giving injections. An area over the vein is clipped and cleaned with spirit, the vein is raised by constricting the limb above the clipped site and the needle, which must be sharp, inserted. The vein should not be kept raised for long before sampling, and if the flow is satisfactory a better sample of blood is obtained without keeping the vein raised. However, in small dogs the flow rate may be slow and raising the vein is then necessary. Do not exert excessive suction and remove the needle before transferring blood from the syringe to the bottle or tube to prevent haemolysis. (If the sample needed is whole blood, the receiver must be gently shaken to mix the blood with the anticoagulant; if serum is wanted, shaking must be avoided.) When sufficient blood has been collected the assistant should put a thumb over the shank of the needle, thus preventing leakage from the vein when the needle is withdrawn. The needle should never be withdrawn while the vein is still raised. After the needle is out a small pledget of cotton wool may be placed over the site and held firmly in place with sticking plaster. This should be removed within a few hours.

If serum is required the receiver is put on one side to allow the clot to form and shrink. If there is an incubator available, 30 minutes at 37°C, followed by 30 minutes in a refrigerator will help the process. This should leave quite a large amount of serum which can be carefully poured off into another clean bottle or tube. If there are some red blood cells that are not trapped in the clot it is better to remove the serum with a narrow glass pipette. If a centrifuge is available, this can be used to get the last of the serum from the clot or to remove any red cells that may have been decanted with the serum. Do not spin blood samples for longer than 10 minutes or at more than 3000 rev/min.

If "clotted blood" is to be sent away for analysis it is wise to allow the serum to separate and send this. A few red cells do not matter since these can easily be spun down by the laboratory. If the blood, clot included, is sent through the post, considerable haemolysis frequently occurs.

### Collection of urine

If the animal is an in-patient, a sample can usually be collected when it is taken out first thing in the morning. Practically anything can be used, but for bitches a small shallow dish or saucer is best and a saucepan or a can, firmly wired to a pole, is very useful for dogs. A kidney bowl can be used for both sexes.

If the patient is presented at surgery and there is space available it can be "walked", though this method is rarely successful. Dogs in particular, and sometimes bitches, will urinate on the floor of the waiting room or surgery; provided that the floor is clean the urine can be salvaged with a pipette or old syringe. The same applies to kennel floors or yards.

If none of these methods is satisfactory the patient can be catheterized. This method is not without drawbacks; it may result in cystitis and damage to the urethra, and in some cases it is impossible to pass even the smallest available cathether (p. 325).

It is wise to have two containers for the urine since the first few drops may be contaminated with preputial and prostatic fluids. This is collected into one container and saved in case there is insufficient urine in the bladder. The main portion is collected into the second bottle; it may be necessary to squeeze the bladder gently through the abdominal wall in order to get sufficient urine for testing, though under no circumstances should undue pressure be applied. Bitches with vaginitis or open pyometra should only be catheterized in an emergency, since the risk of infecting the bladder is very great (p. 333).

A fairly close watch should be kept for 2 or 3 days on any animal that has been catheterized. The frequent passage of small quantities of urine, sometimes even blood in the urine, may indicate that there is an infection present and this should be reported.

If a bacteriological examination is required, catheterization is, of course, the only acceptable method for collection of urine. It may be possible to collect a "midstream" specimen of urine satisfactorily in the dog which can be used for bacterial culture.

### Collection of faeces

This normally presents little difficulty. The simplest method is to provide the owner with a suitable container and ask him to collect a sample.

If a dog is a boarder, faeces can be collected from the run, using a wooden spatula or palette knife. If it is a communal run, however, it is important that the run is clean and that the dog is watched. This will avoid the possibility of material from the wrong dog or stale faeces being collected. It may be possible to collect a sample directly from the dog as it defaecates and this should be attempted if the patient has severe diarrhoea.

If neither of these methods is satisfactory it may be possible to extract a small quantity of faeces from the rectum. Using a finger-stall or disposable glove, lightly lubricated, the middle finger is gently introduced into the rectum. As with catheterization, this is a two-person procedure and must be done gently to overcome constriction of the anal sphincter muscle. It may be necessary to do this two or three times to get sufficient material for analysis.

Store faeces in a wide-necked jar or plastic container.

### Collection of vomit

This will usually have to be collected from the bedding or floor of the kennel. A wooden spatula, or better a palette knife, or preferably two, will do this job satisfactorily. The sample is transferred to a suitable container.

Occasionally it is necessary to make a dog vomit and a variety of emetics may be used; in these circumstances the sample can usually be collected directly into the container. (See also section on Preservation of Material (p. 456).

### Collection of samples from cases of skin disease

*Skin scrapings.* The mites which cause some skin diseases live in the deep layers of the skin and to be of any value the material should be primarily from these layers.

*Reagent.* Ten per cent potassium hydroxide solution or liquid paraffin.

*Equipment.* A used knife blade (too sharp a knife does not scrape well).

*Procedure.* Always take the scraping from the edge of the lesion as it is here that the mites are likely to be commonest. Moisten the area to be scraped with a little potassium hydroxide, anchor the skin between finger and thumb of one hand and gently scrape the lesion until pinpoints of blood develop. The more material collected the better the chance of seeing the parasite. Transfer the material to a suitable labelled container; a small glass jar or test-tube will do.

If a scraping does not provide an answer a small portion of skin may be removed surgically (biopsy). The site is shaved, cleaned and disinfected and infiltrated with local anaesthetic. A small slice is then removed, either with a scalpel, a pair of curved scissors or a special skin biopsy punch. The biopsy is fixed in 10% formaldehyde.

*Hair.* If it is suspected that the skin condition is due to ringworm the patient should be examined under the Wood's lamp (a source of ultra-violet light) (see later).

*Skin brushings.* The method of brushing the skin surface with a stiff nylon brush so that the material can be collected on black plastic or card may be used. It is often used for the more superficial skin parasites; the material can then be examined fresh under the microscope and then treated with potassium hydroxide as for the skin scraping.

### Collection of material for bacteriological examination

The bacteriological examination of blood is a specialized job and microscopic examination of even a thick film is unlikely to be of value since very few organisms will be present. The organisms have to be incubated in a suitable medium to allow them to reach sufficient numbers to be readily examined. The sample should be taken into a sterile syringe and immediately transferred to a suitable medium (this will be supplied by the laboratory that has agreed to make the examination). More satisfactory are bottles containing a special medium into which blood is collected directly.

A slide can be held against some purely superficial lesions; possibly a gentle squeeze will help to express pus from a furuncular lesion.

The *bacteriological swab* is a small pledget of absorbent cotton wool or alginate wrapped firmly round a stick, usually about 15 cm long. This is stored in a testtube with a bung of, usually, nonabsorbent cotton wool. The whole has been sterilized. It is important that the absorbent cotton wool is firmly adherent to the stick, otherwise it may fall off while being used. Sterile swabs are now cheaply available and are economic if large numbers of samples are to be taken. For swabbing many lesions, the usual length is unnecessarily long and sticks about 7.5 cm long are sufficient.

If the lesion is exposed, no preparation is necessary. The swab stick is withdrawn from the tube taking care that it does not touch the neck, which may not be sterile. The cotton wool is then worked well over the surface to be examined until it has picked up sufficient material to be well damped. It is then returned carefully to the tube. The tube is labelled, stating the reference and the site of the lesion, and stored in the refrigerator until examined or dispatched.

If the lesion is less open it may be necessary to reduce contamination by cleaning the surrounding skin. This is particularly so in the cases of furunculosis and some ear conditions. Here, any scabs or debris should be removed and the area cleaned with cotton wool before the swab is used.

It is important that enough fluid is taken up on the swab to prevent it drying out before examination, but if there is likely to be any delay in dispatch or transit, the swab itself can be put into a small container of Stewart's transport medium, which will ensure safe arrival.

The bacteriological loop can be used to make smears directly from infected sites. it may sometimes be necessary to dilute the material with a small drop of sterile saline solution in order to make a good smear.

### Collection of material for cytology

Microscopic, chemical and bacteriological examination of fluid from the pericardial sac, pleural and peritoneal cavities, joint (synovial) and nasal cavities, bronchial tree, stomach, cerebrospinal space and even the eye have all proved to be of diagnostic value.

*Paracentesis* is the name given to the aspiration of material from natural or unnatural accumulations of fluid. The sample must be taken with a sterile dry syringe using a wide bore, 1–2 in. needle, depending on the size of the dog. The site is clipped and cleaned with disinfectant and, if necessary, infiltrated with local anaesthetic. The needle is introduced, at least 10 ml withdrawn if possible (the bacteria are likely to be well diluted and the larger the volume examined the higher the chance of demonstrating their presence), and transferred to a sterile container. A non-sterile dish should be available in case it is necessary to withdraw more fluid as part of the treatment of the condition. Label the bottle, again noting the source. This method can also be used for withdrawing pus from a closed abscess. Pus is very viscid and a wider bore needle is usually necessary. In some cases the pus is so thick that the method fails.

The fluid is transferred to a tube after collection and centrifuged to concentrate cells and bacteria. Most of the clear supernatant is decanted and the sediment resuspended. Some is used for bacteriology and from the rest is prepared a number of films which are then treated, as are blood films.

### Preservation of Blood, Urine and Pathological Material

Optimally blood, urine and other body fluids should be tested virtually immediately after the sample is taken.

### Blood

Preservation in this case is associated with the anticoagulant used. EDTA (versenate) is the best anticoagulant, causing least distortion of cells, but even with this anticoagulant changes occur in the leucocytes, and films made as little as 12 hours after sampling show degenerative changes. Refrigeration at 4°C is important, but on no account should the sample be frozen or should films be put into the refrigerator; the condensation that occurs on the cold glass ruins the cells.

Prevention of glycolysis to maintain a blood glucose value at the level it was when the sample was taken, is usually achieved with the oxalate-fluoride anticoagulant, but if there is likely to be a delay it should also be kept cool.

Plasma or serum, or in some cases whole blood, can be kept for weeks to months in the freezer compartment of a domestic refrigerator ($-10°C$) or for years at $-70°C$ or less. There is considerable variation in the period that enzyme activity can be preserved. Some enzymes deteriorate very rapidly while others are more robust.

Chemically clean, disposable, plastic containers can be used for storing plasma or serum.

### Urine

Again urine should be tested as soon as possible after collection. This is particularly important for sediment. Failing this, refrigeration overnight is satisfactory except that this may cause the formation of many crystals which can interfere with the microscopic examination of sediment. For longer periods urine can be preserved by adding a crystal of thymol, a thin layer of toluene over the surface or 1–2 ml of formalin to 15 ml of urine. This latter is particularly satisfactory for preservation of the sediment.

### Faeces

In warm weather faeces should be examined immediately, particularly if egg counts are to be done.

**Other body fluids**

Fluids should be centrifuged to separate cells and the supernatant fluid can then be frozen. Films of the cells should be made immediately.

It is sometimes recommended that body fluids be mixed with an equal quantity of 50% ethanol as a fixative. Alternatively, films may be prepared in the usual way and then fixed and "stuck" to the slide with one of the proprietary agents (such as "Spraycyte").

**Post-mortem material**

There are three important points to remember; firstly, that it takes a lot of formalin to fix tissues; that it takes formalin a long time to penetrate tissues (even though the outside of a large piece of tissue may be well fixed, the inside will continue to decompose); and, thirdly, that while fixing is going on the tissue becomes very firm and rigid. Soft tissues pushed into a narrow-necked bottle and then fixed can frequently only be removed by breaking the bottle.

Therefore there are three rules to be observed when preserving post-mortem material:

(1) *Use plenty of formalin*, say 20 volumes of formalin for every one of tissue.

(2) *Cut large organs open* so that the formalin penetrates more quickly. Better still, remove a piece which is big enough to show all the abnormalities but no more (it may be necessary to cut more than one piece from an organ).

(3) *Fix the tissues in a bowl first.* When they are well fixed transfer to a wide-necked bottle.

For a small piece of tissue, fixing will be complete in about 24 hours but larger ones may take 2 to 3 days, even longer.

Vomit needs no preservation; its high acidity prevents bacterial action.

If there is any likelihood of the material having to go to an analyst for examination for poison and there is the possibility of a lawsuit, it is as well to keep with it a bottle of the same batch as that in which the vomit is stored. This will answer any suggestion that the bottle was contaminated before the material was put into it. If the vomit was collected from bedding some of this should also be saved.

### Despatch of Samples to Outside Laboratories

This activity is covered by quite strict postal regulations and all packages must be labelled "Pathological specimen". In addition "Fragile with care" may help to ensure safe arrival.

The first thing to ensure is that all bottles are adequately stoppered. A waterproof screw-cap tightly screwed is the best, but corks pushed well home and secured with "Sellotape" are satisfactory.

The next most important precaution is sufficient packing; at least three thicknesses of corrugated cardboard should be used, or, if the container is a small one, cotton wool in a small box will suffice. As a final safety precaution, a polythene bag will prevent any leakage.

Always include with the specimen a note giving details of the case, nature of the specimen, any preservative used and a reference. All containers should be clearly labelled and the labels must be well secured. Where possible avoid having samples in the post over the week-end; if there is any doubt about their arrival by Saturday morning, keep them in the refrigerator until Monday morning and post then. Pathological specimens must be

TABLE 7.2.   *Normal values in haematology*

| | | Dog | | Cat |
|---|---|---|---|---|
| Haemoglobin | g/100 ml | 12-18 | | 8-15 |
| ESR | mm/h | 0.0-1.0 | | 0-8 |
| PCV | % | 37-55 | | 24-45 |
| Buffy coat | mm | 0.5-2 | | 0.5-1.5 |
| Total white-cell count | thousand/mm³ | 6-18 | | 7.0-20.0 |
| Total red-cell count | million/mm³ | 5.5-8.5 | | 5.0-10.0 |
| | | | | |
| Differential count | | | | |
|   Juvenile polymorphs | /mm³ | 0-200 | (0.8%) | 0.5% |
|   Polymorphs | thousand/mm³ | 5-10 | (70%) | 60% |
|   Lymphocytes | thousand/mm³ | 1.8-3.8 | (20%) | 32% |
|   Monocytes | /mm³ | 250-1050 | (5.3%) | 3% |
|   Eosinophils | /mm³ | 200-1000 | (4.0%) | 5.5% |
|   Basophils | | Rare | | 0% |
|   Reticulocytes | | 0-1.5% of | | |
| | | red cells | | 0.2% |

sent by first class letter post to comply with UK postal regulations.

## Examination of Blood

Blood consists of fluid matrix in which are suspended or dissolved a large number of chemical substances and the blood cells. These cells and chemical substances do not vary a great deal in the normal dog, but in disease there is frequently a marked increase or decrease in their numbers or concentration. The degree of change frequently reflects the severity of the condition (Table 7.2).

The study of the cells is called haematology.

## Haematology

Clotted blood is valueless for haematology and therefore an anticoagulant must be used. Different laboratories like different anticoagulants, and if the sample is to be sent away it is as well to find out which anticoagulant is preferred. For most purposes **sequestrene** (known also as EDTA or ethylene diamine tetraacetic acid or dipotassium versenate) is the best. This is readily soluble, and little difficulty should be experienced with clotting if reasonable precautions are taken. One to two mg/ml of blood is sufficient and more than this should not be used. The tube or bottle should be shaken gently to ensure mixing while the sample is being taken; if there is a mark to which the bottle should be filled do not overfill or clotting may result due to insufficiency of the anticoagulant. As soon as sufficient blood has been withdrawn, remove needle from syringe, transfer blood to bottle, cap and mix well by rotating. Do not shake vigorously as this will cause haemolysis. Heparin should not be used as an anticoagulant for haematology. Remember to always mix the sample well before removing an aliquot for examination.

### Preparation of Blood Films

Blood films should be made with absolutely fresh blood and this can really only be done satisfactorily if there are three people available: one to hold the dog, one to bleed, and the third to make the films from blood directly from the needle. If this is not practicable, smears can be made from the collected blood, but this should be done immediately, particularly if anti-coagulants other than sequestrene are used.

There are three precautions to observe when making blood films:

(1) *The slides must be cleaned really well*; particularly they must be free of grease.

(2) *A suitable spreader should be used* (Fig. 7.5).

(3) *Not too much blood should be used,* for a thick film is valueless for differential counts.

Preparation of films on coverslips is recommended. A small drop of blood is placed upon the coverslip and a second coverslip placed on top. The coverslips are then *slid* apart just before the blood stops spreading. Films prepared in this way have usually a much more even spread of leucocytes. After staining and drying the coverslips are mounted face downward.

Put a small drop of blood on to the slide at one end and draw the spreader into this. Allow the blood to spread along the spreader. If the drop is too large, lift the spreader up (this will take sufficient blood with it) and put it back on a clean portion of the slide. Push it gently and firmly along the slide; this should give a good even spread with possibly some tailing at the further end. It is most important that the **blood be pulled along behind the spreader**, not pushed along in front of it. Blood cells are fragile, and if pushed in front of the spreader many will be destroyed.

Always prepare three or four films at a time; this allows for failure in staining, breakages and second opinions.

Wave slides gently in the air or lay on the bench in front of a source of warm air until they are dry and then store face downward on a piece of clean blotting paper. Once again, label the slides clearly. Wax pencil is suitable, or the films can be labelled by writing in the centre of the film with an ordinary pencil (Fig. 7.6). This is probably the best method since there is little likelihood of the "label" coming off during staining.

There are many staining methods for blood films each of which has its advantages and disadvantages. Perhaps the simplest is "Difquik"* which requires 5-second immersion in three solutions, washing in water and drying. The results are only slightly inferior to some of the other techniques (better than others) and the saving in time considerable.

*Harleco, Philadelphia, PA, United States.

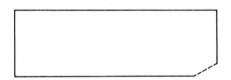

F$_{\text{IG}}$. 7.5.   A spreader. The corner of a slide is scored with a glass file and broken off.

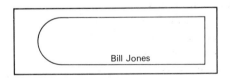

Bill Jones

F$_{\text{IG}}$. 7.6.   Method of labelling blood film with a lead pencil.

In examining blood samples one is looking for changes in numbers, size and shape of the cells; these facts will give some indication of whether there is an anaemia, the type of anaemia, whether the patient is making an attempt to overcome it, whether there is an infection and, if so, whether acute or chronic.

## Estimation of Haemoglobin

Haemoglobin is readily measured in the colorimeter which is used for the clinical chemistry tests. The technique involves mixing 0.02 ml (20 $\mu$l) with 5 ml of Drabkin's solution and allowing the mixture to stand for 15–20 minutes (reading too soon results in erroneously high values) and reading in a colorimeter.

The concentration of haemoglobin is determined from a calibration curve constructed previously from solutions of known haemoglobin concentration.

## Measurement of the ESR (Erythrocyte Sedimentation Rate)

If a sample of unclotted blood is allowed to stand the cells will, due to gravity, sink through the plasma. Certain diseases may accelerate this fall, and the rate at which it occurs can often give some indication of the severity of the animal's condition. This test is done in a special tube (Wintrobe or Westergren tube) which must be carefully filled and then fixed upright. The tube is graduated in millimetres and the distance that the erythrocytes have fallen in 60 minutes is recorded.

## Measurement of the Packed Cell Volume (PCV)

For this test (haematocrit) an electric centrifuge is necessary.

The Wintrobe tube, after the ESR has been measured, is spun at 3000 rev/min for 30 minutes and the level again recorded. This is the PCV.

It is usually possible to see **three distinct layers** after spinning. The largest is the erythrocytes, and is deep red, the next is paler, and this is the **buffy coat**, which consists of the platelets (thrombocytes) and different types of white cells. (The size of this layer is a rough guide to the number of white cells in the blood.) The thrombocytes are arranged at the very top of the buffy coat with the leukocytes below.

The **PCV**, with the total erythrocyte count, gives a measure of the size of the cells or, with examination of the films to give some idea of the size, an indication of the number of cells present. A buffy coat of less than 0.5 mm would suggest a shortage of white cells, while more than 1.5 mm indicates a leukocytosis—increased white cells.

## Total Cell Counts

Special pipettes are usually supplied with the equipment, but these are not absolutely essential since the dilutions can be done with ordinary laboratory pipettes. It is essential to have a counting chamber; this is a thick glass slide with a central platform which is usually 0.1 mm lower than the rest of the slide. There is a channel on each side of this area which prevents seepage of the blood mixture.

On this platform are very accurately engraved a series of squares whose pattern and size vary according to the type of chamber. The best is the **Improved Neubauer**. The chamber and coverslip must be completely free of grease and, in view of the delicate nature of the apparatus, only the softest material should be used for cleaning.

*White-cell count.* The pipette is carefully filled to the 0.5 mark with well-mixed blood and then to the 11 mark with a special fluid (2% acetic acid with 0.01% gentian violet); this gives a dilution of 1 in 20. This fluid destroys the red cells and stains the nuclei of the white cells so that they are more easily seen. The blood and fluid are carefully and thoroughly mixed in the bulb by rotating the pipette. There is a small white bead in the bulb which helps the mixing. (So that no mistake is made the bead in the pipette used for erythrocyte counts is red.) The pipette should be put on one side for about 5 minutes to make sure that all the red cells are destroyed. After this period the pipette is rotated well again to make sure that the leucocytes are equally distributed throughout the fluid. The first three drops, i.e. the fluid in the capillary stem which contains no cells, is discarded and then the tip of the pipette is placed on the counting chamber and a little of the mixture allowed to flow under the coverslip. This requires care and the troughs should not be allowed to fill. The chamber is put on to the microscope stage and the $\times 10$ objective lens used. Counting should be delayed for a few minutes to allow the cells to sink; they will then all be in focus. There should be no movement of the cells; this will occur if there is too much fluid present. If the light source is too hot or too close to the chamber this will cause evaporation.

When all the movement has ceased the count can be made using the $\times 10$ objective lens. Start at the top left-hand small square and proceed along to the right, drop down a row and move back along this row and so on until one big (1 mm) square is completed. Make a note of the number of cells counted at the end of each line of small squares. Count at least four large squares.

Cells on, or touching, a line should be included in the square to the right or below. In this way they will be counted once only. It is necessary to count more than one large (1 mm) square since there is a considerable variation in the cells per square from the same mixture; this is due partly to faults in mixing and partly to chance; counting four squares overcomes this variation. The improved Neubauer has an area of 9 mm$^2$ engraved; this is subdivided into nine large squares (1 mm$^3$ area). The four corner squares are further divided into sixteen squares and the centre square is divided into twenty-five squares which themselves are divided into sixteen small squares (1/400 mm$^2$). The four corner squares should be counted for white cells.

It is important to remember here that the pipette must be absolutely clean and dry before use and must be cleaned immediately after use. Wash well in cold water until all the blood is removed, rinse in hot water and shake dry, rinse in methylated spirit and, finally, acetone and allow to drain. If needed in a hurry the pipette can be warmed on the microscope lamp but if dried in this way it must be allowed to cool before further use.

The calculation of the total white-cell count from the actual count. Let $X$ be the number of cells counted in 4 large (1 mm) squares, then

$\frac{1}{4}x =$ the number of cells in one square.

The depth of the chamber is 0.1 mm, therefore the volume for each square is 0.1 mm$^3$.

Therefore, there are $\frac{1}{4}x \times 10$ cells per mm$^3$, but the blood was diluted $\times 20$.

Therefore,

No. of cells per mm$^3$ of blood $=$

$$\frac{x \times 10 \times 20}{4} \quad \text{or } x \times 50.$$

This calculation obviously only applies to counts with chambers of 0.1 mm depth and with large squares of 1 mm$^3$ area.

Usually sufficient information upon which to base calculations is etched on the chamber.

A very simple diluting technique ("Unopette"*) is available. This consists of a length of capillary tube of known volume which fits a small plastic bottle containing a fixed volume of diluent. The capillary tube is filled with blood which is then transferred into the plastic bottle. The mixture is allowed to stand, then resuspended and transferred to the counting chamber. The capillary and bottle are then discarded. This is infinitely easier and in many cases more accurate.

The red-cell count is even more time consuming than the white-cell count, and until considerable experience has been gained the results are very unreliable. More accurate information can be gained from the PCV, and estimation of the size of the cells from examining the film.

### Examination of Blood Films

In order to examine the cellular elements of blood it is necessary to stain the cells. Special stains are used to show the differences in the cells; these stains are the Romanowsky stains and are a mixture of dyes which stain different portions of the cells different colours. There are a large variety but the simplest stain to use is **Leishman's stain**, and this gives very satisfactory results.

*Procedure.* The dried film is flooded with Leishman's stain for 2 minutes; this fixes the film. After this time, double the volume of buffered distilled water** is added and the slide rocked gently to mix the stain. It is left 5–7 minutes to stain and then washed in buffered distilled water

*"Unopette", Becton Dickinson, Wembley, Middlesex, UK.
**pH 7.0. Proprietary tablets are available for the preparation of this solution

until the film has a pinkish tinge. This should take no longer than 2–3 minutes. It is then rinsed rapidly in water and dried. The back of the slide can be wiped dry and most of the moisture shaken off the front. The slide can then be stood on its sides to drain or it can be carefully blotted with filter paper.

A new stain ("Diff-quik") has been developed which requires 5 seconds only in three solutions. This gives results comparable with the more widely known stains.

Coverslips are stained in special containers for this the May-Grunwald Giemsa method is best. This requires 5 minutes in May–Grunwald fixative and stain, a rinse in phosphate buffer pH 6.4 and 15 minutes in diluted Giemsa. The films are then washed, dried and mounted face downward.

The film should be examined with the low-power lens to get an overall picture of distribution of the cells and the quality of staining. If the film is a reasonable one and staining is satisfactory, a more detailed examination can be made with the highpower lens. This lens can be used for differential counts and for an appreciation of changes in red-cell shape and size. The oil-immersion lens should be used to examine unusual cells. If the film shows a lot of small black granules the stain needs filtering.

*The differential white-cell count* is the most important examination carried out on a blood film since the relative percentages of the different types of white cells are a valuable diagnostic aid. The leucocytes are not evenly distributed throughout the film; lymphocytes are commoner in the body than elsewhere and polymorphs accumulate in the tail. All forms are commoner at the edge of the film than in the middle. This has led to the developments of three methods for doing counts. Of these three the **"battlement method"** is

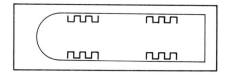

FIG. 7.7.   "Battlement" method of counting; each "step" represents two fields.

a satisfactory method (Fig. 7.7). Each "step" is two fields long; in this way a reasonable area is covered and the sites chosen for the count to some extent counteract the variations in distribution of the different types of cell.

When doing a differential count the more cells counted the more accurately will the count reflect the true picture. Count 100 cells for each 10,000 cells in the total white-cell count.

Banks of counters make counting considerably easier but another method uses squared paper; mark off blocks ten squares by ten squares. For each cell counted put a letter in each small square, N for neutrophil, L for lymphocyte, M for monocyte and E for eosinophil. When two blocks are filled, 200 cells have been counted. Count the number of each type of cell noted and express them as numbers/mm$^3$.

The commonest white cell is the neutrophilic polymorphonuclear leucocyte commonly known as the **neutrophil** or **polymorph**. This cell has relatively little colouring matter in the cytoplasm (minute red granules may be seen occasionally) and a nucleus which varies from a horseshoe shape in the young forms through two, three and four lobes up to twelve to sixteen lobes in very old cells. High numbers of these cells (neutrophilia) are seen as a response to bacterial infection, either general or local. A reduction in number (neutropenia) is sometimes seen in virus diseases.

Fairly closely related to the neutrophil

is the **eosinophil** which has large red granules in the cytoplasm except in the adult greyhound in which the cell has a pale blue cytoplasm which is vacuolated. This cell is relatively uncommon and an increase (eosinophilia) is seen in allergy, worm infestation and in insufficiency of the adrenal glands. A decrease (eosinopenia) is rare and may be seen in hyperactivity of the adrenal glands or in severe distemper.

The **basophil**, with blue-staining granules in the cytoplasm, is extremely rare in the dog.

Myeloid leukaemia is rarely seen in the dog; in this condition cells, which are the early stages in the development of these leucocytes, and which are normally confined to the bone marrow, occur in the blood. There is often also a very high total white-cell count.

Agranulocytosis, or granulopenia, that is a reduction in all these forms of leucocytes, may occur in the dog (as it does in man) as a result of treatment with a drug which depresses the bone-marrow activity.

After the neutrophil, the commonest cell is the **lymphocyte**. Sometimes this type is subdivided into large and small lymphocytes, but for routine purposes this is not necessary. These cells have relatively little cytoplasm, the large form having relatively more than the small. The significance of changes in numbers of these cells is not always certain but an increase (lymphocytosis) is frequently associated with a chronic infection and with some virus diseases. Lymphatic leukaemia is occasionally seen in which cells normally confined to the lymphoid tissues appear in the blood. A lymphopenia sometimes occurs in hormonal diseases, particularly where there is excessive production of adrenal hormones, in distemper, in chronic interstitial nephritis and in "stress".

The **monocyte** is an even more enigmatic cell than the lymphocyte. It is found in increased numbers in chronic disease.

The film will also show some very small blue "cells" with red granules; these are **platelets**. The number of platelets can be crudely assessed by examination of the film, and with experience it is possible to say whether the count is high, normal or low. Less crudely, an indirect count can be made by counting the number seen for every hundred white cells. The direct method is best done using the appropriate "Unopette" for dilution and counting on the haemocytometer.

*Reticulocyte Count*

In cases where there is anaemia it is worth knowing whether the bone marrow is active or whether the anaemia is due to a failure of the marrow to produce new cells. This can be done with a technique known as supravital staining.

Newly produced red cells contain the remnants of the intracellular organelles as a network of basophil, i.e. blue-staining material. This material cannot be demonstrated by the usual staining techniques, but if a drop of fresh, and therefore living, blood is mixed with stain, the network, or reticulum, takes up the stain. This reticulum can be stained with New Methylene Blue, a small drop of this stain is placed on a slide. A dried film is placed face down into the stain, stood for 5–10 min-

utes, and then examined. The result is reported as a percentage of the total red cell count.

**Clinical chemistry**

It is wise, when bleeding a dog for chemical tests, to avoid sampling within 8 hours after a meal. This ensures that for all practical purposes all the constituents are at the "baseline" or "fasting" level for that patient.

For most tests the presence of the blood cells is undesirable and they are eliminated either by spinning "whole blood", i.e. blood which has been taken into an anticoagulant, and recovering the clear plasma, or by allowing blood to clot and removing the serum. These two fluids differ in that plasma contains the clotting protein fibrinogen, but serum contains none. The first method has the advantage that the plasma can be separated from the cells within 15 minutes of sampling, and there are some tests which can only by carried out on serum.

*Anticoagulants*

The clotting process is a complicated one which depends on a number of enzymes and, at one step in the process, the presence of calcium.

Anticoagulants fall into two groups:
(1) Those which "block" calcium; EDTA, oxalates, citrates and fluorides.
(2) Those which interfere with an enzyme system; heparin and fluorides. For most purposes heparin is the best anticoagulant to use (2 mg/ml blood), but for glucose estimations fluoride is used.

For the following tests serum is usually used (but plasma may be)

*Enzyme tests (transaminases, alkaline phosphatase).*

*Sodium and potassium.* (In man plasma is used for potassium estimations; this is unnecessary in the dog since the concentration of potassium in the cell is low whereas in man it is high and rapidly leaks out of the cells.)

*Protein tests* (including tests for specific antibodies). If *total protein* is requested serum must be used.

### Calcium and Magnesium

In these tests plasma may be used:

*Inorganic phosphate* (though, provided that no undue delay occurs, serum or whole blood can be used).

*Cholesterol.*

*Glucose.* For glucose it was customary to use whole blood, but now plasma is frequently used; erthythrocytes are living cells and will continue to use glucose after blood has been withdrawn. It is therefore necessary to prevent this glycolysis if accurate results are wanted. For this reason a **fluoride anticoagulant** (sodium fluoride 10 parts, thymol 1 part; 10 mg/ml blood) is used. The fluoride destroys the enzyme systems concerned and the thymol prevents any bacterial growth. The concentration of glucose is higher in plasma than in the cells, and therefore higher results will be obtained than with whole blood.

*Urea* also may be estimated, depending on the technique used, on whole blood, serum or plasma, but as with glucose, plasma and serum values will be slightly higher than whole blood values.

### Constituents of Blood

Normal dog serum is usually quite clear or only slightly opaque and practically colourless. A pink or red colour shows that the sampling technique is faulty or that the equipment is dirty or wet and that haemolysis has occurred. Some samples, particularly if taken too soon after a meal, are cloudy, sometimes as dense as milk; this is due to fat and is called **lipaemia**. The serum may be yellow and this suggests **jaundice**, though very occasionally the colour may be due to a pigment related to vitamin A. The urine test for bilirubin will differentiate between them.

The compounds existing in the highest concentrations in the blood are the **proteins**. These are placed into two main groups:

(1) *Albumin*: this is a single compound whose properties and functions are very similar in all species but whose chemical composition varies slightly from one species to the next.

(2) The *globulins*: a very complex group in which at least twenty-eight different proteins have been identified. Fibrinogen is present also.

Albumin acts mainly as a means of maintaining the fluid content of the blood at the normal level through its osmotic pressure. It can also act as a transport mechanism for fats, calcium and bilirubin.

The globulins act as transfer systems for fats, copper and iron and the globulins include the **antibodies** to infectious agents. Among these proteins are the enzymes—proteins which assist some vital reactions to take place. A large number of enzymes are present in blood and only a few are of known clinical significance. Most of the clotting factors are enzymes.

Possibly next in importance to the proteins is **glucose**. Glucose is the prime source of energy for all tissues, and if the level in the blood drops too low there is an interference with brain function and fits will result. Insulin is a hormone produced in the pancreas and is necessary for the use of glucose, and where insulin is in short supply, as in diabetes mellitus, the level in the blood rises. On the other hand, if the pancreas is producing too much insulin glucose is used too quickly and the level in the blood falls below the normal level.

The estimation of blood glucose is therefore valuable in both these conditions. Diabetes mellitus can be diagnosed on urine tests alone, but estimating blood glucose will help to assess how severe the condition is and how it is responding to treatment. The excess of insulin can frequently only be differentiated from brain disease by showing that blood sugar level is very low.

Probably the most important constituent of blood from the practical aspect is **urea**. The body is unable to store protein in excess of its needs and therefore any digested protein that cannot be used immediately is excreted. It is converted to urea by the liver, transported in the blood to the kidney and there passed out with the urine. In kidney disease, and one or two other conditions, there is an inability to remove the urea from the blood and the level rises. The degree of increase is a reasonable measure of the severity of the condition, and routine testing for urea is a very good guide to the progress being made by the patient. Frequently related to the failure of kidney function is the level of inorganic phosphate in the blood. Phosphates are very important substances in the body, not only as part of the bone but also as an important compound in the chemical changes occurring in the cell. Excess phosphate is excreted by the kidneys and when the kidneys begin to fail the phosphate level begins to rise. The rise in phosphate and urea is paralleled by a rise in the serum creatinine level; creatinine is a breakdown product of protein metabolism.

It must be emphasized here that the mechanism of illness in **uraemia** is not fully understood. Urea itself is not very poisonous in dogs as they can tolerate large doses of urea given intravenously. It is thought that the illness is due to the failure of the kidneys to excrete substances like the phenols, sulphates and phosphates. Urea is, however, easier to measure than these, and for this reason it is used as an indicator of kidney disease.

The urea level can rise above normal in some conditions that are not primarily due to kidney disease. Poor heart function, with insufficient blood reaching the kidneys, will put the urea level up, and excessive water loss (e.g. after severe vomiting) will have the same effect.

The electrolytes (sodium, potassium, calcium, magnesium, copper, cobalt and iron) are important in a variety of ways but complicated to estimate.

### Chemical Methods

The methods of estimating these compounds are varied but the majority are colorimetric and depend on reacting the substance under test with another substance to produce a third coloured substance. The amount of colour produced is proportional to the amount of test substance.

The simplest methods for assaying urea are "stick" methods, but they sacrifice some degree of accuracy for simplicity and speed. "Azostix" (Ames Co.) and "Urastrat" (Warner) are both satisfactory. More accurate colorimeter methods are available, and very satisfactory enzymatic test kits are available. These require a water bath and colorimeter but give more accurate results. Both the "stick" tests and the enzyme test kits should be used according to the makers' instructions.

Glucose can also be assayed by simple though less accurate stick methods and enzymatic test kits. **Dextrostix** (Ames Co.) will help to demonstrate whether the blood glucose level is high or low, which is all that is needed for initial diagnosis. However, stabilization of diabetics has proved easier using one of the semi-automated instruments for blood glucose than using dip-stick methods. These methods are very good for glucose tolerance tests. The more accurate methods (as, for example, Boehringer and Serometer glucose assay) should be used if day-to-day checks are required.

Commercial kits are now produced for a wide variety of tests which make them suitable side-room techniques. A range of serum enzymes can now be easily estimated and these are useful for checking for liver and pancreatic diseases. Chemical supply houses should be consulted as to what is available.

*Quality control* is an important part of laboratory management. A check should be run frequently on any chemical tests that are in use. For this it is possible to buy control sera whose constituents are accurately known. These are treated in exactly the same way as the unknown sera and the calculated value compared with the value given. Such sera are marketed by Dade, Warner and others.

*Units of measurement.* As clinical pathology has developed, new tests introduced and old ones updated, there has been a proliferation of units in which the results are reported. There is no scientific rationale behind the different results, and in many cases results in one test have no correlation with results from others. In order to rationalize this variation the *Système International* (SI) has been developed. In some there will be no problem in converting from present values to SI units, the normal values will be the same in both sets of units, but with others there will be considerable changes. To assist in this period of change two tables (Tables 7.3 and 7.4) are included (by kind permission of the editor of *The Veterinary Record*).

### Method for the Estimation of Urea

There are many methods for the estimation of urea, of greater or lesser accuracy and simplicity. If one of the kit methods is being used the maker's instructions must be followed carefully.

Without doubt the two "stick" tests are the simplest to use but some accuracy is lost.

### "Azostix" (Ames Co.)

1. Freely apply a large drop of blood and spread to cover entire reagent area on the printed side of the strip. Refrigerated blood must be warmed to room temperature (variable colour development and inaccuracies may arise from the use of an insufficient amount of blood).

2. Wait exactly 60 seconds (use sweep second hand on stop-watch for timing).

3. Quickly wash blood off strip with sharp stream of water from wash bottle

TABLE 7.3.  *Normal haematological values—SI units (adults)*

|  | RBC (x $10^{12}$/1) | PCV (1/1) | Hb (g/dl) | WBC (x $10^9$/1) | Platelets (x $10^9$/1) |
|---|---|---|---|---|---|
| Dog | 6.4 | 0.450 | 15 | 10.1 | 300 |
|  | 5.5–8.5 | 0.370–0.550 | 12–18 | 6.0–18.0 | 200–500 |
| Cat | 7.5 | 0.370 | 12 | 12.5 | 400 |
|  | 5.0–10.0 | 0.240–0.450 | 8–15 | 7.0–20.0 | 300–600 |

TABLE 7.4. *Normal biochemical values—SI units (adults). All values for serum unless otherwise stated*

|  | Dog | Cat |
|---|---|---|
| Bilirubin | 1.71 | 1.71 |
| μmol/l | 0–6.84 | 0–6.84 |
| Calcium | 2.6 | 2.6 |
| mmol/l | 2.3–3.0 | 2.1–2.9 |
| Chloride | 106 | 120 |
| mmol/l | 99–115 | 117–140 |
| Cholesterol | 5.18 | 2.50 |
| mmol/l | 3.80–7.00 | 2.00–3.36 |
| Creatinine | 50 | 120 |
| μmol/l | 0–106 | 40–177 |
| B Glucose | *4.0 | *4.4 |
| mmol/l | 3.0–5.5 | 3.3–5.5 |
| Inorganic phosphate | 1.19 | 2.00 |
| mmol/l | 0.87–1.60 | 1.40–2.50 |
| Potassium | 4.2 | 4.3 |
| mmol/l | 3.6–5.6 | 4.0–5.0 |
| Total protein | 63 | 70 |
| g/l | 53–73 | 65–75 |
| Albumin | 36 | 40 |
| g/l | 31–40 | 35–45 |
| Globulin | 27 | 30 |
| g/l | 18–38 | 25–35 |
| Sodium | 146 | 153 |
| mmol/l | 139–154 | 145–156 |
| Urea | 4.98 | 4.98 |
| mmol/l | 1.66–7.40 | 1.66–7.40 |

B = blood                              *Fasting samples

directed just above reagent area. Shake off excess water (incomplete removal of blood or excessive washing will cause inaccuracies).

4. Read immediately after washing. Place strip at top of appropriate colour block and read from colour block to test area.

5. Interpolate if the colour obtained is between two colour blocks.

The makers emphasize that this is a screening test only and does not substitute for precise analytical procedures.

### "Urastat" (William R. Warner)

1. Using a long tip pipette, place 0.2 ml of plasma or serum in a $100 \times 7.5$ mm test-tube. Do not moisten the tube sides but place the fluid at the bottom of the tube.

2. Place the yellow end of the "Urastat" strip at the bottom of the tube so it dips in the fluid. Make sure the strip is vertical or fluid will creep up between the edge of the strip and the glass tube, then the whole test is ruined.

3. Leave for exactly 30 minutes at room temperature, away from draughts. A timing clock may be used in a busy practice laboratory so the reading time is not missed.

4. Remove the strip and measure the height of the colour change on the indicator band of the strip. A ruler with a millimetre reading or a special measure card may be used. The height of the colour change is multiplied by 5 and 10 added to give the urea nitrogen concentration in mg per 100 ml.

The makers state that the test is accurate for concentrations between 10 and 75 mg per 100 ml; a dilution method using standard serum would be necessary for animals with high urea levels.

### Conversion of urea nitrogen to total urea

The RANA should be aware that urea is reported as either mg blood urea per 100 ml or mg blood urea nitrogen (BUN) per 100 ml. As the nitrogen content of urea is very nearly 50% the results are easily converted by multiplying BUN levels by 2.14 to give a blood urea value.

If SI units are reported by a laboratory this figure has to be multiplied by 6.01 to give the more familiar urea in mg per 100 ml. Nurses and laboratory workers should get used to thinking in SI units as rapidly as possible.

### Examination of Faeces

The examination of faeces can be of value in the differential diagnosis of wasting diseases. As with urine, it is important to examine the sample as fresh as possible.

### Physical examination

*Macroscopic.* Take note of the colour, consistency and smell, and look for blood or mucus and adult worms (Figs. 7.8 and 7.9). Drugs will affect the colour; iron treatment will cause very black faeces, so will bleeding from the small intestine. Much fat, or the absence of bile, will cause pale faeces. Fatty faeces are usually very bulky and often smell of rancid butter.

*Microscopic.* Mix a small amount of faeces on a slide with a drop of Lugol's iodine using the bacteriological loop. Carefully lower a coverslip over the suspension avoiding air bubbles as far as possible. Examine under low power and look for:

*Muscle fibres*: the degree of digestion can be assessed by the structure. If digestion has failed, the muscle fibres stain brown and will be clear cut, the striations visible and the nuclei well preserved. "Blurring" of the nuclei, striations and edges of the fibre indicate that some digestion is occurring (Fig. 7.10).

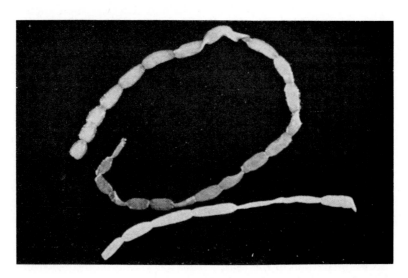

FIG. 7.8.  Tapeworm.

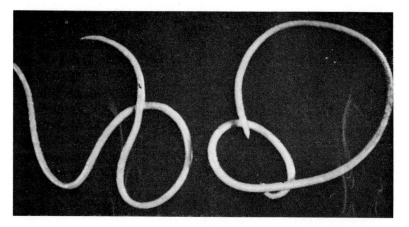

Fig. 7.9.   Roundworm.

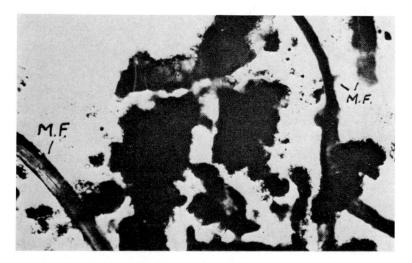

Fig. 7.10.   Suspension of faeces with iodine showing muscle fibres (MF): note striations in the fibre in the bottom left corner.

*Starch granules*: stain vivid blue or black with iodine and this colour change can sometimes be seen with naked eye (Fig. 7.11).

*Fat globules*: these are present in normal faeces and it is only safe to say that they are in excess in extreme cases (Fig. 7.11). If preferred, Sudan Red can be used instead of iodine; this stains the globules red.

Worm eggs may be seen at this stage but if they are not, further concentration methods have to be used before saying that they are absent.

**Chemical tests**

It is sometimes worth testing faeces for the presence of digestive enzymes and of these the easiest to measure is the protein-digesting trypsin.

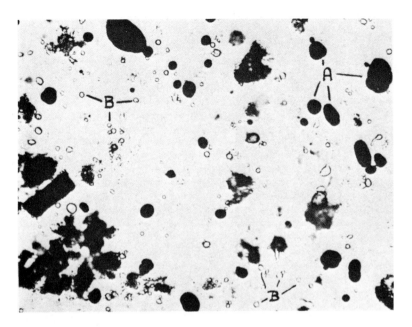

FIG. 7.11. Suspension of faeces with iodine showing black or dark blue starch grains (A), and clear, fat droplets (B).

*Film Test for Trypsin*

Mix well 1 g of faeces with 10 ml of a 1% solution of sodium carbonate, transfer one drop to a piece of X-ray film (undeveloped). Make sure that the drop is applied to the gelatin emulsion of the film. Place in a small dish and cover with a piece of moistened filter paper or blotting paper. Do not allow this to touch the film. Incubate at 37°C for 30 minutes and then rinse gently in cold running water. If trypsin is present the emulsion will have been digested and washed away in the rinse, leaving a clear area. If none was present the emulsion will have remained intact though swollen due to the action of the fluid.

*Tube-test for Pancreatic Trypsin*

(1) Enough faeces are added to 9 ml of 5% $NaHCO_3$ to make a final volume of 10 ml. Mix well.

(2) Warm 2 ml of 7.5% gelatin to 37°C, add 1 ml of faecal suspension.

(3) Incubate at 37°C for 1 hour or at room temperature for $2\frac{1}{2}$ hours.

(4) Refrigerate for 20 minutes and observe. Failure to gel indicates the presence of trypsin.

Consistently positive results (no gelation) rule out the possibility of pancreatic enzyme deficiency. Consistently negative results (gelation) may suggest pancreatic enzyme deficiency. Trypsin inhibitors in the faeces or secretion of only enough trypsin for adequate digestion may give false negatives. False positives may be due to bacterial proteolytic enzymes; however, the clearing time or digestion time is generally prolonged.

The tube-test is more accurate than the film test; the former has an accuracy of 99% as against only 75% in the latter. Occasional false negatives do occur, and if there is doubt the test should be repeated.

Trypsin is present in the normal dog to a dilution of at least 1 in 10 (frequently as high as 1 in 2000); values lower than this are strongly suggestive of reduced digestive function, but **too much reliance should not be put on this particular test.**

## Test for Occult Blood

Bleeding into the alimentary canal is easily diagnosed if there is much blood being lost. If the blood comes from high in the system it will give the characteristic black tarry faeces or if it is from the large intestine it will be obviously red. If the concentration is less than can be determined by unaided eye examination it is called occult blood. B.D.H. produces a test ("Peroheme 40") which will demonstrate the presence of blood in these low concentrations.

Unfortunately most dogs are fed a **diet which contains meat which will give a positive reaction.** A patient should be fed an all bread diet for 3 days before the test can be considered to be absolutely accurate.

## Demonstration of worm ova and coccidia

*Concentration method.* Reagent. Strong sugar solution (133 g sucrose in 100 ml water with 1 ml liquid phenol BP).

Put 1–3 g of faeces in a screw-capped bottle containing a few glass beads and add about 30 ml of water. Shake well until the faeces are completely dispersed and then filter through some coarse muslin or a small coffee strainer. This will hold back the larger debris but allow the eggs through. Centrifuge the fluid for 5 minutes at 1000 rev/min; discard the supernatant fluid. Replace with sugar solution and mix deposit and sugar solution well. Cen-

trifuge again for 2 minutes at 1500 rev/min; this will bring the worm eggs to the surface.

Just touch the surface film with a flat ended glass rod (this will pick up a drop of fluid containing the ova) and transfer to a slide. Apply coverslip and examine under the low power for worm eggs and high power for coccidia. Note presence of eggs or coccidia and relative proportion of each type (Figs. 7.12 and 7.13).

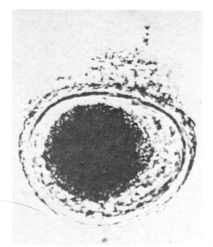

FIG. 7.12.   Roundworm ovum.

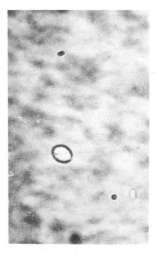

FIG. 7.13.   Coccidial oocyst.

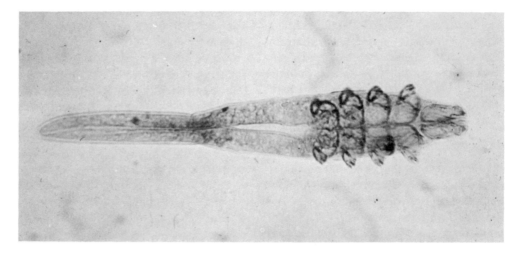

Fɪɢ. 7.14.   Demodex mite.
(by courtesy of M. Geary)

### Examination of Skin

### Demonstration of mites

In some cases of demodectic mange, where there is a secondary bacterial infection, it is worth examining the pus without staining. The lesion is raised between finger and thumb and some of the pus transferred either directly or with a loop or pipette to a slide. A coverslip is applied and the material examined for the presence of long-bodied (*Demodex*) mites (Fig. 7.14).

If there is a particularly heavy infestation of round-bodied (*Sarcoptes*) mites the direct examination may be of value (Fig. 7.15). If there are no mites to be seen by this method it is possible to concentrate them by centrifugation. A generous portion of skin and hair is transferred to a centrifuge tube and about 10 ml of potassium hydroxide solution added. This is then gently heated over a Bunsen burner (it should not be allowed to boil) for 2 or 3 minutes and allowed to cool. It is then centrifuged and a sample taken from the bottom layer transferred to a slide, covered and examined under the microscope. Look for the presence of round-bodied or long-bodied mites, and the presence of ringworm (fungal) spores in or round the broken hairs.

### Demonstration of fungi

**Wood's lamp.** The infected hairs may fluoresce a brilliant yellow-green, this must not be confused with the bluish-white and reddish-fluorescence which is due to a variety of materials. Not all cases of ringworm fluoresce and if there is no fluorescence or there is no Wood's lamp the lesions should be examined closely with a magnifying glass, and hairs (often broken) near the edge of the lesion should be pulled with forceps and examined microscopically.

The material can be examined microscopically either stained or not. Some broken hairs are transferred to a slide with a drop of 10% potassium hydroxide, allowed to stand for 10–15 minutes or

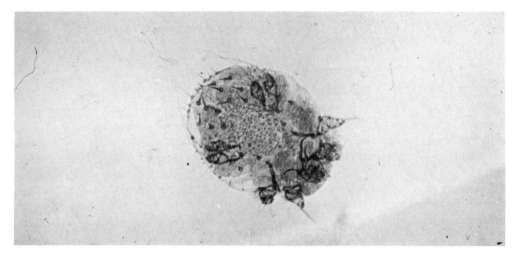

FIG. 7.15. Sarcoptes mite.
(by courtesy of M. Geary)

warmed gently. With illumination low the hairs are examined ($\times$400 magnification) for the presence of spores.

Otherwise hairs may be mounted in lactophenol-cotton blue which stains the fungus.

In unstained preparations the spores are small, round refractile bodies which frequently completely surround the hair shaft. Less commonly they may be seen within the shaft.

Ringworm in spite of its name is a **fungal infection** of the skin, hairs or nails. Fungi grow only slowly in culture and cultures should be kept for at least one month before classed as "no growth", they require special media for growth. The skin and hair are normally contaminated with non-pathogenic fungi and the certain identification of the causal agent requires much experience.

### Microbiology

It is sometimes possible to diagnose a specific condition by demonstrating the presence of the causal organism whether bacterial, viral, protozoan, fungal or parasitic.

In the practice, simple techniques can be usefully employed in showing the presence of significant bacteria or viruses. Examination can be either of the living or of the dead stained organisms; this latter method is used particularly in bacteriology.

### Examination of material for bacteria

The techniques used for the demonstration of bacteria are very similar, regardless of the material examined. It is particularly important to observe cleanliness in all techniques. Some of the organisms involved are transmissible to man and care must be taken to avoid this. It is important to examine all material as fresh as possible.

A wide-necked jar of 2% lysol should be available for the disinfection of used slides and pipettes and a second bottle for disinfection of the bench in case of accidents. Even better is the use of either a clear soluble phenol disinfectant or a hypochlorite bleach.

be obtained ready prepared from a number of sources.

### Staining techniques

*Swab and loop.* If the swab is very moist a direct smear is satisfactory; if the material does not spread well or the swab is rather dry, a drop of sterile saline may help.

Dry the smear at room temperature and fix by passing through a flame two or three times. Fixing is complete when the slide, when held against the back of the hand, is just too hot for comfort. It should never be overheated. The smear is now ready for staining.

*Fluids.* In these the bacteria should be concentrated by centrifugation at 1500 rev/min for 15 minutes. This applies to urine and pleural and ascitic fluids. After centrifugation the supernatant is discarded either by pouring or with a pipette; a few drops should be left. The sediment is resuspended in this fluid and a loopful transferred to a slide and a smear made. If tuberculosis is suspected some of the material should be saved in case animal inoculation experiments are necessary.

Some information about the type of organisms present can be gained by noting their shape and arrangement in the material, and this can be done with a very simple single-stain technique. Further identification can be made with a differential stain which depends on the chemical characteristics of the bacterial cytoplasm.

Certain bacteria, including *Mycobacterium tuberculosis*, have a high concentration of waxy substances which makes them resistant to staining. However, they can be stained using heat and a strong stain, and the stain is then very difficult to wash out. This property is used in looking for these organisms which are called acid-fast organisms. The stains mentioned can

*Methylene Blue*

*Reagent.* One per cent methylene blue. This is the simplest stain to use.

*Procedure.* To save stain and fingers, with the wax pencil draw a circle around the smear which holds the stain. Stain for 3 minutes and then wash with tap water. Shake excess water off the slide, wipe the back clean and blot the front with filter paper or fluffless blotting paper. This procedure requires care, since it is very easy to wipe the material off the slide. Alternatively, the slide may be stood on end to drain or warmed very gently over the Bunsen burner. Discard paper used for blotting. When the stain is dry it is ready to examine.

*Gram's method.* This method depends on the fact that certain bacteria which are treated with methyl violet and then iodine and finally with acetone or alcohol retain the dye while others do not. Those that do retain it are called Gram-positive and those that do not are Gram-negative. The Gram-negative organisms are stained with a red stain so that they can be readily differentiated.

The technique requires considerable practice but will give useful results.

*Reagents:*
(1) methyl violet—0.5%; filter before use;
(2) iodine solution (Lugol's iodine);
(3) acetone;
(4) 0.05% basic fuchsin

*Procedure.* Stain in (1) for 20–30 seconds and pour off excess stain. Hold slide at an angle and wash off rest of stain with (2), allow iodine to act for 30–60 seconds. Wash off iodine with water and treat with acetone for 1 second. Wash with water. Stain with basic fuchsin (4) 2–4 minutes;

wash with water and dry. The slide is now ready for examination.

The Gram-positive organisms stain deep blue-purple while the Gram-negative organisms are red.

*Examination of the Stained Smears*

Examine as for blood films using the low power first, then the high power and, finally, the oil-immersion lens.

## Examination of material for the presence of virus

Sometimes in the course of virus disease there develop within the cell accumulations of material called inclusion bodies. They may occur in the cytoplasm (cytoplasmic) or within the nucleus (intranuclear) and they cause marked changes in the disposition of the cell or nuclear contents.

In virus hepatitis these inclusion bodies sometimes develop in the nuclei of some of the liver cells and in distemper in the cells of the conjunctival and bladder mucous membranes, blood cells and elsewhere. Unfortunately, their absence does not rule out the possibility of either of these diseases, and occasionally inclusion bodies have been seen in the bladder of dogs not known to be suffering from distemper.

*Reagent.* Leishman's stain or other blood stain.

*Procedure.* For liver disease, a small portion of liver (1 cm³) is cut out and dabbed on to a slide several times. This is called an impression smear. For distemper, the lining of the bladder is scraped with a not too sharp scalpel, the material is then transferred to a slide and mixed with a drop of saline and spread.

When dry, the smears are stained with methylene blue or Leishman's stain as for blood films. The nuclei of the cells in the liver are examined for the quite marked changes which accompany the inclusion body. Normally, the coloured material (chromatin) is fairly evenly spread throughout the nucleus, and the nucleolus is centrally placed, but with the development of the inclusion body this chromatin is concentrated round the outside of the nucleus and stains very intensely, and the nucleolus is pushed to the edge. This leaves the centre of the nucleus clear and within this clear area can be seen the inclusion body (Fig. 7.16). In distemper, the development of the darkly staining inclusion body within the cytoplasm will push the nucleus to one side and may distort the cell wall; distemper inclusions in blood cells stain reddish but are very rarely seen.

## Urine

The composition of urine varies considerably according to the animal's diet and needs, and also varies during the course of the day. To obtain the maximum amount of accurate information from urine examination these tests should be carried out on a 24-hour sample, that is, all the urine passed during a 24-hour period. This, however, is not possible in practice and provided that the limitations of the method are appreciated, the "grab" sample method is satisfactory. Care must be taken in interpreting some tests, and some should be repeated on a second sample before using the result to establish a diagnosis. As with examination of blood, tests on urine are either physical or chemical.

## Examination of Urine

### Physical properties

*Colour.* This may range in the normal

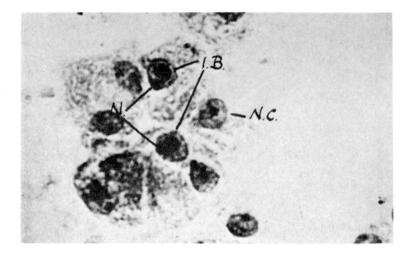

Fig. 7.16.   Impression preparation of liver showing normal cell nucleus with central nucleolus (NC) and two nuclei with inclusion bodies (IB) and nucleolus displaced to edge of nucleus (N).

animal from pale yellow or almost colourless to dark brown. The natural colour in the urine is due largely to urochrome, a pigment of endogenous origin. The variations in colour of the urine in a normal animal depend on many factors, including species, concentration, diet and exercise.

Abnormal colours are due to bile pigments, haemoglobin, blood, myoglobin—this is seen during azoturia and imparts a coffee-brown colour to the urine—and drugs, e.g. methylene blue a blue colour. Greenish fluorescence is occasionally seen in dog urine and this may be associated with colouring matter in the food.

*Turbidity.* Carnivore urine is usually clear, but becomes cloudy on standing, this is often accompanied by an increase in pH due to the presence of microorganisms that can decompose urea into ammonia, and the alkalinity then causes the precipitation of phosphates. Abnormal turbidity may be due to the presence of pus, mucus, bacteria, prostatic or vaginal secretions.

*Odour.* This varies with species and condition; the odour is sourish in dog and cat.

*Consistency.* This varies according to species, condition, diet and fluid intake. Inflammatory changes in the urinary tract may give rise to urinary mucoproteins, which may make the urine viscid.

*Reaction.* (Acid or alkaline). When fresh, normal carnivore urine is acid (pH 5–7); changes of pH may occur in abnormal metabolic conditions. A lowered pH may result from increased acid secretion in diabetes mellitus and other conditions involving increased fat metabolism. An increase in pH results from the activity of urease positive organisms (that is those which can turn urea into ammonia); a high pH in a fresh sample of dog urine indicates cystitis, but, if not fresh, may indicate bacterial contamination. It is rare to find acid urines with pH values below pH 5.

Tests for pH may be made with wide- and narrow-range indicator papers.

*Specific gravity.* This varies widely with time of taking sample, health, fluid intake, degree of exercise and sweating. It is inadvisable to draw conclusions from an observation of the specific gravity of a single urine sample; more than one sample should be examined. The normal range in the dog is 1.012–1.060 and in the cat 1.020–1.040.

Values are low in polyuria, for example, in chronic interstitial nephritis in the dog, and in diabetes insipidus (1.001–1.005): high values (but not outside the normal range) may be found in acute nephritis in the dog, in various fevers and often in diabetes mellitus. A so-called "fixed-level" value of about 1.008–1.012 may be found in severe cases of renal insufficiency when this value remains constant irrespective of diet and fluid intake. This corresponds to the specific gravity of protein-free plasma filtrates. Specific gravity is measured with a urinometer or refractometer.

**Chemical tests**

*Proteins.* Recent developments in analytic technique have revealed that **most normal urines contain traces of protein** although these are in quantities that are too small to be identified by normal chemical techniques. Small quantities of protein are known to pass the normal glomeruli and there is good evidence for reabsorption of albumin and globulin in the proximal tubule.

Protein is pre-renal (haemoglobin, myoglobin), renal (acute fevers, nephritis), or post-renal (lower urinary or genital tract) origin. Spermatozoa are frequently found in male dog urine, and this indicates that there is a leak of seminal fluid into the urinary tract. This fluid is protein rich and will give positive results with protein tests. Severe cystitis will cause an exudation of serum into the bladder and this will also give positive results. In cases of nephritis, where there is little glomerular damage and, therefore, little protein

loss, the urine will be free from protein as shown by the usual tests. It is obvious, therefore, that one must be careful in assessing the significance of proteinuria, and it is worth examining the urinary sediment microscopically for spermatozoa and for bacteria which may be causing cystitis.

*Sulphosalicylic acid test.* In a small test-tube or on a piece of black perspex place one drop of 20% sulphosalicylic acid. This is followed by one drop of urine. Protein is indicated by a faint turbidity (0.01%) to a discrete heavy precipitate (possibly as high as 1%); compare with normal urine. Report as + to + + + + +.

*"Albustix".* These are strips of plastic, one end of which is impregnated with tetrabromphenol blue buffered to approximately pH 3.0 with a citrate buffer. Urine containing protein gives a colour change —yellow through green to blue—depending on the concentration of protein. This test is not satisfactory with urines of high (alkaline) pH.

*Reducing substances.* Most normal urines when boiled with an alkaline solution of a copper salt cause no change; a few, however, reduce the salt. Depending on the amount reduced, a colour change from pale green to bright yellow/brick red occurs. (It is very unusual for a normal urine to contain sufficient reducing substances to produce the complete reaction.) **Glucose will produce this colour change** and so will lactose or milk sugar. Glucose is found in the urine in diabetes mellitus and in very small quantities in occasional cases of kidney disease and occasionally due to a high carbohydrate meal; lactose is sometimes found in the urine of lactating and suckling animals. Lactose is not used by the animal; if, therefore, any be absorbed, as occurs if the mammary gland becomes distended, or if the alimentary mucosa is disrupted, then it is excreted unchanged.

Several substances, other than glucose and lactose, reduce these reagents and may be responsible for false positives. These substances include creatinine, uric acid, glucuronic acid and glucuronides. Pentoses and fructose also reduce copper, but as yet they have not been positively identified in animal urines. The use of certain drugs increase the normal output of glucuronides and may result in a definitive "positive".

*"Clinitest" tablets.* Using the "standard" dropper provided, put five drops of urine and ten of water into a tube, and add one tablet and allow to react, watching all the time. Fifteen seconds after the reaction has ceased, shake the tube and compare with colour chart provided. When the concentration is high, the final colour may be brown rather than orange, but orange colour will have occurred during the reaction, and for this reason the test must be watched throughout.

*Demonstration of glucose in urine.* It is important to show whether or not the reducing substances in the urine is glucose. For this purpose the test papers containing the enzyme glucose oxidase ("Clinistix") are used. These are dipped into the urine. If glucose is present the enzyme reacts with it, liberating oxygen in an active form which turns an indicator in the strip purple within 1 minute. This test is given by glucose only, but if the strip is allowed to stand for a long time after dipping the atmospheric oxygen may turn it purple. It is not sufficient to rely only on "Clinistix", but this *and* "Clinitest" should be used. Alternatively, "Diastix" alone may be used.

*Ketones.* The most satisfactory test for ketones in urine is that of Rothera and its developments. The ketone bodies usually encountered are acetone, acetoacetic acid and betahydroxybutyric acid. Transient false positives may result from the presence of organic sulphides (mercaptans)

and excessive pyruvate will give a very blue reaction. These are yet of no known clinical significance in small animals. Ketone bodies occur in urine as the result of carbohydrate starvation, e.g. in diabetes mellitus.

*"Acetest" tablets.* These are a modification of Rothera's mixture. Place one drop of urine on a tablet, allow to stand for 30 seconds and compare with colour chart provided. Report as trace (+), moderate (+ +) or strong (+ + +). Alternatively, "Ketostix" may be used.

*Blood and blood pigments.* There are **several tests for the presence of blood in urine**. The three most important are (a) the identification of red cells microscopically, (b) spectroscopic examination, and (c) the *o*-toluidine test. There are several modifications of the last. Blood may be present either as haemoglobinuria or as haematuria. Haematuria may become haemoglobinuria as a result of degeneration of red cells. (Haemoglobinuria, or myoglobinuria which also gives a positive reaction with *o*-toluidine are pre-renal conditions, that is to say, they are present in the blood before it reaches the kidney.) Haemoglobinuria or haematuria can be differentiated by microscopic examination of the sediment. Absence of debris or cells indicates pure haemoglobinuria; erythrocytes or debris indicates haematuria. A previously red sample, which becomes clear on spinning, with a red deposit is normally haematuria. Haematuria indicates haemorrhage at some point in the urinary tract, e.g. bruising of the kidneys, inflammation or tumour of the bladder and wounds of the urethra (usually the result of catherization).

*"Occultest".* Put two drops of urine on the filter paid, put a tablet on top and flood the tablet with two drops of water. Watch for speed of development and intensity of the blue colour. Report + to + + + + +. Alternatively, use "Hema-

stix". Haemoglobin may be distinguished from the myoglobin by spectroscopic examination.

*Bile salts and bile pigments.* Bile pigments appear in the urine of animals suffering from various disorders affecting the pigment (haemoglobin) metabolism of the body. It has long been held that the presence of bilirubin in the urine is a good indication of obstructive liver disease, but it is becoming increasingly obvious that this is not the case in the dog. Bilirubin, which is insoluble in water, is transported from the reticulo-endothelial system to the liver as a complex with serum albumin. In the liver this complex is broken down and bilirubin converted to the water-soluble glucuronide. In man this is apparently the only site of production of a water-soluble bilirubin compound. In haemolytic jaundice there is an increased production of the glucuronide excreted in the bile, but there is no regurgitation into the vascular system. In obstructive jaundice, conjugation occurs normally but owing to the obstruction the bile cannot reach the intestine, and bilirubin-glucuronide and bile salts are regurgitated into the vascular system and are excreted by the kidney. Testing for bilirubin is therefore a useful procedure in the diagnosis of these two conditions. However, in the dog this happy state of affairs does not exist, serum bilirubin being in a much lower concentration than it is in man, which suggests a more efficient excretory mechanism. The enzyme necessary for conjugating bilirubin has been shown to exist in the kidney and up to 20% of dogs which show no impairment of their liver function by other tests excrete detectable quantities of bilirubin in their urine. Presumably conjugation is occurring in the kidney. In addition, there are a number of cases in which liver function, as estimated by serum changes, is severely impaired but in which no bilirubinuria occurs. The kidney

can also convert haemoglobin to bilirubin. It has also been shown that 5% of normal cats excrete bilirubin.

It may or may not be justifiable, but it is assumed that trace and even mildly positive reactions are without clinical significance in the dog. However, strongly positive reactions may indicate an obstructive condition, either intrahepatic or in the extrahepatic duct system or an increase in haemolysis. Hayes test (for bile salts) should be positive only in obstructive conditions but positive results occur in normal dogs.

In the absence of information to the contrary it is assumed that species other than the cat and dog simulate man in their metabolism of bilirubin.

*Ictotest tablets.* Put five drops of urine on the special mat provided, put a tablet on the mat and flood it with two drops of water. Note the intensity of the purple colour developed within 30 seconds.

**A wide range of tests can now be performed with one dipstick.** "Multistix" have a patch for detecting and at least giving a semiquantitative value for:

(1) Urobilinogen.
(2) Bilirubin.
(3) Protein.
(4) Glucose.
(5) Ketones.
(6) Blood.
(7) pH.

It is doubtful that the added information afforded by having the urobilinogen patch is worth the added expenditure. The interpretation of other results from the dipstick is the same as that for the "Labstix" test stick.

**Microscopic examination of urine**

Considerable information can be gained about the state of the urinary tract by examination of the sediment in urine. For satisfactory results this must be done on fresh urine.

Put 10 ml of urine in a centrifuge tube and spin at 2500 rev/min for 5 minutes. Discard most of the supernatant fluid (or use for the chemical tests) and mix the sediment gently but well with two or three drops of "Sedistain".*

There may be no deposit, but usually some bladder epithelium cells will be present and crystals are common. "Casts" occur also; these are cylinders of material, protein, fat or cells, which have been washed down from the kidney tubules where they are formed (Fig. 7.17).

Urinary deposits may be divided as follows:

*In the United Kingdom obtainable from Arnold R. Horwell Ltd., 2 Grangeway, Kilburn High Road, London NW6 1YB.

*Deposits*

| *Cellular* | *Inorganic/organic* |
|---|---|
| Excess of these nearly always associated with disease | Rarely pathological, normal result of metabolism. May increase, e.g. alkaline phosphate in infected urine (see above) |

| *Acid* | *Alkaline* |
|---|---|
| Urates | Phosphates |
| Cystine | |

*Cellular Deposits.*

*Epithelial cells.* These are present normally in small numbers, some from the vaginal epithelium in females. Transitional epithelial cells may be seen in cystitis; cells from the kidney tubules may be seen in nephritis.

*Polymorphs.* These look very similar to those seen on blood films. If the urine is also rich in protein and casts, the pus is

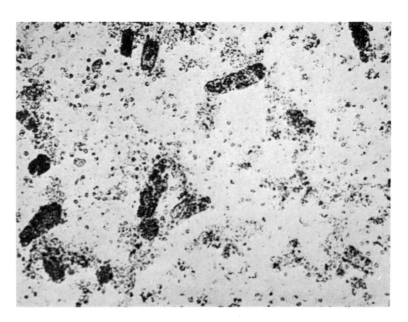

FIG. 7.17.   Urinary sediment showing casts and cells, mostly polymorphs.

likely to have come from the kidney. Pyuria is also seen in prostatitis, metritis and vaginitis. In haemorrhage, red and white cells are present in the proportion in which they are found in the blood.

*Erythrocytes.* Nearly always pathological (but remember that oestrus in the bitch will give haematuria). If from the kidney the cells may form cylinders.

*Spermatozoa.* In urine from males.

*Parasites. Capillaria* spp., in foxes and foxhounds.

*Bacteria. Cocci, coliforms, Proteus.* Urine sometimes contains contaminants; bacteria are present but there is no other evidence of inflammation in the tract.

*Tumour cells.* For example from papilloma of bladder.

*Casts.* These are structures moulded into the renal tubules; look for parallel sides. Hyaline casts are simple protein and indicate a leak of protein in the glomerulus. This protein precipitates as the concentration and acidity increase, therefore the more severe the disease the more casts. Epithelial casts may retain their cellular structure or degenerate and form granular casts; lipid casts also occur. All these forms may be stained with bilirubin. Erythrocyte casts are indicative of glomerular bleeding and on degeneration form copper-coloured haem casts.

### Crystals

*Uric acid.* Usually tinged brown. Rhomboid plates, rosettes of spindle-shaped crystals, clusters of parallel crystals.

*Amorphous urates.* In strongly acid urine, Resemble red, yellow or brown sand in miniature (dissolve on warming). There is a predisposition to these in Dalmatians. They are present in cases of severe liver disease.

*Calcium oxalate.* A small amount in all urines. The crystals are four-sided or dumbbell-shaped. They are soluble in hydrochloric acid, but not in acetic acid.

*Cystine.* Flat regular hexagons. Associated with increased cystine in the urine.

*Triple phosphate.* Magnesium ammonium phosphate. Prismatic crystals with oblique ends (knife rests, coffin lid) or feathery or leaf-shaped, often agglomerated into star-shaped bodies. If found in fresh urine, they indicate retention or alkaline fermentation (pyelitis, cystitis). They will deposit if the urine is allowed to stand.

*Calcium carbonate.* Crystals dissolve in acid giving bubbles of carbon dioxide. They are usually yellowish spheres with radial striation; these crystals are rare in small animals.

*Sulphonamide crystals.* These are sometimes seen in patients that are being treated with sulphonamides. The shapes vary very much according to which drug is being used.

Many other crystals not readily identifiable may be seen in urine but can be ignored as their significance is uncertain.

### Urinary calculi

The factors involved in the development of urinary calculi are not fully understood, but a knowledge of the composition of the stones is sometimes of value in treatment.

*Phosphate stones.* These are the commonest stones. They are found particularly in bitches and in certain breeds which have a tendency to develop them. They may be large or small, rough or smooth, single or multiple. Usually the single stones are rough, two or more are smooth. They are not infrequently associated with an alkaline urine.

*Test for phosphate.* Scrape a little of the stone into a tube and add a drop of concentrated nitric acid, follow this with a drop of 10% ammonium molybdate and warm gently. A yellow precipitate indicates phosphate.

*Cystine stones.* There seems to be little connection between the amount of cystine in the urine and the development of cystine stones. These are usually small, round and smooth and yellowish in colour and cause obstruction of the urethra. Occasionally larger stones confined to the bladder are seen.

*Test for cystine.* Scrape a little of the stone into a test-tube, add a drop of 10% sodium cyanide and a drop of 20% ammonia solution. Allow to stand for 5 minutes and then add a very small crystal of sodium nitroprusside. The development of a magenta colour indicates the presence of cystine.

*Urate stones.* The Dalmatian has a high excretion of urates and has a tendency to develop stones of this type. Again they may be small or large, are usually smooth and are pale green or brown. The larger stones are frequently markedly laminated.

*Test for urate stones.* A little of the stone is treated with concentrated nitric acid, warmed gently until the residue is dry and allowed to cool. A drop of 20% ammonia solution is added and if urates are present a purple colour develops.

*Oxalates stones.* These stones are readily distinguishable by their very crystalline structure and considerable hardness. They are perhaps the least common stone.

*Test for oxalate stones.* Crush a little of the stone into a tube, add a drop of concentrated sulphuric acid and a few grains of resorcinol. Allow to stand up to 3 minutes when a greenish-blue colour develops if oxalates are present.

Frequently calculi are not composed entirely of one substance. For example, many cystine stones contain some phosphate, and for this reason tests for all common constituents should be carried out on each stone.

These compounds described are not the only ones which cause urinary calculi. If further tests are necessary the calculus may be sent away or other textbooks consulted for methods.

## Further Reading

Baker, F. J., Silverton, R. G. and Luckcock, E. D. (1966) *An Introduction to Medical Laboratory Technology,* 4th edn., Butterworths, London.

Bush, B. M. (1975) *Veterinary Laboratory Manual,* Heinemann, London.

Duncan, J. R. and Prasse, K. W. (1977) *Veterinary Laboratory Medicine, Clinical Pathology,* Iowa State University Press, Ames, Iowa.

Kaneko, J. J. (1980) *Clinical Biochemistry of Domestic Animals,* 3rd edn., Academic Press, New York.

Medway, W., Prier, J. and Wilkinson, J. S. (1969) *Textbook of Veterinary Clinical Pathology,* Williams & Wilkins, Baltimore.

Schalm, O. W., Jain, N. C. and Carroll, E. J. (1975) *Veterinary Haematology,* 3rd edn., Baillière Tindall, London.

# CHAPTER 8

# Medical Nursing

## (a) Medical Disorders

F. W. G. HILL

### Introduction

The function of a RANA is to assist animals both sick and healthy whilst they are under the care of a veterinary surgeon. They are to do this in such a way as to help the animals gain independence, confidence, comfort and normal health as rapidly as possible. An ANA should have a caring sympathetic disposition and want to work with animals. She will need to develop an understanding of animals and remember that each one is an individual, whose reaction to the surgery premises and hospitalization may vary considerably. Much of this understanding comes from experience, but some of it can be learnt by giving forethought to each situation as it arises. Most of the medical nursing duties will be with the hospitalized animals. Usually these are dogs and cats plus the occasional exotic species. Animals are hospitalized for the following reasons:
1. surgical procedures and post-operative care. 2. clinical investigation and diagnostic-aid procedures, and 3. special care, where a patient is very ill and needs constant monitoring, attendance to changing needs and support of physiological and metabolic functions.

From this it is very evident that the RANA or ANA trainee performs a vital role in the running of a small animal veterinary practice and provides the essential link between the patient and the veterinary surgeon.

### Nursing guide-lines for the very ill animal

The RANA will be required to have a good knowledge of the serious and common emergency disorders which occur in dogs and cats. This will enable her to anticipate the requirements of the veterinary surgeon dealing with such a case and when necessary to make the initial nursing procedures and initiatives without supervision thus saving very valuable time.

The very ill patients which are admitted and hospitalized represent a wide spectrum of disease, but almost certainly over 50% will be the result of some form of trauma. Of the remainder pyometra, obstructive urolithiasis, neurological disease

483

particularly from intervertebral disc protrusion, haemorrhagic gastrointestinal disorder of dogs, cases of poisoning, renal failure, and severe cardiopulmonary diseases are likely admissions. The most important aspect of the care of the very ill patient is good nursing.

A veterinary practice or hospital may adapt an area adjacent to the kennel treatment area and operating theatre, where critically ill animals may be cared for and at the same time be under constant supervision. This is the equivalent of the **intensive care unit** of a human hospital. Intensive care in general veterinary practice does not necessarily mean sophisticated monitoring techniques, but more appropriately simple clinical procedures such as the measurement of vital signs and appreciation of the need for frequent monitoring and recording the re-evaluation of the findings, and close supervision by veterinary nurses.

## Medical Disorders

The description of some common medical disorders of dogs are of those which a RANA should be aware of and with experience be able to recognize. They are diseases which are unlikely to warrant hospitalization, particularly those of an infectious nature, and more likely the treatment and nursing will be confined to the consulting room and home environment or in exceptional cases an isolation kennel.

## Canine Infectious Diseases

### Distemper

Canine distemper was the commonest infectious disease of dogs. Many different species in the Order Carnivora are susceptible to the infection, including the fox and ferret, and the mortality rate varies greatly between species. It manifests as an acute or sub-acute contagious febrile disease with nasal and ocular discharges, respiratory and gastrointestinal signs. A variable proportion of affected animals develop nervous manifestations, which may occur during the acute phase of the disease or several weeks or even months later. This complication is particularly common in the pedigree breeds of dog. Hyperkeratosis of the foot pads and to a lesser degree the nostrils is seen in some cases.

### Aetiology

Distemper virus (CDV) is a member of the paramyxovirus group and is closely related to the measles and rinderpest viruses. It is a comparatively fragile virus, inactivated by light, heat, and most common disinfectants. It survives freezing, a property used for the preservation of live vaccines. There is only one antigenic type of distemper virus, although variations in virulence may occur.

### Pathogenesis

The natural route of infection appears to be aerosol or droplet exposure into the respiratory tract. The primary routes will be (1) nose to nose contact, (2) inhalation of droplets suspended in air of closed spaces or environments, (3.) droplets from nose and mouth to nose, mouth or conjunctiva. The virus replicates in local macrophages which transport it to lymphatic tissues and subsequently within a few days to the spleen, thymus and bone marrow. Now one of two things can happen. Firstly, if neutralizing antibodies against distemper appear in the tissues within one week of the infection commencing, then the infection remains inapparent and virus can no longer be isolated from tissues. Secondly if the dog fails to develop protective levels of neutralizing antibody by 14 days post infection, the virus continues multiplying and spreads to the epithelium of many organs including the brain, resulting in the clincal disease with a high mortality.

Other agents may complicate an infection. These include bacteria such as *streps, staphs, mycoplasma* and importantly *Bordetella bronchiseptica,* which colonize and set up secondary infections in the respiratory tract. Dual infections with infectious canine hepatitis (CAV) virus and distemper are recognized. As are distemper virus and toxoplasma, where it has been suggested that in the dogs the virus activates the co-existing latent protozoan infection.

*Clinical Signs*

Canine distemper produces a variety of clinical signs ranging from no apparent disease to severe illness with high mortality. This inconsistency exists between and within litters of puppies which have been exposed to the same strain of virus, and is thought to be due to a number of factors including; varying existing immune status and the ability of individuals to develop antibodies; different nutritional states; and the interaction with other agents, i.e. viruses, bacteria and parasites.

The incubation period is 3 to 10 days, after which there is an initial temperature rise 39 to 40°C lasting 24 to 48 hours. If present at all, clinical signs are very mild and transient. Dogs that develop antibodies now show no further signs and recover.

A second temperature rise occurs after an apparently normal period of 1 to 4 days (**Diphasic temperature rise**) and may either persist for the duration of the disease or fluctuate somewhat. Now come the characteristic signs, dominated by secondary infection, and treatment for the dog is sought by the owner.

Anorexia, tonsillitis, conjunctivitis—first watery, later a purulent ocular discharge.

Respiratory signs: rhinitis with watery, later mucopurulent nasal discharge; pneumonia, first viral later secondary bacterial.

Gastrointestinal signs: diarrhoea is common, vomiting occasional.

A gradual loss of body condition, leading to emaciation and dehydration.

Less consistent signs are skin lesions, keratitis, retinitis, and keratitis sicca (may appear after recovery). Later hyperkeratosis of foot pads and nose may take place.

Later signs are from the Nervous System. They can be inconsistent and usually develop in affected animals 3 or more weeks post exposure to the virus. Nervous signs depend upon the particular nerves damaged and may be summarized as follows.

(1) Cranial Nerve lesions: Abnormal pupillary light reflex, optic neuritis and blindness.

(2) Meningeal signs: Hyperaesthesia, hyperthermia.

(3) Cerebral signs: Incoordination, pacing, circling, convulsions—tonic, clonic or grandmal seizures which initially occur sporadically, but in some become more frequent and violent.

(4) Spinal signs: Encephalomyelitis produces posterior weakness or ataxia and leads to paresis and posterior paralysis with faecal and urinary incontinence. "Chorea" (myoclonus) is an involuntary regular movement or twitching of isolated muscle groups, usually in the legs or abdominal wall, and commonly in the temporal muscles of the forehead.

(5) Cerebellar signs: Incoordination, hypermetria, dysmetria, head tilt, nystagmus, circling and rolling over.

The onset and development of nervous signs warrants a grave prognosis.

Distemper is a crippling and despairing disease as it runs its course. Even in the event of recovery from the initial acute disease and less frequently from the neurological disease there is always a possibility of one or more of the following delayed effects; chorea, posterior paresis, seizures, personality changes, retinal atrophy and pitted enamel on unerupted permanent teeth of puppies.

*Excretion of Virus*

From the point of view of control and spread of infection it is as well for the RANA to realize that dogs with the acute systemic infection and generalized distribution of the virus throughout their body will shed virus in practically every excretion, i.e. nasal and conjunctival exudates, saliva, urine and irregularly in faeces.

*Diagnosis* by the veterinary surgeon may be difficult in the untypical dog affected with distemper.

The acute clinical signs, and later the presence of "chorea" is diagnostic. In the laboratory confirmation of the diagnosis is made from (a) ferret inoculation, (b) virus isolation in tissue culture, (c) a fluorescent antibody test, (d) the identification of inclusion bodies in surface epithelial cells such as conjunctiva, nasal mucosa, tongue and vagina. The RANA employed in the practice laboratory may be asked to perform this latter diagnostic test and it is worth noting that the results are inconsistent because the inclusion bodies are not found in all cases of canine distemper and they may only be present at certain stages of the infection.

*Treatment and Nursing Action*

(1) Check record card for any previous vaccination history.

(2) Prepare to disinfect consulting room and any contaminated areas after the infected animal leaves the premises.

(3) Change apron after holding an infected dog.

(4) Treatment is entirely symptomatic and supportive; plus chemotherapy for secondary bacterial invaders.

    (a) Prepare antibiotic therapy as directed i. systemic ii. eye ointment.

    (b) Put up antidiarrhoea therapy.

    (c) Prepare anti-emetics as directed.

    (d) Fluid therapy as directed.

    (e) Put up anticonvulsants as directed (Dilantin, dilantin and phenobarbital, primidone).

(5) Advise the owners on nursing care. Infected dogs require rest, warmth, isolation and cleanliness. Exercise in public places should be stopped and the dog only allowed access to its own garden. Keep the eyes and nostrils clean and free from discharges. Protect the nostrils with petroleum jelly.

(6) Make further appointments for the patient to be seen out of regular surgery hours so that contact with other dogs at the surgery is minimized. A veterinary surgeon may decide to visit an infected dog at the owner's home to minimize the risk of cross infection at his surgery premises.

(7) Warn owners of in-contact susceptible dogs and recommend vaccination.

*Epizootiology*

There is a seasonal incidence of distemper cases in the Autumn and Winter. It occurs in puppies and young dogs under a year of age, when their immunity is minimal. The disease is still common in some urban communities. There is maximum susceptibility at 4 to 5 months of age, when all pups have lost their colostral or maternal antibodies and they are released to the town environment and exposed to the distemper virus for the first time. The disease is always present because of the continuing introduction of new susceptible puppies.

## Control

The control of distemper is by vaccination, which is discussed in a later section (p. 542).

## Canine Adenovirus (Infectious Canine Hepatitis ICH)

Infectious canine hepatitis is a sporadic disease of dogs and foxes. The clinical disease varies between species. Neurological signs predominate in the fox. The disease is distributed world-wide with an approximate 50% incidence amongst dog populations, which is much higher than the incidence of the clinical disease. The severity of the clinical illness decreases as age increases, such that severe clinical disease or death from ICH is rare in dogs over 2 years of age.

### Aetiology

It is caused by an Adenovirus—canine adenovirus type-1(CAV–1). It is more resistant than the distemper virus and survives outside the body for up to 11 days. The virus may be easily destroyed by heat, drying and common disinfectants. It is resistant to solvents and freezing.

### Pathogenesis

The natural route of infection is by the ingestion of infective alimentary secretions from either active clinical cases or infective urine from recovered cases. Adenovirus shows an affinity for reticuloendothelial cells, vascular endothelium and hepatic cells, resulting in the well-known clinical disease of "canine hepa-

titis". This can be reproduced experimentally by the Iv or oral administration of the virus to susceptible dogs.

When the virus is administered by aerosol to the respiratory tract, it causes necrotizing lesions in the lungs and clinical respiratory disease which in turn may be transmitted from infected to susceptible dogs by coughing. The relative importance of the two routes in naturally occurring disease has yet to be determined.

In the early stages (viraemia) of the classical systemic infection, virus is limited almost entirely to the vascular endothelium (liver, lymphoid tissues), and the kidney glomeruli (proteinuria and virus shedding occurs into the urine).

After recovery the virus disappears from most body tissues, but persists in the eye and the kidney (recovered carrier animals).

This persistence of virus in the eye can result in oedema and clouding ("Blue eye") of the cornea 7 to 28 days after the initial infection. In the vast majority of cases this reaction resolves spontaneously without apparent sequella (p. 543).

Dual infections with canine distemper can occur, usually resulting in more severe disease. Unlike distemper secondary bacterial infections do not play an important role in the clinical disease.

### Clinical Signs

The incubation period is 5 to 9 days after which a variety of clinical forms occur, ranging from the most common— very mild or subclinical to a fulminating hyperacute form with high mortality. Usually only dogs with the more severe forms are presented for treatment, creating a false impression that ICH has a high mortality.

1. *Fulminating-hyperacute form.* Neonatal puppies may die suddenly without

clinical signs of disease. Weanling puppies and young adults under one year of age show a temperature rise, 40° to 41° lasting for 24 to 48 hours before dropping. It may either rise again (diphasic rise) for another 2 to 5 days or may drop to subnormal. The puppies have: anorexia, depression, shock, haemorhagic diarrhoea, vomiting blood, intense abdominal tenderness and pain, and possibily haemorrhages on visible mucous membranes. A sudden collapse, resembling haemorrhagic shock occurs and death ensues 24 to 72 hours after the onset of signs.

2. *Severe, non-fatal form.* This is the most usual form presented for treatment.

There is the initial temperature rise, again usually diphasic, anorexia; thirst; enlarged reddened tonsils; prominent peripheral lymph nodes; congested mucous membranes sometimes with haemorrhages visible, and abdominal pain. The anterior abdomen (liver) is tender to the touch, and the swollen liver extending distally beyond the costal arch may be palpable. The dog may have a tucked-up appearance, be reluctant to move, and may from time to time adopt a praying posture.

Less commonly seen are vomiting, diarrhoea, subcutaneous oedema from the ventral neck to thorax and haemorrhages on the skin of the abdomen and inner thighs.

The disease follows a course of 4 to 7 days after which there is a rapid recovery.

3. *Mild clinical form.* This is common with very minimal clinical signs lasting 1 to 2 days. Depression, a slight temperature rise and anorexia, followed by a rapid recovery. These cases are seldom presented for treatment.

4. *Inapparent or transient sub-clinical disease* is also common.

During the convalescent period for any non-fatal cases, 20% may develop corneal oedema ("blue eye"), 1 to 3 weeks after the ICH infection. In the sub-clinical forms of the disease this may be the only sign and may provide a retrospective diagnosis or, if the animal has not previously been presented for treatment, questioning the owner may reveal a few days of malaise, about 1 to 2 weeks previously. The corneal oedema is frequently unilateral, but occasionally is bilateral. It is transient and clears spontaneously in 3 to 7 days in most instances without treatment.

Acute febrile diseases of young dogs must always be differentiated from canine distemper.

1. Clinical signs may distinguish between the two virus infections.

2. Clinical pathology: markedly elevated liver enzymes (SGPT) with adenovirus, infection and an increased bleeding and clotting times are seen.

*Treatment and Nursing Action*

There is no specific treatment. Supportive therapy and nursing care are indicated, depending on the form of clinical disease.

1. Whole blood transfusions—for the hyperacute fulminating form. Where there is extreme blood loss and shock.

2. Fluid therapy—for the severe forms, where haemorrhage is not a problem. (a) Ringers (b) lactated Ringers (c) 2.5% Dextrose + N/2 saline.

3. There is little indication for antibiotics.

4. Vitamins and supplements. B vitamin range either combined with extensive fluid therapy or alone, when anorexia lasts for several days.

5. Check vaccination records.

6. Carry out disinfection of the consulting room and waiting room.

7. Change clothes.

8. Warn owners of the risk to other susceptible puppies and isolate dog at home.

9. Arrange for vet to see the patient either out of surgery hours or at home as directed.

## Canine leptospirosis

This disease is known also as canine typhus, Stuttgart disease, Yellows and Weil's disease in man.

### Aetiology

The organisms responsible belong to the family of bacteria called *Leptospira*. Commonly in disease they are *Leptospira canicola* and *Leptospira icterohaemorrhagiae*. Occasionally *Leptospira pomona* is implicated. Leptospira are not very resistant, being readily destroyed by sunlight, acids and alkalis, chemical disinfectants and extremes of temperature. Their survival outside the body is helped by moisture, moderate temperatures and organic matter. Their incidence is variable throughout the world and many sub-clinical infections occur. The disease is reported only rarely in cats.

### Pathogenesis

Dogs are exposed to the disease through contact with infected urine from recovered dogs (*L. canicola*) and rats (*L. icterohaemorrhagiae*). The leptospira get into the body following ingestion or by penetrating intact skin or mucous membranes. There is a higher incidence of disease in male dogs. In general *L icterohaemorrhagiae* attacks the liver and circulation, causing (1) an acute haemorrhagic syndrome and (2) an acute jaundice syndrome. Whilst *L. canicola* produces predominantly renal lesions, (1) an acute systemic disease and (2) acute or chronic nephritis. The incubation period is 7 to 21 days.

### Clinical Signs

The clinical signs are variable and it is not possible to determine conclusively the aetiological agent from the form seen in the clinical syndrome.

1. *Peracute haemorrhagic syndrome.* (usually *L. icterohaemorrhagiae*).

In this form, the disease is rapidly fatal, running a course of only a few hours in puppies, to approximately 10 days in adult dogs. Jaundice and uraemia are usually absent. There is the sudden onset of high temperature; depression; stiff muscular movements; thirst; vomiting and diarrhoea; both with or without blood; haemorrhage from the nose (epistaxis) and small haemorrhages (petechia) in the skin, sclera and conjunctiva of the eye. The onset of dehydration is rapid and death supervenes.

2. *Acute jaundice syndrome.* (Either *L. icterohaemorrhagiae* or *L. canicola*).

A sudden to gradual onset of high temperature, depression, anorexia, thirst, vomiting, and **jaundice** in affected dogs. The disease runs a course of one to three weeks.

3. *Uraemic syndrome.* (Usually *L. canicola*)

This may be an acute, sub-acute or chronic disease. It can follow an acute systemic infection or possibly occur without any prior illness. The signs are thirst and polyuria, vomiting, weight loss, dehydration, pain in the lumbar region with the spine arched and a stiff gait. In the later stages of the syndrome very little urine is produced and the mouth and tongue become inflamed and even ulcerated.

### Clinical Pathology

This is variable and dependent very largely on the predominate clinical syndrome occurring in an affected dog.

*Haematology*

(a) Leucocytosis (left shift). (b) Anaemia and thrombocytopaenia—haemorrhagic form.

*Urine*

(a) Proteinuria. (b) Bilirubinuria—jaundice form.

*Chemistry*

(a) Elevated blood urea and acidosis—uraemic form (b) Elevated liver enzymes and direct bilirubin—jaundice form.

*Diagnosis*

This will be made by one or more methods.

1. Clinical signs and clinical pathology; a liver and kidney infection; frequently in a young dog.

2. High magnification dark field examination of urine or blood for leptospira.

3. Blood and urine cultures.

4. Serum agglutination—lysis tests. 50% of cases show a positive result within 2 weeks of infection, with a peak antibody level at 4 weeks. Paired blood samples taken at 14 day intervals will demonstrate the rising antibody level (titre).

*Treatment and Nursing Action*

1. Check records for any vaccination history.

2. Prepare to vaccinate any incontact dogs.

3. Give antibiotics as directed. High doses of penicillin/streptomycin given intramuscularly for at least 7 days.

4. Blood transfusions may be required to treat the severe haemorrhage form. (Alert owners of donor dogs).

5. Fluid therapy as directed to combat, water loss—lactated Ringer's solution, calorie deficit—dextrose saline, acidosis—sodium bicarbonate in fluid or orally.

6. Prepare for peritoneal dialysis in the uraemic form of the disease.

7. **Remember the disease is transmissible to humans.** This means *you.* Organisms are shed in the urine from 10 to 14 days post infection for as long as 1 year.

(a) Disinfect all contaminated areas —waiting room, consulting room.
(b) Wear rubber gloves.
(c) Handle urine and blood with care.
(d) Wear plastic overall when handling infected animal

8. Liaise with veterinary surgeon for suitable venue and time for follow-up examination—out of surgery hours at the surgery, or a home visit.

9. Inform owner of health hazard and risk to children.

10. Control measures.

Where appropriate rat eradication and the control of urine, using solid kennels and run partitions.

*Vaccination and Control*

—see later in this section (p. 544).

**Canine infectious respiratory disease**

This is a complex, poorly understood, highly infectious disease syndrome with the following essential features.

*Clinical Syndromes*

1. **"Kennel Cough"** Dogs of any age develop a harsh dry hacking cough, easily stimulated by palpating the trachea. The disease is confined to the upper airways. Rarely is there an elevated temperature and an affected dog continues to feed. It is seen commonly during the summer

months in dogs either in-kennels or shortly out of kennels. The disease runs a self-limiting course of 10 to 14 days. The cough may persist for 6 weeks or more.

2. A distemper-like syndrome with coughing, serous ocular and nasal discharges, elevated temperature, tonsillitis, occasional pneumonia and anorexia. The disease runs a course of 1 to 2 weeks.

Organisms isolated may be one or more of the following:

1. *Canine herpes virus*—causes fatal disease in neonatal puppies.

2. *Canine adenoviruses*
Canine adenovirus type 1 (ICH), infecting the respiratory tract.
Canine adenovirus type 2.

3. *Parainfluenza virus*—causes pneumonia type of kennel cough.

4. *Mycoplasma.*

5. *Bordetella bronchiseptica*
This bacteria is an important cause of kennel cough infection.

### *Treatment and Nursing Action*

1. Antibiotics as directed.
Although kennel cough disease is self-limiting, antibiotic therapy does appear to shorten the course of the illness and reduce the possibility of the complication of chronic bronchitis in older dogs following infection. *Bordetella bronchiseptica* is sensitive to antibiotic therapy.

2. Cough suppressant.

3. Disinfect all contamined areas of the surgery.

4. Arrange with the veterinary surgeon to have any subsequent examinations of infected dogs outside surgery hours.

5. Warn the owners of the highly infectious nature of the diseases and confine the dog to the garden.

6. Advise vaccination of any incontact dogs (p. 544).

7. After handling an infected dog, change clothes and wash hands.

### *Vaccination and Control*

See later in this section.

## Canine parvovirus infection (CPV)

Canine parvovirus is a new disease appearing for the first time in 1978 in America, Australia and Europe. Subsequently it has become a major life-threatening disease of dogs associated with two distinct clinical syndromes. First, and most commonly, an acute gastroenteritis in weaned pups and older dogs; secondly a myocarditis in young pups, which weakens the heart and results in death from heart failure.

### *Aetiology*

It is caused by a small parvovirus closely related to the feline parvovirus (FPV) responsible for panleucopaenia or infectious enteritis in cats. The virus is antigenically distinct from all other previously described non-pathogenic dog parvoviruses, and antibodies to it have not been found in dog sera collected before 1978. The virus is extremely resistant and can survive on the ground for over a year. It is resistant to disinfectants such as phenols and quaternary ammonium compounds, but inactivated by formalin and common bleach.

### *Pathogenesis*

Infection occurs either by direct contact between dogs or by indirect contact with infected faeces. The incubation period is approximately 5 to 6 days. After ingestion the virus passes into the intestines and circulation. It can grow only in actively dividing cells. In young puppies 1 to 4 weeks old, the heart cells are actively dividing and provide a good site for the virus, whereas the intestinal cells are dividing comparatively only very slowly. Infection with CPV in the perinatal period is therefore likely to result in myocarditis and severe damage to the heart. Dogs over 7 weeks in age, when infected, have a gastroenteritis, because by this time in development the multiplication of the heart cells has stopped and mitotic activity of the intestinal cells has increased markedly, as a result of weaning, alterations in the diet, and the intestinal bacterial flora. As a result, the virus is attracted to the intestine and not the heart. The two clinical forms taken by the infection reflect the different growth rates of heart and intestinal cells at different ages in the growing pup.

## CPV enteritis

This is a common form of CPV infection. It is most frequently found to be a major problem in large kennels or breeding units. Additionally it occurs from time to time in small kennels and in the household pet dogs which have little direct contact with other dogs.

### Clinical signs

Dullness, depression and anorexia are the common initial signs. Persistent vomiting becomes the first major sign of illness with the production of a frothy yellow or bloodstained gastric juice and the onset of diarrhoea is 24 hours later. The loose faeces are pasty grey or beige in colour often flecked with blood. Some dogs produce a thin watery reddish brown fluid whilst in the very severe case, the faeces are haemorrhagic. The fluid loss, from the vomiting and diarrhoea results in the affected animal becoming dehydrated.

Pyrexia is usual in the younger dogs, but is not a consistent sign in older animals. It is important to realize that not all infected dogs are equally affected. Within groups some may be asymptomatic, others show transient illness, whilst others experience vomiting and diarrhoea of varying duration from 48 hours to 12 days. Young dogs are the most severely affected. The mortality in weaned pups is around 10%, but in fit, healthy adult animals receiving fluid therapy mortality may be as low as 1%.

### Clinical Pathology

Initial white blood cell count below 3000/cu.mm—leucopaenia.

Later there is a reactive leucocytosis with monocytes and blast cells.

### Diagnosis

By the veterinary surgeon on

1. Clinical signs.
2. The demonstration of the virus in the faeces, by direct visualization or haemagglutinin titration.
3. Specific antibody response in the serum 7 days after infection. Take one blood sample at first signs of illness.

## CPV Myocarditis

Myocarditis was originally seen as a problem in large breeding units. Since most bitches are now immune to the infection and provide their puppies with colostral antibody immunity in the first few weeks of life, CPV myocarditis tends to be only rarely found in pups, from the isolated non-immune bitch which is brought into an infected premises in the later stages of pregnancy or for whelping. The susceptible pups from such bitches meet infection in the vital peri-natal period, when the virus is able to multiply in the heart and myocarditis develops. Depending upon the severity of infection and the degree of damage to the heart, the pups will either die very quickly in acute heart failure or survive for several weeks or months before succumbing to heart failure.

### Clinical Signs

This can take several forms. The most dramatic was sudden death in a previously normal puppy, usually after a period of stress or excitement. Often there was pallor of the mucous membranes. Other pups develop obvious acute heart failure with collapse, respiratory distress, cyanosis, and a fast weak irregular pulse. Death supervenes within hours. Most deaths within a litter occur in one of the above ways, usually between 3 and 6 weeks of age. Unfortunately, apparently normal survivors from affected litters may develop sub-acute heart failure, weeks or months later. These dogs are between 2 and 12 months of age. They present with one or more of the following signs; exercise intolerance, respiratory distress, ascites and enlarged liver. The pulse is weak and rapid. The heart shadow is enlarged on X-ray and ECG examination shows abnormal complexes and extra-systoles. Affected dogs die over a period of days or weeks. For the average affected litter mortality is 70% by 8 weeks of age, and the remaining 30% with varying degrees of cardiac damage may subsequently develop heart failure. Consequently once myocarditis is confirmed in a litter, it is impossible to certify or sell as normal any of the surviving litter mates.

### Treatment and Nursing Action

1. Instructions are as for the other infectious canine and feline diseases with regard to cleanliness and disinfection and contact with susceptible animals.
2. Treatment of CPV gastroenteritis is entirely symptomatic and supportive
    (a) Vigorous daily fluid replacement therapy—lactated Ringer's solution, for badly shocked dogs plasma volume expanders.
    (b) Prepare as directed CNS anti-emetic—Chlorpromazine, Maxalon, gut anti-spasmolytic—Isaverin.
    (c) Put up as directed anti-diarrhoeal therapy.
3. Advise owners on nursing care as for distemper. Diet on recovery is important.
4. Treatment of myocarditis is unsuccessful.
    (a) Advise rest.
    (b) Diuretics for ascites.
5. Remember that this virus is extremely resistant and can survive outside the body for long periods.

### Control

Adequate control has been attained by correctly timed and effective vaccination programmes (p. 544).

## Feline Infectious Diseases

### Toxoplasmosis

A protozoan parasite, *Toxoplasma gondii* is responsible for the disease which can occur in all animals including man (an example of a zoonosis). It is recognized that the cat is the final host for the parasite and the potentially infective oocysts are passed in the faeces of this animal. Oocysts are shed in the faeces of infected cats for approximately 14 days, and they need to be outside the body at room temperature for 1 to 5 days before they become highly infective for other animals and man. Normal attention to personal hygiene after handling cats and their excreta, and disinfection of cat cages, feeding bowls, and litter trays should exclude any risk of infection to the nursing and veterinary staff (p. 386).

*Clinical Signs*

Cats

1. Asymptomatic infection is common.
2. Acute infection, which may be primary infection or activation of a chronic or latent infection, usually runs a short course of less than 2 weeks. Signs are seen most frequently in young cats; pyrexia, anorexia, dyspnoea and pneumonia, occasional diarrhoea and vomiting, myositis, myocarditis, jaundice, enlarged mesenteric lymph nodes.
3. Chronic infection: Occurs more often in old cats. Usually takes a prolonged course over several months; an intermittent pyrexia resistant to antibiotic therapy; vomiting and diarrhoea, which may be related to intestinal, hepatic, pancreatic or mesenteric lymph node lesions taking the form of granulomas; dyspnoea and pneumonia; neurological signs of ataxia, convulsions and blindness; ocular lesions; myocarditis; anaemia; abortion and death in neonatal kittens.

Dogs

1. Asymptomatic infection is very much more common than clinical disease. Younger dogs under 4 months of age are more likely to show illness due to toxoplasmosis alone, whilst in older dogs toxoplasmosis usually occurs concurrently with other disease, frequently distemper.
2. Acute infection **resembles canine distemper** with respiratory, gastro-intestinal and variable nervous signs.
3. The chronic infection takes a similar form to that seen in cats with ocular lesions, retinitis and anterior uveitis, occasional hepatitis, myositis, abortion and neonatal death.

*Investigation*

In cats the disease may resemble lymphosarcoma, feline infectious peritonitis or bacterial septicaemias, whilst in many cases in dogs, the disease is indistinguishable from distemper.

The diagnostic procedures used, will depend on the organs affected and the duration of the disease.

(a) Biopsy of affected organs, fluids and lymph nodes.

(b) Radiographs of the chest in cases with respiratory signs may show up a characteristic pneumonia.

(c) Various tests on the serum for detection of antibodies—for this is necessary to have paired samples at a 14 day interval to demonstrate a rising titre. The acute disease may not allow sufficient time for a titre to develop.

*Treatment and Nursing Action*

Since this disease is a zoonosis, the advisability of treating known infected animals is questionable. Chemotherapy is inhibitory and acts only to control disease until the animal's own immunity develops. It will not eliminate latent infection or heal tissue destroyed in the eye and brain.

1. Drug therapy—A combination of sulphonamide and pyrimethamine (Daraprim B.W.).

Treatment should be continued until clinical signs regress, which is for approximately 2 weeks. When longer periods of Daraprim treatment are necessary, it is advisable to do periodic white blood cell and thrombocyte counts. Folinic acid and yeast are antagonists is cases of Daraprin toxicity.

2. Cleanliness and disinfection as for canine distemper.

3. **Public health aspects.**

(a) After primary infection, cats shed oocysts for 10 to 14 days. These oocysts sporulate after 1 to 5 days and are then highly infective for other animals and man. Depending upon environmental conditions, these remain infective for a prolonged period in excess of one year.

(b) Cats found to be shedding oocysts should be confined to a cage until faeces are negative for 3 consecutive days.

(c) Cat litter trays should be emptied everyday and disinfected. Infected faeces should be burnt or treated with boiling water and disposed of in a toilet.

(d) Children and pregnant women should avoid, soil contaminated with cat faeces, handling cat litter trays and the ingestion of raw meat.

(e) Cats should be fed only cooked or previously deep frozen (for at least 11 days) meat. Cats should be discouraged from eating birds, mice and other potential transport hosts.

Remember that cats do not present a human health hazard if reasonable precautions are taken (p. 388).

## Feline panleucopaenia (Feline infectious enteritis)

This is a highly contagious viral disease affecting all members of the cat family. It is mainly a disease of young kittens but can affect cats of any age.

### Aetiology and Epidemiology

This virus belongs to the parvovirus group. The incidence, morbidity and mortality of the disease varies considerably depending upon the natural and vaccination immunity of the cat population. Infection is either by direct contact with infected cats or ingestion of their infected urine, faeces, saliva and vomit. Fleas may transmit the virus. The virus attacks the small intestinal cells, the bone marrow and lymphopoietic tissues. The virus is resistant to heating at 75°C for 30 minutes and is not destroyed by chloroform, ether,

phenol, acids and alkalis. It can survive for up to one year on infected premises.

### Clinical Signs

Sub-clinical or mild infections can occur. In the more typical case, there is a sudden onset of severe depression, anorexia, pyrexia (40°C or higher), and persistent vomiting. The pre-eminent sign is vomiting and not diarrhoea, but the latter sign may appear in the later stages of the disease. Severe dehydration and electrolyte imbalance occurs, and death may result within the first 5 days of illness. The mortality rate can be 75%. Occasionally in an epidemic, death may occur in cats without them showing any clinical signs.

The virus is able to cross the placental barrier of pregnant queens damaging the cerebellum of embryo kittens. Whole litters may be affected to a greater or lesser extent with cerebellar hypoplasia and signs of ataxia and intention tremor.

### Investigation

1. The characteristic finding is a leucopaenia (1 to 4000/cu.mm).

2. Virus isolation from swabs of the pharynx and rectum (use transport media).

### Treatment and Nursing Action

1. Check vaccination records and take the hygienic and disinfection precautions as described previously for other infectious diseases.

2. Antibiotic therapy to control secondary and opportunist bacterial infections.

3. Replacement and maintenance fluid therapy. Many cases can be saved with rigorous and regular fluid therapy. Lactated Ringer's solution given by subcutaneous or intraperitoneal injection.

4. Vaccination of all incontact susceptible cats.

*Prevention*

The virus of feline panleucopaenia is a very good antigen and the immunity following infection is of a high titre and long persistence. This means that vaccines produced to protect kittens from the disease are efficient (p. 544).

### Feline leukaemia virus (FeLV) infection

*Aetiology*

This is an *Oncornavirus* which is transmitted in the circulation to the bone marrow where it replicates. A persistent viraemia results and the lungs, upper airways and salivary glands become infected and shed the virus. Virus damage is seen in haemopoietic cells. Cells infected by the virus are not destroyed, so that persistent virus infection is established, which may persist for the cat's life.

**Diseases associated with FeLV infection** are of some importance:

1. *Neoplasms*: various types in haemopoietic and lymphoid tissues.
2. *Anaemia.*
3. *Glomerulonephitis.*
4. *Osteosclerosis.*
5. *Immunosuppression.*

*Feline infectious peritonitis.*
*Myeloproliferative disease.*

6. *Abortion and neonatal death.*
7. *Chronic relapsing stomatitis.*

*Investigation*

1. *Fluorescent antibody test.*
2. *Virus isolation* in cell culture from blood or pharyngeal swabs.
3. *Electron microscopy.*
4. *Antibody titres.*

*Epidemiology*

1. Incidence of infection.

(a) In random cat populations (that is urban or suburban single cat households with an average single cat-to-cat contact); there is found a 0.1% infection of FeLV in cats; but 10 to 50% show a titre of protecting neutralizing antibodies against FeLV.

(b) In high-contact population (catteries and multiple cat households) 33% of cats are infected with FeLV and therefore have a much greater chance of developing leukaemia compared to cats in the random group.

*Transmission*

Horizontal transmission of the virus from cat to cat through contact with infective saliva, urine, faeces and possibly blood-sucking parasites. Vertical transmission of the virus occurs (from mother to off-spring) via the gametes. To date there is no evidence of natural transmission to other species, including man.

*Control*

1. In random populations control is probably unnecessary.
2. In an enzootic situation control of the disease may be achieved by combined testing and elimination of sick cats (and possibly healthy positives); disinfection of the premises and a strict control and screening of new cats brought onto the premises.
3. Vaccines being tested, may be available in the future.

### Feline lymphosarcoma

This is probably the commonest neoplasm in cats. The Siamese breed has a high incidence. All age groups are affected.

*Clinical Signs*

The initial signs are variable, but the disease may be associated with one or any of the following signs: lethargy and depression, weight loss, pyrexia (±), anorexia, vomiting and diarrhoea.

The disease will develop into one of the four major clinical forms.

1. Thymic or anterior mediastinal form. Here there is an intrathoracic space occupying lesion and pleural effusion. The signs are coughing, gagging, vomiting, dyspnoea and severe respiratory distress with open mouth breathing. Commonly seen in cats between 6 months and 2 years of age. The diagnosis is established from chest radiographs and cytology of the pleural effusion.

2. Alimentary. The main tumour mass involves:

(a) the terminal ileum, caecum and colon giving annular thickening and leading to either signs of partial obstruction (vomiting) or ulceration and dilation (diarrhoea).

(b) the mesenteric lymph nodes—palpable through the abdominal wall.

(c) liver—enlarged and possible jaundice.

(d) spleen—enlarged and irregular in outline on X-ray.

3. Renal. The kidneys are irregularly enlarged, sometimes several times normal size. The cat presents with signs of renal failure; vomiting, anorexia, anaemia and thirst.

4. Multicentric. There is enlargement of the peripheral lymphnodes (rare in cats), internal lymph nodes, spleen, liver, kidneys. The clinical signs are referable to the organs involved. The diagnosis is made from a lymph node or organ biopsy.

*Clinical Pathology*

1. Pleural effusion—cytology.
2. Anaemia—haemolytic or aplastic.
3. WBC. leucopaenia to leucocytosis, 50% have a lymphopaenia; abnormal lymphocytes are found in many; leukaemia is uncommon.

4. Bone marrow biopsy often has a neoplastic infiltration of lymphocytes.

5. Biopsy—of lymph node or organ involved.

*Treatment*

Treatment is not advisable since an affected cat, shedding FeLV, is a source of infection for other cats. Many authorities regard the present knowledge of the virus as incomplete and the risk to humans is not fully understood. Affected cats should be euthanized.

**Myeloproliferative disease in the cat**

FeLV has been demonstrated in the bone marrow of cats with this disease, but a definite aetiological role has not been established. The disease takes the form of a primary bone marrow dysplasia.

*Clinical Signs.* A variable temperature, anorexia, weight loss, anaemia, and enlarged spleen.

*Clinical Pathology.* Anaemia, abnormal red cells in the blood smear, and bone marrow.

*Treatment.* Transfusions, steroid and/or cytotoxic drugs may induce a remission.

**Feline infectious peritonitis (FIP)**

Originally this disease was described as a diffuse and fibrinous peritonitis, but other "forms" have been reported with a wide range of lesions in the pleura, brain meninges, lungs and eyes and without the typical peritoneal or pleural exudate. Many species of domestic and wild cats are susceptible to the disease. The route of transmission is not known; usually young cats between 1 and 3 years of age are affected, but the disease is reported to have an age range from 1 month to 15 years of age. Males appear to be more frequently affected.

### Aetiology

A viral agent resembling a coronavirus is responsible. There is evidence of a relationship to FeLV infection. FeLV is found in many cases of FIP. FIP is found in clusters of feline leukaemia and other FeLV diseases.

### Clinical Signs

After a suspected incubation period of 4 to 5 months, there is the insidious onset of clinical signs: chronic loss in weight, anorexia, lethargy, pyrexia, and a poor response to any treatment.

In the common form *peritoneal* lesions predominate with ascites, anaemia, jaundice and in some orchitis. Pleural involvement is less frequent and may or may not occur with the peritoneal lesions. The disease is nearly always fatal, running a course of up to 6 weeks.

### Clinical Pathology

A depression anaemia, leucocytosis and lymphopaenia are often found. Hyperproteinaemia (hypergammaglobulinaemia).

Peritoneal exudate, a clear straw coloured fluid, which clots on exposure to air SG1.017 to 1.047, high protein content many globulins, low cell count, no bacteria.

### Investigation

The typical peritoneal lesions and ascites are consistent for the common form of the disease. The other forms (particularly "dry") present difficult diagnostic problems.

### Treatment

Supportive treatment including steroids and various antibiotics may prolong life for short periods.

## Feline upper respiratory disease (FURD) (cat flu')

Present indications are that numerous agents acting singly or in combination are able to produce clinical signs of acute disease in the upper respiratory tract of cats. The two commonest agents are the viruses Feline Viral Rhinotracheitis (FVR) and Feline Calicivirus (FCV). FCR is clinically the most important, but FCVs are more common and some strains are quite pathogenic.

## Feline viral rhinotracheitis (FVR)

### Aetiology

The causal agent is a herpes virus. Only a single serotype is known to exist and it is infectious for felids alone. The virus is very labile surviving only for a few days outside a cat. Transmission from cat to cat is by direct or close contact. The incubation period is from 2 to 10 days depending upon the infecting dose of virus.

### Clinical Signs

These depend upon the immune status, age and general health of the animal. Typically an infected cat will show lethargy and occasional sneezing. The latter becomes more marked and there is pyrexia, conjunctival oedema, ocular and nasal discharges which are at first serous, and later become copious and invariably purulent. Coughing may be a feature with gagging and retching. Saliva drools from the mouth, and occasionally pin-point ulcers are visible on the tongue. There is complete cessation of food and fluid intake and dehydration occurs. Although the clinical signs of FVR are often severe, mortality is not high except in kittens, old and debilitated animals, and some Siamese. Recovery may be expected to begin after 7 to 10 days, but in more refractive cases it may be several weeks before a marked improvement occurs.

## Control

The epidemiology of FVR is dominated by a carrier state in which true latency of the virus, which means it is undetected by conventional means, is the normal state, interrupted by short periods of virus shedding usually at times of stress. The great majority of cats recovering from FVR infection seemingly are carriers but probably only a small proportion shed virus regularly.

1. Effective proprietary vaccines are available.

2. An adjunct to a vaccination policy is attention to management, which aims at reducing the concentration of virus in the environment and minimizing opportunities for transmission.

    (a) Minimize population density.

    (b) For indoor cats ensure a ventilation of 20 air changes per hour.

    (c) in boarding situations, have separate caging which avoids direct contact.

    (d) Disinfect gloved hands, between cages.

    (e) Rear kittens in other accommodation and consider early weaning and separation at 5 to 6 weeks of age.

## Feline calicivirus disease (FCV)

There are a lot of strains of feline caliciviruses, but because there is widespread antigenic cross reaction between them, it is currently considered unrealistic to distinguish more than one serotype. However there is considerable difference between strains in their pathogenicity. Some are non-pathogenic, while others produce severe illness, so that a broad spectrum of clinical signs are possible.

## Clinical Signs

These are pyrexia, general malaise, and ulceration of the tongue. Frequently there is either anorexia or an affected cat wants to eat but is unable to do so because of the tongue lesions. Complete recovery is usual in 5 to 7 days.

## Control

Infected cats shed large quantities of virus in their ocular, nasal and oral discharges. The virus is stable in the environment for several days and it is readily transmitted to cats in close contact or on the hands of attendants. FCV frequently achieves a carrier state in infected cats where there is continuous shedding of virus from the oropharynx area for weeks, months or even years before ceasing. The control of FCV in catteries is similar to FVR. Effective vaccines are available.

*Diagnosis* by the veterinary surgeon in cases of feline respiratory infections is based on the clinical signs, particularly tongue ulceration, and submission of an oropharyngeal swab in transport medium to a specialized laboratory.

## Treatment and nursing action for FVR and severe FCV (cat flu):

1. Combat secondary bacterial infection—Antibiotic therapy as directed by the veterinary surgeon.

2. Counteract dehydration.

Prepare replacement fluids as directed to be given orally, subcutaneously or intraperitoneally—lactated Ringer's solution.

3. Aid healing. Vitamins A, B and C.

4. Good general nursing.

Clear airways with steam vaporizer or a mucolytic agent. Moisten and clean the eyes, avoid the eyelids becoming glued together. Feed highly scented or flavoured foods, which have been previously chilled.

5. Advise vaccination of any healthy incontact cats.

6. Disinfect surfaces and surgery premises and take hygienic precautions as for canine distemper.

## Rabies

Rabies is a virus disease affecting the central nervous system of dogs, cats, foxes, man and many species of wildlife. Dogs are a very important host for the virus and constitute the greatest danger to man. In dogs the disease takes two main forms, "furious" and "dumb".

### Aetiology

Rabies belongs to the Rhabdovirus group. The disease is not present in the United Kingdom, but is common throughout Europe, America and Africa. There are minor differences between strains of virus found in different species and different continents, but for this discussion they may be considered as one.

The pathogenesis of rabies is not fully understood, but it is thought that virus replication occurs in the muscle fibres and connective tissue cells at the site of infection and that the virus may remain there for some time. Then the virus enters a nearby nerve, and moves towards the central nervous system, when further proliferation of the virus occurs throughout the system, and outward along nerves to other parts of the body including, and in particular, the salivary glands.

### Clinical Signs

The incubation period depends upon, the site of infection, severity of the bite, and the dose of virus inoculated, and is usually between 10 days and 4 months. The initial signs in dogs are a change in temperament and pyrexia. The saliva of dogs may contain large amounts of virus up to 3 days before the onset of clinical signs. The hazard of contact with these cases is obvious, and dogs in known enzootic and infected areas or those which are in quarantine or recently released from it, and which show sudden changes in temperament should be handled with caution and treated with suspicion.

In approximately 25% of cases there is gradual marked hyper excitation, (the furious form) and affected dogs become highly restless and irritable. They may show a depraved appetite and swallow stones, chew wood, carpet or straw. They may bite cage bars and wire, breaking their teeth and lacerating gums. The periods of excitement are broken by periods of quiescence, when animals may be friendly. Gradually generalized signs develop as weakness in the limbs and tail, difficulty in swallowing, drooping jaw and eyelids. Dogs may either die in a convulsive seizure or more commonly from a paralytic coma. Great care should be taken in handling such animals and they should be securely caged and confined pending examination by a Ministry Veterinary Officer.

The dumb form of rabies is more common in dogs and may be difficult to diagnose. The signs are congestion of the conjunctiva, sagging of the lower jaw with drooling saliva, difficulty in swallowing, choking (because of food trapped in the pharynx), drooping eyelids, eye squint and a generalized progressive muscle paralysis. Death supervenes within 15 days of the onset of signs.

The RANA must suspect cats and dogs with unexplained nervous signs including unexplained paresis. Animals should be confined and the Ministry of Agriculture informed when rabies is suspected.

If a suspect case dies or is killed, the head is removed by a Ministry Veterinary Officer and transported intact to a diagnostic laboratory. At the laboratory the brain is removed under conditions designed to protect the staff from possible rabies infection, and tests are carried out to determine the diagnosis.

### Control

Modern vaccines, properly used, are capable of inducing a high degree of protection against rabies. Rabies is not present in Great Britain and the vaccination of resident dogs is not permitted. Special permission must be obtained from the Ministry of Agriculture to vaccinate dogs, either in quarantine or to be exported (p. 167).

### Respiratory System Diseases

### Acute respiratory failure

Acute respiratory failure is an extreme emergency resulting from many different clinical disorders. The following is a summary of the general aspects, treatment and nursing considerations for the condition followed by a description of specific causes. Pneumonia or pneumonitis, as an inflammation of the lungs, is an uncommon respiratory disorder seen by RANAs.

### Description

In acute respiratory failure the normal concentration of arterial blood gases can no longer be maintained.

### Causes

*Trauma*, (ruptured diaphragm, pneumothorax, hydrothorax, haemothorax).

*Airway obstruction*, (vocal fold paralysis, congestive heart failure and pulmonary oedema, blood and secretions in airway) (p. 252).

*Drugs*, (anaesthetic overdose).

*Toxins*, (Tetanus, botulism).

*Pulmonary Neoplasia.*

*Pulmonary embolism or thrombus.*

*Pneumonia*, (nocardia).

*Restrictions of thorax* by non-respiratory disorders, (peritonitis, ascites).

*Exudative pleurisy*, (FIP infection).

### Clinical Signs

Hypoxia and later cyanosis.
Increased respirations.
Continual open-mouth breathing.
Elbows abducted, dog-sitting position.
Tachycardia and later Arrhythmias.
Anxiety.
Drowsiness and confusion.
Unconsciousness.

### Treatment and Nursing Actions

The care of patients with acute respiratory diseases and the prevention of secondary respiratory diseases are extremely important aspects of veterinary nursing. **Improve and support respiratory function.**

### 1. Oxygen Therapy

Oxygen is indicated when hypoxia is present. This is when there is a decrease in the amount of oxygen available at the cellular level. Clinical signs of hypoxia are not apparent in the caged dog until the $PaO_2$ falls below 55 to 60 mmHg and are seen as: dyspnoea, tachycardia, heart arrhythmias, drowsiness, and cool extremities.

An oxygen concentration of 30 to 40% only is necessary and advisable for therapy. The oxygen is first humidified by bubbling through water or half strength normal saline.

Techniques for oxygen administration include nasal catheters, masks, intra-tracheal catheters and oxygen cages. The latter may be adapted from a holding cage, replacing the metal door with one made from a clear plastic or perspex sheeting and edged with foam rubber to make a seal against the edges of the cage.

*2. Maintain a Patent Airway*

Deficient ventilation and the onset of hypoxia are the major factors contributing to respiratory failure in the veterinary patient.

Use suction and/or swabs to remove accumulations of blood and secretions from the oropharynx.

*3. Pulmonary Physiotherapy is especially important in good veterinary nursing*

Stimulate the animal to cough by tracheal compression.

Regularly turn immobile animals.

Perform percussion and vibration of the chest wall.

Sling large dogs in an upright position.

*4. Restoration of Pleural Integrity*

Prepare for an appropriate thoracentesis technique (in cases of pneumothorax and haemothorax).

**Improve and support cardiac function** Monitor heart action for arrhythmias (resulting from hypoxia) oxygen therapy may quickly reverse and correct this state.

Treat cardiac disease as directed (e.g. congestive heart failure).

**Closely monitor vital signs** and if necessary the levels of consciousness.

Auscultate heart and lung sounds.

Watch the quantity and quality of respirations.

Notify veterinary surgeon of adverse changes.

**Maintain fluid and electrolyte balance** Monitor electrolytes and PCV.

Record fluid intake and output.

Check skin turgor.

Administer intravenous fluids as prescribed.

**Prevent or treat infection** Administer antibiotics as prescribed to prevent or treat infection.

**Pneumothorax**

An accumulation of air in the pleural cavity causing some degree of lung collapse, dependent on the amount of air that escapes from the lung.

*Causes*

Trauma—hit by car; a fall; penetrating chest injury, fractured ribs.

Complications from thoracentesis.

Thoracic surgery (entering the pleural cavity).

*Types*

**Open pneumothorax (sucking chest-wound).** Air passes freely in and out through an opening in the chest wall (bite wound).

**Closed pneumothorax.** Air enters the

pleural space internally. There is no communication with the outside. Air entering the pleural cavity is trapped and can cause a large build up of pressure in the pleural space.

### Main Clinical Signs

Severity of signs depends on the degree of lung collapse.

Apprehension and reluctance to move.

Dyspnoea and acute respiratory distress.

Hypoxia.

Cyanosis.

Rapid pulse.

Shock.

Audible passage of air during respiration (with open pneumothorax).

Animal adopts dog-sitting position.

### Diagnostic Tests

Drum-like resonance on percussion of the chest.

Chest X-ray film establishes the diagnosis.

### Treatment and Nursing Action

1. Notify veterinary surgeon of chest emergency.

2. Monitor vital signs (every 15 minutes to ensure the animal has stabilized).

3. Confine the animal—cage rest.

4. Prepare for emergency oxygen therapy as directed.

5. Prepare for emergency thoracentesis as directed.

6. Prepare for emergency surgery.
Ensure owners are kept informed.
Admission forms completed.
Premedication as directed.

7. Treatment for pain and shock as indicated and when directed.

8. Prepare antibiotic therapy to prevent secondary respiratory infection.

Where animals present with a sucking chest wound (open pneumothorax) try to make the wound airtight by applying a sterile dressing over the wound and seal it into position with tape.

9. Post-thoracentesis and surgery patient needs total cage rest. Haemothorax and pneumothorax frequently occur together.

## Haemothorax

An accumulation of blood in the pleural cavity.

### Causes

Trauma to the thorax.
Warfarin poisoning.

### Main Clinical Signs

Apprehension and pain.

Dyspnoea.

Cyanosis and or pallor.

Shock.

Bruising and skin contusion over the chest.

Frothy blood sputum.

Fast thready pulse.

Respiratory sounds decreased or absent over affected chest area.

Rapid shallow respirations and limited chest excursion (depending on the amount of blood in the pleural space).

### Treatment and Nursing Actions

As for pneumothorax.
Special Considerations.

Veterinary surgeons may perform an emergency thoracentesis as a diagnostic measure. Blood aspirated from the pleural space indicates haemothorax.

Blood replacement therapy may be

indicated. Warn owners of donor dogs to be prepared: Warn laboratory of possible need of emergency cross-matching and haemogram (haemoglobin and PCV).

Prepare donor blood collection bags.

When blood is aspirated from the pleural space, measure volume.

Prepare Warfarin antidote Vit. K1.

Prepare antibiotic therapy to prevent secondary respiratory infection.

Warn owners to look for source of Warfarin bait.

## Ruptured diaphragm

A surgical condition, is included for comparison with the other medical conditions (p 600).

### Causes

Chest Trauma
Abdominal Trauma    } Commonly road
Multiple Trauma     } traffic accidents

### Main Clinical Signs

These are dependent on the position and length of the tear in the diaphragm musculature and the extent of herniation of the abdominal viscera.

Acute respiratory distress.

Dyspnoea.

Cyanosis.

Dog-sitting posture adopted.

Absent or diminished respiratory sounds over affected area.

Mediastinal shift may occur so that heart sounds are louder on the right chest.

Dullness or tympany on percussion of affected side.

Bowel sounds may be auscultated within the chest.

### Diagnosis Confirmation

Chest X-ray.

### Treatment

Surgical repair.

Positive pressure ventilation from a closed or semi-closed anaesthetic machine is required.

## Acute pulmonary oedema

Acute pulmonary oedema occurs when lung congestion causes the escape of serous fluid from the capillaries into the interstitial tissues and alveoli.

### Causes

Left ventricular heart failure (the common cause).

Chest trauma.

Uraemia.

Inhalation of chemical irritants (ammonia and chlorine gas and hot fumes in house fires).

### Main Clinical Signs

a) *First stage* (Fluid leaks into the interstitial spaces).

Dyspnoea on exertion.

Persistent cough.

Restlessness.

Anxiety.

Râles on auscultation at the base of the diaphragmatic lobes of lung.

Hyperventilation.

b) *Second stage* (Fluid moves into the alveoli).

Respiratory distress.

Acute shortness of breath.

Hyperventilation.

Laboured breathing.

Audible râles and wheezing.

Persistent productive coughing (large amounts of sputum).

Cyanosis.

Hypotension.

Tacchycardia.

Cardiac arrhythmias.

c) *Third Stage* (Fluid moves into the bronchial tree).

Very acute respiratory distress.

Coarse and bubbling râles.

Decreased consciousness.

Signs of cardiac shock.

Breath sounds diminish.

Death is imminent—metabolic and respiratory acidosis.

*Treatment and Nursing Actions*

1. Observe the animal, try to anticipate the early stage. Since the disorder can progress rapidly to the third stage. The quicker the detection the better the chance of survival.

2. Administer 100% oxygen therapy (humidified) by face mask.

3. Anticipate intensive care nursing.

4. Support left side heart action. Prepare to administer rapid acting digitalis preparations orally or intravenously depending on stage of the failure. Repeat doses of digitalis are given until the patient is digitalized. A maintenance dose for digitalis is then worked out. Prepare to administer aminophylline intravenously.

5. Prepare to administer rapidly acting diuretics. Usually Frusemide is given intravenously.

Make a note of increased urine production and notify veterinary surgeon if this does not occur.

6. Provide cage rest. Animal will adopt dog-sitting position with elbows abducted to facilitate breathing.

7. Monitor vital signs frequently. Provide good nursing care.

8. If possible weigh the patient and use repeat weighings as a guide to the effectiveness of treatment.

9. Avoid sodium in the diet.

## Urinary System Diseases

### Chronic renal failure

Chronic renal failure is an insidious disease involving progressive renal deterioration which may be undetected for months or years.

*Causes*

Congenital anomalies of the kidney.

Glomerular nephritis.

Interstitial nephritis.

Metabolic disorders.

*Clinical signs*

Anorexia.

Thirst.

Vomiting.

Lethargy.

Anaemia.

Halitosis—uraemic breath, ulceration of the oropharynx.

Weight loss and gradual physical deterioration.

*Treatment*

Treat the underlying cause.

There may be no cure.

Control vomiting.

Attempt to preserve any remaining functional kidney tissue by instituting a low protein diet, with not more than 0.5 g protein/—Kg/bodyweight daily.

Vitamin B therapy.

Correct any fluid or electrolyte imbalance and add salt to the diet.

Utilize peritoneal dialysis to remove nitrogenous waste products from the body and stabilize the patient.

Prepare for kidney biopsy.

If untreated or if treatment is ineffective

the disorder will progress to uraemia and the eventual death of the animal.

### Diets in Chronic Renal Failure

The dietary management of renal insufficiency is directed towards a limitation of protein intake to meet amino-acid requirements only, or as near to this as practical. The kidney has a great reserve of function, when there is extensive loss of kidney tissue hypertrophy of the remaining nephrons occurs to compensate for the loss of effective tissue. This is usually enough to allow the dog to lead a comparatively normal life if the workload of the kidney is kept to a minimum. Although the protein intake should be restricted in chronic renal failure, it is important to remember that some protein will be needed in the diet as the metabolic requirement is still present and all urinary protein losses will have to be replaced.

For practical purposes, protein intake should be regulated to the level that maintains body weight without raising the blood urea level. A suitable diet* for a 14 kg dog with chronic renal disease might be

(a) 115 g of good quality cooked meat, including the fat; (or 115 g of fish or chicken)

(b) 2 cooked eggs or ½ pint of milk as a milk pudding (or 14–28 g of creamed cheese)

(c) 85 g of biscuit.

This mixture will supply about 45 g of protein, that is about 3.3 g per kilogram body weight and about 1000 to 1200 calories which would meet the calculated energy requirements without using excess protein for energy purposes. An 0.5 g per Kg diet would need one seventh of this protein intake and for this reason is unpalatable and difficult to maintain a dog on.

A vitamin B supplement is advisable as water soluble vitamins will be lost by a damaged kidney. Salt is lost in the same

*The information for this diet was supplied by A. T. B. Edney

way and should be added to the diet at the rate of 2.5 g per 0.45 Kg of the diet. This diet is also likely to be low in calcium, so a mineral supplement will also be necessary. If the amount of energy available as carbohydrate or fat is reasonably generous, less protein is broken down for energy purposes and the products of deamination will not contribute to the uraemia.

The prepared canned nephritis diet is a readily available diet that can be used in impaired kidney function and has the great merit of being a convenient food for the dog owner who does not have the time to weigh out small portions of individual foods.

## Acute renal failure

### Causes

Acute glomerulo-nephritis.
Severe dehydration.
Circulatory failure.
Kidney trauma and haemorrhage following a road traffic accident.
Nephrotoxic agents, some antibiotics, chemotherapy agents.
Pesticides, organic solvents.
Obstruction of the urinary tract (Calculi in the urethra and kidney pelvis).

### Clinical Signs

Sudden onset of illness.
Oliguria (small volume of urine produced) or Anuria (no urine produced).
Vomiting.
Lethargy, confusion and disorientation.
Diarrhoea.
Halitosis (uraemic breath).
Neurological disturbances, convulsions.
Signs increase as the retention of the

nitrogenous waste products increases within the circulation and body tissues.

*Phases of Acute Renal Failure*

(a) Oliguria phase.
Vomiting, lethargy, little or no urine production.
Elevated blood urea, creatinuria, and potassium.

Complications at this phase are hyperkalaemia (increased blood potassium), acidosis, uraemia, death.

(b) Diuresis phase.
Urinary output gradually increases, up to normal levels. The output will depend on the degree of fluid overload present from the oliguric phase.
Diuresis may last for several days.

Complications are excess loss of sodium ion in the urine and dehydration.

Remember that renal function is not normal at this stage.

(c) Recovery phase.
Where renal function is gradually restored, although it may not return to prefailure levels, it takes several weeks for the kidneys to fully recover.

*Treatment and Nursing Action*

1. Monitor vital signs at regular intervals.
Heart sounds—arrhythmias and failure.
Chest sounds—pulmonary oedema.
Report any changes to the veterinary surgeon.

2. Check neurological state.

3. Monitor and correct fluid and electrolyte imbalances.
Care is needed during the oliguric phase to avoid over hydration resulting from sodium and water retention leading to pulmonary oedema and cardiac failure.

4. Daily monitoring of fluid intake and loss, keeping records and measuring specific gravity of any urine produced.

5. Treat and correct the underlying causes.

6. Administer diuretics during the oliguric phase as ordered. (i.e. Frusemide, Mannitol).

7. Provide a low-protein diet.
High calorie content low in potassium and phosphorus.
Give high multi-vitamin supplement.
If necessary prepare for either total parenteral nutrition by drip or pharyngostomy tube insert.

8. Antibiotic therapy to prevent infection.
Administer medications with care because of the impaired kidney function.
Antacids containing magnesium are contraindicated; use aluminium hydroxide.

9. Prevent pulmonary infections. If the animal is immobile turn regularly.

10. Provide cage rest—therefore lowering metabolism and the production of waste products.

11. Prepare for peritoneal dialysis.
If an animal fails to recover from acute renal failure, chronic renal failure may result.

**Peritoneal dialysis technique**

The end-products of metabolism and excess fluid are removed from the body by osmosis and diffusion using the peritonium as a semi-permeable membrane.

*Equipment*

Standard surgical instrument set, drapes and swabs, suture materials.
Local anaesthetic.
Trochar set and peritoneal dialysis catheter.
Peritoneal dialysis giving set.

Sterile dialysis solution heated to slightly above body temperature.

*Preparation*

Clip hair and clean abdomen from umbilicus to pubis.

With patient in lateral recumbency, the veterinary surgeon will infiltrate with local anaesthetic, the mid line abdomen, behind the umbilicus.

Connect up and prime dialysis giving set and dialyser fluid.

*Procedure*

The abdomen is draped and an incision made through the skin in the mid-line below the umbilicus.

The trochar is inserted into the peritoneum through the incision. After the guide is removed, the catheter is inserted through the trochar, which is removed in turn and the catheter sutured into place.

The dialysis giving set is connected to the indwelling catheter and the dialysis fluid allowed to flow into the peritoneal cavity. The flow continues approximately for 5 to 10 minutes depending upon the size of the animal. The patient may require some restraint and reassurance during this period.

Following infusion, the tubing is clamped and the dialysis fluid left in the abdomen for approximately 20 minutes. The animal is allowed to change position during this period.

It is usual to use the solution bottle for drainage. Simply lower it to the floor and allow the dialysis fluid in the abdomen to drain out by gravity.

Measure the volume of dialysis fluid recovered and continue with the next exchange using fresh dialysis fluid.

It is usual to repeat the technique until the blood chemistry levels are brought to the desired levels.

Points to remember.

1. If the dialysis fluid does not flow in quickly, then repositioning of the catheter may be indicated.

2. If the dialysis fluid does not flow out well turn the animal from side to side, and raise the chest and sternum.

3. Keep an accurate record of inflow and outflow. They should be almost equal.

4. Keep the catheter insertion site clean.

Blood chemistry is checked prior to and during the procedure.

The following may be added to the dialysis fluid:

Antibiotics to prevent infection.

Heparin to prevent clot formation in the catheter.

Xylocaine to lessen abdomen discomfort.

The procedure may have to be repeated every 24 to 48 hours to maintain the patient and until kidney function improves.

**The nephrotic syndrome**

*Causes*

Glomerulo-nephritis.
Amyloidosis.

*Clinical Signs*

Lethargy.
Weight Loss.
Thirst.
Widespread oedema and ascites.

The oedema arises as a result of the massive loss of protein in the urine (albuminuria). This loss is reflected in the blood with a loss in osmotic pressure.

## Treatment

Give a high protein diet provided that the blood urea is not too high.

Restrict salt intake.

Give corticosteroids and diuretics as directed by veterinary surgeon.

## Cystitis

Cystitis in dogs and cats is a common disorder, particularly of bitches. The inflammation may result from an ascending infection or may be exacerbated by, urinary obstruction, urinary retention and trauma.

## Clinical Signs

1. Frequency of urination with straining (tenesmus)
2. Passage of small quantities of urine —blood stained (haematuria).
3. Small thickened bladder on palpation.

## Investigation

1. Urinalysis: collect a specimen into a clean container while the patient is urinating. Catheterize patients from whom it is impossible to obtain a urine sample. Cats will have to be given empty clean trays into which they can pass urine with minimal contamination of the sample. The RANA should ensure that urine is being passed by the patient, as cases of urethral obstruction are urgent and potentially life threatening (see acute renal failure).

(a) Alkaline pH.
(b) deposit, red and white blood cells and bacteria.
(c) blood and protein present.
(d) urine normal concentration (S. G.)
2. Urine culture and sensitivity:—

streptococci, staphylococci, klebsiella, E. coli, Pseudomonas, Proteus spp.

3. Radiology of the bladder: plain and contrast studies. A pneumocystogram helps to identify the prostrate gland and calculi and to exclude other diagnoses.

## Treatment and Nursing Action

Cases of cystisis may be admitted for full investigation and observation, but are seldom hospitalized for treatment.

1. Antibacterial Chemotherapy: Agents must be given frequently and for a prolonged period. Potentiated sulphonamides initially and then according to sensitivity tests. In acid urine, erythromycin is used and in alkaline urine penicillin and tetracyclines.
2. Alkaline urine may be acidified using ascorbic acid (vitamin C).
3. Encourage an adequate flow of dilute urine by:

(a) encouraging the patient to urinate; frequent walks on grass etc.
(b) provide ready access to water at all times.
(c) Feed a moist diet; dry diets are contra-indicated.
(d) add extra water or gravy to food.
4. Soiling of the skin and hair around the urinary orifice may cause scalding and often there is a foetid odour due to the alkaline nature of the urine. Careful and frequent cleansing and drying of the area may be necessary. Cats and long-haired dogs are especially liable to blow-fly strike in this region during hot weather, unless kept scrupulously clean.

## Acute Abdominal Disorders

Frequently the RANA will be involved in disorders which are termed, acute abdomen or an abdominal catastrophe.

Usually these result from severe abdominal injuries, acute intestinal obstruction, gastrointestinal ulceration, neoplasia and bleeding, acute pancreatic necrosis, torsion of a retained abdominal testicle, acute gastrointestinal haemorrhage syndrome and gastric tympany and torsion.

**Abdominal injuries**

*Causes*

Trauma.
Road traffic accidents.
Penetrating foreign bodies—sticks, gunshot bullets.

*Clinical signs*

1. Ruptured liver.
Shock.
Tenderness and pain over the anterior abdomen.
Abrasions and bruising to the skin covering the abdomen and thorax.
Evidence of fractured ribs.
Evidence of any intra-abdominal haemorrhage may not be obvious.
2. Ruptured spleen.
Tenderness and pain over the abdomen.
Shock.
Evidence of internal haemorrhage may not be obvious for 24 hours or longer.
Apprehension and dullness due to progressive peritoneal irritation.
*Diagnosis* by the veterinary surgeon may include the use of:
1. Abdominal X-rays.
2. Abdominal paracentesis.
3. Complete blood count (PCV, Haemoglobin).
4. Electrolytes, BUN estimation.

*Nursing Care and Treatment*

1. Monitor vital signs particularly the pulse.
2. Prepare for blood sample (in EDTA) for PCV.
3. Prepare for abdominal paracentesis.
4. Treat shock if present.
Prepare for blood transfusion as directed. Use lactated Ringer solution if blood, plasma, or plasma substitute are not available.
Cross match blood if facility is available.
5. Prepare for emergency surgery, as indicated and as directed.
6. Measure abdominal girth to establish a base line for comparison and then recheck frequently for any increase.
For animals with obvious penetrating trauma wounds.
1. Minimize all movements made by the patient.
2. Monitor vital signs.
3. Inspect animals for puncture wounds. i.e. penetrating bite wounds.
gunshot wounds.
knife wounds.
4. Apply direct pressure to wound with a sterile dressing to prevent external bleeding.
5. When the bowel is protruding, cover with sterile saline dressings and keep wet to prevent drying of the bowel. Also try to avoid contaminations of the bowel and peritoneum.
6. Administer antibiotics as directed to prevent possible infection from contamination.
7. Prepare for emergency surgery as directed.

**Acute intestinal obstruction**

*Causes*

1. Foreign body (stone, plastic toy, sock, string, rubber ball, erasers, coke, coal, sweet corn cobs etc. etc.)

2. Malignancy.

3. Intussusception (p. 595).

*Clinical Signs* (depend on the degree of obstruction, location and cause)

1. Vomiting food.

No faeces produced.

Bloody faeces with intussusception.

2. Dullness, apprehension.

3. Intense abdominal pain.

4. Elevated temperature.

5. Toxicity.

6. Dehydration.

7. Oliguria. The higher the obstruction the more acute the signs.

*Nursing Care and Treatment*

1. Monitor vital signs.

2. Institute saline or glucose saline intravenous drip as directed.

3. Obtain blood for CBC, PCV and haemoglobin. (CBC = complete count)

4. Monitor fluid input and output.

5. Note quality and quantity of any faeces produced.

6. Prepare for emergency abdominal surgery.

*Post-operative Care*

Following gastrotomy, enterotomy, and enterectomy operations, the patient will require a fluid diet for the first 5 days post-surgery. A food blending or homogenizing machine is ideal for this purpose. The daily diet is given as several small meals throughout the day.

**Oesophageal foreign body**

*Cause* Invariably vertebral bones ingested but unable to reach the stomach.

*Clinical Signs*

Dullness, apprehension.

Regurgitation of food—water may be retained.

Elevated temperature.

Palpable foreign body in oesophagus immediately in front of the ribs.

X-ray examination of the thorax will confirm a foreign body is present. Oesophagoscopy may be performed as a further aid to diagnosis.

*Nursing Action and Treatment*

1. Monitor vital signs.

2. Prepare patient for endoscopy as directed and indicated to remove obstruction.

3. Fluid replacement therapy will be indicated.

4. Administer antibiotics as directed to prevent or control possible complications. i.e. mediastinitis and pneumonia.

5. Obtain PCV and haemoglobin estimation.

6. Monitor fluid intake and urine output closely.

**Gastric tympany and torsion**

This disorder is an extreme emergency and should be always treated as such.

*Causes* not fully clear and debatable.

Deep chested breeds, greedy feeders and dry food diets are predisposing factors. Dogs that swallow excess air as they feed are especially liable to tympany (p. 249).

*Clinical Signs*

Suddenly, usually a few hours after a meal, the patient is found to be very dull, apprehensive, and trying to vomit.

Shock, listlessness, unable to move, crying out in pain.

Rapid and progressive abdominal distension.

*Nursing Action and Treatment*

1. Monitor vital signs.
2. Prepare for intravenous fluid therapy N. Saline or lactated Ringers.
3. Prepare an appropriate size dog stomach tube.
4. Prepare for emergency surgery

If patient is not too shocked full-scale laparotomy, gastrotomy and reduce torsion.

If patient is too shocked, then gastro-epidermal-fistula may be performed under local anaesthetic. Full scale surgery when the patient is stable.

5. Antibiotic therapy to prevent a possibility of peritonitis.
6. Monitor CBC and electrolytes.

*Post-operative Care*

As for intestinal obstruction.

Fluid diet, feed small quantities frequently.

**Acute gastrointestinal
haemorrhage syndrome**

This is believed to be an allergic or anaphylactic disorder of usually the smaller breeds of dogs.

*Causes* Unclear, but possibily associated with an overproduction of gram-negative bacteria in the bowel and excess endotoxin production which in turn sets up portal anaphylaxis. There is a massive build up of blood in the portal circulation.

*Clinical Signs*

Dullness and abdominal pain.
Pale mucous membranes.

Tachypnoea.
Thin rapid pulse.
Haematemesis.
Tar-like bloody stools.
Shock.
Rapid deterioration in animal's general condition.

*Nursing Action and Treatment*

1. Monitor vital signs frequently.
2. Prepare for intravenous fluid therapy.
Ringers, Glucose Saline. Blood if available and directed.
3. Prepare intravenous steroid therapy to combat anaphylactic reactions.
4. Prepare covering antibiotic therapy as directed.

**Neurological Problems**

**Increased intracranial pressure**

*Causes*

Trauma and cerebral oedema.
Brain tumour.
Haemorrhage.
Meningitis.

*Clinical Signs*

Evidence of head pain, glazed eyes and drying out of conjunctivae.
Increased respirations.
Decreased pulse.
Moderate rise in body temperature.
Vomiting.
Decline in the level of consciousness to a comatose state.
Pupil changes—fixed uni or bilateral dilatation, unequal size.
Hemiparesis.
Hemiplegia.
The level of consciousness is the single

most important indicator of brain function.

## Nursing Action and Treatment

1. Monitor the level of consciousness. Wake the animal to make certain it is sleeping rather than unconscious.

2. Monitor pupil size and shape.

3. Provide total cage rest.

4. Prepare treatment to reduce intracranial pressure and inflammation.

Mannitol infusions ⎫ Diuretics to
Frusemide ⎭ reduce cerebral
oedema

Dexamethasone steriod to reduce inflammation.

Phenytoin, Diazapam to stop convulsions.

Antibiotics to prevent secondary infection.

5. Provide fluid and electrolye maintenance therapy.

6. Patient care.

Keep unconscious animal in lateral recumbency.

Change the position of the animal every 2 hours.

Moisten and clean eyes as necessary.

Empty bladder and rectum as necessary.

Keep the animal clean, change bedding as it becomes soiled.

Watch for urine scalds and dermatitis.

Remember that an animal unconscious for more than 24 hours will very probably show permanent brain damage on recovery.

## Spinal cord injury

*Causes* Trauma

Intervertebral disc protrusion.

## Clinical Signs

Loss of sensation and motor paralysis below the level of injury.

Loss of bowel and bladder control (faecal and urinary retention).

Spinal shock.

## Nursing Action and Treatment

Monitor vital signs.

Monitor neurological signs.

Report any adverse changes to veterinary surgeon.

Total cage rest.

Try to keep the vertebral column straight, and the animal as still as possible.

A lesion in the spinal cord at:

cervical level may give quadriplegia.

thoracic level may give paraplegia.

lumbar level may give paralysis of the hind limbs and tail.

Prepare treatment to reduce intravertebral pressure and inflammation.

Promote and encourage proper nutrition.

Provide patient care (as for increased intracranial pressure).

## Seizures

For all seizures there is excessive paroxsysmal neuronal discharge in the brain. When seizures recur and when recurrent seizures are not caused by some short term or readily recognized disease, the disorder is called **epilepsy**.

## Clinical Signs

Some or all of the following may be seen during a seizure episode.

1. Tonic (extension) spasms of the limbs initially, then clonic spasms (paddling movements). Tonic/clonic phase may last from a few seconds up to 4 minutes.

2. Brief loss of consciousness.

3. Salivation, urination, defaecation.

4. Either before or after a seizure—Hallucination, chewing, howling, barking, changes in eating and drinking habits, hunger following seizure.

Sometimes ataxia and compulsive walking may persist for hours after a seizure.

*Aetiology*

Anything that alters nerve function is potentially seizure producing. The cause may be either extracranial or intracranial. Both should be considered in the differential diagnosis of canine seizure disorders.

A. EXTRACRANIAL CAUSE seizures and fits due to disturbances outside the brain:

1. *Low blood glucose* (hypoglycaemia) Often due to indiscriminate insulin production from an islet cell tumour.

2. *Hypoxia*
Due to (i) congestive heart failure (ii) aortic stenosis (iii) carbon monoxide poisoning.

3. *Liver disease and kidney failure* (uraemia).

4. *Low blood calcium* (hypocalcaemia) (Eclampsia p. 666).

This situation occurs frequently in lactating bitches of toy breeds in the first 10 to 21 days, after whelping. When the puppies are making most demands on the dam's milk supply. It occurs with large litters.

Initially the bitch is restless, panting, whining, muscle twitching, limb ataxia, jaw champing, salivating, tonic seizures, elevated temperature. The bitch is conscious.

*Treatment and Nursing Action*

1. Prepare 10% Calcium Borogluconate solution for intravenous and subcutaneous injections.

2. Separate and wean pups to avoid the recurrence of the syndrome.

5. *Toxicoses.*
Many insecticides, herbicides and heavy metals are toxic for animals and produce nervous signs and seizures.

B. INTRACRANIAL CAUSES are those which occur within the skull.

1. *Encephalitis*
Distemper virus is the commonest cause.

2. *Neoplasia of the brain*

3. *Trauma*
Scarring as a sequel to head injury may be an epileptiform focus. There can be a long period between the injury and the onset of seizures.

4. *Hydrocephalus*
Seen in small breeds of dogs with domed skulls and open fontanelles.

5. *Cerebral abscess*
Middle ear infection may spread to the brain.

6. *Thiamine defficiency*

C. IDIOPATHIC EPILEPSY—FUNCTIONAL EPILEPSY

It is likely that inheritance (single autosomal recessive gene) plays a major role in the pathogenesis of this form of epilepsy i.e. a lowered threshold to fits. In many cases generalized seizures commence at 6 to 10 months of age. They are of a short duration with few residual after effects. Episodes may occur at regular intervals. Hereditary epilepsy is proven in three breeds—Beagles, Keeshund, German Shepherds, and possibly for Toy Poodles, Cocker Spaniels and W.H. Fox Terriers.

*Differential Diagnosis*

The veterinary surgeon will attempt to determine the underlying cause of the seizure. A negative result may be indicative of idiopathic epilepsy.

1. History.

2. Physical examination.

3. Laboratory tests. Haemogram, blood **urea,** blood **glucose,** serum calcium, blood ammonia, SGPT/SAP/BSP.

4. Neurological examination—localizing signs.

5. Electroencephalography.

6. Cerebrospinal fluid (CSF) analysis and pressure.

*Treatment and Nursing Action*

1. Specific treatment for many of the causes of seizures is available.

2. Sedation to reduce and ideally stop the seizure episodes. Drugs used: Phenobarbitone, prominal, mysoline, dilantin.

When a patient is experiencing continuous seizures (status epilepticus), i/v valium is used to control the condition, it is best given in the first 20 minutes.

3. A RANA will be involved in the management of the patient having a seizure. As a general rule **the animal is best left alone.** On no account should physical restraint be applied during the seizure and in the post-seizure phase, while an animal is still dazed.

Frequently the RANA will be called to give advice over the telephone to an owner whose dog or cat is having a fit for the first time. Such an owner needs assurance that the animal is not dangerous and on no account should it be restrained. The episode will last only a few minutes at the most. The light should be subdued and all sharp or projecting objects moved out of the way of the animal. Epileptiform seizures usually commence with the patient at rest or while asleep.

Occasionally a patient may be hospitalized for investigation and observation of the seizure episodes reported by an owner. The RANA should observe closely and record all physical signs shown by the patient, particularly during a seizure episode. These observations may be of assistance to the veterinary surgeon trying to establish a diagnosis, the frequency of attacks and timing of drugs used must be recorded.

## Skin Disorders

This is a very wide and complex subject, and here it is possible to discuss only briefly some of the more common complaints and to list others.

## Ectoparasites and Parasitic Dermatoses of Dogs and Cats

### Fleas

The most common external parasite of dogs and cats:

*Producing:* nuisance, scratching, fleabite dermatitis (with or without hypersensitivity), transmission of the tapeworm *Dipylidium caninum* and other diseases; human flea bites.

*Treatment*

Animal: insecticidal bath and dip followed by insecticidal powder every 4 days.

Bedding: washed, changed and treated with insecticide every 4 days.

Premises: Insecticidal spray or powders every 14 days. Vacuum carpets thoroughly afterwards.

Cats: Use insecticides with care. Pyrethrum and carbamates suitable.

Kittens: Dip in a warm, weak detergent solution up to the neck for 2 to 3 minutes. Saturate the fur on the head, fleas will drown. Treat bedding and their Queen.

*Flea Allergy Dermatitis*

Results from hypersensitivity to flea saliva. Occurs in cats and dogs.

*Producing*: pruritus and superimposed skin trauma, particularly at the base of the tail and lumbo-dorsal area. During the summer months and in winter to a lesser extent.

*Treatment* 1. Intensive flea control, 2. Systemic corticosteroids, 3. Topical antibiotics/corticosteroid ointments, 4. Shampoos to remove excessive crust and scales. 5. Progestagens in cats.

### Lice

Two biting species and a sucking species affect dogs, while biting lice usually affect cats (p. 368).

*Producing*: irritation, blood loss and anaemia in extreme cases, tapeworm transmission.

*Treatment*: Susceptible to the common insecticides—dips and baths most effective —repeat every 14 days. Clean bedding and equipment. The entire life cycle of the louse is spent on the host.

### Flies

1. Bites may affect the ear tips and face. Crusts of blood with sometimes secondary infection. Apply fly repellants to the ears and head for treatment and prevention (take care with cats). Corticosteroid lotions will reduce irritation after fly and mosquito bites.

2. Myiasis

Most commonly occurs in aged and debilitated animals especially rabbits unable to get away from flies, and especially the uncared for, with matted hair, faecal soiling of the perinaeum or open wounds. Always check anus and ventral neck areas. Maggots and or fly eggs are seen in the lesions. Treat by clipping the hair from the lesion and washing the area with an antiseptic solution. Spread the wound and remove or flush out *all* larvae.

Antibiotic therapy for the wound, wound margins and systemically.

### Ticks

*Ixodes Ricinus* commonly become attached particularly to the head and neck (p. 369).

*Producing*: Irritation, blood loss, disease transmission.

*Treatment*: by first soaking the tick in either oil, alcohol or ether. Then firmly grasp the head near the skin with forceps and pull off. Insecticidal sprays and powders for prevention. Advise owners to cut back any overgrown parts of their garden which might harbour ticks.

### Bee and wasp stings

May have a variable effect, from minimal swelling to widespread oedema of the head and body generally. An anaphylactic reaction is possible. Remove sting and prepare antihistamine or corticosteroid therapy as directed (p. 229).

### Skin mites

There are seven species noteworthy. Most live permanently on the host animal.

1. Ear mites *Otodectes cyanotis*—live on ear wax in the external ear canal of dogs and cats, producing ear irritation and otitis externa.

2. Poultry mite *Dermanyssus gallinae* —Dogs and cats infected incidentally, causing intense pruritus along the back and legs. Treat with insecticidal baths.

3. Harvest mite *Trombicula sp.*—Dogs and cats infected incidentally in the summer, pruritic lesions around the toes and feet.

4. *Cheyletiella sp.* Different species infect cats and dogs. Live off dog in corn

stubbles, rabbits and guinea pigs. Producing excessive scaling (scurf and dandruff effect), hair loss and variable pruritus. Most severe in young pups. Treatment: Insecticidal bath, once weekly for 3 weeks.

5. *Notoedres cati* Head mange—affects principally cats, highly contagious. Ear margins, face, eyelids and neck have dry crusted grey lesions, partial alopecia and intense pruritus. Treatment by bathing ears and head to remove scales and then apply usual parasiticide. Repeat every 10 days. Treat all in-contact cats.

6. *Sarcoptes Scabiei*—Affects primarily dogs, occasionally cats and *humans*. *Producing*: Intense pruritus, reddening, crusting and alopecia, later wrinkling of the skin, a mousey distinctive smell. Lesions are distributed primarily at the elbows, hocks and lower limbs and ear-flaps, eventually whole body is involved. Mites may be difficult to demonstrate in skin scrapings.

*Treatment*

(i) Clipping hair is helpful (ii) Parasiticidal baths weekly for 3 weeks (iii) Additional topical treatment with benzyl benzoate (iv) Treat all in-contact dogs (v) Possibly initial systemic corticosteroids, to reduce pruritus and hypersensitivity reaction. Watch for resistance to conventional parasitic applications.

7. *Demodex*—normal inhabitants of the skin of most dogs. Suckling pups acquire mites from the dam during the neonatal period. Mites colonize the hair follicles feeding on sebum.

In a few dogs mites multiply to large numbers to produce skin lesions on the host. These are predominantly young dogs, from the short-haired breeds. An immunological fault is thought to be present in these animals, allowing the mite to proliferate, particularly at times of stress.

1. *Localized form* (squamous) common and seen as: (a) Focal lesions, mild erythema, partial alopecia, fine scales and skin folding, around the face, mouth, forehead and forelegs. (b) No pruritus.

2. *Generalized form* (a) An extension of the localized form, with lesions appearing all over the body with skin thickening and wrinkling. (b) Secondary bacterial infection (*staphylococci*) of the parasitized skin and hair follicles (pustular form). Abscessation, pyoderma, lymph node enlargement and a systemic reaction may occur. This was known as the pustular form of mange or red mange.

When skin scrapings are taken from this form, mites are easily recovered.

*Treatment*

(1) Localized form, topical treatment with benzyl benzoate, or Necci soap, once daily. Check diet and general health. Usually clears in 2 to 3 weeks.

(2) Generalized form. (i) Topical 8% organophosphate solution. Use gloves and avoid over treatment. Ectoral solution. (ii) Parenteral organophosphates combined with topical treatment. Ectoral tablet. (iii) Wash with a Keratolytic shampoo (Seleen) frequently to remove as much skin debris as possible and open hair follicles. (iv) Antibiotics for pustular form, cepoxillin, potentiated sulphonamide. (v) Amitraz is very effective against demodectic mange but is only available in the U.K. as 'Ficare'.

**Hookworm dermatitis**

Primarily a problem of kennelled dogs i.e. greyhounds (p. 378). When the third larval stage of the hookworm penetrates the skin of the pad and interdigital spaces and lower parts of the body, to gain entrance to the host.

*Signs* 1. Hair loss, thickening and reddening of the skin, where in contact with the ground. 2. Pads become soft and spongy around the edge.

*Treatment* 1. Anthelmintic for hookworms. 2. Treat skin and pad lesions. 3. Avoid using grass exercise runs.

### Dermatomycosis (Ringworm)

The majority of cases in dogs and cats are caused by *Microsporum canis*. Others identified are *Microsporum gypseum* and *Trichophyton mentagrophytes*. Humans are susceptible to the infection.

*Lesions*

Mild: small patch of scales and a few broken hairs.

More severe: large areas (circular, irregular or diffuse) of broken hairs, scales, crusts and sometimes secondary bacterial infection. Pruritus variable. Initial lesions are usually found on the face and/or forepaws (especially cats), but any part of the body may be affected.

*Diagnosis* will be made by one or more of the following.

1. Woods lamp (ultra-violet) *M. canis* lesions fluoresce yellow-green.

2. Skin scrape and KOH preparation.

3. Hair culture for long-term positive diagnosis.

4. Skin biopsy and PAS for difficult diagnosis.

*Treatment*

1. Clip hair from on and around lesions (disinfect clippers). Infected hair is a source of re-infection and a public health hazard.

2. Wash area with antiseptic soap.

3. Bath or dip the animal in a fungicidal agent, especially where multiple lesions are present—(Defungit). Repeat once or twice weekly as directed.

4. Local topical treatment for single lesions. Whitfields ointment, Conoderm, Tinaderm.

5. For diffuse or rapidly spreading lesions use oral griseofulvin, and continue treatment for at least 3 weeks. Warn owners of the danger of teratogenic effects when given to pregnant queens.

6. Isolate infected animals away from other animals and children. Clean bedding, disinfect with an antifungicidal agent. Spores may survive for over 6 months.

7. Prophylaxis for incontact animals, use oral griseofulvin at ten times the calculated daily dosage for a single treatment.

### Pyoderma

Inflammation of the skin frequently resulting from staphylococci, normally present on the intact skin's surface, gaining access to the deeper layers of the skin and subcutaneous tissues. The treatment and nursing actions are listed for each specific area where a pus forming skin infection is found.

*Acute Moist Dermatitis*

May occur at any site on the body, mainly in dogs.

1. Find the cause and treat it. Frequently the lesion is aggravated and enlarged by self-inflicted trauma.

2. Clip the area.

3. Wash gently in a mild antiseptic solution and dry thoroughly (soft paper towels).

4. Treat topically with i. astringent solution (i.e. Eusol) and continue with ii. antibiotic/corticosteroid lotion, three times daily.

5. Systemic antibiotics and corticosteroids are indicated sometimes for a short period to treat lesions that are severe and widespread.

6. During healing an emollient is useful (i.e. vaseline or zinc preparation).

### Lip Fold Pyoderma ("Cocker Spaniel mouth").

Dogs are presented for halitosis and/or drooling. Either one or both lower lip folds are seen to have evil-smelling moist dermatitis.

1. For mild cases, wash the lip fold daily and apply an astringent fluid, dry well, apply a topical ointment containing antibiotics or antibiotics and corticosteroids. Attention to the teeth is advised.

2. Surgical removal of the lip fold for severe and resistant cases.

### Facial Fold Pyoderma

A problem of the extreme brachycephalic breeds of dogs, i.e. Pugs and Pekes.

1. For temporary relief and in mild cases; treat as for lip fold dermatitis, but take care to avoid the eyes. Clip hair away to ventilate the skin.

2. Severe cases and for permanent relief: surgical removal of the folds.

### Vulva Fold Pyoderma

Usually seen in bitches that have been spayed young (infantile vulva) and with obesity allowing urine scalding of the immediate area of skin next to the vulva.

1. Attempt to reduce body weight.

2. Treat as for lip fold dermatitis.

3. Bacterial culture and sensitivity tests are useful for this site.

4. Cosmetic surgery, to eliminate the folds around the vulva, may provide the only satisfactory cure. Scalding by urine should be prevented by barrier ointments.

### Juvenile Pyoderma (Head/gland).

Seen in puppies, 2 to 4 months old and commonly the short-haired breeds. Often only one puppy of a litter is affected. Lesions are due to a staphylococcus and break out around the lips, eyes, ears and feet. The subcutaneous regional lymph nodes become enlarged and may abscessate. There is a temperature rise, anorexia and a cellulitis. Hypersensitivity and immunological incompetence are reported to play a role in the disorder.

The infected skin is oedematous, and a purulent exudate oozes from numerous breaks and ulcers. The disease may last for several weeks. The prognosis is guarded. Permanent scarring and hair loss may result, particularly around the muzzle.

1. Local treatment; **gentle bathing and cleansing;** apply antibiotic lotions, sprays or soluble powders, not ointments.

2. Systemic antibiotics (high doses). Take swabs for bacterial culture and selection of a suitable antibiotic.

3. Good diet with vitamin supplements.

4. Topical and systemic corticosteriod therapy is advocated by some authorities, particularly if culture and sensitivity have been performed and the puppy has shown a response to the appropriate antibiotic therapy.

### Interdigital Pyoderma

Occurs predominantly in short-haired breeds of dogs and sometimes cats. Pustules and draining sinus tracts empty dorsally or ventrally in one or more interdigital spaces. Discrete cysts may form in some dogs, with little or no change in the overlying skin. This disorder always must be differentiated from interdigital abscesses due to grass seed foreign bodies.

1. Bacterial culture and sensitivity (*staph. sp*).

2. Wash feet daily in an antiseptic solution—Hibitane, phisohex, penotrane.

3. Drainage of the abscesses, curettage of the sinuses and removal of necrotic skin; cysts will require surgical removal.

4. Systemic antibiotics.

5. Use of an autogenous vaccine should be considered. The disorder can be very resistant to treatment and recurrences are common.

### Callous Pyoderma "Bed Sores"

Secondary bacterial infection of a pressure callous that is normally found on the elbows and hocks of many dogs, especially large breeds sleeping on hard surfaces.

1. Local and systemic antibiotic therapy.

2. Provision of soft bedding.

3. Surgical removal may be necessary, but the disorder can be a recurrent and chronic problem.

### Generalized Deep Pyoderma

Cellulitis, pustules and draining sinus tracts in various areas of the body, especially at pressure areas, i.e. feet, knees, hocks, elbows. Usually *staphylococci* or *streptococci. Pasteurella* is isolated from cat skin infections.

With time the skin becomes thickened and fibrotic, making it extremely difficult to treat. It can be concurrent with systemic illness; debilitating disorders, where there is lowered resistance. In cats the cellulitis may spread widely under the skin before the abscess bursts and drains.

1. Systemic antibiotics, culture and sensitivity testing.

2. Local treatment; clip away hair, daily wash with hibitane or phisohex solutions, topical treatment with astringents, antibiotic lotions, soaking feet and legs in antiseptic solutions.

3. Autogenous vaccines.

A guarded prognosis as treatment is often prolonged and recurrence common.

### Acral lick granuloma

A single thickened firm oval plaque located on the anterior surface of the lower limbs in large breeds, and caused by the dog's persistent licking. The initiating cause is not understood, but boredom is a factor.

1. Correct any predisposing causes and break the licking cycle.

2. Corticosteroid therapy. (a) topically, cover the lesion with either a plastic sheet or melolin dressing and another dog-proof protective bandage. Repeat the procedure every 3 to 4 days. An alternative to ointment is the intralesion injections of long acting corticosteroid and bandaging.

(b) systemic—oral prednisolone therapy.

3. Sedation and protective devices to stop the dog biting the bandage.

4. Surgical removal of early small lesions.

### Eosinophilic ulcer

Seen in cats, the aetiology is not understood, but persistent licking is incriminated as a cause.

*Oral lesions*: commonly in the upper lip but also seen on gums, palate and tongue.

*Cutaneous lesions*: on abdomen, posterior thigh, digital pads—may occur concurrently with an oral lesion.

Treatments that may be used are:

1. Corticosteroids systemically or injected directly into the lesion.

2. Surgical excision—where possible.

3. Prevent self-trauma in cases of skin lesions. Recurrences may appear after 6 to 12 months.

## Canine and feline acne

A skin disorder where papules, pustules and small cysts form under the skin on the chin and around the lip margins.

*Treatment*

1. Systemic antibiotics—culture and sensitivity if appropriate.
2. Daily washing with dilute hibitane, dry and apply alcohol.
3. Topical antibiotic/corticosteroid cream.

Frequently it occurs in adolescent dogs (3 to 12 months old) and is located along the lip margins and muzzle. It may be also seen on the hairless parts of the skin of the abdomen.

## Nasodigital hyperkeratosis

Commonly occurs in canine distemper. Occasionally only the nasal pad is affected. Sometimes it develops on the nose pad following persistent or severe trauma. Otherwise the aetiology is unknown. The affected areas become cracked and painful and the skin has raised edges.

There is a choice of non-specific treatments. Corticosteroids and long courses of antibiotic may help the nose to heal.

1. Keratolytics i.e. Salicylic acid, pragmatar, and ichthamol ointments.
2. Hydration and softening of the keratin by soaking in water and applying petroleum jelly.
3. Topical corticosteroids, panalog ointment.

## Feline miliary dermatitis (miliary eczema)

This disorder has been attributed to fish diets, a vitamin B deficiency, an endocrine disorder (particularly in neutered cats), most frequently a flea allergy.

The lesions are multiple, scaly papules scattered over the back and neck, but also found over other parts of the body. They may be obscured by fur but are easily felt. The coat hair thins. The pruritus of the affected skin causes licking, scratching and super-imposed self-inflicted trauma of the skin.

*Treatment*

1. Control any fleas.
2. Alter the diet—added vitamin B complex.
3. Corticosteroids provide temporary relief.
4. Progestagen tablets are the therapy of choice. Some cases remain cured, many recur once treatment ends or is discontinued and permanent maintenance therapy is needed. Progesterone can be given parenterally.

## Seborrhoea

A chronic skin disorder of unknown aetiology, but often associated with dermatoses due to endocrine disorders. There is abnormal sebaceous gland activity (p. 48) and accumulation of scales on the skin.

It is seen most often in Cocker and Springer Spaniels.

*Lesions*

May appear very dry and scaly or very greasy.

1. Dry—white, grey or silver scales scattered in the coat.
2. Oily—greasy scaly patches; discrete, circular or irregular in shape anywhere on the body; rancid fat odour; greasy crusts may adhere to the hairs. A ceruminous otitis may be present.
3. **Seborrhoeic dermatitis**—The oily form plus inflammation and pruritus.

*Treatment*

1. Check for any associated endocrine disorder.

2. Treat and *control* symptomatically by: removing scales and crusts; reducing oilyness; controlling odour relieving pruritus and inflammation.

   (a) frequent keratolytic shampoos —Seleen

   (b) topical keratolytics—pragmatar ointment

   (c) corticosteroids—topical and systemic

3. Ceruminous otitis: frequent cleaning, and corticosteroid/antibiotic ointments.

4. Low doses of oestrogens.

### Endocrine based skin disorders

**Hypothyroidism**—decreased thyroid activity may affect the skin.

*Clinical Signs*

In dogs skin signs are: bilateral symmetrical thickening of coat or alopecia on neck and trunk; thickened skin; hyperpigmentation; brittle coat hairs; dull coat.

Other clinical signs that have been associated with hypothyroidism are: lethargy and mental dullness, cold intolerance, decreased exercise tolerance, depressed sexual activity, obesity, diarrhoea, slow heart rate.

*Treatment*

Thyroid hormone replacement therapy for life. Tablets of desiccated thyroid extract are not very stable, now replaced by l-thyroxine—very effective, but possible toxicity and signs of: tachycardia, restlessness, nervousness, diarrhoea and weight loss.

### Acanthosis nigricans

A skin disorder of unclear aetiology seen mainly in Dachshunds. Possibly several different endocrine factors are responsible. It may be a response to trauma. The skin in affected dogs shows a black colour at friction areas.

Hyperkeratosis, lickenification, seborrhoea and pigmentation in the skin are seen in the axillae and later on the flexor surfaces of all legs and ventral body. Secondary infection and pruritus may occur.

Accompanying clinical sign of hypothyroidism in some cases.

*Treatment*

The disorder is usually incurable and at best only controlable.

1. Treatment for hypothyroidism.

2. Reduce any over weight.

3. Corticosteroids.

4. Symptomatic therapy:—Keratolytic shampoos, pragmatar ointment, topical corticosteroids/antibiotic ointments.

### Hyperadrenalocorticalism (Cushing's syndrome).

Excess and indiscriminate production and release of corticosteroids by the adrenal gland. As a result of one of the following: a pituitary neoplasm or dysfunction; an adrenocortical neoplasm; adrenal hyperplasia; iatrogenic (unknown).

*Skin signs:* Bilateral symmetrical alopecia or thinning of the coat hair on the trunk, neck and chest.

Skin is thin and cool with prominent veins.

Calcinosis cutis appears as chalky deposits in the skin.

*Clinical Signs*

Increased thirst and polyuria; increased appetite; pendulous abdomen; muscular weakness.

*Treatment*

1. Symptomatic relief with keratolytic shampoo.
2. Primary treatment aimed at the lesion using cytotoxic drug therapy (o:p—DDD) must be given with caution.

## Male feminizing syndrome

This may be associated with castration, testicular atrophy, abnormal testicular hormone production and Sertoli cell tumour.

Signs are bilateral alopecia; hyperpigmentation; hyperkeratosis in the flanks, thighs, posterior abdomen and perineum; decreased libido; testicular tumour; cryptorchidism.

*Treatment* (1) Castration of entire males followed by (if necessary) supplementary testosterone therapy. (2) symptomatic treatment, keratolytic shampoo.

## Ovarian "imbalance"

Either an excess or deficiency of several hormones may be involved. There is alopecia and hyperpigmentation, mainly on the flanks, genital areas and perineum. Further variable skin changes are enlargement of the vulva, lickenification and generalized seborrhoea. An important clinical sign is a loss of regular oestrus cycles.

*Treatment* (1) Spay entire females. (2) Low doses of oestrogens for spayed females.

## Feline endocrine alopecia

There is progressive symmetrical thinning of the hair coat over the ventral abdomen from the sternum posteriorly, to include the inner thighs, flanks and perineum. Otherwise the skin is normal, occasionally there is mild pruritus present. The aetiology of the disorder is not understood but it is usual for castrated males and to a lesser extent spayed females to be affected.

*Treatment* (1) Thyroid supplementation. (2) sex hormone supplementation given intermittently to avoid signs of sexual activity in the neutered animals.

## Allergic Skin Disorders

There are three main groups.

**A. Flea allergy dermatitis**—discussed earlier under Fleas (p. 515).

## B. Atopic dermatitis

In affected dogs, there is **an inherited predisposition** for the formation of skin sensitizing antibodies in response to either inhaled or ingested substances, which are otherwise harmless in normal dogs.

Terriers (particularly West Highland White Terriers), Poodles, Dalmatians and Beagles are the breeds frequently involved.

The disorder develops in young dogs (1 to 2 years of age). If plant pollens are the allergens, then dogs show signs in the summer months. Generalized pruritus is the over-riding clinical sign. Biting at the feet, face rubbing, sneezing, rhinitis and lacrimation are frequent concurrent signs.

*Treatment*

The disorder is impossible to cure. Only control is feasible but some dogs show reduced skin sensitization after 5 years or more.

1. Inform and educate the owners of the nature of the skin condition. The RANA has an important role in keeping the owner instructed about this type of disorder.

2. Identify and avoid allergens—Intradermal or subcutaneous allergy tests may be of use.

3. Corticosteroid therapy.

4. Hyposensitization injections

## C. Allergic contact dermatitis

Occurs mainly in dogs as a delayed type hypersensitivity to contact allergens to which the body has previously become sensitized. This skin disorder is different from primary irritant contact dermatitis in which irritating substances produce dermatitis upon initial contact with the skin.

Examples of allergic contact substances: Flea collars, plastic feeding dishes, carpets, medications, leather, wood preservatives, pollen and plant extracts.

*Clinical Signs*

1. Affected areas of skin correspond to areas of close contact with the skin (usually hairless areas) i.e. ventral abdomen, inner thighs, perineum, interdigital areas, muzzle and lip margins or other localized areas of contact (collars on the neck etc.).

2. Acute inflammation with papules, then oozing and crusting.

3. Intense pruritus leading to self trauma.

4. The lesions are produced 12 to 96 hours after exposure to the provoking allergen.

5. Repeated exposure leads to chronic hyperkeratosis, pigmentation and fibrosis.

*Treatment*

1. Identify the offending substance and either eliminate or avoid it.

2. Symptomatic treatment with systemic corticosteroids.

3. Local treatment of the inflamed skin—wash and dry the areas, apply soothing lotions and topical corticosteroids.

## Autoimmune skin diseases

It is necessary only for the RANA to be aware of this group of dog diseases. The most important autoimmune conditions of the skin are the bullous diseases (pemphigus and pemphigoid), characterized by the development of blisters (bullae) in the skin and/or mucous membranes associated with the presence of autoantibodies against certain skin components. Skin lesions can also occur as part of the SLE (systemic lupus erythematous) disease complex, and a form of panniculitis in the dog may also have an autoimmune aetiology.

## Endocrine Disorders

Hypothyroidism and Cushing's disease are described under skin disorders. The RANA is most likely to be concerned with the treatment and management of diabetes mellitus.

## Diabetes mellitus

The disorder is due to insufficient insulin in the body. There is either a failure of insulin production, associated with pancreatic disease or the ineffectiveness of insulin which is produced in quantity but antagonized. Heredity, **obesity**, age and the sex of an animal seem to play a part in the aetiology of the disorder.

Diabetes occurs occasionally in cats, but it is a common disease of dogs. Bitches over 8 years of age are frequently affected. Dachshunds, Samoyeds and King Charles Spaniels are breeds affected beyond normal expectation. About 40% of cases are associated with a history of recent oestrus.

Insulin allows the entry of glucose into cells, its combustion in tissues, the formation of glycogen in liver and muscles, the formation of fat and protein synthesis. When insulin is deficient, the metabolism of carbohydrate, fat and protein is disturbed. **Excess sugar accumulates in the blood,** and is excreted by the kidneys, its osmotic attraction preventing reabsorption of water by the kidney tubules. The altered glucose metabolism damages the liver, lens of the eye, heart and blood vessels, kidney glomeruli and nervous tissue.

*Clinical Signs*

The major signs are polydipsia, polyuria, polyphagia, ketotic breath, obesity (later wasting), cataracts and liver enlargement (hepatomegaly).

*Diagnosis*

Diagnosis by the veterinary surgeon may be by:
1. Estimation of "fasting" blood and urinary glucose.
2. Assay of plasma insulin.
3. Glucose tolerance test.

*Treatment and Nursing Action*

1. Daily injections of insulin.—Several preparations are available, veterinary surgeons differ in their preference (note that 100 i.u. per ml strength will be standard in future).

2. A diet based mainly on protein foods fed at least twice daily. Bran may be given to provide bulk.

3. Owner co-operation and instruction is essential, if success is to be achieved. The owner is taught how to administer the insulin and monitor the dog. A good guide is the presence or absence of thirst. A RANA may be the best person to inject insulin daily into a dog.

4. Regularity of the dog's daily routine is essential. Insulin injection and meals given at the same time each day. One meal is fed to correspond to the peak effect of the insulin injection in the body.

Exercise should be a little and often and the same amount each day.

5. Regular urine and blood testing is essential initially until the animal's serum glucose level is stabilized and a suitable daily dose of insulin is established. A dog may be hospitalized whilst stabilization is achieved.

6. To achieve stabilization, the dose of insulin should be gradually built up and the blood or urine monitored each day. The aim is to produce and maintain a normal blood glucose level at the time of maximum blood insulin level and minimal glycosuria in the morning urine sample, collected prior to the insulin injection. Protamine Zinc (PZ1) has a duration of action of 24 to 36 hours with a peak activity at 14 to 20 hours. Zinc lente insulin has a shorter duration of 18 to 24 hours with a peak activity at 10 to 12 hours.

7. Problems with stabilization occur when:
    i. An animal is elderly and has advanced secondary pathological changes.
    ii. Bitches in oestrus—always advise spaying entire bitches.

iii. Resistance develops to one insulin (a change to monovalent (Novo) insulin may be tried).

Occasionally cases of diabetes present with Ketodiabetic acidosis and coma. They require immediate intensive therapy. The nurse can give very small quantities of oral glucose solution in first aid, then

(a) Intravenous soluble insulin injection.

(b) Intravenous fluids: 0.9% Saline and bicarbonate. Rehydration is most important.

(c) Oral potassium supplementation for a few days.

Then commence usual stabilization procedure, converting to one of the longer acting insulins.

Diabetes mellitus is a killing disease of dogs. Approximately 40% of cases die or are destroyed within a month of being presented at the surgery and a further 20% within 6 months. With insulin treatment, at least 15% survive over 1 year and a few up to 5 years. Much depends on the age of the dog at the time of onset of the disease, good nursing and advice will prolong the dog's life.

It is important to be able to recognize the difference between collapse due to diabetic coma, from that due to hypoglycaemia (insulin shock). The following signs may be helpful to the RANA when dealing with this emergency.

## Secondary hyperparathyroidism

Occurs in dogs and cats fed solely meat diets, which tend to be low in calcium and rich in phosphorus. For the healthy development and maintenance of bone, calcium and phosphorus need to be fed in a ratio of 1:1 with some vitamin D. The excess phosphorus and low calcium stimulates the parathyroid gland to release hormone which in turn releases calcium from the bone. This results in poor bone development in puppies, particularly in the giant breeds, and the demineralization of bone in adults.

Clinical signs are of skeletal pain, lameness, reluctance to stand and walk. With X rays, lack of skeletal density and, pathological fractures may be seen.

*Treatment*

1. Calcium supplementation: Calcium Carbonate powder.

2. Oral aluminium hydroxide preparations.

3. Rest and analgesia.

Owners of puppies should be advised by the veterinary surgeon, and when appropriate by the RANA, of the importance of a correct diet plus mineral and vitamin supplements to achieve optimum growth and development (p. 190).

| | Hypoglycaemia (Insulin shock) | Hyperglycaemia (Diabetic coma) |
|---|---|---|
| Seizures | Present | Absent |
| Nervous reflexes | Brisk | Diminished |
| Respiration | Normal | Exaggerated |
| Mouth | Moist | Dry |
| Breath | Acetone absent | Acetone present |
| Pulse | Full | Weak |
| Urine | Sugar and ketones negative | Ketone positive |
| Vomit | Sometimes | Often. |

Table 8.1

### Common Gastrointestinal Parasites

#### Helminths

*Nematodes*

(a) **Ascarids** Dog and cat ascarids (roundworms) are the commonest of small animal helminths. They are commonest in puppies and kittens, from 2 weeks to 2 months of age, although animals over 1 year may be infected (p. 374).

Clinical signs depend upon the severity of the parasite burden. Cases with only a few adult ascarids in the intestine show no illness, whilst those with heavier infections have an unthrifty appearance and pot-bellies. Extreme cases may show vomiting, diarrhoea, anaemia, partial intestinal obstruction intestinal rupture, and seizures. Larval migration in young puppies, is usually symptomless, but coughing and even pneumonia can occur.

(b) **Uncinaria stenocephala** (hookworms).

Adult dog and cat hookworms live in the small intestine. They are found in all ages of dogs and cats, but they are not as common as ascarids (p. 378).

The life-cycle is direct. Hookworms, unlike ascarids, require a free-living period as larvae before developing to the infective stage. Dogs and cats that have been imported to the British Isles may have become infected with Ancylostoma spp.

Anaemia is the main clinical sign, usually more severe in puppies and kittens, bloody mucoid diarrhoea, anorexia, poor growth and hair coat.

Infective hookworm larvae can penetrate human skin and migrate indiscriminately producing inflamed erythematous tracts—cutaneous larva migrans.

(c) **Trichuris vulpis** (whip worms)

The dog whipworm occurs in the caecum and large intestine. Trichurids are rare in cats. The life-cycle is direct. Dogs become infected by ingesting infective larvae. Whipworms are primarily blood feeders. Infections are seen in older dogs, occasionally showing clinical signs including profuse haemorrhagic diarrhoea, anaemia and weight loss.

(d) **Filaroides osleri** (lung worms)

This is a slender round worm (1 cm. long) found in the dog grouped in fibrous nodules at the bifurcation of the trachea. Clinical signs of coughing, respiratory distress and even death, depending upon the severity of the infection. Treatments evaluated so far have not given consistent results. Bronchoscopy is advised for the diagnosis.

#### Cestodes

*Dipylidium Caninum, Taenia spp., Echinococcus spp.*

These are the common tapeworms of dogs and cats. When mature they are elongated, segmented flatworms that parasitize the small intestine. The tapeworms have an indirect life cycle. The intermediate or larval form of the worm undergoing some development in a second vertebrate or invertebrate host.

**Dipylidium caninum** passes double-pored cucumber seed-like gravid segments that contain many eggs. If and when ingested by fleas or lice, eggs develop to the larval stage within these hosts. If this intermediate host is then eaten by a dog or cat, the tapeworms mature in the small intestine.

It is unnecessary to differentiate between the different *Taenia* **spp.** Each gravid segment has one lateral genital pore and the eggs are characteristic. The intermediate larval stage of *Taenia* **spp.** is called "bladderworm" and found in a wide variety of intermediate hosts including sheep, rabbits, rats and mice. Intermediate hosts become infected by ingesting eggs, and dogs and cats are infected by eating the intermediate host.

*Echinococcus* **spp.** are tapeworms of major public health importance. Usual intermediate hosts are wild and domestic ruminants (sheep) and rodents, but humans may be infested. The larval stage is the hydatid cyst. Depending upon the species of *Echinococcus*, invasive or non-invasive hydatid cysts will be produced in various organs of the intermediate host, and can lead to severe illness. *Echinococcus* **spp.** are not likely to infect urban or suburban dogs and cats unless fed uncooked offal containing hydatid cysts.

## Protozoans

### (a) *Giardia* spp

These are flagellated protozoans sometimes "incriminated", when found in the faeces of young dogs and cats with diarrhoea. However they can be recovered from animals with normal consistency stools. Humans may be infected and it may be assumed that **Giardia** may be transmitted from one species to another.

### (b) *Isopora* spp (Coccidiosis)

*Isopora* **spp.** are the most commonly diagnosed protozoan parasites in puppies and kittens. They parasitize the epithelial intestinal cells, and can cause watery bloody diarrhoea, dehydration and anorexia. Often coccidiosis is associated with overcrowded and unhygienic conditions.

### (c) *Toxoplasma gondii* (Toxoplasmosis)

See infectious diseases (p. 384).

## Medical nursing and parasites

Anthelmintics may be regarded as having either a "broad" or "narrow" spectrum of activity. Examples of broad spectrum compounds are nitroscanate (Lopatol), fenbendazole (Panacur) and mebendazole (Telmin KH). They are used where multiple parasitisms are known or suspected to occur. The use of narrow spectrum products is restricted to situations where a definitive diagnosis is made of the parasite involved.

Table 8.2 lists some of the dog and cat wormers available in the U.K. and gives their spectrum of activity.

| Product | Ascarids | Hookworm | Whipworm | Tapeworms | | |
|---|---|---|---|---|---|---|
| | | | | Echinococcus | Taenia | Dipylidium |
| Piperazine | + | 1.5x normal dose | − | − | − | − |
| Droncit | − | − | − | + + | + + | + + |
| Lopatol | + + | + + | − | + | + + | + + |
| Yomesan | − | − | − | − | + + | + + |
| Panacur | + + | + + | + + | − | + + | − |
| Telemin KH | + + | + + | + + | + | + + | − |
| Scolaban | − | − | − | + | + + | + + |

Table 8.2

The products, when used at the normal dose rate, are effective only against worms in the gastrointestinal tract. They do not kill somatic or visceral larvae of Toxocara in the tissues of the bitch. Pre-whelping treatments are ineffective in eliminating transplacental infection of the unborn puppies. Similarly there is no control of larvae migrating through the liver and lungs of young puppies.

By far the most important source of *Toxocara* infection for puppies is the dam. Killing the somatic larvae dominant in the bitch would reduce the worm burden of the pups considerably and it has now been shown that Panacur (fenbendazole) will do this. The dose rate is 50g./Kg./day from day 45 to 50 or earlier of pregnancy (22 to 27 days before whelping) to 12 to 18 days post whelping.

### Disorders of the Alimentary Tract

Many of the disorders will be covered in Chapter 10. From a medical point of view it is convenient to consider the common clinical signs of vomiting and diarrhoea.

### Vomiting

Disorders affecting the stomach directly or indirectly are likely to show vomiting as one, if not the main, clinical sign. Veterinary surgeons examining and investigating a dog or cat that is vomiting will pay particular attention to the following.

*History*: diet; age; vaccination history; ingestion of garbage and foreign bodies; description of vomiting episodes; nature of the vomiting; animal's willingness to re-ingest vomited food (food from the oesophagus (regurgitation)), not acidified by stomach acid, is usually re-eaten by the patient. Typically acute gastritis produces frequent **episodes of vomiting after drinking;** presence or absence of faeces and its consistency.

*Physical Examination*: Abdominal disorders are responsible for the majority of the causes of vomiting. Careful and systematic abdominal palpation is required for every case. A note is made of the animal's state of hydration since serious fluid and electrolyte loss may occur from frequent vomiting.

*Investigation*: A lot of cases of vomiting, such as acute non-specific gastritis, require no diagnostic or investigative procedures, and are confirmed by the good response to symptomatic therapy. In contrast the dog with severe vomiting and systemic illness is a real diagnostic challenge to the veterinary surgeon, often requiring extensive investigation.

*Laboratory tests*: Complete blood count; biochemical profiles may be necessary for adrenocortical insufficiency, renal failure, diabetic keto acidosis, pancreatic necrosis; pH of the vomitus.

*Radiology*: Radiographic evaluation of the abdomen is a very important diagnostic tool in the "workup" of a vomiting patient. Contrast radiography using micropulverized barium sulphate suspension either as the fluid or mixed with a meat meal provide a basis for the diagnosis of megalo-oesophagus and delayed stomach emptying.

*Endoscopy*: This is a valuable non-invasive technique to visualize and evaluate the gastric mucosa. It is used when abnormal radiographic findings need to be confirmed or when radiology fails to demonstrate a lesion. During the procedure, gastric fluid, brush cytology, and mucosal biopsies can be obtained.

**Medical Nursing Conditions** that will have to be recognized or distinguished

## A. *Gastric Disorders*

Dogs vomit readily and the vomiting reflex is easily excited.

### Acute Gastritis

A broad clinical term given to syndromes producing gastric mucosal injury. These may be physical agents, corrosive compounds, viruses, aspirin, phenylbutazone.

### Chronic Gastritis,
### Chronic Hypertrophic Gastritis,
### Eosinophilic Gastritis

Uncommon disorders requiring investigation. The cause of most cases is seldom determined.

### Pyloric Stenosis

This is the predominant cause of delayed stomach emptying. It usually results from hypertrophy of the circular muscle fibres in Boxers and Boston Terriers and Siamese cats (p. 594).

### Gastric Ulcers and Neoplasia

These disorders present with blood in the vomitus (haematemesis) and stool (melaena).

### Bilious Vomiting Syndrome

Early morning vomiting of bile on an empty stomach in an otherwise healthy animal.

*Gastric Dilation and Torsion Syndrome* this sudden and acute emergency is dealt with in First Aid (p. 249) and in Surgical Nursing (p. 594).

## B. *Abdominal Disorders*

Almost any abdominal disorder particularly those in the anterior abdomen will cause vomiting. These include, pancreatic necrosis, liver disease, enteritis (infections, parasitic, inflammatory), colitis, constipation, partial or complete intestinal obstruction, intussusception, peritonitis, pyometra, renal disease, urolithiasis, prostatitis and paralytic ileus.

## C. *Systemic and Metabolic Disorders*

Diabetic ketoacidosis; uraemia of renal failure, hepatic encephalopathy; adrenocortical insufficiency; lead poisoning.

## D. *Neurological Disease*

Diseases of the central nervous system stimulate vomiting through a variety of pathways. Examples are:

Intracranial neoplasia, inflammatory lesions, hydrocephalus, cerebellar or vestibular disorders, idiopathic epilepsy in small breeds of dog.

**Treatment and nursing action**

Vomiting is a clinical sign, not a disease. The veterinary surgeon will devise a therapeutic plan for each vomiting patient. Whenever possible this plan will be directed at correcting the primary cause.

The basic therapeutic regime will be to remove the initiating cause, control the vomiting and to correct any fluid or electrolyte imbalances. Fluid therapy may be asked for and the RANA should have equipment ready and suitable solutions put out for use.

1. *For simple non-specific acute gastritis*—**withhold all food for at least 12 to 24 hours,** and offer only very small volumes of water at frequent intervals.

2. *Anti-emetic drugs* are given to control vomiting. i.e. Chlorpromazine, anti-histamines, anticholinergic drugs used for short periods.

3. *Fluid therapy* to control and correct any dehydration and electrolyte imbalance.

Metabolic alkalosis occurs only in extreme cases of vomiting. When no information on the serum pH and bicarbonate status is available, the replacement fluid of choice is Ringer's solution. When metabolic acidosis is known to be present lactated Ringers is recommended (p. 322).

4. *Oral protection of the gastric mucosa* such as kaolin and bismuth preparations are rarely effective.

5. *Antacid therapy.* They act to neutralize gastric acid and inactivate pepsin. They need to be given every 2 to 4 hours. They are useful for longstanding persistent cases of vomiting, but should be used with caution for only short periods. i.e. Aluminium hydroxide, sodium bicarbonate.

6. *Inhibitors of gastricacid secretion.* These drugs act by blocking the histamine receptor on the parietal cell, stopping the release of acid and its effect on the mucosal surface. i.e. Cimetidine (Tagamet).

7. *Surgery* may be indicated to remove foreign bodies, to relieve pyloric stenosis, and to resect diseased parts of the stomach.

**Disorders of the intestines**

The common clinical sign is diarrhoea which is the frequent passage of loose or liquid faeces. It may present as an acute or chronic problem. Acute diarrhoea in dogs often is the result of scavenging household and garden rubbish (garbage) which either irritates the lining of the intestine or initiates osmotic pressure changes drawing water into the lumen of the intestine. Frequently acute diarrhoeas are self-limiting and require only simple symptomatic therapy. Cases of chronic diarrhoea require a specific diagnosis and present the veterinary surgeon with a real clinical challenge.

The veterinary surgeon will investigate a case using the following guide: A careful history; complete blood count; clinical pathology; faecal examination. From this data it should be possible to differentiate the presence of either a large or small bowel problem. Rarely are both involved simultaneously.

A. **Disorders of the large intestine**

*Clinical Signs associated* with large intestine disorders are

1. *Straining* (Tenesmus) after the passage of faeces.

2. *Increased frequency of defaecation.*

3. *Diarrhoea in small amounts with* **mucus and often fresh blood.**

4. *Abdominal palpation* reveals:

a. Tenderness in distal abdomen.

b. Impacted faecal mass in colon and rectum (particularly cats).

*Diagnosis* by the veterinary surgeon may require the nurse to assist with

1. Clinical Pathology: Faecal examination for parasites (whipworm), bacteria, mucus and blood.

2. Proctoscopy: To examine the mucosa

of the rectum and distal colon and if appropriate to obtain biopsy specimens.

3. Contrast Radiography of the rectum and colon.

*Specific Disorders*

1. Colitis. Idiopathic and ulcerative in many breeds of dog, histiocytic ulcerative colitis in the Boxer breed.

2. Foreign bodies. Needles and bones (frequently macerated).

3. Salmonellae infections.

4. Parasites. Whipworms and Coccidia.

5. Neoplasia.

6. Constipation: Due to, diet, i.e. bones; old age and debility; spinal paralysis; anal and rectal obstruction; pelvic fracture; enlarged prostate gland.

7. Mega colon. Enlarged due to perineal herniation and colon flexure; atonic colon.

*Treatment and Nursing Action*

1. **Colitis**
a. Diet: add bran and bone flour.
b. Often affects nervous dogs. Advise owners to avoid situations of stress. i.e. Kennels.
c. Sulphasalazine tablets, prednisolone tablets and enemas as directed by veterinary surgeon.

2. **Salmonellae infections**
The nurse must be aware of the **public health risk.** Take special cleansing precautions of all areas of potential and known contamination. Await instructions from the veterinary surgeon.

3. **Whipworms**—see section on parasites.

4. **Constipation**
a. Oral liquid paraffin. The prolonged use of mineral oils should be avoided.
b. Laxatives. Mucilagenous bulking agents are also of benefit.

c. Soft soap enema plus manual relief, under general anaesthesia (p. 308).
d. For intractable cases and as a last resort prepare for laparotomy and surgical removal of impacted mass.

B. **Diarrhoea due to Disorders of the small intestine**

*Causes*

1. Enteritis (frequently presents as gastroenteritis (vomiting and diarrhoea)).
a. Scavenging habits, garbage eaters.
b. Infections, Distemper, Parvovirus, Coronavirus, Salmonellae, Shigella, Campylobacter.

2. Haemorrhagic diarrhoea syndrome (Haemorrhagic gastroenteritis).
An acute rapidly fatal disorder associated with an allergic endotoxin shock reaction in the intestines.

3. Dietary upsets and intolerance i.e. lactose in milk.

4. Partial obstruction of the small intestine.
Due to cloth, string (linear foreign body). Flat sided solid foreign bodies producing a valve-like reaction. Intussusception at the ileocaecal colic junction.

5. Severe diffuse changes in the wall of the intestine i.e. lymphosarcoma.

6. Parasites.
a. Very heavy toxocara spp, infections, particularly in the young, producing diarrhoea.
b. Hookworms.
c. Coccidia and Giardiasis.

7. Focal Neoplasms
May cause diarrhoea and eventually weight loss and/or obstruction.

*Investigation*

The diagnosis in cases of small intestinal diarrhoea, particularly those of a chronic nature, is complex and the RANA need know only of the procedures likely to be used.

    a. Complete blood count and blood chemistry.
    b. Detailed faecal examination.
       i. fat, ii. trypsin, iii. parasites, iv. microbiological culture.
    c. Small intestinal function tests.
    d. Intestinal biopsy.
    e. Test therapy.

*Initial General Treatment and Nursing Action*

The majority of cases of diarrhoea in small animals appear to be functional and transient and result from the patient having ingested or being given food to eat, which has either been unabsorbed and fermented in the lumen of the intestine or has irritated the intestine wall. Both situations produce "intestinal hurry".

    1. Starve for 24 hours, and allow only frequent small volumes of water.

    2. Give oral absorbents—Kaolin, bismuth, charcoal.

    3. Gut-active sulphonamide and antibiotic therapy for diarrhoea cases is common in small animal practice. Authorities believe this to be of doubtful value and to be avoided whenever possible.

    4. Intestinal sedatives i.e. Lomotil.

    5. Intestinal spasmolytics i.e. Atropine, Hyoscine (Buscopan) and Menthidizate (Isaverin).

    6. Feed a bland diet i.e. Tripe, chicken, lean mutton and boiled rice.

Request owners not to feed; milk, milk products, any tit-bits, uncooked offal, coarse biscuit meal.

**Stop the patient from scavenging**

    7. Great care is required to ensure that patients are kept clean. Dogs and cats with long coats may need to have their "back end" washed and dried regularly. Ulceration of the anus is common in cases of prolonged diarrhoea, gentle washing and powdering with talc or cream with a zinc ointment or preparation containing a local anaesthetic or cortisone will help to relieve the problem.

**Anaemia**

Anaemia is the clinical sign, when there is a significant reduction in the number of circulating red blood corpuscles (RBC) such that there is a marked decrease in the ability of the blood to convey oxygen to the body tissues.

*Causes*

In small animal practice several different disorders and circumstances can produce anaemia.

    1. *Acute Haemorrhage*

    a. Resulting from severe trauma, when a major blood vessel is ruptured either externally or internally (ruptured liver or spleen).
    b. Blood clotting disorders i.e. Warfarin poisoning; inherited haemophilias in dogs; disorders of the blood platelets.
    c. Tumours of the spleen, liver and lungs. Haemangiosarcomas.
    d. Gastrointestinal haemorrhage syndrome (haemorrhagic gastroenteritis).

    2. *Chronic Haemorrhage*

    a. Haematuria—blood in the urine resulting from, tumours in the bladder and kidney; severe cystic calculi.
    b. Gastrointestinal—changed blood in the faeces (melaena) resulting from peptic or duodenal ulcers and neoplasms. Fresh blood in the faeces

due to colitis, rectal foreign body, large intestine neoplasm.

c. Parasites; severe lice and flea infestation.

d. Less severe blood clotting disorders.

3. *Depression of the Bone Marrow*

a. Failure of vital organs and metabolic toxaemia; chronic kidney and liver failure.

b. Purulent toxaemia i.e. pyometra, pyothorax.

c. Neoplasia—leukaemia, lymphosarcoma, myeloma.

d. Therapeutic drugs with adverse affects on the bone marrow i.e. chloramphenical, phenylbutazone.

e. Poisons i.e. lead.

f. Nutritional deficiences. Vitamin B deficiency due to malabsorption; iron deficiency resulting from chronic haemorrhage and malabsorption.

4. *Haemolysis* (destruction of the RBC within the blood vessels)

a. Autoimmune haemolytic anaemia.

*Clinical Findings*

1. Signs of weakness, dyspnoea with exertion and collapse.

2. Pallor of the mucous membranes.

3. Fast heart rate (tachycardia). Murmur may be present, weak rapid pulse.

4. Haemorrhages in: skin; mouth; joints; urine; thorax and abdomen.

5. Enlarged spleen, liver and lymph nodes.

*Investigation*

The veterinary surgeon will try to establish the cause of the anaemia, as long term symptomatic treatment is of little benefit to the patient. The investigation may be complex and require, bone marrow biopsies; tests to check the validity of the blood clotting and immune competence.

*Treatment and Nursing Action*

1. Transfusion: using blood or plasma expanders as directed by the veterinary surgeon. Blood is the fluid of choice to restore the circulating blood volume prior to surgery; following traumatic haemorrhage; when clotting factors or platelet function is deficient or absent; in severe chronic anaemia patients. Plasma expanders are very good when blood is not available.

Alert owners of donor dogs, that a transfusion is needed. 60% of dogs are A-positive (Universal recipients) and 40% are A-negative (Universal donors). So that where a cross-matching facility is not available, it is reasonably safe to administer one transfusion of unmatched blood. Cross-matching will be essential for any repeat transfusions (p. 318).

2. Corticosteroids (prednisolone 2 mg/kg body weight).

a. to counter hypovolaemic shock.

b. immune disorders.

3. Vitamin $K_1$ (1 mg/kg bodyweight for 5 days) for cases of warfarin poisoning.

4. Where possible eliminate the source of the haemorrhage or bone marrow depression; i.e. medical: parasites, colitis, provide vitamin B and iron. Surgical: panhysterectomy, splenectomy.

5. Provide complete cage rest. Give a good quality high protein diet.

6. Dietary supplements. B vitamins, anabolic steroids, folic acid, iron dextran.

**Exocrine Pancreatic Insufficiency of Dogs**

The disorder results from degenerative atrophy of the gland. It is seen mainly in young dogs particularly German Shepherd Dogs, where it is thought by some workers to have an hereditary link.

*Clinical Signs*

These result from the loss of function of the pancreas, which is the main digestive gland in the body. Affected dogs have voracious, scavenging appetites, and frequently show **coprophagia**. There is a marked loss in bodyweight. Either voluminous yellow-grey putty like faeces or yellow diarrhoea are passed. The hair coat under the anus may be soiled with oily droplets and/or rancid smelly faecal material. Otherwise the dogs are alert and lively.

The diagnosis is confirmed by screening tests. Traditionally the estimation of faecal trypsin has been a simple and popular practice-laboratory test. When used alone, it can give an unreliable result, and should only be used in combination with other screening tests or preferably avoided altogether in favour of the more recent oral BT-PABA test or the canine serum trypsin-like immunoreactivity assay (TLI).

*Treatment and Nursing Action*

The disorder is incurable. Treatment is aimed at controlling the diarrhoea, reducing faecal volume, and feeding diets which do not first require pancreatic hydrolysis for absorption from the intestine.

1. Feed a low-residue protein diet; using meat and tripe as the major dietary constituents and fed several times spaced through the day. Double to treble the amounts of food required for an equivalent size healthy dog will be required. This regime will eliminate the diarrhoea and also the stomach enzyme pepsin may hydrolyze some of the protein allowing absorption from the small intestine.

2. Remove all fat, milk and starch foods from the diet. Provide calories and energy by feeding

    a. glucose and maltose in the main meal.

    b. coconut oil fed separately.

3. Give a little sodium bicarbonate in the food, to buffer stomach acidity, which otherwise tends to destroy pancreatic enzyme therapy. Cimetidine may also be of value.

4. Pancreatic extracts.

Several commercial preparations are available and as cases of exocrine pancreatic insufficiency often respond differently to the same product it is worthwhile trying different products in order to try to obtain the optimal benefit. Enteric-coated or acid-protected preparations may be advantageous. Usually it is necessary to feed large amounts of the extract with every meal and this form of therapy is expensive. As an alternative and whenever available fresh whole pancreases collected from the abbatoir and deep frozen until required may be cut up and mixed in with the protein meals.

## Pyometra

**Description**

In this disorder of the bitch reproductive system, following oestrus, the endometrium turns hyperplastic and subsequently becomes necrotic. There is an intense purulent inflammation and toxaemia.

*Clinical Signs*

10 to 24 days post-oestrus or longer.

Anorexia.

Thirst.

Elevated temperature.

Vomiting.

Purulent discharge from vulva in open-pyometra.

*Confirmation of the Diagnosis*

Elevated white blood cell count over 30,000/cu.mm with neutrophil shift to the left.

X-ray abdomen—enlarged uterine horns.

*Treatment and Nursing Action*

Prepare for surgery: pan-hysterectomy.

Fluid therapy. Ringers solution or Normal Saline. Plasma when available (to replace protein lost in pus).

Prepare antibiotic therapy as directed.

## Acid-base Disturbance

From the point of view of medical nursing the two following states are most important.

### Metabolic acidosis

Occurs when there is a deficit of bicarbonate ions in the circulation.

*Causes*

Disorders where there is excess production or accumulation of metabolic acids.

Cardiac arrest.
Renal failure.
Anaesthesia.
Diabetic Keto-acidosis.
Disorders where there is excess loss of alkali.
Diarrhoea.
Salt poisoning.

*Clinical Signs*

Reduced consciousness.
Coma.
Increased depth of respirations.

*Nursing and Treatment*

Treat the underlying cause.
Prepare bicarbonate replacement therapy.

### Metabolic alkalosis

Occurs when there is an excess of bicarbonate ions in the circulation.

*Causes*

Situations producing a loss of metabolic acid.
Vomiting.
Lowered serum potassium.
Situations leading to excessive intake or retention of alkali (bicarbonate).
Excess administration of sodium bicarbonate.
Diuretics.
Low salt diet and no potassium chloride supplement.

*Clinical Signs*

Shallow respirations—respiratory arrest.
Heart rhythm abnormalities.
Vomiting.
Weakness, confusion and unconsciousness.

*Nursing and Treatment*

Treat the underlying cause.
Prepare to correct electrolyte imbalances as directed.
Give potassium chloride supplement in the diet.

## Heat-stroke

Heat-stroke is a life-threatening syndrome seen mainly in dogs, when the body mechanisms for heat loss become inadequate and fail to keep the body temperature within normal limits.

### Predisposing Factors

1. Hot summer weather.
2. Brachycephalic breeds. Short faces and the tendency for obstructed upper airways.
3. Dogs left in inadequately ventilated environments. i.e. Cars with all the windows shut on hot days.

### Clinical Signs

Panting, salivation, collapse, injected and hyperaemic mucosae, rectal temperature highly elevated (41 to 46°C).

### Treatment and Nursing Action

1. Reduce body temperature rapidly.
   a. Immerse the patient in cold water; if available a bath, otherwise a hose.
   b. Intravenous drip using a pack of chilled fluid (kept in the refrigerator).
   c. Keep the patient in a cool, shady, well ventilated room—an electric fan is useful.

The rectal temperature should be taken every 10 to 15 minutes and as soon as it is falling steadily, the cold water treatment may be stopped.

2. Intravenous fluid therapy to replace water lost from salivation and the respiratory tract.
3. Sedation. Chlorpromazine injection as directed.

## (b) Specific Infections and Vaccinations

A. LEYLAND

### Infectious Disease Control

This section is concerned with certain specific infections of small animals for which vaccines are available.

Infectious diseases are those capable of being transmitted to healthy animals. The micro-organisms involved unlike commensals are not present in normal animals except perhaps in the carrier state. Spread is achieved by close contact or via infected material from affected animals. Where close contact is needed for spread to occur the disease is referred to as contagious. However the words infectious and contagious are not always used with precise meaning, being somewhat interchangeable.

Close contact between healthy and diseased animals is required to transmit feline leukaemia virus whereas some other infections can *also* be transmitted indirectly via clothes and shoes, for example canine parvo virus, or *Leptospira icterohaemorrhagiae* from contaminated rat urine. The vehicle transmitting the virus or bacteria is known as a fomite. Some highly infectious diseases are easily transmitted such as distemper and canine parvo virus, rabies virus is only likely to be dangerous when introduced directly into tissues by a bite from an infected animal, the virus being present in saliva.

A Zoonosis is an infection capable of being transmitted from animals to man. Many micro-organisms fall into this category including *Leptospira icterohaemorrhagiae* from rats or dogs urine causing *Leptospiral jaundice* in man, toxoplasmosis from cats, tuberculosis from cattle or imported monkeys and of course rabies.

### Spread of infections

Bacteria, fungi and viruses which are resistant to environmental conditions including disinfectants can be more easily spread outside the animal body than more susceptible micro-organisms. For infections to be spread, direct contact with the infected dog or cat may occur. Alternatively indirect contact occurs from bedding material, pavements, exercise areas, cages, surgery floors or tables previously contaminated with excreta, urine or other infected discharge. Removal of the excreta may leave behind the microscopic organisms, hence the need for disinfection. Thus canine parvo virus is particularly resistant to disinfection whereas feline leukaemia virus will not survive long outside the animal body. Most other bacteria, fungi and viruses lie between these extremes of resistance.

Spread of infections can occur from the following sources—

1. *Infected faeces,* which may be normal or diarrhoeic containing for example, salmonella, parvovirus, campylobacters.

2. *Urine* contaminated with for example, *Leptospira canicola* or infectious canine hepatitis virus passed from dog to dog or *Leptospira icterohaemorrhagiae* from rat to dog.

3. *Nasal secretions* from animals with respiratory infections which can be sneezed long distances, by becoming small air borne droplets. Such droplet infection could occur for example, with distemper or cat flu. Isolation of infected cases would require separation and intervening impervious walls.

4. *Saliva* which could contain FeLV or rabies virus.

Details of isolation and quarantine are discussed more fully (p. 165.) Disinfection is dealt with on page 403.

It is important to realize that old and particularly very young animals are more prone to infectious diseases. For example infectious canine hepatitis is primarily a disease of young dogs. Older animals have usually been exposed at an early age and become immune, often without showing symptoms.

Any area where there is a concentration of diseased or apparently healthy animals is likely to be a source of infection, especially if hygiene is poor. Veterinary premises can only be kept safe by constant meticulous attention to cleanliness. Ideally only vaccinated dogs and cats would be admitted to the surgery or hospital, but in practice this is impossible, as sick or injured animals cannot be turned away. Stray dog and cat homes, pet shops and to a lesser extent shows and boarding kennels present opportunities for spread of disease. Thus a puppy obtained from a dog's home or pet shop is much more likely to be diseased or have had contact with disease than one having been bred in a private household. Some dealers collect puppies from a wide area which are mixed prior to sale. As conditions of hygiene and feeding on these establishments may be far from ideal, problems can and do ensue. Similarly kittens obtained from farms with large colonies of cats will very often be affected with cat flu. Large breeding kennels may from time to time have outbreaks of diseases such as distemper, parvovirus or infectious canine hepatitis. Introduction of these diseases may have occurred following contact with other dogs at shows, mating or new purchases. Recovered animals may be infectious temporarily or permanently. Such animals are referred to as **carriers**. Canine adeno virus (hepatitis) can be excreted for 6 months in urine following recovery. Some cats having been infected with flu may be persistent transmitters of the disease.

## Incubation periods of infectious diseases

The incubation period is the time lapse between acquiring infection and the presence of symptoms. During this time the bacteria or virus multiplies in the lymphoid or other tissues until sufficient infectious agent is present to attack the target organ for that particular disease. Canine adeno virus attacks the liver, rabies the brain, whilst distemper affects many organs particularly epithelial structures producing respiratory symptoms, gastroenteritis, conjunctivitis, hyperkeratosis and encephalitis. During the incubation period there may be a reduction in circulating white blood cells, but this may not be detected in the naturally occurring case.

The usual incubation periods of some diseases are given in tabular form. (Table 8.3)

## Immunity and prophylaxes

When infection occurs the body responds by producing antibodies specific to that infection. Once recovery is complete the animal is resistant to further infection and is said to be immune. The infective organism may be overcome by this immunity and other defence mechanisms before

TABLE 8.3

|  | *DISEASE* | *INCUBATION PERIOD* |
|---|---|---|
| *Dogs* | | |
| | *Leptospira—icterohaemorrhagiae* | 7 days ± 2 |
| | *—canicola* | 14–21 days |
| | Distemper (CDV) | 3–10 days but often much more |
| | Canine adeno virus (CAV) (Infectious canine hepatitis) | 7 days ± 2 |
| | Canine parvo virus (CPV) | 7 days ± 2 |
| | Rabies | up to 6 months or more |
| | Bordetella (kennel cough) | 4+ days |
| *Cats* | | |
| | Feline infectious enteritis | 7 ± 2 days |
| | Feline rhinotracheitis virus | 2–4 days but can be 10 days |
| | Feline calici virus | 1–3 days |

symptoms occur. As the virus infections of small animals can be difficult to treat, the emphasis is on prophylaxis, that is preventative measures. Immunity is produced by the use of vaccines, (see page 361) or occasionally by hyperimmune serum.

A vaccine is prepared by modifying a bacterial or viral culture in such a way that the animals immunity is stimulated but the agent is incapable of producing the disease. This is achieved by killing the organism or by changing it so that it loses its ability to produce disease but still has the antigenic properties to cause the protective responses required in the animal into which it has been injected.

**Live and dead vaccines**

Both bacterial and viral vaccines can be live or dead, and examples of both are in common use. Dead vaccines are produced from organisms killed by heat or chemicals. An infectious agent treated in this way loses its ability to multiply in the animal's body but will stimulate immunity.

Live vaccines are produced from laboratory cultures, for example viruses grown on chicken embryo cells. The virus gradually changes until it has lost is ability to infect the original host, becoming more and more infective for the tissues in which it is growing. Fortunately it will still live in the animals body until a satisfactory immune response is achieved. This process is known as attenuation and results in an attenuated vaccine (i.e. live). Live vaccines in general produce a strong long lasting immunity similar to natural infection. Dead vaccines can be improved in efficiency by the incorporation of an **Adjuvent**. This is a chemical usually aluminium hydroxide which delays the disappearance of the antigenic stimulus long enough to give a response, but dead vaccines usually need frequent boosting.

## Autogenous vaccines

An autogenous vaccine is one prepared by altering bacteria or virus obtained from an individual animal for injection back into the same animal. They may be used in dogs with chronic staphylococcal skin infections which are difficult to correct by other means. It is illegal to use such a vaccine on an animal other than the one from which the vaccine is prepared.

Bacteria grown on a blood agar plate are suspended in saline, Pasteurized (heated at 60°C for 1 hour), formalin is added and after testing for sterility the suspension is injected. Localized reactions, sometimes mildly painful are more likely to occur with such vaccines, which because of their nature are not able to be tested before being used on large numbers of animals.

## Heterotypic vaccines

Similar viruses affecting a different species can sometimes be used to produce immunity for example, Canine distemper and human measles are caused by closely related viruses. The injection of measles vaccine into puppies produces antibodies closely resembling distemper antibodies giving immediate but short-lived protection against distemper. A follow up injection with distemper vaccine stimulates more long lasting immunity, but this can only be given after antibodies derived from the mother have waned. Canine parvo virus is similar to the parvo virus of cats which causes FIE (panleucopenia). Thus live cat parvo virus vaccine has been used to protect dogs against canine parvo virus. Measles vaccine has been used to confer immediate immunity to puppies passing through stray dog's homes or where a puppy is expected to encounter distemper virus before its maternal immu-nity has worn off. This has largely super-seded the use of hyperimmune distemper serum.

## Maternal immunity and the timing of vaccines

A puppy or kitten will derive immunity from its mother and the content of this immunity will depend on which diseases the bitch has encountered both naturally and from vaccination. The protection conferred may prevent a satisfactory response to a vaccine. Eventually this immunity will wane, and at a certain level of antibodies for a given disease the animal will respond to vaccination. For canine parvo virus, distemper and canine adeno virus this will often be 12 weeks although some puppies may be susceptible at a younger age. Vaccine given at this age will produce a long lasting immunity against all diseases. Similar considerations apply to cat vaccinations. These are general rules and in particular individuals maternally derived antibodies may persist for longer periods, so that there is only poor or short lasting protection. This occurs with parvo virus, so that some veterinary surgeons prefer to give additional injections against canine parvo virus at 16 weeks. Rottweilers and other breeds have been known to carry maternal antibodies for 5 months and therefore further vaccination at this age is recommended. As protection from the mother wears off, there is a danger that any parvo virus in the environment, particularly in breeding kennels will prove overwhelming. In infected kennels it is advisable to move puppies to uncontaminated surroundings such as their new home at 6 to 8 weeks before their maternal immunity has waned; vaccination of pregnant bitches with dead vaccine is recommended 4 weeks before whelping to maximize maternal immunity. In general the use of live vaccines is avoided in pregnancy because of the possibility of abortion. Live vaccines generally give more immediate protection as do vaccines given by the intranasal route as for example in cat flu protection.

### Failure to respond to vaccination

Provided that vaccine has been stored and administered correctly, vaccine failure is rare. However, when it does occur the most likely cause is abnormal **persistence of maternal antibody.** It is always advisable for the animal nurse to closely question the owner of a puppy or kitten brought for vaccination about the animal's exact age. A sick kitten or puppy is unlikely to respond normally to vaccination and it is important that a thorough prevaccination examination is carried out by the veterinary surgeon. Corticosteroids can depress the immune mechanism, and it is generally considered wise to avoid vaccinating animals being treated, especially puppies and kittens.

The administration of vaccine to sick puppies or kittens may sometimes be necessary, it is unlikely to do any harm but it may be too late to prevent disease.

Recent reports from Glasgow Veterinary School suggest that the use of combined vaccines may produce a lower protection against CDV and CPV than when the vaccines are used separately. The small survey reported at the 1984 BSAVA Congress also suggested that some makes of vaccine were producing higher success in establishing immunity in puppies: these varied between 22% with one CPV vaccine to 90% with another brand of vaccine given at 13 weeks of age.

### Vaccines available

Table 8.4 shows the vaccines available to the veterinary surgeon. It will be necessary to make a decision on the range of cover advisable for the individual dog or cat. Usually in dogs, protection is provided against distemper, adeno virus, Leptospirosis and parvo virus. Kennel cough vaccines are often reserved for dogs to be boarded. The use of rabies vaccine is only permitted in quarantine kennels or dogs for export. Tetanus vaccine is rarely used in small animals.

Cats are usually vaccinated against FIE but increasingly also against flu, with FVR and FC component vaccines.

Certain manufacturers include PI3 vaccine with the distemper component and there is a choice of dead or live vaccines against CPV, FIE and CAV.

### Administration of vaccines

It is important that a syringe and needle sterilized other than by chemical means is used. Traces of chemicals or antibiotics could alter the vaccine adversely. Normally an unused disposable syringe is used for each dose. In an animal with clean dry skin, it is unnecessary to use a spirit swab, as some of the chemical disinfectant could be carried through the skin as the injection is made.

Vaccines are produced in solution or a freeze dried pellet which is reconstituted either in sterile distilled water or vaccine in fluid form. The distemper fraction may be dissolved in the Leptospirosis fluid. Reconstituted vaccine must be used within one hour. For subcutaneous administration the neck is used and minimal restraint is needed. Intranasal vaccination is well tolerated by both cat and dog: the head is held to raise the chin and the vaccine administered equally to each nostril allowing time for the solution to be drawn in during inspiration. Sufficient is provided to allow for some spillage. Sneezing may occur for several days following vaccination in certain cats.

### Completion of vaccination cards

Each dog and cat vaccinated should be issued with a certificate. These are produced by the vaccine manufacturer and they can be placed in waterproof envelopes individually printed for the veterinary practice carrying information about surgery hours and telephone numbers. It is important that details of ownership, breed, colour, sex, age and batch numbers are correctly filled in, particularly when several puppies or kittens are vaccinated for a breeder. **Details of ownership must always be completed**, if necessary leaving room for alteration later. This will help to avoid transfer of certificates to an unvaccinated animal. With animals of undetermined breed, it may avoid embarrassment to the veterinary surgeon if the nurse makes the necessary enquiries. The owner should be reminded to keep the card safe to provide evidence of vaccination for kennelling or subsequent booster vaccinations.

### Booster vaccinations

Most practices will send out reminders to clients regarding subsequent vaccinations and this will involve keeping accurate records of primary and subsequent vaccinations. Leptospirosis, kennel cough, parvo virus and cat flu need annual revaccination with a single injection. Distemper and adeno virus vaccines probably confer long lasting immunity, however in the absence of challenge from the naturally occurring pathogen, immunity may wane in the occasional individual and many veterinary surgeons will wish to

provide subsequent cover against these diseases, typically every other year. Where live FIE vaccine has been used, injections every 2 years are advised, in comparison, yearly administration of dead vaccine is needed.

### Storage of vaccines

Vaccines are damaged by warmth. Therefore storage in a refrigerator between +2 to +8°C is essential. If vaccine has to be transported by car the time spent out of the refrigerator should be minimal. A careful check should be kept that stored vaccines have not been kept beyond their expiry date as they may lose their effectiveness. However before discarding expensive quantities of out of date vaccine, a check with the manufacturers may produce assurance that the date can be safely extended.

### Side effects to vaccination

Apart from occasional swelling at the site of the injection which resolves spontaneously, adverse reactions to vaccinations are very rare. As well as their antigenic component vaccines may contain small quantities of chemicals or antibiotics included as preservatives to which an allergic reaction may occur. This is usually treated with adrenalin and may take the form of generalized itching or swelling of the face.

More serious effects may be associated with the use of hepatitis vaccine producing so called "blue eye". This is an opacity due to corneal oedema and can occasionally be long lasting. The side effect is associated with CAV1 vaccines, and will not occur with vaccines utilizing CAV2. Breeders of Afghan hounds seem most aware of this reaction although it may occur in many breeds.

| DISEASE | AGENT | VACCINE | PRESENTATION | ADMINISTRATION | INITIAL COURSE | SPECIES |
|---|---|---|---|---|---|---|
| Distemper (hardpad) | Virus | Live Attenuated virus adapted cell culture | Freeze dried pellet Ready for dissolving in sterile water immediately prior to use | Subcutaneous | Once | Dogs Ferrets (some vaccines only) |
| Contagious hepatitis (I.C.H., Canine viral hepatitis Canine adenovirus—CAV1 or CAV2) | Virus | Dead Grown in cell culture and chemically inactivated | In solution | Subcutaneous | Twice | Dogs |
| " | Virus | Live | Freeze dried pellet | Subcutaneous | Once | Dogs |
| Leptospira icterohaemorrhagiae (Leptospiral jaundice) plus Leptospira canicola (acute and chronic nephritis) | Bacteria | Dead | Solution | Subcutaneous | Twice | Dogs |
| Canine parvo virus (CPV) | Virus | Live Attenuated same as cat Panleucopenia | Freezed dried pellet for reconstitution immediately prior to use | Subcutaneous | Once | Dogs |
|  | Virus | Live Canine cell origin | Reconstitute pellet | Subcutaneous | Once | Dogs |
|  | Virus | Dead From cat or dog virus. | Solution | Subcutaneous | Once | Dogs |
| Panleucopenia Feline infectious enteritis (FIE) | Virus | Live | Freeze dried pellet for reconstitution immediately prior to use | Subcutaneous | Once | Cats |
|  | Virus | Dead | Solution | Subcutaneous | Twice | Cats |
| Parainfluenza (one cause of kennel cough) | Virus | Live | Freeze dried pellet | Subcutaneous | Once | Dog |
| Bordetella bronchiseptica (one cause of kennel cough) | Bacteria | Live | Freeze dried pellet | Intranasal | Once (into the nose) | Dog |
| Tetanus | Bacteria | Dead (Formalin treated toxin) | Solution | Subcutaneous | Twice (2 weeks apart) | Dog |
| Rabies | Virus | Dead | Freeze dried pellet | Subcutaneous or Intramuscular | Twice (14–28 days) | All carnivores including dogs and cats |
| Calici virus FC (one cause of cat flu) Plus | Virus | Live | Freeze dried pellet | Subcutaneous or Intranasal | Twice (3–4 weeks apart) | cats |
| Rhinotracheitis virus FVR (one cause of Cat Flu) | Virus | Live | Freeze dried pellet (Different manufacturers) |  | Once | Cats |
| Measles (for distemper protection) | Virus | Live | Freeze dried pellet | Intramuscular | Once | Dogs |

**Table 8.4**
**Vaccines available in U.K.**

*Notes:* Paramyxovirus vaccine is available for use in pigeons. Myxomatosis vaccine is available for use in rabbits. There is no vaccine against feline leukaemia virus at the present.

**Vaccination of dogs and cats in kennels**

Proprietors of boarding catteries and kennels are well advised to refuse admission to a dog or cat without a current vaccination certificate. It is preferable for vaccination to be completed 2 weeks prior to kennelling. The use of quick acting vaccines should be considered if boarding is imminent, that is measles vaccine in dogs, intranasal flu vaccine in cats. Kennel cough vaccine may be requested by keepers of dogs in kennels that have had previous problems with this illness.

Kennel owners often **require an annual full booster** course before a boarding cat or dog is admitted, since they may have difficulty judging how many components of a vaccine were given to a dog when a vaccination card is presented to them.

## (c) Poisoning

### A. LEYLAND

Cases of poisoning are too often suspected by animal owners but on occasions the signs of poisoning may be missed by veterinary surgeons. Clients may make accusations against neighbours who they think dislike their cat or dog, but these are rarely later substantiated. Poisoning may arise not only from malicious intent but also accidentally. A vast range of compounds present in an animal's environment have been known to produce symptoms, and possible death when ingested. However if the symptoms are not specific for a particular poison (or toxin) and they rarely will be, and there is no circumstantial evidence to incriminate a poison, then suspicions may not be aroused. For example a dog initially had convulsions but was not suspected of being poisoned until a second dog in the same household showed identical symptoms. Laburnum poisoning was diagnosed and it became clear that an overhanging branch had been chewed.

In the literature, cases of poisoning in small numbers of animals only, have been recorded and the symptoms described can not necessarily be regarded as typical. The diagnosis is largely based on circumstantial evidence and therefore a carefully taken history is extremely important. The animal nurse should beware passing an opinion when it is suggested that an animal has been poisoned maliciously.

## Treatment for suspected poisoning

i. *As a first aid measure it may be appropriate to induce vomiting* in a dog known to have ingested a toxic substance using a crystal of washing soda pushed to the back of the tongue. As the stomach takes up to 4 hours to empty, there is little point in causing vomiting beyond this time. Gastric lavage may be considered by the veterinary surgeon attending the case by the use of a stomach tube, washing out the contents of the stomach with water or saline. Charcoal can be administered to absorb further toxin. If malicious poisoning is suspected it is important to preserve the vomitus for possible future analysis. Analysis by a forensic laboratory can be carried out, but a search for a particular toxin should be requested as it would be impractical and expensive to look for all possible poisons. Analysis in general is carried out on vomit, urine and blood in live animals, liver, kidney, stomach and intestinal contents from post-mortem material.

ii. *In the case of contamination of the coat with oil or creosote the application of "Swarfega"* is recommended, (if not available cooking fat can be substituted) subsequently washing off with soap and water. If extensive contamination has occurred it may be necessary to perform this treatment under general anaesthesia, and it is important to be as thorough as possible especially in cats covered in oil or tar, to avoid Phenol poisoning.*

iii. *Supportive treatment can be given according to the circumstances.* Animals becoming hypothermic (for example following alphachloralose poisoning) must be kept warm. Intravenous fluid therapy is often necessary. Intravenous pentobarbitone may be used by the veterinary surgeon to control convulsions. Fullers earth can be given by mouth if paraquat may have been swallowed.

iv. *Specific antidotes should always be used,* but unfortunately these are available for very few poisons, the identity of which must be known. Vitamin K is a specific antidote to Warfarin (rat bait).

v. *The other measures taken will depend on the identity of the poison.* If a drug is involved useful information regarding antagonists (drugs counteracting the symptoms) and antidotes (chemicals specifically replacing the poison) will be found in the Compendium of Data Sheets. Information regarding veterinary drugs will be present in most veterinary surgeries, but where human drugs are involved the equivalent human data sheets are invaluable. In cases of emergency, manufacturers of chemicals or drugs, for example mouse and rat poisons will be able to supply the necessary information. Charts for display in the surgery are available from some vermin control firms. Finally make sure the source of poison is removed to prevent further attacks.

### Species variation

A wide variety of substances in the environment can lead to poisoning and in this section only the more common ones will be mentioned. Dogs are prone to chew almost anything and therefore become poisoned easily. Cats are much more

*A mixture of acetone and Liquid Paraffin (mineral oil) has been used to remove tar in severely affected animals, shampoo well afterwards.

fastidious but because their liver enzyme systems are poorly developed for detoxification the effect of ingestion can be very serious. Dogs or cats which are hunters can be secondarily poisoned by eating mice or rats which have been killed by bait.

### Examples of Poisonous Substances

#### Domestic Poisons

*Fumes* can be very dangerous. Incomplete combustion of methane from gas fired central heating boilers or fires, and *Carbon monoxide* production (also in car exhaust fumes) have proved fatal to caged birds. Overheated fat producing *Acrolein* can produce respiratory symptoms, collapse and death, in cats and dogs unable to escape their effects.

*Ethylene glycol* is used as antifreeze and its sweet taste can be attractive to dogs who obtain access to water drained from car radiators. There is an initial depression of the central nervous system, vomiting and weakness. Subsequently there may be haematuria, or lack of urine production as crystals are deposited in the kidneys. Death may occur. Treatment within four hours may be successful. Ethanol and sodium bicarbonate should be injected every 6 hours for 2 or 3 days. Convulsions can be controlled with pentobarbitone and further absorption prevented by charcoal administered orally.

*Lead* is a common poison for dogs. Sources include red lead, putty, linoleum, metallic lead objects and old flaking paint, all of which may be chewed. Modern paints are low in lead. The symptoms produced can be very variable. Nervous signs include excitement or depression, convulsions, paralysis or blindness. Older dogs may show abdominal pain, inappetance and vomiting. Fits are sometimes seen (specific treatment is available in the form of sodium calcium edetate administration, as well as pentobarbitone to control convulsions).

*Phenolic* compounds contained in rubber toys have caused poisoning in cats. Symptoms were ataxia (inability to stand) hyperaesthesia (excitability) and photophobia (resentment of light).

### Drugs

Poisoning may occur with veterinary drugs administered normally or at inappropriate doses. The animal nurse will have experienced at first hand the variability of the individual dog in its response to acetylpromazine (ACP). Apart from the difference in response of very sick, old or very young animals, the effect of the same dose of ACP on dogs apparently of similar size, health and age can vary from mild sedation to deep sleep. This phenomenon is known as biological variation and to some extent will apply to all drugs. ACP will also occasionally cause fits, particularly in boxers. Usually no treatment is required. The same variability in response can be seen to ACP tablets, which are used as sedatives for travelling and during thunderstorms. Thus the dose needs to be tailored to the individual. An exaggerated or unusual response can be seen with many drugs.

Allergic reactions can follow the administration of antibiotics, particularly penicillin and oxytetracycline. Itching, redness of the skin and swelling of the face are produced. Adrenaline is used to treat these reactions, which occur extremely rapidly following administration usually by injection.

The general public often do not appreciate the species difference between man and animals. Hence *aspirin* and particularly *paracetamol*, considered to be very safe in humans are administered to dogs and cats often at human doses sometimes leading to fatal consequences. Aspirin can cause gastric ulceration and paracetamol methaemoglobinaemia (chemical combination with haemoglobin in red blood cells reducing the oxygen carrying capacity).

In the author's experience medical practitioners are particularly likely to administer drugs to their own animals. Drugs used to treat arthritis may well produce gastric ulceration in dogs.

Therefore **the animal nurse should not advise administration of medicines** intended for human consumption: for example aspirin until such times as the animal can be seen by a veterinary surgeon. Any aspirin ingested by a cat in excess of one tenth of a 500 mg tablet will lead to liver damage.

Accidental access by dogs and cats to their owners or their own veterinary medicines is a common occurrence. Tranquillizers or contraceptives are often involved. Gastric lavage may be performed easily in the over-tranquillized dog whilst no harm ensues from the hormones ingested from contraceptives which are detoxified and excreted.

### Venoms

The poisonous snake which occurs naturally in the British Isles is the adder or viper. Bee and wasp stings are very common. For snake and insect bites, treatment with antihistamines is usually sufficient.

Dogs can be poisoned by mouthing toads which secrete an irritant from their skin producing retching and salivation. Certain exotic toad species if ingested can be fatal. Treatment consists of washing the mouth and administering atropine to control salivation.

## Pesticides

1. **Herbicides** (Compounds used to kill plants)

*Sodium arsenite* is rarely used nowadays and is far less toxic than in organic forms of arsenic, which occurs in wood preservative and fruit tree sprays. Poisoning may be malicious but usually follows careless disposal or spraying. Vomiting, salivation, weakness and abdominal pain lead to profuse bloody diarrhoea and death occurs rapidly.

*2.4.D and 2.4.5.T* (Chlorophenoxy acids) are commonly used lawn weed killers and are selective in their action on plants. They are of very low toxicity, but poisoning has occurred from careless disposal of solutions used in horticulture.

*Diquat and paraquat* are used as weed killers for clearing ground or paths. Once in contact with soil they are harmless, but prove lethal when vessels used to prepare solutions are chewed or used as drinking bowls. Initially there is vomiting and lethargy. Jaundice may be present but the lethal effect occurs from changes in the lung tissue leading to respiratory symptoms. Treatment is unlikely to be successful.

*Sodium chlorate* is used as a total weed killer. If a dilute solution is ingested poisoning may occur, for example drinking from pools formed after spraying. Methaemoglobinaemia occurs causing the mucous membranes to become brown. Symptoms include depression, anorexia, abdominal pain and blood in the urine. The outlook for recovery is poor.

2. **Insecticides** (Compounds used to kill insects)

*Organochlorine compounds* include DDT, benzene hexachloride (BHC, gammexane, lindane) and numerous others used in garden sprays and animal shampoos. Similar symptoms are produced in varying degree by these compounds, that is restlessness, salivation, vomiting and inco-ordination. Treatment comprises controlling the convulsions by pentobarbitone and administering calcium borogluconate. Dieldrin, used industrially as antiwoodworm treatment for house floors has caused acute and chronic poisoning in cats. In the chronic cases, as well as the typical symptoms of organochlorine toxicity, hair loss and emaciation were noted in those cats surviving for several weeks. In one reported case, the cats involved had been denied access to the treated room for six weeks and symptoms developed four weeks after initial contact. All affected cats died.

*Organophosphorus compounds* include many animal and plant insecticides similar to organochlorine compounds. All act by inhibiting cholinesterase and the signs produced are those associated with stimulation of the parasympathetic system and include salivation, abdominal pain, vomiting, inco-ordination and convulsions leading to coma and death.

Treatment comprises **the use of atropine** intravenously. The animal nurse should take particular care to warn owners to use insecticidal shampoos and sprays carefully.

Flea collars incorporate these powerful chemicals in a slow release form which can make subsequent anaesthesia or treatment with certain drugs dangerous. Local irritation has also been seen. Their use is better avoided.

## Molluscicides

*Metaldehyde* is a slug bait (molluscicide) usually incorporated in a bran base which makes it palatable to dogs and cats. Symptoms are convulsions, salivation and hyperaesthesia, (that is increased excitably when stimulated). There is no specific antidote and the convulsions are controlled with xylazine or pentobarbitone or acetylpromazine. Recovery is not very likely but poisoning from this substance is now rare.

### Rat, mouse and pigeon baits

*Alphachloralose* is used to kill mice and pigeons, acting as an anaesthetic, allowing body temperature to drop (hypothermia) leading to coma and death. Excitement may precede the dullness, inco-ordination and hypothermia. Treatment is aimed at providing warmth and the avoidance of sedatives.

*Antu* is rarely used nowadays but is extremely toxic. Dyspnoea, difficult breathing following fluid accumulating in the lungs with salivation, vomiting and diarrhoea are the main symptoms.

*Red squill* is a relatively safe rodenticide which is not used in Great Britain. It is rarely eaten by dogs and cats and if it is, promptly causes vomiting and therefore recovery.

*Strychnine* is not legally available in Great Britain but in those countries including USA and European countries where it is freely used it is the most frequent cause of poisoning. Illegal use certainly still occurs in Great Britain where it is used to poison bait put down for foxes. If consumed by dogs or cats symptoms of excitement, violent tetanic spasms and salivation are produced. The tetany is intensified by external stimulation. Death usually occurs, but if a poisoned animal survives 24 hours the outlook is good as the strychnine is excreted. There is no specific treatment.

*Warfarin* is used as rat bait. It interferes with the clotting mechanism of the blood and the symptoms seen are palor due to anaemia following haemorrhages below the skin, into the mucous membranes, and internally. Other similar compounds are available, for example difenacoum (Neosorexa). Death does not usually follow ingestion of a single dose and as the symptoms are slow in onset, **treatment with vitamin K1 as a specific antidote** is often successful.

Handling of poisoned cases should be minimal to prevent further haemorrhage, and whole blood transfusions may be considered necessary.

*Calciferol* is vitamin D2 which causes calcification of the arteries, and other tissues. Signs of poisoning are depression, anorexia, spinal arching, polydipsia and polyuria.

Treatment is a high fluid intake, high salt and low calcium, Combination with warfarin (neosorexa CR) makes treatment more difficult and recovery unlikely although death may be delayed several days.

### Plants

Plant poisoning is more commonly associated with farm animals. However as dogs and cats will chew almost anything, poisoning has been recorded from laburnum, mistletoe, various mushrooms and undoubtedly many plants could be toxic in certain circumstances. For example some house plants, unsuspected when grown here, are well known as poisons in their own country of origin.

### Further Reading

Chandler E. A. (1984) *Canine Medicine and Therapeutics*. 2nd Edn Blackwell Scientific Publications. Oxford. (see chapter by Clarke.)

Clarke, E. G. C. (1975) *Poisoning in Veterinary Practice*. Association of the British Pharmaceutical Industry. London.

Darke, P. G. C. (1983) *Notes on Canine Internal Medicine*. Wright. Bristol.

# CHAPTER 9

# Radiography

S. W. DOUGLAS

## Introduction

Radiography is employed as a means of investigating disease and injuries in animals in most veterinary practices and is another specialized technique in which RANAs are expected to play an increasing part in assisting the veterinary surgeon. Such assistance can be given more effectively if the RANA understands something of the principles underlying the production of X-rays, the apparatus required and its use (Fig. 9.1). This cannot be explained fully in one chapter, where it is necessary to concentrate on particular details and to employ oversimplification in explaining some technical aspects, and the student is advised to study the subject more fully in *Principles of Veterinary Radiography* (p. 571).

## Elementary Principles of Radiography

There are a wide variety of X-ray machines used in veterinary practice: some are relatively small and simple while others are large and complicated pieces of machinery. However, for the purposes of this chapter each may be regarded as an apparatus in which the electric current from the mains is transformed into a current of high voltage (measured in kilovolts) and low amperage (measured in milliamps). When this new current is passed through an X-ray tube, X-rays are produced which travel in straight lines and can be directed in the form of a beam known as the **primary beam** through the part of the patient which it is desired to investigate. Portions of the beam will be

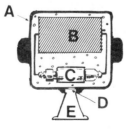

FIG. 9.1.(a)

The structure of the tubehead of an X-ray machine; A, tubehead casing; B, high-tension transformer; C, X-ray tube (together with the transformer; it is surrounded with insulating oil); D, window and filter; E, cone.

obstructed or absorbed by the denser structures within the patient's body, thus causing the beam to cast a "**shadow**" of the various structures penetrated on the film. This **shadow picture** cannot be seen until the film is **processed** by passing it through certain chemical solutions.

If the part of the animal being examined is not likely to produce a distinct shadow, substances of high atomic number, such as iodine or barium compounds, may be introduced into it in order to show the outline more distinctly on radiography. Such substances are known as **contrast agents**.

The properties of the X-rays comprising the beam and their ability to penetrate the patient and affect the film can be varied by adjusting the various dials on the control panel of the X-ray machine and must now be considered in detail.

### Exposures

As already stated, there are a wide variety of X-ray machines, and the nature of the knobs on the control panels and the exposure factors necessary to operate each will vary with machines of different output and of different make. It is to be expected that, in each practice, a chart or table of exposure factors suitable for the apparatus used will be available for consultation before making an exposure. However, if this is to be used intelligently and adjusted for different patients, or in order to improve the radiograph, the significance of the following factors, which contribute to any radiographic exposure, must be clearly understood.

### Kilovoltage

The higher the kilovoltage selected the greater the penetrating power of the X-rays produced. Therefore, when attempting to penetrate thicker and denser areas of tissue the kilovoltage will have to be increased. However, the use of too high a kilovoltage results in over-penetration of all areas of the part being examined, and the radiograph will lack contrast (p. 567).

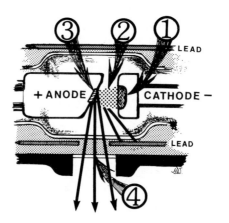

Fig. 9.1(b)

*How an X-ray tube functions:* (1) the filament in the cathode is heated to provide a source of electrons to carry the high-tension current across the tube vacuum to the anode; (2) the electron stream crosses between the cathode and the anode target carrying the high-tension current; (3) the electrons travel at high speed and hit the target (a slip of tungsten set in a block of copper) and their energy is converted into a large amount of heat and a small quantity of X-rays; (4) the rays are only permitted to emerge from the tube in the area of the window. The remainder are absorbed by the lead shielding.

Thus the kilovoltage selected should be the lowest sufficient to penetrate the part under investigation and for most small animal radiography the kilovoltage employed is likely to be between 50 and 70 kV. An exception to this rule is occasionally encountered when, in some circumstances, it is necessary to increase the kilovoltage in order to compensate for the low milliamperage provided by some of the smaller X-ray machines.

It will be found that with some X-ray apparatus the kilovoltage control knob is clearly calibrated in precise figures, but that with other machines it is indicated by a series of letters or numbers, because the kilovoltage output will vary with the amperage output at which the set is being operated.

### Milliamperage

The milliamperage chosen controls the amount of X-rays produced and the blackening effect they have on the radiograph. Thus the choice of too high or too low milliamperage settings results in radiographs which are too dark or too light for satisfactory interpretation. However, the amount of X-rays is also controlled by the *time of exposure* and these two factors should be considered in relation to each other.

### Time of exposure

The time of exposure (measured in seconds) is the period for which X-rays are being produced, and obviously this also controls the amount of X-rays reaching the film. Since there are two factors affecting the quantity of X-rays produced, it is usual to multiply them together and to use the product, which is measured in **milliampere-seconds (mAs)**, as an indication of the amount of X-rays being used.

The advantage of this combination is that one of the factors may be varied to compensate for the other. Thus the following different exposure settings for a particular X-ray machine would all produce the same amount of X-rays:

|     | kV | mA | s(time) | mAs |
| --- | --- | --- | --- | --- |
| (1) | 65 | 10 | 1 | $10 \times 1 = 10$ |
| (2) | 65 | 20 | 0.5 | $20 \times 0.5 = 10$ |
| (3) | 65 | 40 | 0.25 | $40 \times 0.25 = 10$ |

Since veterinary patients will not co-operate by holding their breath or remaining still at the moment of making a radiographic exposure, it is usually important to use the shortest practicable exposure time to minimize blurring from patient movement. To permit this it is necessary to employ comparatively high milliamperage settings (see example (3) above), and most of the small sets are used consistently at their maximum milliamperage output which is usually 20–30 mA.

### The effects of distance from film to tube

The quantity of X-rays reaching the film is also affected by the distance of the film from the X-ray tube, and decreases as the distance increases. So, if the film is placed further from the tube, the mAs has to be increased to compensate for this. Unfortunately, the amount by which this is increased is proportional to the square of the distance, i.e. if the distance is doubled the mAs has to be increased 4 times.

Increases of this magnitude are not practicable with the smaller X-ray machines, and with such apparatus the film is usually placed at a comparatively short distance (75 cm or 30 in.) from the tube (although a longer distance would give a more accurate reproduction of the part being X-rayed).

The important point is to operate each X-ray machine at a constant distance from the film and to remember that, if the distance is varied for any reason, the exposure factors must be adjusted to allow for this.

### The thickness of the subject

The amount (mAs) and penetrating power (kV) of the X-rays required to adequately investigate a patient will vary with the thickness and nature of the part (it is easier to penetrate an air-filled chest than an equivalent thickness of muscle and bone in a limb). When radiographing thick areas of tissue it is usual to increase kilovoltage by approximately 1–2 kV for each centimetre increase in depth. Where the limited kilovoltage output of some of the smaller sets will not permit such an increase, a similar effect can be achieved by raising the mAs by roughly 25% for each centimetre of increased tissue thickness.

### The estimation of exposure factors

*Summary*

The most important factors to be considered in selecting exposure settings have been listed above, and others (the use of grids or of particular films or intensifying screens) will be considered later in the chapter. Because there are a number of factors involved and adjustment of one has an effect on the others, it is important not to change or adjust more of these factors than is absolutely necessary.

### Recording Apparatus

### Films in veterinary radiography

**X-ray films.** The type of X-ray film usually employed is known as **screen type** film because it can only be used in conjunction with intensifying screens (these will be described subsequently). The film and screens must, in turn, be encased in a film cassette to exclude light. This type of film is made in various speeds or sensitivities and each variety is marketed by different firms under different proprietary names (e.g. Kodak's Blue Brand or Agfa-Gevaert's Curix Blue Base). These differences are of importance to the radiographer who must adjust the controls of his apparatus to allow for variations in the film speed. Therefore, if at any time the type of film being used is changed, the radiographer must be informed of this fact.

X-ray film is produced in a number of standard sizes. In most practices only a few of these sizes will be kept and used, but it is important to see that these sizes correspond with the sizes of the intensifying screens, film cassettes and film hangers employed. The sizes commonly employed are:

> 13 × 18 cm
> 18 × 24 cm
> 18 × 24 cm
> 24 × 30 cm
> 30 × 40 cm
> 35 × 35 cm
> 35 × 43 cm

(Other sizes can be obtained for special purposes.)

X-ray film is a particularly sensitive material which can be marked or spoilt in a number of ways, including:

(1) *Exposure to X-rays.* Boxes of film or loaded cassettes must never be left near an X-ray set when it is likely to be used.

(2) *Exposure to light.* Boxes of film and film cassettes must be kept closed and only opened in the dark room with safelight illumination.

(3) *Dirty or greasy hands.* As far as possible film should be handled only through the paper folder which surrounds each film in the box in which it is obtained.

(4) *Chemical splashes.* Hence the importance of separating the wet and dry benches.

(5) *Folding or compression of film.* Boxes of X-ray film should always be stored on end and nothing heavy should be allowed to rest on these boxes.

(6) *Deterioration with keeping.* Most X-ray films can be kept for a year or longer under good conditions of storage. If, however, a box of film is allowed to become damp, is exposed to any fumes, or is left at the back of a shelf and kept indefinitely, it will deteriorate. For this reason all boxes of film should be dated (in the spaced provided) on receipt and used in turn; and they should be stored in a clean, dry situation well away from X-ray apparatus.

(7) *Scratching during processing.* The softened emulsion of the wet film is particularly liable to be scratched and care must be taken to avoid this during processing.

**Intensifying screens**

These closely resemble two sheets of white cardboard and are in fact coated with fine crystals (usually calcium tungstate). These crystals intensify the effect of the X-ray beam on the film because they **fluoresce when exposed to X-rays**. Radiographic film is particularly sensitive to fluorescent light and thus is affected partly by the X-ray beam but mostly by the light produced in the screens. Because of this intensification, a smaller quantity of X-rays are required to produce the necessary changes in the film.

The degree of intensification can be increased by the use of *rare earth intensifying screens*. These incorporate rare earth phosphors and can, in some circumstances, permit the reduction of exposure factors by 15 to 50% of the amount required for calcium tungstate screens. They are, however, expensive and function most effectively only when they can be used in conjunction with the higher range of kilovoltage exposures (this is not always possible with low output apparatus). While some of these screens can be used with ordinary X-ray film others can only be employed if special film and different dark room illumination is available. If rare earth screens are used X-ray film should not be left in close contact with the screens for long periods (as may occur if cassettes are normally kept loaded with film) as they can emit small amounts of light which will result in the appearance of black spots on the radiograph after processing.

Intensifying screens are always used in pairs and are usually kept in film cassettes in such a way that when the film is inserted and the cassette closed, the film is tightly sandwiched between the two screens.

When inserting new screens into a cassette always follow the manufacturer's instructions with regard to fixation, and see that the front and back screens are correctly placed.

Any dirt or marks which occur on the screens will interfere with the fluorescent effect and result in similar flaws being seen on the radiograph. Precautions which can be taken to avoid the development of such screen marks include:

(1) Always keep film cassettes tightly closed, except when loading or unloading.

(2) Never touch the screens with the fingers.

(3) Do not write (for identification purposes) on films which are still in the cassettes.

(By dark room illumination it is only too easy to write on the screen instead of the film.)

(4) Brush out dust and hairs with a fine brush. If necessary the surface of the screens can be gently washed, using damped balls of cotton wool and good quality soap. Use very little water to rinse the soap away, and see that the open cassette is allowed to dry thoroughly in a dust-free place before using again.

**Film cassettes**

These are light-proof metal containers (Fig. 9.2) designed to protect the film and the intensifying screens. Except when inserting or removing film, these cassettes must always be kept closed to exclude light and dirt. Furthermore, since they come into frequent contact with animals and any mark on the cassette may be reproduced on the film, they must be kept scrupulously clean.

**Grids**

It is the fact that X-rays travel in straight lines that enables a beam of X-rays to produce an accurate "shadow" or X-ray image of the part of the patient penetrated on the film. Unfortunately, when higher kilovoltages are used to penetrate thicker areas of tissue, some of the X-rays undergo a complex change within the tissues and emerge as **scattered** or **secondary radiation** (Fig. 9.3). These secondary rays no longer follow the direction of the primary beam and travel in all directions causing a safety risk (p. 568) and resulting in blurring of the X-ray image.

Blurring of the radiograph is only likely to become a significant problem when attempting to investigate portions of the patient which are approximately 10 cm (4 in.) or more in thickness. In these circumstances a **stationary grid** is placed under the patient and on top of the film in order to filter out the secondary radiation before it can have an effect on the radiograph.

A grid is a flat plate made up of thin longitudinal strips of lead which are separated by material (usually plastic) which is easily penetrated by X-rays. The strips of lead may be placed parallel to each other (Fig. 9.4b: *parallel grid*) or angled in such a way as to correspond with the divergence of the X-rays in the primary beam (Fig. 9.4a: *focused or radiused grid*).

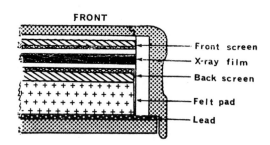

FRONT

— Front screen
— X-ray film
— Back screen
— Felt pad
— Lead

FIG. 9.2.    Cross-section of a cassette.

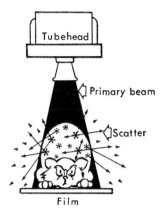

Fig. 9.3. The primary beam and "scatter".

Figure 9.4 shows how the strips of lead obstruct the useless secondary radiation but permit the passage of the primary beam. It can also be appreciated that, because the X-rays of the primary beam travel at an increasing angle towards the edge of the beam, some of these will be absorbed by the lead strips of a parallel grid, and the edge of the film will be underexposed. Similarly, Fig. 9.4a illustrates the fact that a focused grid is more efficient provided that it is placed centrally and the right way up (from Fig. 9.4 the student should attempt to deduce the effect on the film if a focused grid is placed upside down or towards the edge of the beam). It will be found that focused grids are marked in such a way as to indicate which is the upper or tube side.

The use of a grid is important and almost essential when attempting to show fine detail in thicker areas of tissue (e.g. when obtaining radiographs of the pelvis of the larger dogs for submission under the hip dysplasia scheme) but it also suffers from certain disadvantages:

(a) *A grid is expensive* and, although reasonably robust, the delicate alignment of the lead strips can be damaged if the grid is handled roughly or dropped, and care must be taken to prevent this.

(b) *A focused grid must be positioned accurately* in the centre of the primary beam or it will spoil rather than enhance detail in the radiograph.

(c) *It is necessary to increase exposure* because of the lead strips it contains; any grid will absorb some of the primary beam as it passes through it. Thus when a grid is used in radiography the film will be thin and underexposed unless the mAs is multiplied by an amount known as the **grid factor** (this is usually a factor of $2\frac{1}{2}$ or 3).

(d) *The use of a grid results in a series of fine lines* appearing on the radiograph. While this is not a serious defect it can be prevented by the use of a **moving grid** (sometimes known as a Potter-Bucky diaphragm). This is a mechanical device (usually fixed under the X-ray table) which causes a grid to be moved across the film during the exposure, and thus prevents the formation of grid lines on the film. Moving grids are seldom used in veterinary practice.

The greatest and most significant amount of scattered radiation is produced

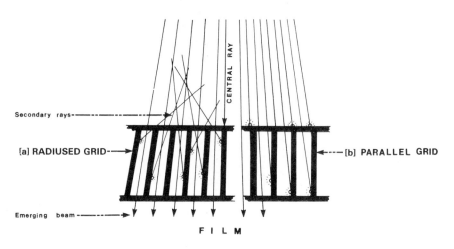

FIG. 9.4.   (a) A radiused grid compared with (b) a parallel grid.

within the tissue of the patient when it is penetrated by the primary beam, and the effects of this on the radiograph can be reduced by using a grid. However, scattered radiation can also be produced if the primary beam penetrates the film and reaches the X-ray table. In most cases any effect on the film is prevented by the fact that the back of the film cassette incorporates a thin layer of lead. When non-screen films are used a piece of lead or lead rubber should be placed between the film and the table.

**Film markers**

It is necessary to accurately identify each film in order to prevent the accidental muddling of two or more patients examined within a short time of each other, and also to permit certain reference, at a later date, to radiographs which may have been taken months or years previously. It is also helpful to be able to include other information on the radiograph (e.g. the right or left side of the animal, the time after administration of barium at which a film was taken, etc.).

The method of identification will vary from practice to practice, but a common practice is to write the necessary information in the top right-hand corner of the film. One suitable system is illustrated (Fig. 9.5), in which the top line represents the serial number of the radiograph, the second line gives the patient's and owner's name, and the third line indicates the date on which the radiograph was taken.

Part, or all, of the information required may be written on the X-ray film in pencil immediately before processing, in order to avoid muddling of films when washing. Ordinary pencil, however, is not suitable for permanent recording, and this identification should be rewritten, when the film is dry and ready for filming, with white (on a dark portion of the radiograph) or black felt pen or ink (on a pale area).

The best permanent method of identifying radiographs is either to place lead letters or suitably inscribed lead tape of the cassette at the time of making the exposure or to use a light contact marker in the dark room immediately prior to processing. It is essential to use one of these methods of identification if the films

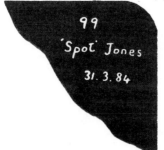

FIG. 9.5. Identification of a corner of a radiograph.

are to be submitted for scrutiny in connection with the hip dysplasia scheme.

## Processing the Film

Processing of the exposed X-ray film is necessary before the image which has been produced on the film by the X-ray beam becomes visible and can be viewed in detail.

The production of a good radiograph requires considerable skill and experience on the part of the radiographer; but it also requires care and attention in processing. Carelessness in this procedure can waste the radiographer's efforts and render the finished radiograph useless.

Since an X-ray film is even more sensitive to light than to X-rays, it can only be handled and processed in a room from which all white light can be excluded —usually known as the dark room. The requirements and equipment of this room must be considered before the details of processing can be discussed.

## The dark room and its equipment

The type of dark room met in veterinary practices will vary very greatly, depending on the space available and the amount of use which is likely to be made of it. Some will be little more than cupboards; others are definite rooms. In all instances they must comprise a working space which can be effectively blacked out, and they are usually fitted with electrical and water supplies.

It is advisable to arrange the equipment of the dark room into two distinct sections:

(1) *The dry bench.* Here the films are stored, handled dry and loaded into and out of the cassettes.
(2) *The wet bench.* This is where the processing solutions are kept and used.

It is important to keep these two sections well apart, otherwise splashes from the processing solutions will reach the dry films and the intensifying screens and produce permanent stains. Ideally the dry and wet benches should be situated on opposite sides of the dark room, but if it is necessary to arrange them side by side, then some form of partition should be erected between them (Fig. 9.6).

The equipment of the dark room will comprise:

*Safelight.* X-ray films can only be handled safely in a dim green or orange light. This illumination of the dark room is provided by a **safelight** which consists of a metal box holding a low-powered electric light bulb and fitted with a specified filter (e.g. Kodak Wratten 6B). These lights are classed as either **direct**, when they are placed immediately over a work point, or **indirect**, when they are hung

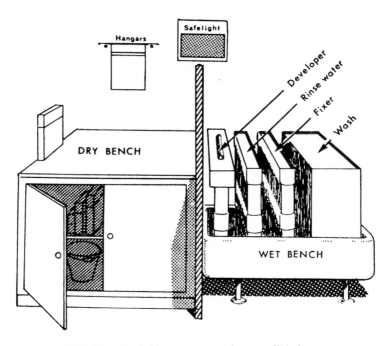

FIG. 9.6.   A suitable arrangement for a small dark room.

from the ceiling with the light directed upwards so that it is reflected off the white ceiling. In large rooms more than one safelight may be required.

It must be realized, however, that these lights are only comparatively safe and that X-ray films can be affected if exposed too closely or for too long a period to such illumination.

*Processing frames.* These are employed to hold the film while it is being passed through the tanks of solutions used in processing. There are two patterns, each with a different method of holding the film.

The channel type is easier to load but more difficult to keep clean (Fig. 9.7). The clip type holds the film more securely provided that one can avoid tearing the film during its insertion (Fig. 9.8).

The above equipment (together with a pencil for identifying films) comprises the equipment of the dry bench.

The wet bench is likely to include the following:

*Processing equipment.* Essentially, this will comprise four containers for (1) the developing solution, (2) water—for rinsing the film, (3) the fixing solution, (4) water—for washing the film.

Occasionally (2) and (4) are combined and only one container used, but this is not very satisfactory. If running water is not available in the dark room, the fourth container may only comprise a means of rinsing the film, and thorough washing will have to be carried out elsewhere.

The containers will either consist of a series of deep tanks into which the film is inserted vertically or else of a number of flat dishes in which the film is placed horizontally.

*Processing tanks.* These are more suitable for a busy unit. The tanks may be housed in a specially constructed processing unit or merely stood in a sink.

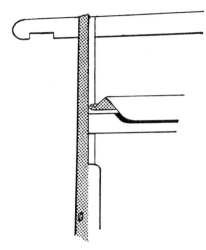

FIG. 9.7.   Channel-type processing frame.

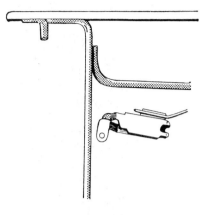

FIG. 9.8.   Clip-type processing frame.

The tank intended to contain developer is fitted with a light-proof lid and also with some means of warming the solution which it contains (Fig. 9.9). The heating may be carried out by means of an immersion heater within the tank or, more frequently, by standing the tank in a larger tank of heated water (usually thermostatically controlled at 20°C (68°F)). The other processing tanks are sometimes also contained in the heated water bath, but this is not essential.

*Processing dishes.* These are flat dishes, similar to those used for photographic processing, but of a suitable size to take the X-ray films being used.

Heating of the developer is carried out by either heating the solution before it is placed in the dish or else by placing the dish on a flat low power electric heating plate.

*Processing solutions.* These consist of the developing solution or developer and the fixing solution or fixer. The exact composition of these solutions is not of importance since they are normally obtained in a prepared form.

*The developer.* This is used to develop or make visible the image produced on the film by the X-ray beam. However, the best results will only be obtained if the film is developed (immersed in the developer) for a certain time at a certain temperature (usually 3 to 5 minutes at 20°C (68°F)). The precise time and temperature will be stipulated by the manufacturers of the developer. This information is usually supplied with the developer and also some indication of how the time of development may be varied to compensate for changes in the temperature of the solution.

Developer may be purchased either in the form of a powder or as a concentrated solution, both of which are made up to a specified volume (9 or 22 l) with water according to the capacity of the developer tanks. The liquid form can be poured directly into the tank and diluted, but the powder form should be well mixed with water in a bucket before adding to the tank.

When the developer is to be used for dish development, it is best stored in concentrated form in a dark, stoppered bottle. When required it is diluted with warm water to produce a solution of an appropriate concentration and temperature. If used in dishes the developer is

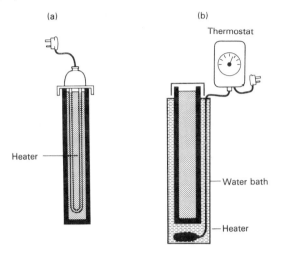

FIG. 9.9. Two ways of heating the developer solution.

particularly liable to oxygenation and should be discarded after use.

When developer is used in a tank the level of the solution will steadily drop as some of the developer is carried away with each film processed. The level of the solution should be maintained by adding a special **replenisher solution** prepared by the manufacturers of the developer solution. The usual practice is to make up a tank full of developer and at the same time to prepare a similar volume of replenisher. The replenisher is stored in dark, stoppered bottles and used as necessary to maintain the level of the developer. When the replenisher has been completely used, the developer is considered to be exhausted and is discarded and fresh solutions are made up. Even if the replenisher is not fully used the developer should be discarded after 3 months, as old developer produces stained, underdeveloped films.

Occasionally assistants have developed a dermatitis of the hands as a result of handling processing solutions. This is usually considered to be a form of allergic reaction to some of the chemical constituents of the developer (particularly the substance known as metol). While this is not a common occurrence, it emphasizes the need for strict cleanliness in handling all processing solutions.

Should any skin irritation be experienced, the use of gloves when handling the solutions may be of assistance. However, if the gloves are allowed to remain soiled with the chemicals, or if they contain holes, they may in fact aggravate the trouble by causing the solutions to make a more prolonged contact with the skin. Some developer solutions do not contain metol, and the substitution of these may also have to be considered.

If any marked skin trouble occurs, medical advice should always be obtained and the doctor informed that the person concerned is handling film processing chemicals.

*The fixer.* Film which has been passed through the developer is still sensitive to light and if exposed to white light would blacken rapidly, completely obliterating the image. This is prevented by immersing the film, after rinsing, in the fixer, which prevents any further action by light rays on the sensitive film and also hardens the film. After the film has been immersed in the fixer for some 30 seconds, it can be examined very briefly in white light, when it will be found that the film shows a whitish opaque appearance. This opacity will clear on further immersion of the film in the fixer. The time taken to achieve this is known as the **clearing time**, and until this has taken place the film should not be exposed to bright light for any length of time. For complete fixation and hardening of the film it should be kept in the fixer for a period at least equal to twice the clearing time.

Fixer is available both in a liquid and a powder form—to be made up to a certain volume according to the manufacturer's instructions. The temperature at which the fixer is used need not be quite so precise as is required for development, but should be kept within the range from 15.5° to 24°C (60°–75°F). The time required for clearing of the film will become progressively longer with use and when the time becomes more than double the original clearing time, the fixer should be discarded and a fresh solution prepared.

Further requirements for the wet bench are:

A *thermometer*—to check the temperature of the developer.

A *darkroom clock*—to control the time of development of the film. Any clock or watch which is readable by safelight can be used for this purpose, but clocks specially made for use in dark rooms and which can be set to ring a bell after the appropriate interval have an obvious advantage.

*Film clips*—by which the films may be hung up to dry, either over a sink or within a heated drying cupboard.

### General care of the dark room

A major requirement in the care of any dark room is to ensure that scrupulous cleanliness is observed, particularly in handling the processing solutions.

If the chemical solutions are splashed on to the surrounding walls and allowed to dry, they will produce dust which may settle on films or on screens and cause screen marks. Furthermore, the chemicals may have a corrosive action on unprotected walls and produce further dust.

Therefore the solutions should be prepared and mixed outside the dark room in clean containers made of glass, plastic or unchipped enamel. Separate stirring rods should be employed for mixing the developer and the fixer, and containers and stirring rods should be thoroughly cleansed after use.

Splashes from the processing solutions can cause permanent stains on clothing, and plastic aprons should be worn whenever these are handled.

Clean paper for wiping the hands should be kept near the wet bench and used each time the hands are wet.

Film hangers and dishes soon become stained by chemical oxidation products and must be kept clean (when necessary, persistent stains may be removed by the use of 5% acetic acid).

### Dark-room technique

Efficient processing of X-ray films requires the adoption of a definite routine at all stages of this procedure. This routine may be subdivided and summarized as follows:

(1) *Keep down dust by* mopping the floor and dusting the walls with a damp cloth. Let in fresh air and sunshine whenever possible.

(2) *Note the temperature of the developer* and adjust the heater if necessary.

(3) *Check the levels of the developing and fixing solutions.* Top up the

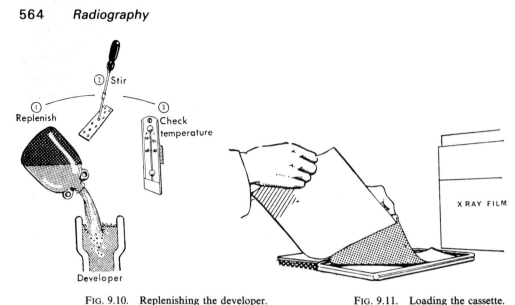

FIG. 9.10.   Replenishing the developer.                FIG. 9.11.   Loading the cassette.

developer with the replenisher as required and see that this is well stirred in (Fig. 9.10). The level of the fixer seldom drops to any significant extent as it tends to be maintained by water carried over from the rinse. However, any marked fall might prevent complete fixation of an edge of the film, and if necessary the level can be maintained by adding further fixer.

(4)  *See that film hangers previously used are clean and dry and ready for use.*

The following procedures must, of course, only be carried out by safelight illumination.

### Loading the film cassette

(1)  *Open the cassette.*
(2)  *Remove a film from the box of X-ray film,* taking care only to handle the film through the paper folder which surrounds (Fig. 9.11).
(3)  *Pull back the upper piece of protective paper that covers the films* then turn it through 180° so that it may be dropped into the well of the cassette with the minimum of handling. Discard the folder.

(4)  *Gently run a finger round the edge of the film* to check that it is correctly placed and will not be bent when the cassette is closed.
(5)  *Close the cassette and the box of film* before *switching on the light.*

### Unloading the exposed film

(1)  *Open the cassette* and gently shake out the film from the front of the cassette until it can be picked up at a corner, using the finger and thumb (Fig. 9.12).
(2)  *Insert the film into a hanger with the minimum of handling.* With the channel type of hanger the film is slid into the channels and the top hinge closed (Fig. 9.13). When using the clip-type hanger, fasten the lower clips first then press down the springs of the upper clips

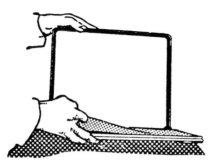

FIG. 9.12.   Unloading the cassette.

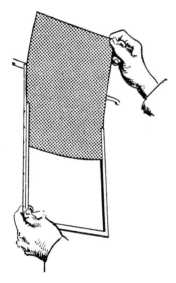

FIG. 9.13. Loading a channel-type processing frame.

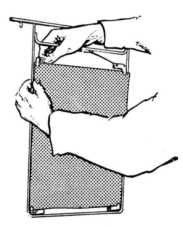

FIG. 9.14.   Loading a clip-type processing frame.

until these can be made to grasp the film and hold it taut (Fig. 9.14).

(3) *Identify the film by writing in pencil* on the top right-hand corner (p. 558).

(4) *Commence processing the film.*

(5) *Reload and close the cassette.*

**Processing the film (tank development)** (Fig. 9.15)

(1) *Insert the film, supported in the*

*hanger, gently into the developer* and raise it vertically two or three times to remove air bubbles from the surface of the film. Immediately **note the time** or set the darkroom clock for the appropriate period.

(2) *Replace the lid on the developing tank* and, making sure that one's hands are clean and dry, reload the film cassette. At the end of the correct period, remove the film

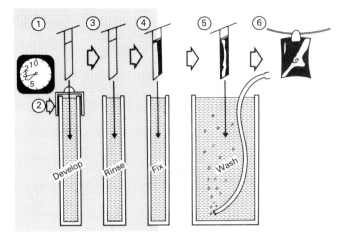

FIG. 9.15.   Processing routine.

slowly from the developer, allowing excess fluid to drain back.

(3) *Place the film in the rinse tank and rinse for some 10 seconds.*

(4) *Transfer the film to the fixing tank.* After it has been in this for about 30 seconds the white light may be switched on, and once the film has cleared it may be examined fully in a bright light. In order that fixing may be complete the film should be left in this solution for at least 10 minutes.

(5) *Wash the film in running water for some 30 minutes* (if running water is not available in the dark room, the film can be transferred to a suitable sink elsewhere).

(6) *Remove the film from the processing frame, attach a film clip and hang it up to dry in a dust free, and preferably warm, situation.*

*Note*: If the film is not left in the developer for the full time, or if the solution is allowed to become exhausted or used at too low temperature, the film will be **underdeveloped—it will appear pale and grey**. If the developer is too hot or the film is left in it for too long it will be **overdeveloped—becoming dark** and losing detail. While comparatively slight under-

development will lower the quality of the radiograph, considerable overdevelopment must take place before its effect can be seen.

## Automatic Processing

Where large numbers of radiographs have to be developed daily (in veterinary institutions and some large practices) automatic processors may be installed. All that is necessary is to insert the exposed film into the apparatus and, after a very short period (usually 90 seconds), it emerges fully developed and dry. Such automation permits the consistent production of very satisfactory radiographs but, because processing takes place at a much higher temperature than that required for hand processing, the radiographs will lack a little of the contrast and "sparkle" that, under ideal conditions, can be produced manually. In addition, such apparatus uses considerable quantities of processing solutions and requires regular cleaning, maintenance and servicing.

## Filing

In a busy practice a large number of radiographs can accumulate in the course of a year, and unless some system of filing is organized, it will not be possible to quickly locate a particular radiograph, particularly if it was taken a year or so previously.

Storage of radiographs can involve the purchase of special X-ray film envelopes and a suitable filing cabinet. However, a satisfactory method, involving no additional expense, is to replace the dry radiograph in the paper folder which protected the unexposed film, and then to store the radiographs in empty film boxes as they become available. If this system is adopted, the identification details which have been inscribed on the radiograph should be repeated on the paper folders and the radiographs placed in the boxes in chronological order. The boxes should be labelled with the date range of the radiographs which they contain. Then, provided that the date of radiography can be obtained from the patient's case history, it should be a simple matter to locate the relevant radiograph, and the owner's and patient's names will confirm the correct identification.

Before filing any radiograph it is essential to see that it is absolutely dry, otherwise it will stick to any folder or film envelope and may be ruined when any attempt is made to remove it for examination.

## Qualities of Radiographs

If a radiographic examination of an animal is to provide the maximum information concerning the patient, it is essential that the film will be of high quality. This will depend on the use of correct technique both in the X-ray room and in the dark room, and the diagnostic value of a radiograph can easily be impaired by mistakes made in either area. Therefore **each** film should be examined critically

for evidence that it is of satisfactory technical standard before submitting to the veterinary surgeon for interpretation. In assessing this standard the following characteristics of the film should be noted and checked.

*Density.* This refers to **the blackness** of the radiograph and is controlled by the quantity of X-rays reaching the film. If the radiograph is too dark the amount of radiation (usually the mAs) should be reduced and, if it is too low, increased. However, if in doubt as to the exact amount of blackening required, it is better to slightly over-expose the film (when detail can usually be shown by viewing the radiograph against brighter illumination).

*Contrast.* This is the difference between **the tones of the various parts of the film**—the dark areas should be as black as possible and the light areas as pale as practicable. Films which lack contrast will appear grey and "lifeless". This can be due to the use of too high kilovoltage exposure factors, or, more frequently, to insufficient development (this is usually associated with stale or cold developing solutions or with too short a development time).

*Definition.* Good definition is shown by the recognition of **distinct fine detail** in a radiograph. Significant loss of definition may be caused by:

(a) *Movement of the patient* (this may be either voluntary or involuntary).
(b) *Fog.* This is an additional density in the radiograph which is not associated with the X-ray image usually results from accidental exposure of the film to radiation or to light.
(c) *Scattered radiation.* The result of radiographing thick areas of tissue without using a grid.

*Extraneous marks on the film.* Small

localized marks on films may result from a number of causes. Those most frequently encountered include:

(a) *Dirt or stains on the intensifying screens.* These prevent the light from the screens affecting the film and produce a corresponding **white defect**, which will be noted every time the same screen is employed.

(b) *Contamination by processing chemicals.* Splashing of the film before processing with developer or fixer solutions will cause black or white **splash marks** respectively. Similar streaky stains around the edge of the radiograph can result from stale chemicals (usually fixer) on dirty film hangers. **Finger prints** can result from similar chemical contamination, or by depositing grease and thus preventing processing chemicals reaching the film.

(c) *Crimp marks* (blacks or white **cresentic shadows**) are caused by crinkling the film by holding it too roughly between the index finger and thumb instead of the forefinger and thumb.

### The Dangers Associated with Radiography

Repeated exposure of the human or animal body to X-rays can lead to injury to the body tissue. This danger is often not realized because (1) the X-ray beam is invisible, (2) the damage to the tissues may not become obvious until a considerable time after the person was exposed to X-rays.

The main effects of X-ray injury are (1) damage to the skin, (2) destruction of certain blood cells, (3) injury to the sex organs, (4) the production of malignant growths.

Injuries of this nature will occur only if the person concerned receives repeated exposure to X-rays, and, **provided that the precautions which are advised are observed**, there is no significant risk.

This aspect of radiography is stressed since the nursing staff may be asked to help in restraining patients for X-ray examination, and it is essential that they should understand how exposure to X-rays can occur, and also the routine precautions to take to avoid this danger.

### The source of exposure

X-ray apparatus will only emit X-rays at the time of making the exposure (i.e. when the radiographer presses the exposure button). Furthermore, since the X-ray tube is surrounded with lead, the X-rays can only emerge from the tube through the aperture provided. The X-rays will emerge as a beam (known as the primary beam), and, although invisible, the size of this beam can be estimated by noting the size and angle of the lead cone which is attached to the X-ray tube or from information supplied with the set. (With some of the larger sets the extent of the primary beam is made visible by incorporating a similar sized beam of light in the apparatus.) Assistants should never place their hands, or any other portion of their body, even if covered with protective clothing, within the primary beam while an exposure is being made.

Unfortunately, avoidance of the primary beam is not sufficient to avoid all exposure to X-rays. This is because of the phenomenon known as scatter (Fig. 8.3), whereby a small proportion of the X-rays that make up the primary beam reach the patient of the table and are then deflected in all directions and may reach those holding the animal.

The amount of X-rays received in this

way is comparatively small and will become progressively less the further the assistant is from the primary beam. Adequate protection will be obtained if assistants stand as far away from the patient as possible and **always wear protective clothing** (lead-lined aprons and gloves).

It is usual to ask the owners of animals to hold them during radiography, so as to restrict the use of assistants for this purpose. But, since the tissues of the young are particularly susceptible to X-rays, no child under 16 or any expectant mother should be exposed to X-rays. Assistant can often help by recognizing those who come within these categories and tactfully removing them from the room before radiography is undertaken.

## Routine precautions

It is the responsibility of the radiographer to ensure that his assistants are protected from all significant irradiation during their work, and he will issue detailed instructions with regard to the particular circumstances under which he and his assistants are working. However, the following precautions apply to all situations and should be observed on all occasions when X-ray exposures are being made.

(1) *Always wear the protective clothing provided,* even though it is heavy and uncomfortable (this will provide protection against scatter).

(2) *Stand as far away from the X-ray beam as is practicable.* (Two people should always be available if it is necessary to restrain the patient since each will then be able to stand at arm's length from the animal; Fig. 9.16).

(3) *See that the task of holding animals is shared by as many persons as possible.*

(4) *Check that protective clothing is stored or hung flat* (the lead lining is easily cracked by frequent folding).

TABLE 9.1. *Maximum permissible doses (MPDs) for occupationally exposed persons*

|  | Old milli-rads | New rems |
|---|---|---|
| MPD to whole body per year | 5,000 | 5 |
| MPD to hands, forearms, feet and ankles, per year | 75,000 | 75 |
| MPD to whole body per calendar quarter | 3,000 | 3 |
| MPD to abdomen of women of reproductive capacity, per calendar quarter. | 1,300 | 1.3 |
| Minimum detectable dose on film badge | 20 | 0.02 |
| Typical natural background dose per year | 80 | 0.08 |

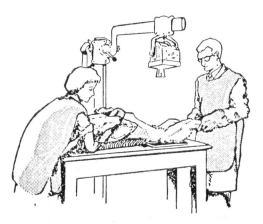

FIG. 9.16. Restraining a patient for radiography.

(5) *Monitoring badges* (small films which, when processed at a special laboratory indicate the amount of irradiation received by the wearer) should be provided. These are pinned to one's clothing, and should be worn whenever radiography is undertaken. (See Table 9.1.)

### The Code of Practice

A document entitled *Radiation Safety in Veterinary Practice* was issued in 1970 by the Ministry of Agriculture, Fisheries and Food and has provided official guidance as to how radiography may be employed safely for veterinary purposes. These instructions will soon be replaced by *Guidance Notes for the Protection of Persons against Ionising Radiations Arising from Veterinary Use,* which is to be published jointly by the Health and Safety Executive and the National Radiological Protection Board.

It is the responsibility of the principal of the practice to ensure that the recommendations contained in these documents are carried out and he will probably issue "local rules" designating those members of staff who may routinely take part in radiography and detailing the precautions they are to observe when doing so. A RANA who has been authorized to take part in radiography should bear in mind that it is her duty to protect herself and others from the hazards associated with this procedure. She should therefore closely observe the rules which have been laid down and, if in doubt, ask for further instructions before taking any risk of exposing herself or others to X-rays.

### Positioning

It is important that the patient should always be positioned in such a way as to facilitate accurate and complete visualization of the part which one wishes to investigate. Suitable positions in which the patient should be placed to permit examination of particular parts of the body are described in detail in standard texts (see **Further Reading**).

It will be necessary for the RANA to be familiar with most of these positions; she will find it easier to appreciate their importance and significance if she fully understands the following basic principles of positioning:

(a) *The structure or part to be demonstrated should always be placed as near to the film* and as far from the X-ray tube as is practicable. Where this is not possible (e.g. when X-raying a bone which is surrounded by a large amount of soft tissue) some magnification of the part is inevitable.

(b) *Similarly, the part must be positioned in the path of the central rays of the X-rays beam* and parallel with the film, or magnification and distortion will occur.

(c) *A radiograph can only give a flat or two-dimensional reproduction of a structure or lesion* (which will have depth as well as height and breadth), therefore it is usually necessary to **make two radiographic exposures**, directed at right angles to each other, in order to fully demonstrate the part.

(d) As animals are unco-operative patients, *some restraint will be necessary* in order to achieve the required positioning. Whether this is undertaken by **general anaesthesia**, by sedation or by manual restraint (or by a combination of methods) must be decided by the veterinary surgeon responsible in the light of his knowledge of all the circumstances, but two considerations will be paramount—the avoidance of pain or suffering for the patient and the safety of all those taking part in the examination.

## Further Reading

B.S.A.V.A. *Guide to Diagnostic Radiography in Small Animal Practice,* Published by the British Small Animal Veterinary Association (1981).

*Code of Practice for the Protection of Persons Exposed to Ionising Radiation from Veterinary Uses,* HMSO, (1970).

Douglas, S.W. and Williamson, H.D. (1980) *Principles of Veterinary Radiography,* 3rd edn., Baillière Tindall, London.

*Draft Guidance Notes for the Protection of Persons against Ionising Radiations arising from Veterinary Use,* HMSO (1983).

*Mosley's Fundamentals of Animal Health Technology. Small Animal Radiography.* The C.V. Mosby Company. St Louis, Toronto, London, 1983.

Ryan, Gerald D. *Radiographic Positioning of Small Animals,* Bailliere Tindall, London.

# CHAPTER 10

# Surgical Nursing

(a) General Surgical Nursing

D. G. EARNSHAW

### Local Inflammation and Wounds

Whenever the body is injured either by violence (trauma), by microrganisms, chemical agents (corrosive burns) or heat (thermal) a defensive response is generally evoked by which the body attempts to curtail the extent of the injury and to initiate reparative measures. This interaction of causal factors and body responses is termed inflammation.

The essential changes occurring in the inflamed region are, firstly, an increase in the number of functioning blood and lymph vessels and dilatation of these vessels. Their walls become more permeable to fluid and cells. Later, cellular changes, such as fibrosis, predominate. The former are defensive measures, the latter reparative.

When the reaction occurs over a short period and is of some severity, the lesion is referred to as **acute inflammation**, whereas if the causal agent is applied over some time and provokes a prolonged but less intense reaction, the inflammation is chronic. These terms are not very precise. An intermediate type of lesion is referred to as subacute. We also use the terms mild, moderate, marked and severe to indicate the intensity of the inflammatory reaction.

The picture of inflammation at the cellular level can be followed in more detail if we consider the case where the skin is broken, the subcutaneous tissues slightly damaged and a number of pyogenic (pus-forming) bacteria enter the gap created. This is what we find in a small infected wound.

Blood vessels, at least of capillary size, may be damaged and there may be a little bleeding. The body defence mechanisms come into play, and at first there is a transient constriction of vessels in the area. Very shortly afterwards the vessels dilate and become more permeable to the passage of fluid and cells. The inflammatory zone becomes inundated by tissue fluid derived from the blood. Cells of various types, particularly polymorphs, invade the area and come into contact with bacteria; later other cells, including histiocytes, play some part in phagocytosis (engulfing bacteria). Pus may be formed from dead and disintegrating bacteria, polymorphs and other cells. In the later phases the outer part of the inflammatory zone is invaded by fibroblasts which produce fibrin and tend to wall off the region.

If early recovery occurs and the bacteria are killed with little or no frank sepsis (pus, suppuration) the products of cellular disintegration, increased tissue fluids, etc., are removed by the increased circulation. In such cases the fibrotic reaction is small and directed to repairing the tissue and everything heals up. Healing is known as resolution.

In the case of chronic inflammation there is a marked increase in the fibrotic reaction, and less evidence of cellular activity.

Inflammation is manifested clinically by "cardinal signs" which may be correlated with the microscopic picture, viz.:

1. *Pain*—due to pressure on nerve ends by the increase in tension of the area produced by infiltration of serum, dilation of vessels, etc., and possibly also by the action of chemical breakdown substances on the sensitive nerve endings.

2. *Heat*—due to increase metabolism in the area and increased blood flow.

3. *Swelling*—due to increase in volume of fluids and cells as indicated in (1) and (4).

4. *Redness*—due to increase in blood in the area. Only seen clearly in animals with non-pigmented skins and where the hairy coat in the area is thin or absent, e.g. ears, under chin, axillae, belly or inguinal region.

5. *Loss of function*—commonly due to increased pain of moving the injured part; muscle spasm in the area may also occur. Injury to important structure (such as nerve and bones) in limbs will produce marked loss of function.

### The results of inflammation

1. *Resolution.* The body defences rapidly overcome the inflammatory cause or causes and the tissues heal and become virtually normal within a short time. Generally, there is little or no pus formation, e.g. aseptic surgical wounds.

2. *Suppuration* (pus formation). Commonly this phase of inflammation ensues where the body defences have not been able to dispose of invading micro-organisms rapidly. Here there is massive cellular mobilization in the area especially polymorphs and other white blood cells. **Pus** is formed as previously indicated. Pus may also contain bacterial toxins, enzymes and products of chemical disintegration of body tissues such as cells. Pus may be mixed with serum, blood, mucus or other body fluids and is described accordingly. Abscesses are common septic lesions caused by bacteria and consist of a mass of pus surrounded by fibrous tissue wall. They may extend internally and involve other tissues or may "point" to the surface of the body, rupture and discharge their contents (pus).

3. *Necrosis* (rotting). This refers to the death of tissue on a larger scale and is seen by the naked eye. Necrotic tissue may come away (slough) from the healthier tissue with which it is continuous and this is one of the means by which healing can proceed. Liquefaction of such tissue does not occur to any extent except at the zone of separation from the healthy tissue.

4. *Gangrene*—refers to gross death of tissue. All the local tissues are affected and they die. The gangrenous region may become extensive unless drastic measures are taken. This phenomenon may ensue when an extremity is deprived of its blood supply, e.g. over-enthusiastic use of tourniquets or when certain bacteria (e.g. *Clostridia*) invade tissues. The latter case is not common in small animals but often ends fatally. The gross tissue destructions is often accompanied by general systemic disturbance due to toxins from the dead tissues and/or the invading bacteria.

5. *Ulceration.* Where the skin or surface of epithelium is broken—but the lesion is shallow and more or less confined to the surface. Ulcers show little or no tendency to heal. Frequently a discharge is shed from the surface of the ulcer.

6. *Granulation* (fibrosis). This is, in essence, chronic inflammation with marked connective tissue reaction. It occurs when the body defences cannot overwhelm the inflammation rapidly or when the inflammation is of low but continuous activity, e.g. continuous rubbing of the skin against a hard object. Pus may be present in pockets in the inflamed tissue. Cold or chronic abscesses are thick walls of granulation tissue enclosing watery sanguineous fluid.

**Healing**

Where inflammatory lesions show early resolution and rapid restoration to the normal we refer to it as healing by **first intention**. This is the way in which most surgical wounds heal. The tissues are closely opposed, the small amount of haemorrhage is rapidly organized and the tissues are rapidly knit together with a minimum of fibrous tissue. The surface wound dries, forms a thin, more or less flat linear scab, and is not painful or irritating.

In the case of large wounds with a gap between each side, or in infected wounds, the tissues are not readily brought together. There may be considerable seepage of tissue fluid or actual bleeding into the gap, and infection more readily gains a foothold. This is what happens with many accidental and neglected wounds.

After cessation of bleeding the zone of tissue adjacent to the gap of the wound becomes invaded by fibroblasts, and new capillaries and a process of organization occurs much the same as in primary healing but far more extensively and, of course, over a longer period. A sheet of smooth but uneven tissue, known as **granulation tissue**, is produced. If this is healthy it is pink and only very slightly moist; if infected, it may be dark in shade,

or grey coloured, and be overlain by a discharge.

Healthy granulation tissue, once formed, is somewhat resistant to infection. It becomes thicker until the wound gap is filled, and then, when the tissue level reaches that of the subcutaneous tissues on either side of the lips of the wound, the skin (epithelium) grows in to cover the surface. This type of healing is by **second intention** or by granulation.

Healing by second intention takes much longer and there is much more scar formation. This process may be complicated by producing too much healing tissue which is then known as proud flesh and it often protrudes beyond the wound margins and above the surface of the epithelium.

The healing of specialized tissues varies —some cells do not regenerate, e.g. nerve cells of the brain and elsewhere. Axon, or nerve-cell processes, can heal, but there may be some interference from the general healing process of fibrosis, and one frequently encounters fibrous tissue formation instead of the normal functional tissue which was originally present. In most wounds, this may not matter very much as the animal body is wonderfully adaptable, but sometimes there is a permanent interference with normal function, e.g. in the case of injured brain cells. Muscles can still function fairly adequately even if there is some fibrotic replacement. Other blood-vessel branches can compensate for loss and damage to the circulatory system. Nerve trunks may show some regeneration, especially if adequate surgical therapy is applied immediately after injury. Glands and glandular tissues frequently show good regeneration, and even where their functioning tissue has been replaced by fibrous tissue there is no apparent disability for a very long time. The body is normally endowed with much more of certain glandular tissues than are actually required, e.g. between 20% and 75% of the liver can be removed and a dog continues to remain healthy, and the liver tissue increases almost to the original bulk in about 2 months. A dog has to lose about 60% of its kidney mass before a serious clinical manifestation is apparent.

## (b) Shock

R. S. JONES

This is rather a complex subject to deal with in detail and in order to offer a comprehensible account it is necessary to over-simplify. It is defined as: a state of progressive circulatory failure in which the output of the heart is insufficient to meet tissue requirements for nutrition, oxygenation or waste disposal. Shock in animals is a condition which is not often recognized. It is **most frequently associated with loss of blood by haemorrhage** either to the exterior or within the body into a body cavity or organ where the blood is effectively removed from the circulation. Other causes of shock are burns and traumatic injury which lead to a loss of circulatory fluid. Antigen-antibody reactions, drug overdose or poisoning with sedative or anaesthetic drugs, are further causes of shock (p. 624). Loss of body fluids, particularly extracellular fluids (see section on fluid therapy p. 315) may produce a state of shock. A bacteraemia can be a very important precipitating factor in shock.

Whilst apprehension of pain and emotional trauma are important in initiating shock in humans and possibly wild animals, they are of little importance in the domestic animals.

Tissue hypoxia (darkening of visible mucosa).
Capillary stasis.
Haemoconcentration.
Reduced venous and arterial blood pressure.

Clinical examination may reveal some or all of the following signs:

(1) *Lack of response to stimuli, apathy and weakness.*
(2) *Weak, rapid and irregular pulse.*
(3) *Cold and shivering with a clammy skin.*
(4) *Paleness of the mucosa* and sometimes a blue tinge to the visible mucous membranes.
(5) *Rapid and shallow respirations.*
(6) *Sub-normal temperature.*
(7) *Thirst and vomiting.* This may produce gastric lavage and loss of electrolytes.
(8) *Dilated pupils and glazed cornea.*
(9) *Fall in venous and arterial blood pressure.*

Considerations of the case history and clinical signs should make the RANA aware of the possibility of shock occurring and report the findings to a veterinary surgeon.

### Signs of Shock

Reduced circulatory blood volume.
Increased pulse rate.

### Types of Shock

Shock may be classified as:

(1) *Impending* (threatened). Clinical signs may not be evident but from

the history of the case one might expect a state of shock to develop.

(2) *Established.* Established shock can be treated by the administration of intravenous fluid plus supportive therapy. Shock is considered to be *irreversible* when it does not respond to intravenous fluids and specific drug therapy has to be resorted to.

(3) *Irreversible* (see above).

### Treatment of Shock

1. *Restore the circulatory blood volume.* Compatible whole blood, warmed to body temperature, is the fluid of choice. If blood is not available, plasma or plasma substitute which is most often recommended is of the modified gelatin type ("Gelafusine" or "Haemaccel"). In an emergency dextran can be used.

2. *Oxygen* administered by a method which is not resented by the animal. A fine bore nasal catheter is probably the technique of choice. If the oxygen therapy is continued over a period of time longer than one hour, it should be humidified by bubbling it through warm water.

3. *Broad spectrum antibiotic therapy* should be instituted to either treat or prevent infection.

4. *Prevention of heat loss.* Do not make the animal warmer than its surroundings. Hot-water bottles and electric blankets may produce dilation of the skin vessels and allow the animal to lose heat and its blood pressure to fall.

5. *Alleviation of pain by analgesic drugs.*

6. *Posture.* The animal's head should be kept low by slightly raising the hindquarters, but the animal should be allowed to lie down and be kept comfortable. The head and neck should be kept in the natural position to ensure a clear airway (p. 641).

7. *When irreversible shock is considered to be present* then specific drug therapy is essential. Cardiac alpha-blockade with large doses of corticosteroids and phenoxybenzamine is recommended. Cardiac beta-stimulation with isoprenaline may also be considered. Medication should only be administered on the direct instructions of the veterinary surgeon.

**The prevention of shock is more likely to benefit the patient than the most enthusiastic treatment**. This can be achieved in a number of ways:

(a) Gentle handling of the animal and the judicious use of premedication with sedative and/or analgesic drugs.

(b) The use of safe and efficient anaesthetic techniques which will produce a rapid and quiet recovery.

(c) Rapid, gentle and efficient surgery will reduce the incidence of shock.

(d) The judicious use of fluid therapy before, during and after surgery is essential. The circulation should be restored to normality before surgery in such conditions as foreign bodies in the gastrointestinal tract and pyometra. Blood loss which occurs during surgery should be replaced both adequately and rapidly.

(e) Pre-operative administrative of glucose water is considered to be useful in the prevention of shock.

### Hyperthermia

The condition of hyperthermia occurs when there is an elevation of body temperature due to excessive heat production or to defective heat loss. Heat stroke is the most commonly encountered physical entity (p. 536–7). The major causes are a raised environmental temperature and/or prolonged muscular exertion especially in fat animals with a hairy coat and during conditions of high humidity. Particular problems occur in animals which are confined in closed cars in summer. Minor causes are brain damage to the hypothalamus and dehydration. The condition may occasionally occur, when the environmental temperature is high, during closed circuit anaesthesia in dogs.

Clinical signs, in addition to a raised temperature, are an increased thirst, a rise in pulse rate and an increase in respiratory rate and depth. When the critical body temperature (of 41–42°C) is exceeded, there is depression of the central nervous system's activity and the respiratory centre's depression causes death by respiratory failure. Treatment is first directed to removal of the cause. Cold applications including immersion in cold water or spraying are often effective. Drugs such as aspirin and chlorpromazine are also considered to be effective. A specific condition of malignant hyperthermia, associated with general anaesthesia, has been described in pigs and in humans. It may also occur in other species. The precipitation factors appear to be halothane and/or the muscle relaxant suxamethonium. The condition is fatal in a high percentage of patients.

## Hypothermia

The condition of hypothermia occurs when there is a fall in body temperature below the normal range for the species (p. 281). This fall may be due to shock, prolonged anaesthesia or inadequate energy intake. In the very young animal there is an inability of the temperature regulation mechanism of the body to function and the young are unable to raise their body temperatures by shivering.

Heat loss in the unconscious patient is best prevented by wrapping the body in blankets and all such animals should be kept in a hospital cage in a warm room. The use of infra-red lamps, heating pads and hot water bottles should be limited to those occasions when the veterinary surgeon in charge of the case thinks them essential. As a general rule, it is better to prevent further heat loss and administer intravenous fluids warmed to blood temperature rather than attempt to artificially warm up the patient. Glucose water may be given by mouth if the patient is able to swallow but other stimulants may be inadvisable. Coma and drowsiness as a result of inadequately treated Diabetes is associated with raised blood sugar and keto-acidosis; in the case where the RANA knows of a history of Diabetes, it is safer to give normal saline intravenously to the hypothermic animal than one of the glucose containing fluids.

## (c) Fractures and Dislocations

## L. C. VAUGHAN

### Fractures

A bone fractures as a result of it being subjected to a particular force or stress. The manner in which it breaks varies greatly and an extensive classification exists by which the different types are described. Many of these terms, however, are largely of academic interest because they merely identify precise details of a fracture. Of more importance are the broad categories into which fractures may be placed, and these should be understood because the management that is appropriate is often related to the basic features involved. The terms **simple**, **compound** and **comminuted** are among the most helpful means of indicating the main nature of the injury.

1. Simple: an uncomplicated break with one fracture line.

2. Compound: a break associated with an open wound leading to the fracture site.

3. Comminuted: involving a number of pieces.

In addition, the term *greenstick* is often used, indicating an incomplete fracture in which the bone bends and the convex side of the curve alone is broken; it is common in puppies and kittens.

When a fracture occurs because of some underlying weakness or disease of a bone it is referred to as a "pathological fracture".

The cause of the fracture should always be noted since it may well have an important bearing on the type of injury to be expected. Road traffic accidents figure prominently as a cause of longbone fractures in dogs and cats but it should always be remembered that other structures are often injured at the same time, ranging from simple abrasions to rupture of the diaphragm. The bone injuries are usually readily apparent but some of the soft tissue complications may pass unnoticed unless careful observations are made. On the other hand, when there has been a relatively trivial accident such as a fall from a chair a simple fracture of the forearm or of a humeral condyle would be suspected. Whatever the cause all cases require thorough observation to determine the full extent of the injury and its effects before any drugs are administered or any form of therapy is embarked upon.

In order that the basic requirements of fracture treatment may be properly appreciated it is essential to have a sound knowledge of anatomy and an understanding of the process of fracture healing.

### Fracture healing

The healing process is complex and comprises a progressive sequence of changes. Although a number of different stages may be recognized they are not clear cut and are subject to considerable overlap. At first there is haemorrhage at the fracture site caused by rupture of blood vessels in the periosteum, bone marrow and adjacent tissues. The

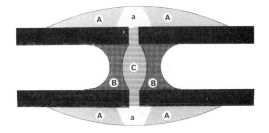

FIG. 10.1. The callus. A, anchoring callus; a, bridging callus; B, sealing callus; C, uniting callus. The solid black blocks are the bone cortices.

haemorrhage coagulates after 6–8 hours and a **haematoma forms** which envelopes the bone ends. Included in the haematoma are fragments of bone and connective tissue which degenerate and are removed by phagocytes.

The haematoma undergoes organization and is replaced by granulation tissue. Fibroblasts at this time produce numerous collagen fibres mostly parallel to the long axis of the bone, and in this way the **fibrous callus** is formed. The fibrous callus forms a spindle-shaped cuff around the fracture ends and in the next stages is replaced by a primary and then a secondary bony callus. Different parts of the callus can be recognized; **anchoring** and **sealing** describe that surrounding the fragments and closing the bone marrow respectively; **uniting** refers to the tissue between the bone ends; **bridging** that encircling the fracture (Fig. 10.1).

The ossification that occurs in the anchoring, sealing and uniting callus is by direct transformation of the fibrous tissue into cancellous bone by means of osteoblasts. The bridging callus is transformed into cartilage and then into bone. The uniting callus is the last to form. The bone first produced is immature (spongy) and this is in due course replaced by adult (lamellar) bone. In the final phase of the reparative process the bone is remodelled over a period of months by the resorption of excess callus until the original contour of the bone is re-established and the medullary cavity is re-canalized.

In an average shaft fracture in dogs after 3–4 weeks there is little movement between the bone ends, handling the leg is not resented and soft tissue swelling has subsided. Limb function may be about 50% of normal. The fracture components are at this time merely enveloped by primary bony callus and it is too early to discard limb supports or remove implants. Consolidation of the fracture may not be complete for 12–16 weeks. If the fracture is not adequately immobilized for a sufficient length of time it may not heal (non-union) or heal in a deformed position (mal-union).

The rate of healing may be affected by a number of factors. It is rapid in puppies in which a fractured radius/ulna may feel firm after 2 weeks. Conversely, in aged animals healing is slower. Fractures in cancellous bone (extremities of long bones) usually heal more rapidly than those in cortical bone (shaft). Union is quicker in oblique fractures because there is a large area to promote tissue growth. Infection interferes with healing but union will occur once it has been overcome.

**Fracture treatment**

The dual objectives of treatment are to return the damaged bone to its normal anatomy and to restore limb function. The means used to achieve these aims must enable the fracture to heal in a reasonable time and with the minimum of adverse effects on the well being of the patient. Fractures require individual consideration to decide which method of management is most likely to achieve the optimum result. Although many methods are available the same basic principles of repair apply, namely, to obtain accurate anatomical reduction of the fragments and to immobilize them until union occurs.

There are two categories into which all the methods of treatment fall:

(1) **closed reduction** (external fixation) which involves either the application of some form of external support or appliance to the limb after manual reduction of the fracture, or an entirely conservative approach of judicious inactivity; (2) **open reduction** (internal fixation) which involves surgical realignment of the bone ends using metallic implants such as nails, plates, screws and wire.

Before deciding which of these approaches to adopt a number of factors have to be considered. The specific bone damaged, the position and type of fracture, have an important bearing on the choice. The size, shape, age and temperament of the animal have to be taken into account, and thought also given to the environment of the patient and the ability of its owner to cope with the aftercare required. Experience has a part to play and a veterinary surgeon may be loth to change from a technique he finds satisfactory notwithstanding the claims of some other approved method.

*1. Closed Reduction*

(a) Conservative measures

It is well recognized that certain fractures heal satisfactorily without either external or internal fixation. Generally speaking this applies to bones in well-muscled regions where it is difficult, if not impossible, to provide external support that does not inconvenience the patient, and where methods of internal fixation are hazardous or are technically inadequate at present.

Pelvic fractures are probably the best example in this category. Although certain types are with advantage repaired surgically, there are some beyond operative repair and many of these heal surprisingly well given the necessary care and attention. For cats and small dogs the method of choice is confinement in a cage, basket or tea-chest, which allows them room to do little more than change position. Analgesic drugs are administered in the early stages. Soft, absorbent bedding is needed, but animals of this size are readily removed for emptying of bowels and bladder, and also to feed and drink, thus reducing soiling. It is more difficult to confine a large dog in this way unless it is in a cage of adequate size to allow manhandling or by keeping it at home in a small downstairs room or in a warm garden shed. For these the avoidance of bed sores is a major priority. The sheer physical stress to the nurse or owner in caring for heavy dogs with such injuries should not be ignored.

The time taken for recovery depends on the severity of the injury and on the weight of the animal. Cats and small dogs respond the quickest and may have improved hindlegs use after 3 weeks, but they should not be allowed freedom for at least 6 weeks. Heavy dogs regain leg use more slowly and may find difficulty in rising for 4–6 weeks.

Other fractures which often heal satisfactorily without immobilization are those of the vertical ramus of the mandible, prominences of the skull, vertebral processes and the body of the scapula. On occasions very severely comminuted fractures of the femur and humerus are best managed conservatively.

(b) External Support

Fractures below the elbow and stifle joints are the most effectively treated with casts or splints. This includes fractures of the shaft of the radius/ulna and tibia, and of the metacarpal, metatarsal and phalangeal bones. In the upper parts of limbs, because of the shape and muscle development, it is difficult to support a fracture adequately, although the Thomas extension splint has advantages for certain fractures of the femur and humerus.

Firstly, the fracture has to be reduced by manipulation and then a closely fitting rigid support is applied to maintain the bone ends in apposition during healing. General anaesthesia is an essential prerequisite for the reduction of major fractures since the muscular relaxation it provides renders powerful traction unnecessary, and additionally it can be done humanely. The difficulty experienced in apposing the bone ends depends on their degree of displacement and their shape. Another important factor is the timing of the reduction; the sooner it is done the easier it will be, and the converse applies. Generally speaking it ought not to be delayed for more than 24 hours, depending on the health status of the patient. Radiographs indicate the direction in which the fragments have to be moved to obtain reduction. In cats and small- to moderate-sized dogs the force needed is not great and is applied by hand. Care must be taken not to add to the tissue damage that is already present. Once

reduction is achieved it is helpful to check the result radiographically.

A variety of materials is available for the construction of casts and splints. **Plaster of Paris** was among the earliest used and was the usual choice until recent years when other products have been introduced. The application of a total cast of any material needs practise to achieve immobilization of the bones and to avoid certain hazards. If too tight it causes pressure sores over bony prominences or, worse, may so constrict the limb as to produce gangrene. If too slack it may lead to non-union or slip downwards and cause pressure or even fall off. Although opinions vary about the methodology of application there are some central points to be borne in mind. If the fur is naturally short a layer of bandage or gauze should first be applied; a layer of tubegauze is ideal for this purpose. Long fur should be clipped to about 1 cm or else it will act as excessive packing and prevent adequate immobilization and, in addition, removing the cast will be difficult and painful. Prominences are padded, and if the foot is included, pledgets of cotton wool are placed between the digits. Ideally the cast should immobilize the joint immediately above and below the fracture but this cannot always be achieved because it is difficult entirely to prevent movement of the elbow and stifle joints.

After reducing the fracture the leg is held by an assistant using gentle traction so that it is in proper alignment. If plaster of Paris is used the layer of gauze is damped, then previously prepared strips of plaster bandage are soaked in tepid water, squeezed to remove excess fluid, and placed longitudinally on the limb. Enough strips are used to encircle the leg, and they are gently squeezed to conform to its shape. Further bandages are wound around the strips until a cast of sufficient strength is produced. The surface of the cast is smoothed by hand until the edges and weave of the bandages are no longer visible. As the cast begins to set the leg is placed on a sandbag under the heat, say, of an operating light until the cast is hard. Further drying must be allowed, at least 2 hours, before the dog is discharged, and at this time a covering of adhesive tape is applied as protection against moisture and licking.

Plaster of Paris bandages must be kept dry during storage. If moisture is absorbed the bandage will feel gritty instead of being creamy during application, and it must be discarded or the resulting cast will be weak. Some manufacturers pack plaster bandages in tins or metal foil to prevent this problem. Owners must be advised about aftercare of the patient. They must ensure adequate restriction of activity, keep the cast dry when out of doors by covering it with a plastic bag and report urgently to the veterinary surgeon about mutilation of the cast, evident discomfort or limb swelling. A weekly re-inspection is advisable.

Removal of the cast is most readily accomplished with a special electric saw which has a reciprocating blade. Shears may also be used, but for very small animals they tend to be unwieldy and the force required often causes unacceptable discomfort. The problems of removal can be greatly reduced by splitting the cast lengthwise along its lateral side just before it sets; the final cover of tape will bind it sufficiently. Alternatively, a half-cast type of shell can be made. In recent times refinements in the preparation of plaster bandages have resulted in the reduction in the weight of casts without any loss of strength.

Other improvements have been made towards making plaster water resistant and more lucent to X-rays, with obvious advantages, as in "Crystona" (Smith & Nephew), and the introduction of resin-plaster with faster setting times as with "Zoroc" (Johnson & Johnson). Another new product consists of a fibreglass fabric impregnated with resin ("Vetcast"-3M) and it has the advantages of being light-weight, strong, radiolucent and porous. These newer products require extensive clinical trial to test their usefulness in small animal orthopaedics but they appear to provide an advance on conventional materials. Meanwhile it must be stressed that the manufacturers' instructions must be strictly followed since the method of application of these products vary and with some of them precautions are needed to avoid the material contacting the patient's bare skin and also the applicator's hands.

Various forms of splint may also be used as supports, and most are made to suit the dimensions of the particular case. Aluminium is commonly employed; obtainable from ironmongers in sheet form, it is light, and easily cut and bent into shape. Nevertheless, it cannot be closely moulded to the limb and has, therefore, to be well padded with cotton wool to protect prominences. Two gutter-shaped splints are required adequately to support a fractured forearm, being secured firmly in place with a layer of adhesive tape. Another type, produced commercially, is a light aluminium strip backed with foam (Zimmer) which is suitable for toy dogs. Many other materials such as laths of balsa wood or fragments of wooden tongue depressors are used as splints occasionally. Thomas extension splints are popular with some surgeons, especially for injuries in the upper regions of the fore or hindlegs where other means of support are not practical. They are constructed to suit the individual case, from malleable aluminium rod, and with practise provide a very satisfactory method of limb support for all sizes of dog. The limb is kept in rigid extension, and this sometimes makes care at home difficult because the dog has difficulty getting about.

## 2. Open Reduction

The choice of implant depends on the site and type of the fracture and on the size and shape of the bone affected. Of the various methods now available wiring was the first used, usually limited to jaw fractures or separated fragments. In the early 1930s attempts were made to repair long bone fractures with metal or bone pegs, but they mostly proved disastrous largely because of infection. It was not until shortly after the Second World War that the surgical repair of fractures of long bones was shown to be practical and successful. Fixation with an intramedullary pin was the first method to be widely adopted, but as experience extended other techniques, employing screws and plates, were introduced. Nowadays fracture sugery is commonplace and a large array of implants and techniques is available. It must be emphasized, however, that none of these procedures should be undertaken lightly because inherent dangers to life and limb are involved. They require technical skill, a sound understanding of the principles of repair, strict attention to asepsis, and a high standard of post-operative nursing. Additionally, the implants must be manufactured of the best quality metals and be stored carefully to prevent surface damage before use.

### (a) Intramedullary Pin/Nail

A cylindrical, solid section steel pin (Steinmann) or a nail with a cross-section of various shapes (Küntscher) is inserted along the medullary cavity of the main fragments with the object of immobilizing them. The pin or nail must closely fit the cavity, be of sufficient length to hold the bone ends securely and be capable of being removed at a later date. Its size is measured from a radiograph of the fractured bone or, better still, of the same bone in the opposite leg. Pinning is commonly used for fractures of the femur and humerus in cats and in small- to moderate-sized dogs. Unless a tight fit is achieved the distal fragment will tend to rotate and a delayed or non-union may result. In active dogs not adequately restrained post-operatively the implant often rides upwards and may lose its hold on the distal fragment, and on occasions it becomes so loose that it has to be removed. In giant dogs two or more pins could be used to obtain a close fit in the medullary cavity, but the application of a plate would provide a more secure fixation.

### (b) Plate

A wide variety of size and shape of plates is available, made of stainless steel or an alloy. Two patterns are used—Sherman and Venable; the latter is rectangular and is the stronger mechanically. It is important for the plate to be of sufficient strength to support the fracture once weight bearing begins, otherwise the plate or screws may break or be torn from the bone. The radius/ulna and tibia are common sites for plate application, but in large dogs they are indicated for most longbone fractures.

The screws used must be of the same metal or else an electrolytic reaction could be set up which might cause loosening of the implant and interfere with bone healing. The self-tapping screws used are made in different lengths from $\frac{3}{8}$ in. (9.5 mm) upwards. Ideally each screw traverses both cortices of the bone and just emerges on the far side. The RANA must know that for screws of 7/64 in. (2.7 mm) and 9/64 in. (3.6 mm) calibre, the sizes of bit used to drill the tracks are 3/32 in. (2.3 mm) and 7/64 in. (2.7 mm) in diameter respectively. Packs containing screws and bits should be always marked accurately to avoid mistakes during surgery.

The further study of fracture fixation has, in recent years, led to the development of new methods of plate and screw fixation.

These so-called ASIF (Association for the study of Internal Fixation) techniques require special equipment and expertise and now they are becoming increasingly used in fracture surgery in animals, Veterinary nurses must become familiar with the instruments and understand the way they are used. A wide range of plate and screw sizes is now available, capable of dealing with virtually any size of dog or cat, and any type of fracture. The precise techniques involved are properly the concern of the veterinary surgeon and courses are available in Switzerland and in the UK where these procedures may be learned under expert guidance. The nurse's involvement is particularly concerned with the care, packaging and sterilization of the instruments and implants, so recognition of the various items is the first essential. A simple approach in practice where a wide range of such equipment is kept, is to maintain the instruments in specific sets according to their size and to have them accurately labelled accordingly. In the near future it is likely that a practice with a large throughput of fractures would stock instruments to cover the use of dynamic compression plates; screw size 4.5 mm, 3.5 mm, 2.7 mm; and miniplates and screws. The sets containing drills, taps, screwdrivers, drill guides, and a range of screws of different lengths should be in separate boxes, sterilized by autoclave and ready for use. The plates are best individually sealed in nylon film and packaged in cardboard boxes. After use the instruments require thorough cleaning of blood and tissue before being re-sterilized in order to keep them in peak working condition. Nurses will find the brochures published by the manufacturers of these instruments helpful with their recognition and those employed where the techniques are commonly practised would be advised to consult AO/ASIF Instrumentation by H. Willenegger (1981) in order fully to understand what the procedures involve.

### (c) Screw

Apart from being used in conjunction with plates, screw fixation alone is indicated for certain injuries such as separation of epiphyses and condylar fractures. In most of these situations the **lag-screw** principle is involved, which basically means over drilling the track in the smaller fragment so that compression is achieved as the screw is tightened. Attention to the size of the screw and bit is important to obtain good fixation.

### (d) Wire

Monofilament steel wire is used for the repair of some jaw fractures, either by winding it around the teeth above gum level or by placing it in the form of a mattress suture across the fracture site. Its use in cerclage form in conjunction with pinning to support separated fragments is a matter of controversy because some authorities believe this may interfere with the blood supply to the bone. Whenever used it must be strong enough to withstand the stress in a given situation, so a range of different sizes has to be kept.

## (e) Half-pin assembly

This method involves inserting two pins at right angles into each half of the fractured bone and linking them up with cross bars outside the body in order to maintain alignment. On occasions it may be done without exposing the fracture, and reduction is achieved by manipulation of the bone ends via the pins. Although popular in North America for many years it has not been generally accepted in the United Kingdom, probably because it has the disadvantages of being readily knocked out of place and the fear that infection might track along the pins into the bone.

The **nursing needed after fracture** surgery is closely concerned with the prevention of infection and restriction of the patient's activity. A course of antibiotics is administered and regular inspections are made to assess wound healing, local swelling and pain which could be indicators of bone infection. Hospitalization is seldom necessary or practical for the whole time it takes for the fracture to heal, but it is beneficial for the first few days especially for very active dogs and when the home environment is not conducive to rest. Advice has to be given about the level of permissible activity; avoid stairs, stop playing with children or other dogs, restrict to a leash when out-of-doors. The use of external support as an adjunct to surgery is to be recommended when it is feasible; firm bandages or light splints are of great assistance for fractures below the elbow and stifle joints and, additionally, they protect the wound from extraneous infection and from self-mutilation.

## Dislocations

The aim of treatment is to reduce the dislocation, preferably by means of manipulation, and thus return the joint to normality. Generally speaking success with reduction depends on the duration of the injury, and the sooner it is attempted the better. After several days the soft tissue structures associated with the joint undergo contraction and this may make reduction difficult or even impossible without surgical intervention.

Radiography is necessary not only to confirm the diagnosis but also to determine whether the bony components have suffered other damage. With hip dislocations, for example, it is important to know if there has been a fracture of the acetabulum or of the head of the femur, because either would cause problems with reduction and the achievement of satisfactory stability afterwards.

General anaesthesia is essential for the reduction of dislocations of the hip, tarsus and carpus in order to overcome muscle action and to perform the procedure humanely. Some other dislocations, for example of the shoulder, patella and phalanges, are usually readily repositioned in the conscious animal.

The way in which the manipulation is applied depends on the joint involved and it requires an understanding of joint anatomy. It is not just a matter of force, although some traction is needed at times, but rather of leverage and pressure in the correct direction. When reducing the hip the femoral head is first raised from its position on the ilium by applying leverage to the femur and is then more readily pushed or pulled into the acetabulum than if traction alone is applied. The elbow can only be reduced when the joint is flexed because otherwise the anconeal process of the ulna will obstruct against the humeral condyle.

After reduction the joint can be tested for stability by moving it manually. It has to be remembered that dislocation implies damage to the supporting structures (ligament, capsule, muscle) of the joint. At the time of reduction, therefore, the joint is invariably potentially unstable.

*Post-operative care* is concerned with the avoidance of forces that could produce a recurrence. Whenever possible external supporting bandages or splints are employed. For the hip the application of a figure-of-eight bandage to keep the leg in full flexion is a very helpful method of maintaining reduction; it is kept on 5–7 days. Additionally the patient's activity should be greatly curtailed for 3–4 weeks, as in the case of fractures.

Surgical measures are indicated if reduction proves impossible and when the joint remains so unstable that it dislocates recurrently. A variety of methods is available for this purpose, most of them aimed at repairing the supporting structures or constructing new ligaments using tissue grafts or manmade materials.

The foregoing applies particularly to dislocations of traumatic origin (acquired). Congenital dislocations also occur and some (shoulder, elbow) cannot be corrected by manipulation or surgical means because the deformity is usually too great. The most commonly encountered congenital dislocation in dogs affects the patella. Its effect on function may be slight so that little treatment is needed, but some dogs suffer a severe disability and require surgery in order to improve their locomotion.

## (d) Common Surgical Diseases

N. J. H. SHARP

### Common surgical terms

You will find that many words used to describe the various surgical procedures in this chapter have similar endings. These endings can be divided into three types:—

1. *Words ending in -otomy:* this means to surgically create a temporary opening into an organ or structure. An example would be urethrotomy, where an incision is made into the urethra e.g. to remove an obstructing calculus; or an enterotomy, where an incision is made into a portion of intestine e.g. to remove a foreign body. Once made, the incision can either be allowed to close of its own accord as is done for example with an urethrotomy, or the edges are sutured together, e.g. enterotomy.

2. *Words ending in -ostomy:* this means to create a permanent opening into an organ or structure. A good example is urethrostomy, where the incision is made in exactly the same manner as a urethrotomy but then, instead of being left to heal over, it is prevented from doing so by suturing the edges of the urethral opening to the adjacent skin surface.

3. *Words ending in -ectomy:* this means the removal of all or part of an organ or structure. For example, enterectomy is the removal of a length of the intestine and the two remaining free ends can then be sutured together by an end to end anastomosis. Ovariohysterectomy is the removal of both ovaries and the uterus.

*Laparotomy:* One of the most common operations in veterinary practice is the laparotomy, which is where the abdominal cavity is opened in order to examine the organs contained within. Depending on the exact reason for the laparotomy, a variety of different incisions sites (called surgical approaches) may be used (Fig. 10.2).

(a) The most common is a midline laparotomy, where the incision is made through the fibrous tissue of the linea alba. This gives excellent access to nearly all of the abdomen and is easy to perform and repair. In the male dog the penis overlies the linea alba towards the caudal end of the abdomen. Here a paramedian skin incision can be made to one side of the penis, which can then be reflected to expose the midline linea alba for access into the abdomen.

(b) If the abdominal cavity is penetrated to one side or the other of the midline, then this is done by either a paramedian or possibly a pararectal laparotomy. In some instances, where access is required to the anterior abdomen or the diaphragm, a paracostal incision is employed.

*Thoracotomy:* Thoracotomy is the creation of an opening into the thoracic cavity. It is usually performed via an incision through an intercostal space, i.e. between the ribs, on one side of the chest, although occasionally better access can be obtained by the removal of a rib.

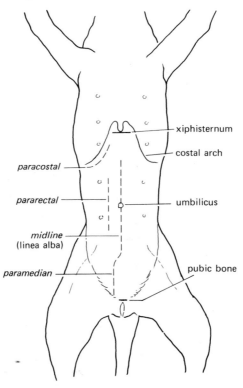

FIG. 10.2.    Surgical Approaches for Laporotomy

## Common Surgical Conditions

ABSCESS: A collection of pus which is separated from the rest of the animal by a capsule of often quite fibrous connective tissue. This can occur in almost any part of the body but is most commonly encountered in the skin following a bite wound. Initially the area will swell and becomes painful and then over several days the infection will be walled off as an abscess. Toxins from the abscess may make the animal feverish and anorexic (due to toxaemia) but this will usually resolve after the abscess points, or softens at one part of its surface, and then bursts to release its contents.

*Treatment* of an abscess is basically to either prevent its occurrence by thorough cleansing and systemic antibiotics in the case of a fresh bite ($<$12 hours old); or to hasten its development once the above process has started. Hot poulticing, either using commercially available products such as Animal Lintex, or by applying cotton wool soaked in a hand hot, concentrated solution of salt and/or Epsom salts will encourage an abscess to point and relieve discomfort. Once pointing has occurred, the veterinary surgeon should make a large opening into the abscess cavity (using e.g. an "abscess" scalpel blade) at its most prominent point. After evacuation of the contents and checking for the possibility of a foreign body, the cavity is flushed with an antiseptic solution e.g. Pevidine. Irrigation should continue through this opening for a day or two, to prevent premature closure of the cavity walling off infection, which will tend to cause a recurrence of the abscess. For a similar reason, antibiotics should only be used in the case of a recent bite or if the animal is obviously sick. Unless the abscess has been drained, antibiotics will sometimes prevent the contents pointing and being released. If this should happen the pus is walled off completely but is never properly cleared up. Such an abscess may flare up periodically and swell but be prevented from bursting by the now thick fibrous wall—this is often called a "**cold abscess**".

HAEMATOMA: This is a collection of blood, usually under the skin, which forms a discrete swelling e.g. aural haematoma on the pinna or ear flap. Haematoma's will usually resolve without problems although they should be checked for any evidence of secondary infection. Should drainage of a haematoma cavity be necessary for any reason, it should be performed once the bleeding source has had time to seal e.g. after 2–3 days. In the case of an aural haematoma, drainage is nearly always necessary so that the pinna is not deformed as the scar tissue of the resolving blood clot retracts.

SEROMA: This is the collection of serum or frequently blood and serum, usually in a surgical wound. Proper closure of a wound by sutures will eliminate any large gaps between the layers of a wound (the so called "*dead space*") where fluid might accumulate. If this is not possible then drainage tubes e.g. Penrose drains should be sutured in place to allow this fluid to escape. A seroma provides the ideal medium for bacterial growth and will therefore predispose a wound to breakdown (**dehiscene**).

ULCER: This is where the skin or epithelial surface has been lost leaving a raw area which is often slow to heal. Ulcers may occur in a number of locations such as in the mouth e.g. due to cat flu; on the lip e.g. "rodent ulcer" in the cat; or the term may be used to describe the "ulcerated" surface of a tumour. Treatment will vary with the specific site involved but the surface of an ulcer should be kept clean and possibly dressed with a suitable antiseptic e.g. Betadine.

FISTULA: This is an opening or canal lined by epithelium, which connects one skin or mucosal surface to another. An example is a **recto-vaginal fistula** a rare congenital abnormality where the animal is born with an opening which connects the lumen of the rectum to that of the vagina.

SINUS: This is a similar opening or canal arising from a skin or mucosal surface but which has a blind ending and is not normally lined by epithelium. A *foreign body* such as a grass seed in a dog's foot will tend to discharge through an opening on the skin surface, but the sinus that it has created will lead nowhere other than to a pocket of pus containing the foreign body.

FOREIGN BODY: This can apply to any structure which is not normally found within the body, including the animals own dead tissues e.g. a piece of dead bone or *sequestrum*. Foreign bodies may either penetrate the skin surface e.g. a grass seed or a fish-hook (the latter should be removed carefully and never simply pulled because of the barb); obstruct a hollow organ e.g. a stone or rubber ball in the intestines; or they may simply cause irritation by their presence e.g. a grass seed lying in the ear canal or nasal cavity.

**Surgical conditions of the gastro-intestinal tract**

*Lips, Buccal Cavity and Pharnyx:*

—*Harelip:* This is a defect between the nostril and the edge of the lip, it can also be associated with a cleft palate. Both abnormalities render sucking difficult and the animal is usually put to sleep at birth, although corrective surgery is possible if it survives to 10 or 12 weeks of age.

—*Labial dermatitis:* Labial dermatitis of the skin fold on the lower lip is seen typically in spaniels. Food debris may accumulate in this fold and cause infection, swelling and irritation.

—*Rodent ulcer:* occurs in the cat, mainly on the upper lip close to the midline, and resembles a flat, ulcerated granuloma. Sometimes associated with excessive licking, the true aetiology is unknown but many cases respond to cortico steroids or "progestogens".

—*Tumours:* Tumours of the lips, buccal cavity or pharynx tend to be malignant but the main problem is of local recurrence rather than spread to distant sites, e.g. lung. Some are amenable to radical surgical excision or possibly radiotherapy.

—*Epulis:* is the one common benign tumour in this region which affects primarily the gums. Once diagnosed an epulis may be simply left alone, or it may be surgically removed if it interferes with chewing or bleeds when the dog eats.

—*Stings:* If in the mouth these can cause severe swelling and especially in brachycephalic breeds e.g. bulldogs, they may cause respiratory problems. If these progress despite steroids, antihistamines and an ice-pack around the throat, then emergency endotracheal intubation or intubation via a tracheotomy opening may be necessary.

—*Foreign bodies:* a bone may lodge between the upper carnassial teeth, or a needle, fish-hook or stick penetrate the wall of the buccal cavity or pharynx. All will cause salivation and difficulty in swallowing (these are also early signs seen in rabies, the possibility of which should first be ruled out). Radiographic diagnosis may be useful before removal under general anaesthesia.

—*The tongue:* can be affected by ulcers, foreign bodies or tumours which will interfere with swallowing and, of great importance in the cat, grooming.

—*Ulceration:* may occur anywhere in the buccal cavity due to a wide range of causes, e.g. cat "flu" viruses, systemic illness e.g. uraemia, or dental disease; these factors should be identified and treated if possible. Some cases, especially cats, may have no obvious cause of ulceration and may not respond to treatment with antibiotic, steroids and even removal of all the teeth as a last resort. In cases where the animal refuses to eat, despite treatment and the provision of tempting aromatic foods, temporary *pharyngostomy* intubation can be useful. This technique is also useful following extensive fractures of the jaw or in any debilitated anorexic animal which is not also vomiting. It entails the surgical implantation under general anaesthesia of a tube passing from the skin surface of the submandibular region through the lateral pharyngeal wall to the oesophagus, and then into the stomach (Fig. 10.3). Fluid (liquidized food and water), amounting to 40–60 ml/kg body weight/day can be provided in 20–100 ml. amounts fed 6–8 times per day, using the water last to flush clean the tube which is then stoppered.

—*Tonsils:* usually become inflamed secondary to disease elsewhere e.g. in the nose or mouth, the tonsils may be the site of neoplasia.

—*Dentistry:* This is very necessary in veterinary practice as teeth may be damaged by a wide variety of causes, e.g. fractures, stone-chewing. The retention of deciduous beyond 7 months of age will cause malalignment especially the canine teeth of toy breeds. By far the most important cause is **periodontal disease**. This starts as a bacterial film (plaque) over the teeth which becomes mineralized by the calcium salts in saliva to form tartar

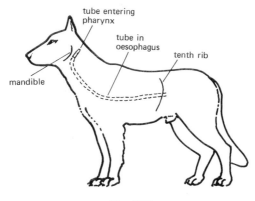

tube entering
pharynx

tube in
oesophagus

tenth rib

mandible

FIG. 10.3.

(calculus). Build-up of this is favoured by a soft diet and dental malocclusion but it is normally worn away by chewing hard foods, e.g. bones or biscuits. If allowed to accumulate the calculus soon inflames the gums (gingivitis) which tend to recede so exposing the periodontal membrane (Fig. 10.4). When this becomes infected (*periodontitis*), the tooth will loosen and the breath will often smell (**halitosis**). Once present this condition is almost impossible to cure but its progression can be slowed by regular removal of all tartar, preferably by ultrasound scaling, removal of loose teeth and correction of the diet. Cleaning of the teeth by the owner, using a soft rag and Chlorhexidine tooth gel or baking soda once a week, can also be very useful and is often quickly accepted by the dog. Before dentistry, the nurse should ensure that an adequate supply of forceps (to remove teeth and/or calculus) and elevators (to breakdown the tooth's attachments) are available, and that she is familiar with the workings of the ultrasonic scaler. The use of this will create a cloud of plaque-laden water droplets so a protective face mask is desirable as are goggles worn to protect the eyes from tooth or calculus chips.

The patient's mouth should be held open by a gag and the head kept clean by being placed on a metal grill over a tray to collect debris and water. An endotracheal tube, with the cuff inflated, is advisable combined with a single large swab to pack the pharynx. This swab should have a length of 1 inch bandage tied firmly to it, to be left protruding out of the mouth so its presence is not forgotten. These precautions will maintain a blood and tooth-free airway. All debris and the pharyngeal pack should be removed before extubation and the animal's head then kept slightly lower than the body to allow free escape of water and blood from the mouth.

*Oesophagus*

*Foreign bodies*—such as a chop bone, may lodge in the oesophagus, usually just in front of the diaphragm. This will obstruct the passage of food, causing regurgitation after eating, and require removal either using long forceps via the mouth or, failing this, via an oesophagotomy incision following a thoracotomy.

*Megaoesophagus*—is a flaccid dilation of the oesophagus; it can benefit from gravity-assisted feeding (feeding from a height and/or then raising the front end of the animal) so that food passes into the stomach more easily.

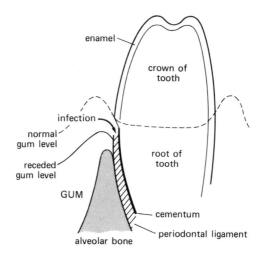

enamel

crown of
tooth

infection

normal
gum level

receded
gum level

root of
tooth

GUM

cementum

periodontal ligament

alveolar bone

FIG. 10.4.   The tooth in periodontal disease

### Stomach

*Foreign bodies*—these usually result in persistent vomiting and require removal by gastrotomy following laparotomy.

*Pyloric stenosis*—is where the pyloric sphincter of the stomach prevents emptying of its contents into the intestine so causing vomiting. It is not uncommon in young dogs and kittens and usually responds to simple surgery.

*Gastric dilation/torsion*—this very important, yet fortunately quite uncommon condition, occurs mainly in deep-chested dogs, e.g. hounds. The history is frequently of recent feeding with a large meal followed by exercise. Food and gas in the stomach cause it to dilate, putting pressure on the diaphragm and embarrassing respiration. The stomach then tends to rotate about itself which causes interference to its blood supply and may result in necrosis of part of the wall. The dog quickly becomes dull, may make unsuccessful attempts to vomit, and classically its abdomen will appear swollen due to distension with gas. This is an emergency condition with a high mortality rate; the dog is in shock and requires rapid

surgical attention. In particular, decompression of the stomach to improve breathing combined with fluid therapy to counter shock are vital. If the animal is dying of respiratory embarrassment, a hypodermic needle inserted through the abdominal wall, into the gas cap of the stomach can give relief until veterinary attention arrives (p 250). Post-operatively fluid therapy should be maintained and oral fluids or food be withheld for 24 hours. Over the next few days small volumes of first water and later food, can be offered and it may be useful to feed the animal from a raised bowl to reduce the amount of air swallowed with the food. Once home the dog should be fed small meals several times a day and then be made to rest afterwards because recurrence of this condition can be a major threat. Cereals should form as small a proportion of the diet as possible and certainly any biscuit fed should be pre-soaked.

### Small Intestine

*Foreign bodies*—such as stones or rubber balls, cloth may cause a complete

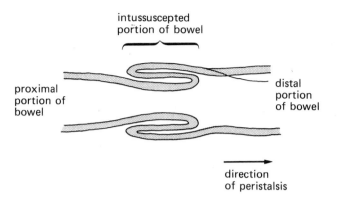

intussuscepted
portion of bowel

proximal
portion of
bowel

distal
portion
of bowel

direction
of peristalsis

FIG. 10.5.   An intussusception

obstruction to the passage of gut contents. The animal will vomit and rapidly become shocked and dehydrated, requiring intravenous fluid therapy before surgical removal by enterotomy.

*Intussusception*—is the telescoping of a portion of bowel (Fig. 10.5), usually due to diarrhoea (particularly in puppies) and this condition also requires surgical correction, often by enterectomy. Following surgery on the stomach or intestines, water is normally withheld for 24 hours and then only soft food offered for the next few days.

### Rectum

*Foreign bodies*—mainly sharp bones, tend to lodge here causing pain and constipation, and often require a general anaesthetic to allow their removal by digital manipulation or by using whelping forceps.

*Chronic constipation*—such therapy may also be required here but often an enema will bring about successful evacuation of the impacted rectum. The enema can either be a proprietary product e.g. "Microlax", or an infusion of a large volume (e.g. 20 ml, for a cat, up to 500 ml for a large dog) of warm soapy water into

the rectum using a soft enema tube. This should be introduced gently using plenty of lubricant to avoid causing damage to or perforation of the rectal wall, especially in cats. The enema fluid can be administered using a syringe for smaller volumes, or by funnel or enema pump for larger volumes, and should meet with little or no resistance. Liquid paraffin (2–10 ml/day) and a bulk laxative, e.g. "Isogel", are useful in the prevention of further bouts. Other possible causes of constipation are prostatic enlargement, perineal ruptures and tumours of the wall of the rectum.

*Anal sacs (glands)*—these may impact, causing the animal to drag its backside along the floor and/or bite at its back end. Digital pressure will empty them and if the problem persists or abscessation occurs, then they can be surgically removed.

*Anal adenoma*—is a large, usually benign, tumour occurring near the anus of old male dogs which respond well to removal and also so castration, since the growth of this tumour is dependent on male sex hormones.

*Anal furunculosis*—here multiple sinuses around the anus cause pain and difficulty defaecating. The condition is usually seen in German Shepherds and requires surgery to remove all the diseased tissue, followed by cryosurgery of the exposed surfaces which are then left open to heal by second intention. Post-operatively laxatives are useful, combined (if possible) with gentle bathing of the area with warm salt water.

*Rectal prolapse*—is the eversion of the rectal wall out through the anus, due to straining because of e.g. diarrhoea, or rectal tumours. This requires prompt protection of the delicate mucosa by obstetrical jelly and/or moist towels and the use of a collar to prevent the animal from licking the area. Surgical replacement or resection is necessary, combined with treatment of the original cause. A temporary purse-string suture in the anus is useful to prevent recurrence but must be removed as soon as possible to allow defaecation.

*Imperforate anus*—or failure of the rectum to unite with the anus during development prevents defaecation, so the animal will present in the first few weeks of life with abdominal distension. Surgical correction is sometimes successful.

## The respiratory tract

### Nasal Condition

*Nasal discharge* is seen in the cat mainly as a feature of cat 'flu, while in the dog distemper is an important cause. Foreign bodies such as grass seeds, will cause an intense discomfort with sneezing and discharge in both species but can often be easily removed using an auroscope and crocodile forceps. **Epistaxis**, or nose bleed, it not uncommon in the cat due to trauma such as an RTA. In the dog it is also seen either in association with a nasal tumour, or due to a fungus, *Aspergillus*, which grows on the delicate turbinate bones of the nasal cavity. Radiography is the most useful method for the diagnosis of nasal conditions although a blood test can be employed in the case of aspergillosis. Surgical exploration of the nasal chambers for any of these reasons is undertaken by performing a **rhinotomy** operation.

### Larynx and Trachea

The larynx in old dogs can become paralyzed, causing difficulty in breathing, this condition being similar to "roaring" in horses. The trachea of certain toy breeds can collapse due to faulty conformation and so result in a peculiar honking cough and respiratory embarrassment.

*Tracheotomy*—can be a life-saving procedure whereby a hole is created in the trachea between its cartilaginous rings, just behind the larynx. In an emergency this can be performed by the nurse using local anaesthetic, followed by a skin incision made immediately behind the larynx in the ventral midline. The trachea lies beneath a pair of thin muscles which can be bluntly separated in the midline to expose the cartilaginous tracheal rings. A scalpel incision is then made between the second or third pair of rings and extended for 180° around the tracheal circumference. This must be kept open by inserting a metal or plastic tracheotomy tube which is then tied in place. In the cat a simpler alternative can be to push a 16 gauge needle through the skin into the trachea at the same level. Tracheotomy is used to bypass the upper airway and so enable an animal with an obstructed pharynx or larynx to breathe, or it can be used to facilitate surgery on, e.g. the larynx. The opening of the tracheotomy tube tends to block with mucus and so must be scrupulously cleaned every 3 hours or so.

### Thoracotomy

This entails surgically opening the chest or thorax, for example to remove an oesophageal foreign body. Following this procedure, the thoracic cavity must be properly sealed against leaks and the remaining air the remaining air and fluid drawn off to allow the lungs to expand properly. A temporary chest drain of sterile tubing is often employed with one end placed inside the thoracic cavity to ensure that further accumulations of gas or fluid can thus be removed. This tube must be kept sealed and protected from dirt or disturbance, and is therefore usu- ally incorporated in an encircling chest bandage.

### Upper Airway Obstruction of Brachycephalic Dogs

One characteristic of all brachycephalic dogs is the foreshortening of the skull bones which crowds together all of the associated soft tissues of the mouth, nose and pharynx. So, for example, the tongue is effectively too long for the mouth and tends to loll out and, more importantly, breathing is made difficult by a narrowed nasal cavity and pharynx. In particular the relatively overlong soft palate tends to obstruct the larynx causing laboured, noisy breathing in most of these dogs and in some individuals may lead to serious respiratory obstruction. Surgery particu- larly to shorten the soft palate, can be very helpful but requires care with anaesthesia especially during recovery. The animal's breathing can then often be helped con- siderably by pulling forward gently on the tongue which is most easily held using tongue forceps, and also by encouraging the animal to swallow occasionally.

### Conditions affecting the urinary tract

*KIDNEY* Rare conditions such as tu- mours or severe infection within one kidney, may require removal of this kid- ney (nephrectomy) provided that the other is functioning normally.

*URETER* *Ectopic ureter* is a condition where one or both ureters empty into the urinary tract beyond the retaining sphinc- ter of the bladder neck and so cause dribbling of urine, or incontinence, from birth. It is mainly seen in bitches and can be corrected surgically.

*BLADDER* Removal of urinary cal- culi, which may cause a cystitis or obstruc- tion is performed by *cystotomy*.

*URETHRA* Blockage by small uri- nary calculi in the male is very important in both the dog and the cat, as obstruction to urination may rupture the bladder and will cause uraemia and rapid death. The

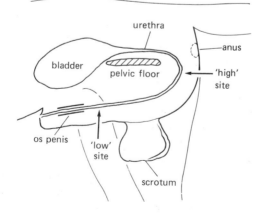

Fig. 10.6.

animal becomes depressed, strains constantly but can pass no urine. If catherization fails to relieve the obstruction, then a *urethrotomy* opening in the urethra, proximal to (above) the obstruction, will allow the animal to pass urine and recover. This opening is best made permanent (*urethrostomy*) to prevent recurrence of obstruction by further calculi. Usually obstruction occurs at the level of the os penis in the dog as so a "low" urethrostomy (Fig. 10.6) is adequate. Some cases will require a "high" urethrostomy; while in the cat the urethra in the penis is very narrow so this portion is simply amputated. Post-operatively a collar is important to prevent trauma to the wound and sutures. Vaseline is useful to prevent excoriation from urine at the surgical site until the animal learns to cope with the situation. See "Medical Nursing" for preventive measures (p. 508).

### The genital tract

### In the Male

*Castration* in the male or removal of the **testes** is, performed to prevent breeding, roaming, spraying (by tomcats) and, sometimes, to treat excessive sex drive (libido) or inter-male aggression. Less common reasons are for treatment of testicular tumours or to remove the source of hormones which stimulate certain disorders of the prostrate gland, and anal adenoma.

### In the Female

To spay or neuter, means to remove the ovaries and uterus (*ovariohysterectomy*) which, as well as rendering pregnancy impossible, will prevent both oestrus and the possibility of future development of pyometra. An animal should not be spayed during an oestrus or if heavily pregnant

and, in the bitch, preferably not before her first season to allow her vulva to mature properly. It is best to avoid metoestrus, as false pregnancy in the recently spayed bitch is undesirable.

*Pyometra*—this is the accumulation of secretions within the uterus. It usually occurs in the older bitch who has never had puppies but may recently have been in season. She is frequently depressed, vomiting and polydipsic and may have a vaginal discharge (open pyometra) or the cervix may be closed (closed pyometra). Both conditions are life-threatening and require ovariohysterectomy (p. 597).

*Hysterotomy*—or *Caesarean section* is performed if the bitch cannot deliver her puppies due to uterine inactivity or foetal obstruction. This procedure has the usual obstetrical requirements of plenty of warm towels and willing hands, preferably also facilities to resuscitate the newborn, such as simple suction, and oxygen; material to tie off the navels and possibly a respiratory stimulant, such as "Dopram". The puppies or kittens should be allowed to suckle as soon as possible after they have been checked for the presence of any congenital abnormalities, such as cleft palate.

*Vulva*—incontinent bitches or those suffering from cystitis may develop a very inflamed vulva. This should be regularly washed, rinsed and then dried, after which a soothing antiseptic ointment should be applied and preferably covered by vaseline. Barrier creams of the type produced for newborn infants will be of value to reduce scalding by urine.

### Hernias and ruptures

Although some books place all of the following conditions together under "Hernias", it is useful to differentiate them into either "Hernias" or "Ruptures".

*THE DEFINITION OF A HERNIA*
—is the protrusion of abdominal contents through a natural opening in the wall of the abdominal cavity. This includes both openings that should have closed before birth, such as the umbilicus; and normal openings that may become enlarged, such as the inguinal canals. Hernias are thought to be often inherited and so, for this reason, affected animals should be neutered.

*THE DEFINITION OF A RUPTURE*—is the protrusion of abdominal contents through an unnatural opening, such as a tear or weakness, in the wall of the abdominal cavity. This includes a tear in the muscle of the diaphragm or diaphragmatic rupture, or the weakening of the pelvic muscles, which occurs in perineal rupture. A rupture occurs due to trauma, although other factors would also appear involved in the case of perineal rupture.

Hernias and ruptures may be classified according to their location, as is shown below, and this can be further qualified by one of the following terms: *reducible* which means that the contents of the hernia or rupture can be replaced back into the abdomen via the opening in the abdominal wall.

*Irreducible* which means that the con-tents cannot be replaced because they have become stuck in position for example due to adhesions. This usually occurs in longstanding conditions or where no peritoneal lining to the defect is present and such a situation may also be termed incarceration. A serious complication of hernias and ruptures is where the contents become **strangulated**. Here the venous return of blood from the contents becomes impaired and so they swell which prevents their replacement. Swelling causes a rise in pressure, which then occludes the arterial supply, and the contents then become necrotic. This is similar to the events occurring if a bandage is applied too tightly around an animal's leg, causing the foot to first swell and, if neglected it may go cold and die. Strangulation is obviously an emergency situation, particularly if a piece of intestine is the strangulated organ.

### Structure of a Hernia

**A hernia is normally lined** by the same peritoneal covering as the rest of the abdominal cavity (Fig. 10.7).

**The neck** of the hernia represents the opening through the abdominal wall, in this instance the still patent umbilicus. **The lumen** of the hernia contains the **contents**

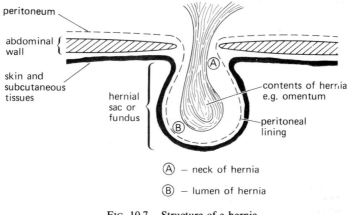

Ⓐ — neck of hernia

Ⓑ — lumen of hernia

Fig. 10.7.  Structure of a hernia.

JAN–MM

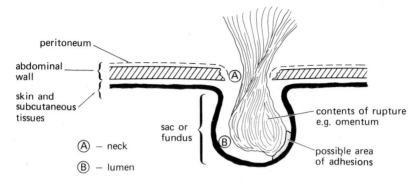

Fig. 10.8.    Structure of a Rupture e.g. Ventral rupture.

of the hernia, which have protruded through the neck. Here is shown omentum, which is one of the most common structures to herniate; others include intestine or, of course, any mobile abdominal organ. The contents of the hernia are contained by a **sac or fundus**, which in this case is made up of the peritoneum, subcutaneous tissues and skin.

*The Structure of a Rupture*

Such as occurs through a tear in the abdominal wall, called a ventral rupture, is essentially similar. However, the peritoneal lining is also torn and for this reason it is more common for the contents to stick to the sac by adhesions and therefore become **incarcerated**. Diaphragmatic ruptures are an exception to the type of structure shown in the diagram because here the contents protrude directly into another body cavity, i.e. the thorax, and no covering sac is present. (Fig. 10.8). Correction of both hernias and ruptures consists of returning the contents back into the abdomen if possible, and then closing off the neck with strong sutures.

**Specific types of hernia**

*Umbilical:* Usually seen in puppies, as a small soft swelling at the mid-ventral point of the abdomen. This can usually be left alone, providing that it is not causing problems because the hernia tends not to grow with the puppy and so becomes smaller and relatively less important; or correction can be performed at the same time as a midline laparotomy, e.g. spaying. Large hernias should, however, be corrected as soon as the animal is old enough because of the risk of strangulation and also for the cosmetic appearance. Some veterinary surgeons employ an encircling abdominal bandage for a few days following repair, as an extra support.

*Inguinal:* This is much more common in the bitch, but in both sexes the abdominal contents enter the hernial sac via the inguinal canal.

*IN THE BITCH*—the contents are usually either uterus (usually enlarged by pregnancy or pyometra), intestine or bladder. These result in a swelling situated in the groin.

*IN THE DOG*—is usually an emergency as small intestine an emergency as small intestine enters the scrotum and tends to strangulate quickly.

**Specific types of rupture**

*Diaphragmatic:* The diaphragm normally separates the thoracic from the abdominal cavity, and assists in respiration. If a tear occurs, respiration is also hindered because protrusion of abdominal organs into the thorax will cause compression of the lungs, so these animals are obvious anaesthetic risks. Repair, performed if possible once the animal has recovered from any initial shock, is usually performed via the abdomen following laparotomy.

*Ventral:* Where a tear occurs in the body wall at any point other than the umbilicus or the inguinal canal. It is usually seen after severe trauma, such as RTA or a mauling by a large dog. The animal again is usually shocked and sometimes an abdominal support bandage can be useful whilst it is awaiting surgery provided, of course, that the contents of the rupture can be fully reduced back into the abdomen beforehand.

*Eventration:* is the term given to the breakdown of all or part of the repair of a laparotomy incision, which allows prolapse of abdominal contents, sometimes on to the floor! In this unfortunate situation, the animal must be prevented from damaging its own intestines.

*Perineal:* This is nearly always seen in old male dogs, which show difficulty defaecating and also have a swelling on one or even both sides of the anus in the perineal region. Although dietary management can help, surgery is nearly always required and an enema is useful on the day preceding surgery in order to empty the rectum. Occasionally the bladder can come to occupy the rupture and become strangulated, which will require emergency treatment. After surgery a diet high in fibre (vegetables, bran, "Isogel") is useful to make defaecation easier.

**Ear and eye**

*The Ear*

Inflammation of the ear, **otitis**, is very common in practice and can have a wide range of causes. The ear flap or *pinna* can be damaged by a bite or it may be the site of haematoma formation where the animal bursts a blood vessel under the skin on the inside of the pinna due to excessive head shaking or scratching. In this situation, the blood clot should be surgically removed once the bleeding vessel has sealed (see Haematoma) and the dead space left behind is then usually obliterated by sutures through the full thickness of the pinna. These sutures can be passed through a button on either side of the pinna to further compress the "dead space" and to prevent the sutures tearing through. *Otitis externa* or inflammation involving the ear canal itself down to the level of the eardrum or tympanic membrane is the usual underlying reason for aural haematoma formation. It can be due to such factors as foreign bodies e.g. grass seeds, the ear mite *Otodectes*, poor conformation e.g. a floppy pinna, and many others. If the cause can be identified, for example **by using an auroscope**, then it must be removed and the associated inflammatory reaction treated. Grass seeds can be removed with the aid of the auroscope and narrow crocodile forceps, ear mites can be killed using the types of ear preparations available to soothe the inflamed ear and treat infection. The nurse should become familiar with the types of preparation used in her practice, their indications, and how to instil them effectively. Some animals will benefit considerably from the use of cerumenolytics to loosen and dissolve excess wax in the ear, or the ear may be gently cleansed using a dilute (0.5%) solution of Cetrimide (Cetavlon) followed by copious lavage with saline. The latter technique can sometimes be performed in the conscious dog but is best combined with general anaesthesia to allow proper cleansing and examination of an often very painful ear.

Cases which do not respond to such medical management require surgery to improve both the drainage and degree of aeration or ventilation of the ear canal. This usually involves removing the lateral portion of the ear canal by performing an **aural resection**. Some dogs may attempt to scratch their sutures and here an Elizabethan collar can be useful although it must be kept clean of blood and exudate. Another means of protecting the ear, which is also useful following surgery on aural haematomas, is to bandage the ear flap(s) to the head.

*Otitis media* or inflammation of the middle ear cavity is a not uncommon complication following rupture of the eardrum due to longstanding otitis externa, or infection may ascend through the *Eustachian tube* from the pharynx. This is often very difficult to cure and it is important to treat adequately cases of otitis externa to prevent them from becoming chronic and resulting in otitis media.

*Otitis interna* or damage to the delicate organs of balance or occasionally hearing, is an uncommon complication of otitis media resulting in usually a loss of balance and head tilt. Similar signs can occur for an unknown reason in cats of any age, or old dogs where the animal is sometimes euthanased with the erroneous diagnosis of "a stroke". In fact many of these cases will recover completely in 1 to 2 weeks.

### The Eye

*The eyelids* may either be rolled inwards, **entropion**, causing the eyelashes to rub against the cornea; or they may roll outwards, **ectropion**, causing a disturbance to the circulation of tears. In a few instances these two disorders may be combined in the same animal resulting in a so-called "diamond eye". The other not uncommon condition affecting the eyelids is the presence of small hairs growing from the lid margin, called **distichiasis**, which themselves abrade the cornea. Each of these conditions is best treated surgically.

*Conjunctivitis*—will be a sequel to these three conditions although it can also result from other disorders such as virus infections particularly distemper, foreign bodies beneath the eyelids e.g. grass seeds, or inflammatory disorders within the eyeball for example following a penetrating wound.

*Trauma to the eye* may cause damage to the eyelids or the cornea, and occasionally dogs particularly those of the brachycephalic group may present with complete **prolapse of an eyeball.** As a first aid measure the eyeball should be prevented from drying out by ophthalmic ointment and/or KY jelly and supported by a saline soaked soft gauze pad. Replacement into the socket should be performed as soon as possible.

A sequel particularly to disorders of the eyelids or foreign bodies is an inflammation of the cornea or **keratitis**, and the surface of the cornea may actually become ulcerated. The normally clear cornea will first become cloudy, an ulcer is present is often very hard to see unless the exposed corneal tissues are stained with fluorescein. In very severe cases or perhaps following an injury to the eyeball, the cornea can rupture which will generally result in blindness.

*Glaucoma* is another disorder of the eye that can result in blindness. The disturbance in the circulation of aqueous humour causes a rise in pressure within the eyeball, which in turn causes irreparable damage to the delicate retina. One possible cause of obstruction to flow of the aqueous is a dislocation of the normally fixed lens into the anterior chamber, commonly seen in the terrier breeds.

Typically the eye will become suddenly very painful and blindness rapidly ensues. Unless medical and usually also surgical therapy is instituted within a very short period of time after onset, then the blindness will be permanent.

*Cataract* is due to the lens becoming opaque, this can arise from a variety of reasons and if complete will result in considerable loss of vision. As well as a keratitis or cataract causing the eye to appear opaque, this can also result from inflammation or pus within the anterior chamber.

The retina may be involved in a number of congenital disorders e.g. Progressive Retinal Atrophy (PRA) and Collie Eye Anomaly to name but a few, and these are the subject of several schemes run by the British Veterinary Association and Kennel Club with which the nurse should become familiar. The nurse should be able to advise dog breeders and owners of the correct ages for presenting dogs for inspection.

## (e) Tumours

D. G. EARNSHAW

### Nature and Significance

All neoplasms (new growths) are commonly referred to as tumours and the term cancer should be restricted to the malignant type of growth. There is a growing awareness of the need to report any unexplained lumps or growths found in animals and the animal nurse may well be the first person to hear about these problems. Some growths are benign and will not grow again if removed.

With advances in the care of domestic pets, longer lives are expected in animals and it is not surprising that neoplasia has become more important as a cause of death in dogs and cats. The nurse should be well informed about the types of tumours, treatments available and any preventive measures to reduce the chances of cancer causing death. It has been recognized for some time that mammary tumours of the bitch will often increase in size during oestrus and immediately afterwards but the nurse must be able to distinguish this type of gland swelling from the generalized enlargement of the mammary glands in psuedo-pregnancy.

There has been no dramatic advance in the knowledge of the causes of tumours but the extensive research programmes are now showing why certain cells of the body start increasing in numbers and are no longer under the control of the homeostatic mechanisms of the body. Recent research points to the importance of oncogenes as being a factor in causing the rapid growth of cells. The work on feline leukaemia indicated a virus affecting the younger cat and the possibility of a vaccine that can be used in prevention of this disease of cats is awaited. There is the possibility of eradicating this tumour of cats since the virus is a fragile one and is easily killed by disinfectants, heat and cold. Unlike other cancers that still need investigation, the virus found to cause cat leukaemia is transmissible to kittens up to 4 months old since their immune systems are not fully developed (p 496).

Tumours may occur at almost any site in the body; the commoner sites are skin, the mammary glands, the alimentary tract (from mouth to rectum), testicle (dog), bones (especially limb bones of the giant breeds—Wolf Hounds etc) and the lymphatic system. The solid enlargements of lymphoid tissue are more common than the circulatory leukaemias in animals. Canine lymphosarcoma is probably the tumour that the RANA will most easily recognize particularly in the form where all the superficial lymph nodes become enlarged. Feline leukaemia is being diagnosed more and more frequently and many cat owners are aware of the blood test for leukaemia in the cat (p 497).

### Benign and malignant tumours

Benign tumours usually grow quite slowly and for this reason may not be noticed by the owners of pet animals until the growth is quite large. The nurse should be aware that the person who has discovered the lump may be in a considerable state of anxiety and tact will be required in advising on whether a growth is benign or malignant. In many instances, the veterinary surgeon will advise surgical treatment so that a biopsy of the tumour can be taken for laboratory examination.

**Benign tumours** are distinguished by their well developed capsules, they are usually easily separated from adjacent tissues and do not usually exert serious pathological effects. They may be dangerous if their position causes pressure on adjacent structures. A swelling under the skin surface may be liable to accidental injury with haemorrhage from the surface of the tumour. Some benign tumours may produce excess hormones.

Lipomas are very common in the older animal especially if there is a tendency to obesity: this suggests that these tumours are merely an overproduction of normal fat cells. A lipoma on the leg may be harmful in that it will interfere with the animal's normal walking.

Adenoma is the name given to a benign tumour of glandular tissue. The tumour found on the perineum of the older dog is one of the most common examples: these are known as Hepatoid gland (perianal) tumours and some of these hepatoid tumours may be malignant. Papilloma is a wart like tumour found in dogs and cats, it arises from epithelial tissues. The papilloma found in the mouths of young dogs is caused by a virus, it may be recognized as small greyish warts on the gums or inside of the lips. The same virus may cause warts on the feet of the young dog, various treatments have been tried and an autogenous vaccine may produce a quicker return to normal than direct applications to the wart. The papilloma found on the ear of the cat should be treated as a potential cancer and total excision of all affected tumour tissue is advised. Multiple wart growths in old dogs are usually another type of tumour, a sebaceous adenoma. The frequency with which warts are met in old Poodles and other breeds that are clipped frequently suggests that mechanical irritation may predispose these breeds of dogs to warts in old age.

Melanomas in the skin of the dog are often benign, usually they will be seen in the older dog as blackish round lumps on the surface of the skin, they grow slowly and there may be very many of them on the body. Melanomas of the mouth are usually malignant in animals. Occasionally a melanoma will be found on a cat's skin which can grow to a size of two centimetres or more. Malignant melanoma is a very dangerous cancer and is notorious for the ease with which its cells invade the blood and are planted at other places in the body. The spread of tumour cells to other sites in the body is called **metastasis**. This spread to the regional lymph node and the lungs is not uncommon in the Scottish Terrier and sometimes the Black Labrador Retriever. It is thought that some of the melanoma cells must migrate towards a blood vessel and they do this in response to laminin, a protein secreted by the basement membrane of the blood vessel. In these malignant melanomas, the dog's urine can be examined for the excretion of excess black melanin pigment. The use of a biopsy to examine these tumours is not without danger as the surgical procedure may make the tumour cells more likely to spread rapidly.

**Malignant growths** are usually known as carcinomas although the type of malignant growth that affects the tissues that originate from the mesodermal layers of the embryo, is called a sarcoma. These malignant growths are usually irregular in shape, often grow quite rapidly and infiltrate into surrounding tissues so that there is no capsule recognizable. The histological appearance of a biopsy taken from a malignant tumour is one with large nucleoli, and many mitotic figures as the nuclei are frequently dividing.

Tumours of the mammary glands may be small enough to be overlooked by the pet owner but when they grow rapidly the skin is stretched so that ulcers form that are recognized as a bleeding or infected area on the animal's abdomen. Metastasis is frequent, either to the regional lymph node or to one of the other filtering organs such as lungs, liver or kidneys. The sarcoma of the mammary gland may have developed from a benign mixed mammary tumour that existed as a small slow growing tumour in the gland. Adenomas and carcinomas of the mammary glands of dogs and cats are also seen. Early excision of small mammary tumours is advised and biopsy material should always be collected. The mammary tumour of the bitch can largely be prevented if spaying is performed before the second oestrous cycle. In the United Kingdom, mammary tumours are almost never seen in the 2,000 or so spayed guide dog bitches. These dogs live and work in a variety of domestic and industrial situations and may be more prone to tumours in old age than non-working dogs, but mammary tumours are rare.

In cats, mammary tumours develop more often in old age and the animal nurse should be aware that these are carcinomas and treatment surgically will be less successful than in the bitch. The tumour that will be most often met in the cat is the lymphosarcoma and can affect cats young and old. When affecting the alimentary canal it may cause diarrhoea with an associated loss of appetite and vomiting (p 497).

The liver and kidneys of the cat may also be infiltrated with lymphosarcoma cells and death may occur soon after the cat is first noticed to be ill. The lympho-sarcoma of the thymus gland of the young cat may first be seen as causing a respiratory problem but X-ray examination reveals the enlarged thymus in the thorax.

Although, there are many other types of malignant tumour such as the osteosarcoma affecting bones and the epithelioma, these are fortunately uncommon. The lympho-sarcoma of the dog is less often seen than the tumour of the cat, when all the superficial lymph nodes are enlarged, it is known as pseudo-Hodgkins disease.

The veterinary nurse as a technician may have an important role in the collection of biopsy material from any tumour excised by the surgeon. She must make sure that the sample contains some of the underlying tumour and a sliver of the normal tissue if possible. Each specimen should not be too large and should be fixed in 10% formol saline or other suitable fixative for 24-48 hours. The specimens should be well immersed in a good volume of fluid in a wide-mouthed container. The fixed specimen, correctly labelled, can then be sent to the laboratory wrapped in cotton wool soaked in the fixative and sealed up in two or three polythene bags, one inside the other. Alternatively, plastic specimen bottles can be used to hold small biopsy slices soaked in fixative (p. 456). It is advisable that the owner of the animal that has an operation involving a biopsy, is informed that there may be 2 or 3 weeks delay when an outside laboratory is used for biopsy examinations. The pathologist should be given as much information as possible about the animal from which the biopsy has been taken as this will be of use in arriving at a diagnosis and prognosis.

The treatment of neoplasms will most frequently be by surgical excision sometimes aided by cauterization. The application of extreme cold (often liquid nitrogen) is a method employed in some veterinary practices. Radiotherapy is of

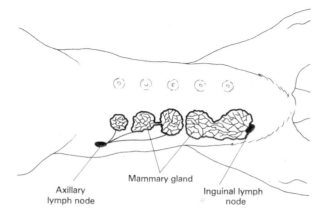

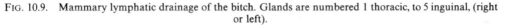

|  | Axillary lymph node | Mammary gland | Inguinal lymph node |

FIG. 10.9.　Mammary lymphatic drainage of the bitch. Glands are numbered 1 thoracic, to 5 inguinal, (right or left).

most value when used after the surgical excision of a malignant growth but it is not generally available except at specialized centres. Chemotherapy is often of benefit in some of the lymphoid tumours in dogs; results are very variable, sometimes the animal lives only 2 to 3 months but others can live 2 or 3 years, the majority fall between these ranges. Hormonal therapy is often used to cause the regression of perianal tumours, oestrogens may be injected at the tumour site or given orally. Corticosteroids are used in the treatment of lymphosarcoma orally or parenterally.

Editor: The help of Dr L. N. Owen is acknowledged in revising this section.

## (f) Anaesthesia in the Dog and Cat

R. S. JONES

### Introduction

The Protection of Animals (Anaesthetics) Act of 1964 controls the administration of anaesthetics to animals in Great Britain. In addition to legal requirements one must always consider the humane aspects of procedures which may be carried out on animals. As a secondary consideration anaesthesia is often required as a means of restraint, particularly in the unco-operative patient. Therefore one of the most important duties of the RANA is to assist the veterinary surgeon in the administration of anaesthesia. Whilst no practising veterinary surgeon or RANA employed by him may be expected to be familiar with every anaesthetic method available, it is extremely important that a range of techniques should be utilized. The importance of the choice of a suitable anaesthetic method to suit a particular animal affected with a certain condition cannot be over-emphasized. This may often mean the difference between the survival of the animal or its death. This approach is to be preferred to the use of the same anaesthetic method for all animals whatever their species or clinical condition. Under the economic conditions of general practice it is essential, however, that the RANA should be familiar with all the anaesthetic techniques that are in general usage in his or her practice.

An anaesthetic agent may be used to produce general anaesthesia, or local anaesthetic agents can be used to produce regional or local anaesthesia. General anaesthesia can be produced by the administration of gases or vapours, by inhalation or by other drugs which can be administered parenterally. If the drugs are of an irritant nature, or a rapid effect is desired, they may be given by intravenous injection.

A tranquilizing drug such as acepromazine can be administered to animals to reduce their awareness of their surroundings, make handling easier and hence enable minor procedures to be carried out. One of the important uses of these drugs is for premedication prior to general anaesthesia. Certain drug combinations of a potent analgesic (pain-killing drug such as fentanyl) with a tranquillizer (e.g. one of the butyrophenone group such as droperidol) are used to produce a state of neuroleptanalgesia. Under the influence of neuroleptanalgesic drugs, examination of the animal and certain minor surgical procedures can be carried out.

### Types of Anaesthesia

#### Local anaesthesia

The drugs which are most commonly employed for this purpose are lignocaine hydrochloride and procaine hydrochloride. These drugs produce a temporary block of the transmission of nervous impulses both in sensory and motor nerves, and hence produce a loss of sensation and of motor power in the area supplied by nerves. It is common practice to add 1 in 50,000–200,000 adrenaline hydrochloride to local anaesthetic solution in order to constrict small blood vessels at the site of injection. This has the effect of reducing the rate of removal of the local anaesthetic drug from the site by the circulation and hence prolongs its action.

It is important to remember that all local anaesthetic drugs are toxic and they should be used in as low a concentration and in as small a volume as possible.

Local anaesthetic drugs can be administered by one of three methods:

(1) surface application;
(2) infiltration anaesthesia;
(3) regional anaesthesia.

### Surface anaesthesia

Surface anaesthesia may be produced by spraying a highly volatile liquid such as ethyl chloride on to the area. The rapid evaporation of the volatile liquid from the skin produces freezing and a localized anaesthesia. If great care is not taken in the use of these substances tissue damage and even necrosis can result. Local anaesthetic agents, either in the form of a gel or in solution, can be used to produce surface anaesthesia of the skin and mucous membranes. However, their value and use is limited. It is probably only **on the cornea** that surface anaesthesia has any real application, and for this cocaine or proparacaine are used. These drugs are too toxic to be used for parenteral administration and, therefore, their use is limited to the eye.

### Infiltration anaesthesia

Infiltration anaesthesia is produced by the injection of a local anaesthetic from a hypodermic syringe and fine-bore needle (22 or 23 gauge). Alternatively, if small areas are involved a dental syringe may be employed. It is important to limit the injection to the site of surgery, and to avoid toxic effects care should be taken to prevent injection into a blood vessel.

### Regional anaesthesia

Regional anaesthesia is produced by either blocking nerves within the bony spinal canal or main nerve trunks before they divide.

In **epidural** (or extradural) anaesthesia a needle is introduced into the bony spinal canal through the lumbo-sacral space. An injection of local anaesthetic solution is made which blocks the spinal nerves before they leave the spinal canal. Varying degrees of anaesthesia of the hind part of the animal can be achieved by varying the dose of local anaesthetic employed. A solution of 1% lignocaine hydrochloride with adrenaline is preferred. This technique can be used in the dog but is rarely employed in the cat, and it is advisable to administer a potent sedative to the animal.

A technique of **blocking the nerve** supply to the teeth in order to carry out dental surgery has been described in the dog and cat. However, the lack of co-operation on the part of the patient means that this technique is of limited value. A technique of brachial plexus block has also been described in the dog. This involves the injection of local anaesthetic into the brachial plexus region in the axilla. Anaesthesia is produced in the forelimb distal to the elbow joint.

One other technique which may be utilized to produce anaesthesia of the limbs, and in particular the forelimb, is intravenous regional anaesthesia. A 1% solution of lignocaine hydrochloride without adrenaline is used for this procedure. A tourniquet is placed on the limb proximal to the area to be operated on. The local anaesthetic is injected into a suitable vein and anaesthesia is evident within 10 minutes and lasts as long as the tourniquet is in place.

### General anaesthesia

The condition of general anaesthesia has been described as a state of unconsciousness produced by a reversible and controlled intoxication of the central nervous system. During this state there is a lowered sensitivity to stimuli from the external environment and a reduced motor response to these stimuli.

General anaesthetic agents can be gases or the vapours of volatile liquids, both of which enter the body by inhalation into lungs, or non-volatile substances which are usually administered intravenously. The latter may be either water-soluble (e.g. thiopentone or pentobarbitone) or lipid soluble (e.g. the combination of alphaxalone and alphadolone acetate).

The action of anaesthetic agents on body tissues is not fully understood, but theories which have been advanced suggest action either inside the nerve cell or on its surface or at both sites. It is the action on the central nervous system which is of greater importance in anaesthesia.

Inhalational agents (gases or vapours) reach the central nervous system in three phases:

(1) The transfer of the gases or vapours from the outside through the respiratory tract into lung alveoli which are lined by epithelium.
(2) The diffusion of the gases or vapours through the alveolar epithelium and through the endothelial cells lining the lung capillaries into the blood of the pulmonary veins.
(3) Diffusion of the anaesthetic agent from solution in the blood via the capillaries and their endothelial lining into the tissues. The actual distribution of the anaesthetic agent into each type of tissue depends on a number of factors, mainly the blood supply and lipid (fat) content. The central nervous system has an extremely good blood supply and a high lipid content, and hence a large proportion of the circulating anaesthetic agent is taken up by the brain.

The process of gaseous absorption depends upon the laws governing the diffusion of gases through membranes. Elimination of the anaesthetic agents also depends on the same principle. It will be appreciated. therefore, that although the blood supply to and the structure of the brain enables rapid and relatively high concentrations of gases to accumulate in the brain, this is governed by the concentration in blood and alveoli which in turn is related to the solubility of the particular agent in blood. If anaesthesia is of short duration, the concentration in the central nervous system will fall rapidly due to the agent passing back into the blood and hence either into the alveoli or into other tissues of the body. The distribution into other tissues depends in no small measure on the lipid solubility of the particular agent. Therefore, in order to achieve a satisfactory and prolonged state of anaesthesia, the concentration of anaesthetic agent in the central nervous system and other tissues must be maintained.

Non-inhalational anaesthetic agents, if they are not administered by the intravenous route, must be absorbed from the alimentary tract, muscle or other sites into the blood and thence to the body tissues.

Inhalational agents (except trichloroethylene) are eliminated almost entirely through the lungs but non-inhalational anaesthetic agents require to be broken down or rendered inactive by the liver and excreted by way of the kidneys. This process can be prolonged and depends a great deal on the proper functioning of the liver and kidneys. In the majority of cases, therefore, recovery from the inhalational agents is much more rapid than from agents which are administered parenterally.

**Anaesthesia is conveniently described as having four stages**, and it is necessary to be aware of this subject in order to understand the action of anaesthetic agents. During the induction of anaesthesia with inhalational agents, particularly diethyl ether (the classification of the stages is based upon the action of this agent in man), it is possible to recognize each stage separately. Induction of anaesthesia with certain agents such as thiopentone sodium produces such a rapid transition from consciousness, through stages I and II to stage III, that these stages are difficult to recognize.

### Stage I

The stage of **voluntary excitement**. This lasts from the beginning of induction to loss of consciousness. During this period the animal may exhibit signs of fear and apprehension, together with a rise in respiratory and pulse rates. It may also hold its breath, particularly if irritant vapours are being administered. Urine and faeces may be voided. The pupils is dilated and the pedal reflexes are still present.

### Stage II

The stage of **involuntary excitement**. It lasts from the onset of unconsciousness to the onset of automatic respiration. During this stage reflex responses to stimuli are exaggerated. The animals may struggle, breath-hold and possibly vomit. Violent and unpredictable movements often occur.

Stages I and II can often be associated with difficulties for both anaesthetist and patient. The untoward effects can be reduced and often eliminated by the judicious use of premedication with phenothiazine derivative tranquillizers (e.g. acepromazine) and/or analgesics (e.g. pethidine).

### Stage III

The stage of **surgical anaesthesia** which lasts from the onset of automatic breathing to the eventual cessation of respiration. It is convenient to divide stage III into three planes of anaesthesia.

*Plane I* is indicated by the onset of automatic respiration and is considered to be light anaesthesia. Respiration is regular, deep and rapid. Limb movements cease and there is no struggling but the pedal reflex is still maintained. As anaesthesia progresses through plane I the movement of the eyeball from side to side is reduced and eventually it becomes fixed. The palpebral and corneal reflexes are also gradually reduced during plane I. Minor surgical procedures and diagnostic investigations can be carried out during this plane.

*Plane II* is indicated by movement of the eyeball to a downward position. Muscular relaxation is more apparent and respiration is regular but becomes slower and shallower. The pedal reflex becomes sluggish and may be absent. This plane is considered to be medium anaesthesia and is adequate for the majority of surgery except for intra-abdominal procedures.

*Plane III* is indicated by an increase in

respiratory rate whilst the depth decreases, and as the depth of anaesthesia increases there is a pause between inspiration and expiration (intercostal lag). The eyeball becomes central and fixed again. The pedal reflex is completely absent and the abdominal muscles are relaxed. This plane is considered to be deep anaesthesia and is adequate for all surgical procedures.

*Stage IV*

This is the stage at which respiratory paralysis occurs. The onset is characterized by the onset of solely diaphragmatic respiration which finally ceases. The pulse is rapid, the pupils dilate, and the eye takes on a glazed appearance. Cyanosis of the mucous membranes occurs and progresses to a characteristic grey colour which indicates cardiac arrest and death.

## General Anaesthetic Agents

For the purposes of description it is convenient to divide the drugs used in general anaesthesia into three separate groups:

(1) premedicant agents;
(2) induction agents;
(3) maintenance agents.

We can also consider three different procedures of premedication induction and maintenance of general anaesthesia. However, it is important to remember that each "state" merges one into the other and also that one drug may be used for more than one of these purposes (e.g. halothane is usually used for maintenance of anaesthesia but can be used for induction, whereas the reverse applies to thiopentone sodium, which is normally used only for induction of anaesthesia but in repeated dosage can be used to maintain anaesthesia).

## 1. Premedicant agents

There are a number of reasons why it is considered desirable to premedicate animals before anaesthesia. The first and main reason is to produce a quiet, calm and relaxed patient for the induction of anaesthesia. Quiet and gentle handling is also extremely important in this respect, particularly as the animal will have been brought into a strange environment. Linked with a quiet induction is the production of a quiet and pain-free emergence from general anaesthesia. Premedication can be used to prevent vomiting both during the induction of and emergence from general anaesthesia. Atropine premedication is used to block the parasympathetic nervous system and hence reduce vagal tone.

A variety of routes can be used for the administration of premedicant drugs. If a rapid action is required then the intravenous route is the one of choice. If, however, speed is not the main consideration and one wishes to obtain the maximum effect in about 30 minutes, then the intramuscular route is the one of choice. In the case of an extremely fractious animal it may be considered desirable for the owner to administer oral premedication, such as acepromazine, before presenting their animal to a veterinary surgeon. The speed of onset of the drug will vary and will depend on a number of factors not the least of which is the state of the stomach. A period of at least 1 hour should be allowed to achieve the maximum effect.

(a) *Atropine sulphate* is a water-soluble alkaloid derived from the "deadly nightshade" (*Atropa belladonna*). The main action of atropine is on the heart rate, which it increases, and hence it offsets the deleterious slowing of the heart which may be produced by some anaesthetic agents (e.g. halothane). A well-known property of atropine is its effect on the reduction of salivary and bronchial secretion during anaesthesia, particularly when irritant agents such as ether are employed. Probably the oldest-known property of atropine is that it dilates the pupil of the eye, but this is only seen in the conscious animal as this effect is overcome by general anaesthetic agents. The dose of atropine in the average cat is 0.3 mg. In the dog the dose range varies from 0.3 mg to 1.8 mg depending on size. It can be given either subcutaneously, intramuscularly or intravenously.

(b) *The phenothiazine derivatives or ataractic drugs* are used extensively as premedicant drugs. They have a number of properties which are common to the large number of drugs in the group. They produce sedation and calm the animals, making them less aware of their surroundings. However, they do not cause drowsiness. The drugs in this group potentiate the action of anaesthetic agents and reduce the total dose administered, thereby reducing the overall dangers from toxicity. By their sedative action they usually ensure a quiet induction and recovery from general anaesthesia. The drugs have an antiemetic action which is useful both immediately before and after anaesthesia. There are a number of drugs in this group which are available for veterinary use. The most important one is acepromazine maleate. The dose of acepromazine in the dog and cat is 0.1–0.2 mg/kg intramuscularly and 1–3 mg/kg orally.

(c) *Analgesic drugs* are used to relieve pain. They are all, however, subject to the Misuse of Drugs Act and hence subject to control which effectively reduces their use to the veterinary surgeon or under his direct supervision. There are three drugs which can be considered for use in veterinary practice. It is well to remember that whilst they may be very effective in reducing the effect of pain these drugs can cause a **profound depression of respiration**, which can be extremely serious in the sick or injured animal.

(i) *Pethidine* is a synthetic drug, which is used primarily as an analgesic, in the cat and dog. It does, however, have a sedative action in the cat. An intramuscular dose of 1–2 mg/kg is considered to be effective. At a lower dose it can be combined with a tranquillizing drug for premedication or sedation. Its administration is compatible with that of atropine. Overdosage rarely occurs, but if it does the signs include hyperaesthesia, disorientation and incoordination; convulsions are rarely seen.

(ii) *Morphine* is a plant alkaloid obtained from the opium poppy. It is a powerful analgesic drug but it also produces vomiting and has a powerful respiratory depressant effect. Its use is limited to the dog only at a total dose of up to 10 mg. In the *cat morphine* causes maniacal excitement and is *contraindicated*.

(d) *Xylazine* is a synthetic non-narcotic sedative compound with mild analgesic and muscle-relaxant properties. It can be used in both cats and dogs at a dosage rate of 1.0–4.0 mg/kg, and the degree of sedation achieved appears to be dose-related. It produces emesis in a considerable proportion of cases. The intramuscular route of administration is the one of choice.

## 2. Induction agents

The main drugs which are used for the induction of anaesthesia belong to the barbiturate group. There are a large number of drugs in this group but only three will be considered here: thiopentone sodium, methohexitone sodium and pentobarbitone sodium. These three are all water soluble and are normally administered intravenously in both cat and dog. They are all primarily hypnotic (sleep producing) drugs and have little or no analgesic properties.

(a) *Thiopentone sodium* is the most widely used drug for the induction of anaesthesia in both man and animals. It can also be used as a sole agent to produce anaesthesia of short duration for minor surgical procedures. Occasionally the intermittent injection technique may be used to produce anaesthesia of prolonged duration, but this is not to be recommended as it can lead to a number of complications including prolonged recovery. A concentrated solution is irritant, and if it is accidentally injected extravascularly can cause tissue necrosis and sloughing of the area. A solution of 2.5% is recommended for dogs over 5 kg in weight, and for cats and dogs under 5 kg a 1% solution may be employed. When the drug is to be used as an induction agent a dose of 20 mg/kg is drawn up into a syringe and up to half of this amount (i.e. 10 mg/kg) is given by rapid intravenous injection. The actual amount injected will depend on the clinical condition of the patient, the rate of injection and the skill of the anaesthetist. Pre-medication can also reduce the amount of thiopentone or other induction agent due to a potentiation effect. It will, therefore, be obvious that it is difficult to be specific on dosage.

(b) *Methohexitone sodium* is considered to be twice as potent as thiopentone and hence is usually at half the concentration and half the dose is required. Its action is similar to thiopentone but recovery is more rapid. It is considerably more expensive than thiopentone, but its main advantage lies in the rapid recovery in animals (e.g. Greyhounds and Whippets) which

tend to "sleep" for a prolonged period after thiopentone administration and in animals which are to be returned to their owners after a short period of anaesthesia.

(c) *Pentobarbitone sodium* has been used for many years as the sole anaesthetic agent in dogs and cats. However, its use has been superseded by more modern techniques. There are a number of disadvantages in its use including a prolonged recovery period. A dose of 30 mg/kg is usually considered to be necessary although this may be variable. In contrast to thiopentone the injection of pentobarbitone should be made slowly and the depth of anaesthesia assessed by testing reflexes such as the pedal as small incremental doses are given. Its long duration of action can be utilized in the treatment of convulsions produced by such poisons as strychnine.

(d) *A combination of steroid anaesthetics, alphadolone acetate and alphaxalone* have recently become available for veterinary use. It is unique in that it is insoluble in water; the solvent is polyoxyethylated castor oil in saline. It is used in cats and laboratory animals but not in dogs. It is used at a rate of 9 mg (0.75 ml) per kg intravenously either as an induction agent or for operations of short duration. It is non-irritant if given extravascularly and can be used for sedation and possibly anaesthesia by the intramuscular route. A dose of 12 mg (1 ml) per kg is recommended by the intramuscular route, but up to 18 mg ($1\frac{1}{2}$ ml) per kg can be used. The intramuscular route can sometimes give variable results, and the intravenous mode of administration is preferred. The administration of "Saffan" can sometimes produce an anaphylactoid reaction in the cat. This is shown as hyperaemia of the ears, nose and paws with occasional oedema of the ears and interdigital areas. Such reactions are usually of little consequence.

### 3.  Maintenance agents

The drugs in this group are either gases or volatile liquids with boiling points lower than that of water (with the exception of methoxyflurane).

(a) *Diethyl ether* (commonly known as ether) is probably the most commonly used anaesthetic agent in veterinary practice. It is a colourless liquid with a boiling point at 35°C and a vapour heavier than air. When the vapour is mixed with air or oxygen it is inflammable and can be explosive, and extreme care should be taken with the use of electrical appliances in its presence. Nakes flames should be extinguished and it is important that diathermy should not be used during surgery. It should be stored in dark bottles away from sunlight and sources of heat, and it is inadvisable to use it in the vicinity of X-ray machines. Ether vapour has a characteristic smell and during anaesthesia produces salivary and mucous secretion due to its irritant effect on the mucosa of the mouth, pharynx and respiratory tract. This effect can be avoided by the prior administration of atropine. Ether is considered to be a very safe anaesthetic agent as there is a wide margin between the anaesthetic and toxic doses. It is also considered to be a compound of low potency and without premedication induction of anaesthesia tends to be relatively slow and accompanied by considerable excitement. Ether may be administered by any of the common inhalation methods employed in anaesthesia.

(b) *Halothane* is widely used in veterinary anaesthesia. It is a colourless liquid with a boiling point of 50°C and is non-inflammable and non-explosive. It is considered to be **four times as potent as ether**, and a vapour concentration of up to 4% is recommended for the induction of anaesthesia and of 1–2% for maintenance. It has

a safety factor that has been shown to be twice that of ether. Recovery from halothane anaesthesia is rapid, and where no other agents are used animals can walk normally within 30 minutes of cessation of administration Halothane administration tends to slow the pulse rate and to reduce blood pressure. It can be administered by all of the common methods used for inhalational agents, but on the grounds of economy and ease of administration it is best administered with oxygen, or oxygen-nitrous oxide in a semi-closed or closed system utilizing anaesthetic equipment. Whilst a number of reports have occurred in the medical literature of so-called "halothane jaundice" a considerable amount of controversy surrounds this subject. There is no real evidence to suggest that under conditions of clinical anaesthesia that a similar condition occurs in domestic animals.

(c) *Methoxyflurane* is a colourless liquid with a characteristic heavy fruity odour and a boiling point of 104°C. It is non-inflammable and non-explosive. Due to the high boiling point of methoxyflurane and its low vapour pressure at room temperature it is not a satisfactory agent for the induction of anaesthesia. Its main use is in the maintenance of anaesthesia after induction with an intravenous agent such as thiopentone sodium. Recovery from methoxyflurane anaesthesia is relatively prolonged when compared to other inhalational anaesthetic agents. It can be used in any type of anaesthetic circuit and method of administration, but on the grounds of economy it is best administered in a closed or semi-closed system.

(d) *Trichlorethylene* is a liquid with a blue dye added to distinguish it from chloroform. It has a characteristic smell and is non-explosive and non-inflammable in the concentrations used in anaesthesia. It has a boiling point of 87°C, which is relatively high, and gives it a low vapour pressure, and, like methoxy-flurane, it is difficult to induce anaesthesia with it, and to give high concentrations which increases its safety. When one attempts to deepen anaesthesia with this drug in the dog and cat, a rapid increase in respiratory rate is often seen which is a distinct disadvantage. Its main use is in supplementing nitrous oxide/oxygen anaesthesia in a semi-closed circuit after induction with a barbiturate. Trichlor-ethylene **should not be used in a closed circuit as it reacts with soda lime to produce toxic products**.

(e) *Cyclopropane* is a colourless gas with a characteristic odour and is available commercially in orange-coloured cylin-ders. It is heavier than air and is a potent anaesthetic agent but is both inflammable and explosive when mixed with air or oxygen. Whilst it can be used for the induction of anaesthesia its main use is in the maintenance of anaesthesia with oxy-gen in a closed circuit in order to reduce the risk of explosions by preventing its escape to the atmosphere. (Note: cyclo-propane is rarely used these days in veterinary practice).

(f) *Nitrous oxide* is a colourless gas with only a faint smell and is available as a compressed liquid in blue-coloured cylinders. It vaporizes on release from the cylinder. Nitrous oxide is relatively non-toxic but is only a weak anaesthetic and usually requires supplementation with one of the volatile agents in veterinary anaesthesia. It is usually administered in a semi-closed circuit and should be administered with at least 30% oxy-gen.

### Basic Anaesthetic Equipment

(a) *Cylinders* which are available both for veterinary and medical anaesthetic purposes are classified by letters from size AA to size J.

Oxygen is supplied in black cylinders* with white necks and the ones commonly used in veterinary anaesthesia are size E (680 L; 24 ft³) and F (1360 L; 48 ft³).

Carbon dioxide for anaesthetic pur-poses is supplied in grey cylinders. Sizes D and E are used commonly.

Nitrous oxide cylinders are blue in colour and sizes D (900 l; 200 gallons) and E (1800 l; 400 gallons) are used com-monly.

Cyclopropane is available in orange cylinders and sizes A (90 l; 20 gallons) and B (180 l; 40 gallons) are usually employed.

(b) *Combined reducing valves and pres-sure gauges* are attached directly to the cylinders in order to reduce the pressure of gas leaving the cylinder and ensure a constant pressure of the gas delivered to the flowmeters. The pressure gauge is required to give an indication of the pressure in the cylinder and hence in the case of oxygen the quantity of gas in the cylinder. No reducing valve is necessary in the case of cyclopropane.

(c) *Flowmeters* are required to control the flow of gas to the patient. A number of types of flowmeter have been described but only the rotameter in common use. Each rotameter is specific to a particular type of gas (e.g. oxygen). It consists of a graduated glass tube (usually in litres or parts of a litre) in which a bobbin is kept afloat by the flow of gas. The higher the flow of gas the higher the bobbin passes up the tube.

(d) *Vaporizers* are required when vola-tile liquids are employed. A large number of different vaporizers have been de-scribed but the Boyle's bottle is the most commonly used in veterinary anaesthesia.

*Nurses should be aware that oxygen cylinders are green in the United States and blue in certain European Countries.

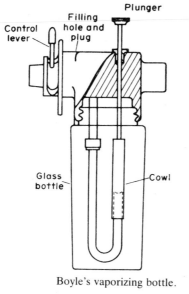

Boyle's vaporizing bottle.

Fig. 10.10.

By means of a control lever it is possible to direct a variable amount of the carrier gas into the bottle and allow the remainder to bypass the bottle. In the ether bottle, there is in addition a cowl which can be raised to a variable distance above the level of or lowered below the surface of the ether to allow higher concentrations to be delivered (Fig. 10.10).

A number of temperature compensated and accurate vaporizers are now being used in veterinary anaesthetic practice. The one which is most commonly used is the "tec" type. The "Fluotec" for use with halothane is the most generally used. These vaporizers are extremely accurate and have dial settings which read directly in percentages of the vapour in the carrier gas or gases.

### Method of administration of inhalational anaesthetic agents

Inhalational agents may be administered to animals by way of one of four systems.

(a) *The open method* is one which is rarely used but may be utilized in emergencies if equipment is not available. It consists of placing lint or similar material near to the animal's nose and dropping the volatile anaesthetic agent on to it. The depth of anaesthesia is controlled by the rate of the drops.

(b) *The semi-open method* again involves the use of lint or a similar absorbable material in a mask through which all the inspired air is made to pass. These two techniques have serious disadvantages and hence they are not employed to any extent at the present time.

(c) *The semi-closed method* of administration requires the use of an anaesthetic machine together with an anaesthetic circuit. The important point about a semi-closed circuit is that it does not involve the use of soda lime to absorb the carbon dioxide exhaled by the animal. In a semi-closed circuit the flow rate of gas has to be high enough to wash all of the expired gases out to the atmosphere. Two types of a semi-closed circuit are in general use in

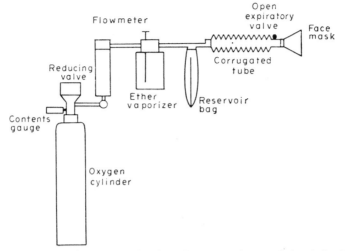

A method of administering ether oxygen in a semi-closed circuit.

FIG. 10.11.

veterinary anaesthesia: (i) Magill circuit, and (ii) Ayre's T-piece.

(i) In the **Magill circuit** the anaesthetic mixture passes from the machine to a reservoir bag and then down a wide bore corrugated tube attached to either a mask or an endotracheal tube. The expired gases pass partly out to the atmosphere through an expiratory (Heidebrink) valve and partly back up the corrugated tubing. During the expiratory pause (i.e. after expiration and before the next inspiration) the flow of gas from the machine forces the rest of the expired gases out to the atmosphere through the expiratory valve. A flow rate equal to the animal's minute volume (i.e. the amount of air breathed per minute) is required to ensure adequate carbon dioxide removal. A typical circuit is shown in Figs. 10.11 and 10.12.

(ii) The **Ayre's T-piece** is recommended especially for small dogs and cats in that it has no valves and hence very little resistance to breathing. A typical Ayre's T-piece with an open-ended bag mounted on the expiratory limb is shown in Fig.

10.13*. The principle of its use is similar to that of the Magill circuit.

(d) **The closed method** of administration of inhalational anaesthetics involves the use of an anaesthetic machine and an anaesthetic circuit (Fig. 10.14). The anaesthetic circuit contains soda lime in order to absorb expired carbon dioxide. As high flow-rates are not necessary to remove the carbon dioxide it is an economical method of administering anaesthetic agents. It should not, however, be used in cats or dogs under 10 kg in weight due to the resistance to respiration which is produced by the soda lime. The anaesthetic agent is administered with oxygen and this mixture is inhaled by the animal. The exhaled gases contain an increased amount of carbon dioxide, but if the mixture is passed through soda lime to remove the carbon dioxide and into a reservoir bag, it can be re-breathed. Small amounts of oxygen are required to supply the animal's

*The figure shows a Jackson Rees modification of the Ayres T-piece. This is the commonest of a number of modifications of the original Ayre's T-piece.

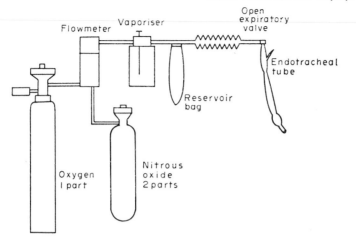

A method for administering trichlorethylene with oxygen/nitrous oxide in a semi-closed circuit.

FIG. 10.12.

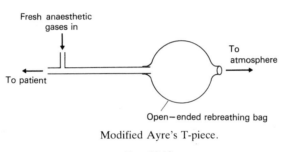

Modified Ayre's T-piece.

FIG. 10.13.

metabolic requirements. Whilst theoretically more anaesthetic agent is not required it has to be added to make up for leaks, passage into rubber and uptake by the body. Soda lime is used in granular form to absorb carbon dioxide by a simple chemical reaction. It consists of 90% calcium hydroxide, 5% sodium hydroxide and 5% silicates and water to prevent powdering. It usually incorporates a dye in order to indicate when its absorbent capacity has been exhausted.

In veterinary anaesthesia two types of closed circuit are employed.

(a) *To and fro system.* In this system the *soda lime canister* (**Water's**) is interposed between the animal and the rebreathing bag (Fig. 10.15).

The fresh gas supply enters the near the animal in order to enable the anaesthetist to effect rapid changes of concentration in an emergency.

(b) *The circle system.* This is more complex and involves the use of *unidirectional valves, a reservoir bag and soda lime* **canister** (Fig. 10.16). This equipment is more expensive and is in limited use in veterinary practice. It is, however, extremely efficient in removing carbon dioxide from anaesthetic mixtures.

Gases are supplied from closed circuits to the patient by mask or more often by endotracheal tubes.

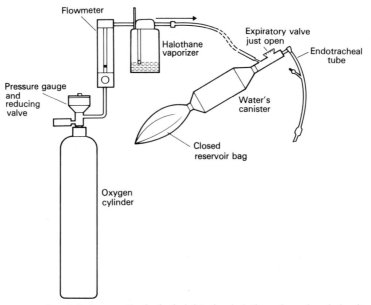

A satisfactory method of administering halothane in a closed circuit.

FIG. 10.14.

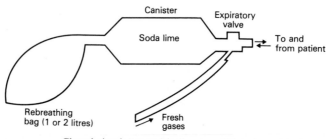

Closed-circuit "to and fro" system (Water's canister).

FIG. 10.15.

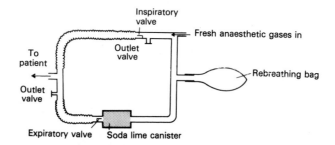

Diagrammatic representation of circle absorber.

FIG. 10.16.

## Miscellaneous Agents

There have been introduced into veterinary practice in the last few years a number of new techniques and drugs which have different effects on the central nervous system from those of conventional anaesthetic agents. These are:

(a) Neuroleptanalgesic agents;

(b) Dissociative agents.

(a) *Neuroleptanalgesia* is produced by administration of a combination of a neuroleptic (or tranquillizer) drug and a powerful analgesic (pain-killing drug). The commonest neuroleptic used are the butyrophenone drugs such as a droperidol or haloanisone. Occasionally the conventional phenothiazine derivative tranquillizers are used. The analgesic drugs which are used are either fentanyl or etorphine. There are three combinations which are used in veterinary practice:

(i) fentanyl and droperidol at a ratio of 50 to 1 and in a dose of 1 ml per 9 kg;

(ii) fentanyl and haloanisone at a dose of 1 ml per 2.3 kg;

(iii) etorphine with methotrimeprazine at a dose rate of 1 ml per 9 kg.

In the first two combinations the analgesic component can be reversed by lethidrone and etorphine is reversed by diprenorphine.

These techniques are useful for minor procedures such as removal of foreign bodies from ears and X-ray examination in fairly healthy animals; but they have serious side effects such as cyanosis, convulsions and whining which makes the exercise of care in their usage essential. It is usually necessary to give atropine before these drugs in order to offset their effect on the heart.

Extreme care is essential in the handling of potent analgesic drugs such as fentanyl and etorphine. The manufacturer's instructions should be studied and, when an emergency occurs, acted upon immediately. **After initial first aid has been carried out then medical attention should be sought as quickly as possible** either by summoning a doctor or an ambulance.

(b) *Dissociative* anaesthesia is a term borrowed from human anaesthesia where patients remain unconscious but retain certain reflexes and where muscle relaxation is not present. The compound which is recommended for use in cats is ketamine hydrochloride at a dose rate of 20–30 mg/kg by intramuscular injection. The effect is rapid and certain but muscular rigidity is a problem, which can usually be overcome by premedication with xylazine.

## Technical Procedures for RANA

There are two important technical procedures in anaesthesia which the RANA may be required to assist with or carry out alone and with which she should be completely familiar. These are to give an intravenous injection and to pass an endotracheal tube.

*In order to give an intravenous injection* it is first essential that the animal should be restrained in the correct manner on a table or trolley. The assistant should stand on the animal's left side. The area over the vein is clipped and the site cleaned with spirit. The vein is then raised by the assistant applying pressure with her thumb at the elbow if the cephalic vein is to be used. The leg should be held in full extension and the right leg is used for a right-handed operator. The operator grasps the animal's leg and tenses the skin over the vein. An eccentric nozzled syringe and a sharp needle of appropriate size are selected. Disposable needles are preferable as they are readily available, sterile and sharp. The needle, attached to the syringe, is introduced through the skin and through the wall of the vein. The plunger is withdrawn slightly to draw blood back into the syringe barrel indicating satisfactory venipuncture. The injection into the vein should not be made until a good flow of blood is observed. The assistant then releases the pressure on the vein but continues to hold the leg in the extended position as the injection is made (p. 305) and Figs. 5.16 and 5.17.

*Endotracheal intubation* is a relatively simple technique in the dog but requires more skill in the cat. When the dog is anaesthetized either with an intravenous or inhalational agent the mouth is opened and a gag is placed between the canine teeth. The head is held up by an assistant and the right-handed operator places the lubricated tube of suitable size in his right hand and pulls the tongue out of the dog's mouth with his left hand. The tube is then introduced into the mouth and the soft palate, which usually lies below the epiglottis, is pushed upwards and backwards. The tip of the tube is used to depress the epiglottis and the entrance to the larynx is observed. The tube is then advanced down the trachea until its tip lies midway between the larynx and the first rib. Care should be taken in the positioning of the endotracheal tube because if it is not inserted far enough then inflation of the cuff may damage the larynx. If the tube is inserted too far into the trachea it may enter one of the bronchi and produce

collapse of the rest of the lungs. The cuff is inflated once the endotracheal tube is in place to produce an airtight seal. Care should be taken to ensure that the cuff is not over-inflated as this may damage the wall of the trachea. The tube is then connected to an anaesthetic apparatus (Fig. 10.17).

In the cat it is necessary to suppress the extreme nervous activity of the larynx either by spraying it with local anaesthetic or by administering a muscle relaxant such as suxamethonium to paralyze the animal and hence its larynx. The technique of introducing the tube is similar, although a laryngoscope may be used to illuminate the pharynx and a stilette may be used to give rigidity to the flexible small endotracheal tube.

### Anaesthetic Monitoring

Whilst there is a considerable amount of sophisticated monitoring equipment produced for use in anaesthesia it is possible to use the human senses and simple equipment to give reliable information regarding the status of anaesthetized patients.

In veterinary anaesthesia the RANA can be responsible for the monitoring of the heart and circulation, the respiratory

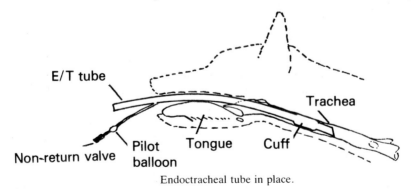

Endoctracheal tube in place.

FIG. 10.17.

system and body temperature without too much sophisticated equipment.

## (1) *The heart and circulation*

(a) Heart. The function of the heart can be monitored by a number of different techniques. The simplest technique involves counting whilst palpating the pulse in the facial, femoral or labiol arteries. Stethoscopes can also be used to detect the heart beat, which can then be counted, either by strapping the instrument to the precordial area or by inserting it into the oesophagus. Oesophageal stethoscopes are available in three different sizes and are positioned within the oesophagus, over the base of the heart. A simple pulse meter attached to the distal part of a limb may be used to give an audible and/or visual indication of the presence or absence of a pulse together with its rate. Electrocardiography can also be used to measure the pulse rate either by the use of a built-in-rate meter or by direct counting of the complexes.

(b) Circulation. Information on the state of a patient's circulation can be obtained from the monitoring of a number of parameters e.g. the nature of the pulse, capillary refill time and venous pressure. The pulse volume reflects the output of the heart. The capillary refill time can be measured by applying pressure with a finger to a visible mucous membrane such as a gum which produces blanching. The time taken for its return to its previous colour is noted. Central venous pressure can be measured using relatively simple equipment (p. 319).

The monitoring of arterial blood pressure is somewhat more sophisticated and beyond the scope of this textbook on veterinary nursing.

## (2) *Respiratory system*

Under normal circumstances in the anaesthetized patient it is common for respiratory depression to occur before cardiovascular depression. It is relatively easy to monitor the rate and nature of respiration and tidal volume can be measured. The rate and nature of respiration can be measured readily by observing movement of either the rebreathing bag or the thoracic wall. A temperature sensor has been used to monitor respiration. It is based on the changes in temperature between inspiration and expiration. The temperature changes can be converted into an audible tone which changes with respiratory movements.

## (3) *Temperature*

Body temperature is one of the most simple and effective parameters to measure. Measurement with a clinical thermometer is difficult and cumbersome and does not provide a continuous record.

Thermistors are most suitable for temperature measurement during anaesthesia; oesophageal measurement gives the best indication of body-core temperature although other sites can be used.

## Pre- and Post-Anaesthetic Care

Before any animal is anaesthetized it is essential that the possible risks of anaesthesia are explained fully to the owner and that the owner or their agent should have signed a consent form giving permission for the animal to be anaesthetized. Except in the case of emergency it is desirable that all animals undergoing general anaesthesia will have been starved of food and water for 12 hours which usually means overnight. If there is any doubt about this and the operation is not a life-saving one, then the animals should not be anaesthetized until a further period of 6 hours has elapsed. Before an animal is anaesthetized it is essential that the veterinary surgeon should carry out a full clinical examination after first obtaining a careful history from the owner. Particular attention should be paid to the circulatory and respiratory systems, and any abnormalities should be fully investigated.

It is essential that all animals should be kept warm both during and after general anaesthesia. However, care should be taken to ensure that animals are not burnt by electric blankets or heating pads or by the over-enthusiastic use of electric heaters. The animal should be left in a lateral recumbency and covered with a blanket. Constant and careful observation is essential until the animal is able to sit up. A quiet environment is important for animals recovering from anaesthesia, particularly in certain excitable breeds, and on recovery from anaesthesia produced by certain agents (e.g. methohexitone).

If recovery is delayed the animal should be turned over at least every hour until recovery is complete in order to prevent respiratory complications such as hypostatic pneumonia.

If an endotracheal tube has been used it should be left in position until the animal shows signs of rejecting it either by swallowing or retching movements. In addition, if gentle traction applied to the tube causes the animal to "cough" it should be removed. It is particularly important in brachycephalic dogs (e.g. Boxers) to leave the tube in place as long as possible in order to prevent asphyxia. Once the endotracheal tube has been removed the head should be placed in its natural position and tongue pulled well out of the mouth.

## Anaesthetic Accidents and Emergencies

In veterinary anaesthesia a number of accidents and emergencies can and do occur. It is extremely important that anyone who is involved in the use of anaesthetic techniques should be able to anticipate the onset of problems and deal effectively with them when they occur. One of the most important ways in which a RANA can contribute to the reduction of the incidence of anaesthetic accidents and emergencies is by **careful preparation before anaesthesia**. It is essential to ensure that anaesthetic machines are working correctly, cylinders are full and an adequate supply of drugs, syringes and needles are readily available. Cuffs of endotracheal tubes can be checked by inflating them in a closed glass vessel such as a test tube.

**Respiratory arrest** occurs quite commonly in anaesthesia due to either an overdose of anaesthetic agent or respiratory obstruction. The treatment is by endotracheal intubation and artificial ventilation with 100% oxygen.

*Hypoxia* occurs when the oxygen content of the inspired atmosphere is low. This can occur due to oxygen cylinders running out or when lungs collapse or there are large masses or fluid in the thoracic cavity. Treatment is aimed at correcting the hypoxia by *ventilation with 100% oxygen.*

*Respiratory acidosis* or carbon dioxide build-up occurs when respiration is depressed or when gas flows are too low in a semi-closed circuit or soda lime is exhausted in closed circuit. Treatment is by artificial ventilation with a carbon-dioxide-free atmosphere.

Hypoxia and carbon dioxide build-up are the commonest causes of the most serious anaesthetic accident—**cardiac arrest**. This can also be caused by either a gross or a relative drug overdose. The signs are cyanosis of the mucous membranes, cessation of pulse and dilation of the pupils. The first action is to cease administration of the anaesthetic agent and, if one is not already in place, to insert an endotracheal tube and ventilate the lungs with oxygen. Closed cardiac massage may be instituted, but if this does not restore a spontaneous beat an **emergency thoracotomy and open chest massage** must be carried out at a rate of about 60 per minute. Cardiac arrest can either occur in asystole or fibrillation. **In asystole** it may be necessary to inject adrenaline or calcium chloride into the circulation by way of the left ventricle. **In the case of fibrillation** an electric defibrillator or an intracardiac injection of procaine is used to abolish the fibrillation. If an effective beat is restored the chest must be kept open for at least 15 minutes to ensure that all is well.

**Laryngeal spasm** is a not uncommon emergency in the cat. It is most often seen under ether anaesthesia when high concentrations are being administered. The best treatment of this condition is to administer a muscle relaxant drug, pass an endotracheal tube and carry out artificial ventilation.

*Vomiting* or passive regurgitation can occur either at the induction during the course of, or during recovery from anaesthesia. When the active process of vomiting occurs the protective reflexes are present and, therefore, the pharynx must be cleared of this material and the head and neck kept lower than the rest of the body. The signs of passive regurgitation which are first seen are often respiratory in nature. Treatment consists of aspiration of the respiratory tract. Oxygen and antibiotics should be administered in order to reduce the risk of aspiration pneumonia.

*Anaesthetic explosions* and fires may occur in veterinary anaesthesia and are best prevented by avoiding the use of agents (e.g. cyclopropane and ether) which are inflammable. However, commonsense measures such as the banning of smoking and open fires and reduction of static electricity can go a long way to reducing the problem. Efficient fire-fighting equipment should be readily available.

*Accidents are sometimes associated with the extravascular injection* of irritant anaesthetic agents such as thiopentone. If this should be seen to happen, the thiopentone must be diluted by the injection of relatively large volumes of saline at the site to reduce the local irritant action.

*Note:* A number of pathological changes have been attributed to working in the environment of a medical operating theatre, although the evidence of this is still in dispute. There is no definite evidence to link these changes with the inhalation of waste anaesthetic gases or vapours. As a number of these changes have been associated with possible abnormalities of female reproduction then it is desirable for any woman who is concerned about the problem to take medical advice, preferably from a gynaecologist.

## (g) Theatre Nursing

## I. O. KNAPP

### General Considerations

Surgery has been defined as the treatment of accident or disease by manual or mechanical means, that is cutting into or removing tissue. Surgical operations may be (i) Operations of choice, when time is available to plan the operation and prepare the patient. (ii) Operations of necessity, which are essential to the well being of the patient but must be performed at once. (iii) Emergency operations, which must be performed immediately as the patient's life is in danger.

The success of most operations depend largely upon the thoroughness of preparation. This may take far longer than the operation itself, but operative time is vital to the patient and anything which will make the surgeon's task easier and quicker should be included in the preparation. It is a fallacy to think that animals are less susceptible to infection than humans or that their tissues heal any quicker. Even one infected wound is too many. There is no point in commencing surgery if one does not intend to maintain rigid asepsis throughout. Careless mistakes such as touching the edge of an undraped operating table while scrubbed up, picking up an instrument which has fallen on to the floor, or allowing an operation to take place under a dusty operating lamp must be anticipated and avoided.

### The duties of the operating theatre nurse

1. *Scrupulous cleaning of the operating theatre.*
2. *Preparing and checking the anaesthetic equipment.*
3. *Sterilizing instruments, gowns, drapes and gloves.*
4. *Preparing the patient.*
5. *Preparing the theatre.*
6. *Setting out of the instruments required.*
   (a) in the preparation room.
   (b) in the theatre.
7. *Preparing the surgeon and assistant.*
8. *Assisting at the operation.*
9. *Immediate post-operative care of the patient.*
10. *Cleaning and routine maintenance of the instruments.*

### The Surgical Unit

The surgical unit includes a sterilizing room, preparation area, operating theatre and recovery area. These should be near together and should at all times be kept clean and tidy and prepared to receive the emergency case. Although the unit must be properly ventilated, doors and windows must not be left open to allow a cross flow of air which may introduce dust and other sources of contamination.

## The Sterilizing Room

In many practices the sterilizing room is also used as a laundry and washing area. If this is so it should be divided into a clean area and a dirty area. There should be cupboards for storing the sterile packs and clean laundry. In this area drapes, gowns and instruments should be prepared, packed and sterilized ready for surgery.

## The Preparation Area

This area should be close to the operating theatre. Here the patient will be given the anaesthetic and the surgical site prepared. In this area the theatre staff will change into appropriate protective clothing prior to entering the operating theatre. Nobody should be permitted to enter the theatre unless **properly dressed** in theatre clothing.

## The Operating Theatre

This will include a scrub-up area communicating with the theatre. Here the surgeon, assistant and scrub nurse will scrub-up, gown and glove prior to entering the theatre perhaps through a swing door. The operating theatre itself must not be used as a store room and there should be no shelves or cupboards in it. Free standing items should be kept to a minimum.

## Care of the Operating Theatre

1. All theatre equipment, lamps, tables, anaesthetic machines and trolleys should be dusted daily using a damp cloth soaked in an antiseptic solution. Trolleys should be covered with a surgical drape when the theatre is not in use. When cleaning the theatre particular attention should be given to extractor fans, ceiling fittings, door handles and window fastenings. A vacuum cleaner fitted with a bacterial filter is recommended for cleaning the theatre.

2. Floors and walls should be washed daily using a disinfectant solution in the concentration recommended by the manufacturers for this purpose. Ideally the theatre should be mopped out after each operation although this is not always possible.

3. Swabs for bacteriological examination should be taken at regular intervals from various points within the theatre to check for the presence of contamination. The sources of such contamination should be sought and if possible eliminated.

4. A temperature of about 20°C should be maintained in the theatre.

## Recovery area

This area should be near the theatre and should be warm and quiet. The patient can be put here and observed while it is recovering from anaesthesia prior to returning to its kennel.

## Sterilization

## Preparation and sterilization of instruments and materials

All materials and equipment used during a sterile procedure must be sterilized. Methods of sterilization are classified according to the agents used, heat, chemical agents, gas and irradiation. These methods vary in efficiency and have both advantages and disadvantages (p. 412).

## 1. *Boiling*

All pathogenic organisms in the vegetative form and many spore forms are killed by 5 minutes immersion in boiling water, but there are resistant spores which will withstand longer periods of boiling. If the water is made slightly alkaline its lethal effect is increased. Hence a 2% solution of sodium carbonate (washing soda) should be added. This retards rusting and reduces the blunting of instruments. When boiling, make sure that all the instruments are covered with the water and fast boil for 5 minutes by the clock. If more instruments are added after commencing boiling, timing must begin again.

## 2. *Hot Air Oven*

This is a useful method of sterilization for fine and sharp instruments as these may be laid out on a tray in the oven and not packed together where sharp points can get damaged if they are not protected. The method is quick. Temperatures of 180°C for 60 minutes are required. The tray becomes very hot and must be removed from the oven with care.

## 3. *Ethylene Oxide Sterilization* (The Anprolene method)

Ethylene oxide is a highly penetrating but toxic gas (p. 408) that is effective in the sterilization of surgical equipment. The materials to be sterilized must be dry and clean. They may be wrapped in paper packages or nylon bags. The most convenient method is the seal and peel polythene wrapping which produces a transparent long lasting sterile pack.

The sterilizer consists of a small plastic container or a large metal box with a time lock, within which is placed a liner bag of thick polythene. All packs to be sterilized are loaded into the liner bag. Without opening the bag in which it is contained, the ampoule containing the Anprolene is broken at the prescored neck and placed in the centre of the load. The time lock is set for 12 hours so sterilization is best done overnight with the materials ready to be unloaded next morning. Following sterilization the packs must be allowed to stand in a well-ventilated area for some time to ensure that the toxic gases are diffused. An indicator tape is available for use with this gas.

## 4. *Cold Chemical Sterilization*

This method may be used for perishable goods or instruments which cannot be exposed to high temperatures required for the other methods of sterilization. Disinfection by chemicals is effective only if articles are thoroughly cleaned and free of debris, blood, pus, oil and grease. The presence of any organic matter greatly reduces the efficiency of the chemical and may inhibit its action altogether. Whenever possible instruments should be taken to pieces for chemical sterilization. Care should be taken to use the specific concentrations and times stipulated by the manufacturers. Some chemicals can cause skin irritation so that instruments should be rinsed with sterile normal saline solution before using on tissues. Solutions such as chlorhexidine, iodophors and 70% alcohol are used.

## 5. *Autoclave*

Steam under pressure is the most widely used and most efficient method of sterilization and kills organisms by coagulation of the cell proteins. The steam must be under pressure, dry and saturated. It will condense when it meets the cooler surfaces of the articles in the autoclave and the latent heat released penetrates and kills the organisms present.

Three main types of autoclave are available.

1. The simplest operates by boiling water in a closed container like a household pressure cooker, and it will operate at 15 psi. These autoclaves are fairly small but useful for a few instruments packs.

2. A larger horizontal or vertical autoclave which provides downward displacement of air, with the air outlet valve at the bottom and the steam outlet at the top. By this method the air is driven out of the autoclave more effectively but the packs may often remain wet if incorrectly used.

3. A vacuum assisted autoclave works on the same principal but is fitted with a vacuum and air filter which allows clean cool air into the autoclave to replace the steam in the final cooling stage, which will dry the packs. It is important that the contents of packs become dry, as bacteria may more easily contaminate a moist environment and wet drapes may act as a wick to draw bacteria into a pack.

## Using an Autoclave

1. The jacket should be filled with water, to the indicated level.
2. Taps should be set and valves set.
3. Heat is applied and the valve is not closed until the steam is escaping freely.
4. The valve is then closed and pressure allowed to build up to the required pressure.

5. It is held at this setting for the required time.
6. The valve is opened, the water drained off, and the heat lowered but not turned off.
7. Heat is maintained for a further 10 minutes to drive off any moisture (this is not necessary in a vacuum assisted autoclave).
8. When the pressure has dropped the lid should be opened, and left to cool, before removing the contents.

Autoclave at a pressure of—

15 psi (1.2 kg/cm²) at 121°C for 15 min
20 psi (1.4 kg/cm²) at 126°C for 10 min
30 psi (2 kg/cm²) at 134°C for 3 min

It is recommended that rubber articles, endotracheal tubes, catheters and gloves be autoclaved at 15 psi at 121°C for 15 minutes as at this temperature and pressure the articles will not be damaged.

It should be noted that these times are holding times only and do not take into account the time taken for the autoclave to reach the operating temperature.

## Packing instruments, gowns, drapes and swabs for the autoclave

All materials to be autoclaved must be carefully packed into either drums or autoclave bags of paper or an autoclavable nylon film from which bags of different sizes can be made. Otherwise they may be doubly wrapped using a surgical drape. If bags are used the opening must be correctly closed using a double fold at each end and sealed with autoclave tape, paper clips or a stapling machine. Paper clips have an advantage in that the bags can be easily and quickly opened without damage so that they can be used again. Disposable paper autoclave bags may also be used but involve expense and cannot be recycled.

## Drums

Autoclave drums are very useful as they may be packed with all instruments, drapes, gowns and gloves that are required for an operation. When packing the drum the instruments should be placed at the bottom followed by the drapes, leaving the gowns at the top as they will be required first. Drums should not be packed too tightly to allow the steam to penetrate all the contents.

There are different types of drums. For use in a vertical autoclave the drums should have openings at the top and bottom. For a horizontal autoclave the openings are at the sides. This facilitates the displacement of air and the penetration of the steam.

When using drums make sure to open the air vents before placing them into the autoclave. The vents should be closed as soon as the drums are removed to prevent contaminated air being drawn in as the contents cool.

## Gowns

The gown must be folded correctly (see Fig. 10.19) and a towel placed on top followed by a second gown and towel. These are doubly wrapped in a surgical drape and sealed with a small piece of autoclave tape. Record the contents of the pack clearly on the tape with a "biro" pen. The date should also be included as properly stored packs remain sterile for up to 3 weeks.

## Drapes

These should be folded (see Fig. 10.19) and wrapped in a similar way to the gowns. It is suggested that four small drapes are packed together with a split or window drape in each pack. Record the contents of the pack on the sealing tape.

## Swabs

Surgical swabs may be packed in the instrument pack, but it is advisable to have other swabs packed separately in autoclave bags. These bags should always contain a standard number of swabs, say ten, so that at the end of the operation the number used can be counted easily to make sure that none are missing. The number of swabs used also gives some indication of the blood loss during surgery.

## Instruments

A standard pack is made up of those instruments which are used during most operations. The instruments are placed on a doubly folded drape and wrapped into a neat parcel closed by a small piece of autoclave tape. Sharp instruments should be protected by covering the points with a small piece of swab or cotton wool attached with autoclave tape. This avoids damage to the instruments and perforation of the wrapper.

Extra instruments may be individually wrapped using autoclave bags of nylon film or paper.

## Monitoring sterilization

The efficiency of sterilization can be monitored using indicator tape, Brown's tubes and spores.

## Indicator Tape

Incorporates a series of chemical stripes which become visible provided steriliza-

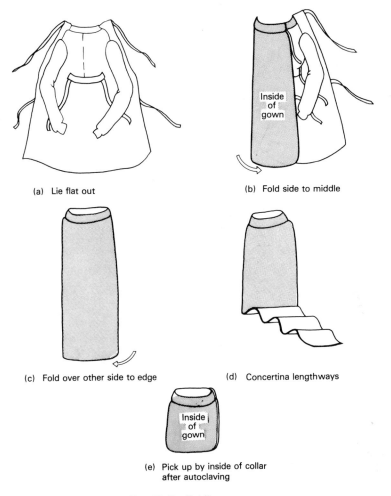

(a) Lie flat out

(b) Fold side to middle

Inside of gown

(c) Fold over other side to edge

(d) Concertina lengthways

Inside of gown

(e) Pick up by inside of collar after autoclaving

FIG. 10.18. **Folding a gown.**

tion has been adequate. These tapes are available for use in autoclaves, ethylene oxide sterilization systems and hot air ovens. The correct indicator tape must be used for the specific type of system used.

### Brown's Tubes

Are small glass tubes filled with a dark green liquid which changes colour to a brown colour when exposed to tempera-

ture and pressure. These are useful and accurate indicators of the autoclave cycle as they are placed within the packs. Different tubes are available for use in autoclaves and ethylene oxide gas sterilizers.

### Spores

Small sealed packets of spores can be placed within the packs. When removed

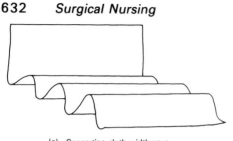

(a)  Concertina cloth widthways

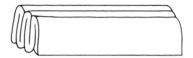

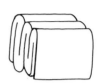

(b)

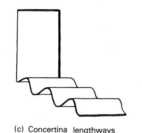

(c)  Concertina  lengthways

(d)  Pack cloths in autoclave drum or autoclave
.bags sealed with indicating tape

Folding surgical drapes.

FIG. 10.19.

from the autoclave, the spore packs are cultured to ensure that all the spores have been killed.

## Preparations for Surgery

### The operating list

The daily operating list should be planned so that the theatre is used first for the "clean" surgery such as intra-abdominal and orthopaedic procedures. These are followed by those that are "dirty" or infected, such as pyometritis, oral and anal work.

### Operating room technique

#### Surgery Attire

Theatre clothing should consist of a loosely fitting, cotton two piece scrub suit or scrub dress. Clean scrub suits should be worn every day.

#### Footwear

Antistatic footwear is essential in an area where anaesthetic gasses are used. This should be cleaned frequently and be worn only in the theatre. In some theatres plastic shoe covers are worn.

#### Surgical Caps

All persons entering the theatre should wear a surgical cap and face mask. Caps are made of cloth or paper which provide ventilation and are comfortable to wear. The cap must completely cover all the hair. Hair which is worn long should be tied up first. A clean cap should be used each day.

#### Face Masks

Are made either of cotton or paper. Masks should cover both nose and mouth and be snugly tied since air is intended to filter through rather than escape around them. Masks should not be kept in pockets or allowed to dangle around the neck or chin, but left in place and then discarded.

*Scrub-up Procedure*

1. *Change into theatre wear.*
2. *Put on surgical cap and mask.*
3. *Ensure that nails are short* and nail polish removed. Take off all rings and jewellery.
4. *Regulate the hot and cold water taps.*
5. *Either a sterile scrub brush or one which has been kept in an antiseptic solution should be used* together with an antiseptic soap or a surgical scrub such as Betadine.
6. *Wash hands and arms up to the elbows.* Keep arms flexed so that hands are always above the elbow level.
7. *Rinse, removing all soap and lather* by allowing water to flow down hands and off elbows.
8. *Using the scrub brush and surgical scrub, systematically scrub the arms and hands* using a circular movement taking care to scrub the finger nails and knuckles. Scrub for 5 minutes by the clock.
9. *Discard the brush and rinse well.*
10. *Dry hands and arms using a sterile towel* or a hot air drier. If using a towel use a different part for each hand and arm, working from the wrist to the elbow.

## Gowning procedure

1. Stand well back from the table or trolley on which the opened gown pack has been placed. Pick up the sterile gown holding it by the shoulders and allow to fall open. The gown has been folded so that the inside only is exposed. (Fig. 10.18e). Slip one hand into each sleeve.
2. An assistant will tie the tapes firmly at the back.
3. It is important not to touch the outside of the gown.

## Gloving procedure

1. *After scrubbing and drying hands, the gown is put on,* then the sterile surgical gloves.

## Gloving procedure

1. *After scrubbing and drying hands, the gown is put on,* then the sterile surgical gloves.
2. *The glove pack is opened by an assistant.* The gloves should be folded correctly with their cuffs turned down (10.20(a)).
3. With the left hand *pick up the right glove by the turned down cuff,* handling only the inner surface of the glove. Draw on to the right hand directing the fingers into place. Do not unfold the cuff at this stage.
4. *Place the gloved fingers of the right hand* under the cuff of the left glove and draw on to the left hand, handling only the outer surface of this glove (10.20d).
5. *Draw the cuff of the left glove over the wristlet of the gown* using the fingers of the right hand (10.20f).
6. *Repeat for the right glove* (10.20g).
7. Now *massage the glove fingers* making sure that the finger tips fit snugly.
8. *When the hands are gloved they are clasped together,* as in prayer, away from the gown, in front of the chest and held until ready to commence surgery.

## Preparation of the patient

The patient is a potential source of contamination and particular care should have been taken to prepare the patient well.

1. Ideally the patient should be admitted 24 hours prior to the operation. A blood sample and any X-rays that may be required should be taken, and the animal fasted prior to anaesthesia.
2. On admission details of case history should be recorded on a hospital

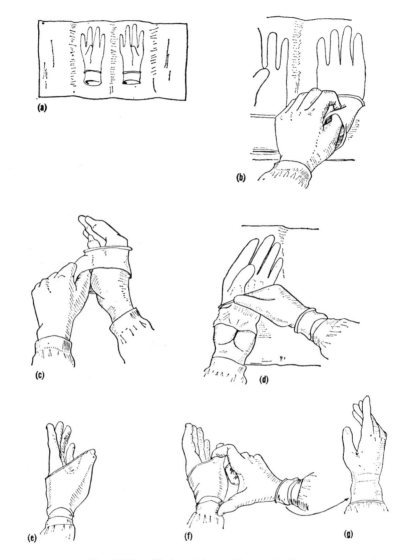

FIG. 10.20. Gloving. After putting on sterile gown.

card which is fixed to the kennel door. (see practice organization ) (p. 272).

3. The owner must be asked to sign a consent form giving permission to administer an anaesthetic and to perform surgery.

**Preparation of the operation site**

1. Using a fine clipper blade, *close clip a generous area* around the operation site.

2. *Scrub the site well with a brush,* using a suitable surgical scrub solution and warm water.

3. *Wipe away the scrub using a swab.* The area should be swabbed along the line of incision and then outwards from this site towards the periphery of the prepared area. Do not return to the incision site again unless a clean swab is used.

4. *Rinse the site well with surgical spirit.*

5. *Wipe again using a sterile swab.*

6. *Finally use a skin preparation such as Betadine Skin Preparation or Tincture of Iodine with surgical spirit as a 50% solution.*

**Position the patient on the table**

Position the patient on the table and secure in position with the use of ties, sandbags or inflatable supports. In doing so give the surgeon easy access to the site of operation, and make the animal as comfortable as possible. Do not overstretch the limbs and do not abduct forelegs as this can cause radial paralysis. The three positions most often used are the sternal position, the dorsal position and the lateral position. By tilting the operating table, the head or tail can be raised or lowered. This is useful for operations on the anal sacs or the repair of a perineal hernia.

**The duties of the surgical assistant**

1. *Draping the patient.* The surgical area is draped using four sheets. The first drape is placed between the assistant and the patient. The second drape is handed to the surgeon and placed between himself and the patient. The third and fourth are placed on top of these covering the head and tail. These are secured in position using four towel clips. In this way a longitudinal incision can be ex- tended without gross disturbance of the drapes. Finally a split sheet is placed on top.

2. *Sort the instruments.* Always lay out instruments in the same way, so that you automatically know where each instrument is on the tray. In this way you can save time and always have the next instrument ready as required.

3. *Swab firmly using a dry gauze swab.* Always dab but never wipe as this disturbs blood clots and fine capillaries and increases bleeding.

4. *Pass the instruments as required to the surgeon* and always try to anticipate requirements, and have the next instrument ready promptly. Always return used instruments to their position on the tray after use.

5. *Keep the instrument trolley tidy at all times.*

6. *Take care* that sharp instruments do not perforate and damage gloves or drapes. Should this occur it must be recognized and precautions taken to maintain asepsis by changing the gloves or drapes if they become contaminated.

8. *Always have suture material ready with needle threaded.* Take the loose end of the suture material between the fingers and thumb, so that the thread is not pulled off the needle, when passing it to the surgeon.

**Post operative theatre procedure**

1. *Remove all drapes.*

2. *Always check the instruments and count the swabs* to see that none are missing.

3. *Clean around the surgical wound* and remove any clots of blood.

4. *Check the wound* for haemorrhage, the colour of the mucous membranes, also take the pulse and res-

piration rate. These checks should continue at regular intervals until the patient has regained consciousness.

5. As soon as the patient regains its swallow and cough reflex, *remove the endotracheal tube,* remember to deflate the cuff before removing the tube. Ensure an airway is clear and the patient is comfortable (p. 641).

6. *Apply a dressing* if required.

7. *Return to a warm kennel* on a stretcher before the patient attempts to walk.

8. *Ensure that operation records have been completed* as these are important for future reference, for issuing reports and making up the account.

9. *Obtain all necessary information* from the veterinary surgeon so as to be able to advise the owner on aftercare, treatment, special diets and protection of the wound. The danger of a patient licking the wound, nibbling the sutures or taking too much exercise should be emphasized. The owner must contact the surgery, after the operation case is discharged, if problems develop.

**Care and maintenance of the instruments**

Thorough and careful cleaning of instruments is the key to optimum conditions of asepsis and the long life of the instruments. Organic materials left on the instruments inhibits sterilization, while blood acts as a corrosive agent on stainless steel.

Instruments should be cleaned using a brush and washing well under cold running water. Cold water is best as hot water causes blood to coagulate. A blood solvent such as Grotonat may be used. Instruments may also be washed by using an ultrasonic cleaning machine. If using a

chemical detergent always rinse in cold water afterwards.

After washing the instruments must be dried, taking special care to dry the joints well. This gives the RANA a chance to check the instruments prior to repacking. If using a hot air drier leave the instruments open in order to dry the joints. After drying make sure that all the instruments close properly and that they have not been bent or damaged. Joints should be lubricated occasionally using an instrument oil. One of the instrument milk preparations used following washing, helps to keep the instruments in good condition.

Instruments are expensive and they can last for years if properly looked after. Instruments should be stored in a cupboard on glass shelves, or hanging so as to minimize damage and scratching.

**Suture Materials**

Suture materials are divided into two groups: absorbable sutures and non-absorbable sutures.

**Absorbable suture materials**

*Cat Gut and Collagen*

Cat gut is made of twisted collagen derived from the submucosal layer of bovine intestine. Cat gut is available as plain cat gut or chromic cat gut. Plain cat gut begins to lose its tensile strength on about the fifth day and then is absorbed fairly quickly. Chromic cat gut is plain cat gut which has been tanned with chromic acid, this makes it slower to be reabsorbed. Chromic cat gut lasts up to 21-days. Hence is known as 21-day cat gut. Collagen is used for suturing the cornea.

## Polyglycolic Acid Suture.
## (Dexon)

This is a synthetic suture material. It is inert, braided and its absorption time has been prolonged to take place at about 30 days. It is easy to work with and will hold a stable knot. It can be used as a buried suture or when used as a skin suture and kept dry, it will not need removal.

## Non-absorbable Materials

(a) nylon
(b) polypropyl-
ene
(c) polyester
Dacron
(d) silk
(e) stainless steel
(f) linen

### Nylon

Monafilament is a synthetic suture with a smooth surface which does not injure tissue as it passes through. It is slightly elastic and causes minimal tissue reaction. It is available in various size ranging from 10/0 to 3.

In general surgery for dogs sizes 2/0, 0 & 1. are most commonly used. For cats sizes 3/0 & 2/0 are the most common.

### Braided Nylon

Available in various sizes 2/0 to 3. It is also available with swaged needle. Because of its braided properties it can cause tissue reaction and acts like a wick which can cause infection. It is used in eyelid suturing.

### Polypropylene Monofilament Suture

A synthetic, relatively inert material, which is easy to handle, knots hold well, it can be used as a buried suture as can monafilament nylon. It is available as Supramid and Vetafil.

### Dacron Polyester Suture

A synthetic braided suture material of uniform size and tensile strength. It is easy to handle being very pliable, Knots must be carefully tied and the loosening of knots can occur. It is available in various sizes, also with swaged needle attached.

### Silk

A natural suture material that is principally a polypeptide. Individual silk fibres are relatively short and must be braided to provide adequate tensile strength and length. Because of the braided nature of the silk, organisms and debris penetrate the suture material. Also silk sutures tend to loosen after they have been in the tissue for a short period of time, they rarely break and cause little tissue reaction. Sutures are often left *in situ* for up to 14 days before being removed. But if they are left in an incision for 21–28 days they can cause a chronic inflammation with micro-abscesses.

Silk sutures are available in various sizes also as swaged needles, the material is used in eye surgery and in aural haematome suturing.

### Stainless Steel Suture

A strong suture, which can be difficult to work because of its springy nature. It is liable to kink if the sutures are not guided carefully. It is available in various sizes on reels and with swaged needle attached. Sizes from 7/0 to 5 are available and may be used for orthopaedic surgery and occasionally as a strong buried suture.

### Linen Thread

This was used extensively in veterinary work in place of cat gut for internal and muscle sutures. It is cheap, and can be boiled to sterilize it, but now has been replaced by other materials. It is available in sizes from 3/0 to 0 also on reels from which lengths can be taken off for sterilizing. It causes a little tissue reaction which has been of use in hernia repairs to provide a long lasting suture material.

Most suture materials are now available on reels which come already sterile complete with sterilizing fluid in the pack. It is important to keep a check on the level of the sterilizing fluid as in a warm atmosphere this can and does evaporate. Most suture materials are now available with swaged on needles in various sizes. Individual sterile suture packs are recommended.

### Instrumentation

#### Suture needles

These are classified according to whether they are cutting or non-cutting and by their shape.

*Plain suture needles* are separate suture needles, which have an eye for threading, and are available in packets of different sizes. These needles are described according to shape. There are straight needles, and half curved needles. All needles are either traumatic, with a cutting edge, or autraumatic, which are round-bodied. Needles range in size from larger sizes 1, 2 down to fine needles sizes 20–22. For small animals the most popular sizes for dogs are sizes 12–14. For cats sizes 15–17.

*Swaged needles* are needles attached to the suture material. These needles are used for the repair of skin, internal organs, viscera, and other repairs which require as little trauma by the needle as possible. The diameter of the thread and needle are the same with no double fold of suture material from threading the needle.

In general, traumatic or cutting needles are used for skin, dense tissue and facia. Autraumatic or non-cutting needles are used for delicate tissues, viscera and muscle. Swaged needles for repair of intestine wall, vascular and ophthalmic use are favoured by the surgeon.

### Instrument packs

For all routine operations a basic instrument pack is used. This includes a standard set of instruments which are used for all operations, for specialized operations the basic set is used together with extra instruments for the operation in question.

The standard or basic pack should always be made up to include the same number of instruments. In this way it is easy to check the pack after the operation to see that none of the instruments or swabs are missing.

#### *A Standard Pack*

1   No. 4 knife handle.
1   Mayo scissors, straight.
1   Mayo scissors, curved.
1   Rat-toothed dissecting forceps.
1   Smooth dissecting forceps.
4   Allis tissue forceps.
6–8 Artery forceps make up the number to include some straight and curved forceps.
    (fine mosquito forceps may be added).
6–8 Towel clips.
1   Needle holder (e.g. Gillies).
Suture needles, and suture material.
Swabs. ×10 or 20.
Scalpel blades ×2.

*Specialized Instruments:* additional instrument packs may be prepared.

*Abdominal Surgery.*

Extra scalpel handle and blade.
Metzenbaum scissors.
Retractors, self retaining.
Pair Doyen's bowel clamps.
Sterile kidney dish.
Turkish towels.
Sterile normal saline solution.
Suction apparatus with appropriate attachments.
Electro-cautery and attachments if required.

*Thoracic Surgery*

Retractors.
Rib cutters.
Rib spreaders.
Chest drain.
Strong suture material for chest repairs.
Include instruments as for abdominal surgery.

*Orthopaedic Surgery*

Listers bone cutting forceps.
Rongeur or bone nibblers.
Farabeuf's periosteal elevator.
Bone holding forceps.
Osteotomes or bone chisels.
Orthopaedic saw.
Gigli wire and handles.
Bone curettes.
Retractors.
Orthopaedic ruler.
A selection of these may be required depending upon the operation.

*Bone Pinning*

Jacobs chuck and key.
Pin cutters.
Selection of intramedullary pins. These can be measured from the X-ray.

*Bone Plating*

Orthopaedic drill and key, with suitable twist bits.
Plate benders.
Reamer.
Screw depth gauge.
Screwdriver (e.g. Lane's).
Selection of suitable plates and screws.

*Wiring*

Selection of wires.
Wire cutters.
Wire tightener or pliers.
Aneurism needle.
Selection of Kirschner wires if required.

*Obstetrical Instruments*

Vaginal speculum.
Whelping forceps.
Vulcellum forceps.
Sterile kidney dish.
Sterile normal saline.
Turkish towels.
Puppy resuscitation equipment.

*Dental Instruments*

Mouth gag.
Dental scalers.
Selection dental forceps.
Dental elevator.
Dental chisel.
Kidney dish and warm normal saline.

*Ophthalmic Instruments*

A basic pack of fine instruments including.
No. 3 knife handle, with No. 11, 12 or 15 blades.
Mosquito forceps, curved and straight.
Adson forceps.

Small fine scissors.
Towel clips.
Keratome.
Self-retaining lid retractor and speculum.
Vectis.
Capsule forceps.
Iris scissors.
Iris spatula.
Entropion clamp.
Chalazion clamp.
Iris forceps.
Corneal forceps.

Lid-holding distichiasis forceps.
Ophthalmic needle holder.
Anterior chamber irrigation cannula and syringe.
Small stainless steel dish.
Normal saline solution.

All surgeons have their individual preferences with regard to the instruments they use, so these lists are a guideline. Drawings of many of these instruments may be found in the catalogues available from surgical instrument manufacturers.

## (h) Post-operative Care

### NICOLA PRICE

The post-operative supervision of the patient is frequently the duty of the RANA from the moment the patient leaves the operating table. The animal should be carried so that no stress is put on the wound, and care should be taken not to bump the patient into walls or doors on the way to the kennels. The anaesthetized patient is unable to feel pain and therefore is unlikely to cry out if hurt.

The patient should be placed in a warm kennel, with a front opening door for easy access. It should be positioned with its head down, neck extended and its tongue pulled forward to prevent choking. The endotracheal tube (if used) should be removed as soon as a cough reflex is obvious. In the case of the brachycephalic dog, a close watch should be kept on its breathing; these dogs are susceptible to choking, and any excess mucus should be removed from the mouth and pharynx to prevent interference with the breathing. Collars should be removed from all anaesthetized patients and bandages applied after head and neck surgery, should be as loose as possible compatible with efficiency.

If the kennels are adequately heated and restful, the patient may then be left to recover quietly. However, in the case of old and very young patients, a heated pad or infra-red heating lamps may be utilized. As an alternative, padded hot-water bottles or blankets placed over the patient's body are often sufficient to retain its body heat.

Surgical patients should have constant attention in the immediate post-operative period. The nurse should be on hand and within hearing distance to cope with frightened or struggling patients or any post-operative emergencies that may arise.

### Post-operative Emergencies

Included in the duties of post-operative care is the awareness of and coping with post-operative emergencies.

If the patient begins to vomit, the head should be lowered below the rest of the body to prevent inhalation of the vomit, and mouth and pharynx should be swabbed out. In the case of respiratory obstruction, the cause should be located and rectified. The common causes are:

(1) The base of the tongue may be blocking the larynx, especially in brachycephalic breeds of dog. The head and neck should be straightened and the tongue pulled forward out of the mouth.

(2) If an endotracheal tube is still in place, this may be kinked due to the animal biting on it.

(3) Mucus may be blocking the airways, in which case the head should be lowered and the mucus removed.

(4) Foreign bodies, especially after dental attention, e.g. blood, swabs,

teeth, tartar, may be the cause. These should be removed and the head lowered so that any debris can drain away.

Haemorrhage is an important emergency. External haemorrhage is rare, but internal haemorrhage may occur in the case of a slipped ligature. The animal will probably show signs of shock and the mucous membranes will be pale. In these cases veterinary attention should be sought immediately. The cause may then be located and fluid therapy administered as considered appropriate (p. 318).

During the early recovery period it is necessary to observe the well-being of the patient. A check should be made on the respiration and pulse rates, temperature and the condition of the mucous membranes. It is good practice to note these observations on a chart. Most patients recover quietly, but in some cases they may become violent during recovery. This often occurs if inadequate or no premedication has been administered. It is the nurse's job to restrain and comfort these patients and prevent physical damage.

**The duties of the RANA continue even when the patient has regained consciousness.** During the period that follows a careful watch should be made and the animal's progress reported:

1. *Temperature, pulse and respiratory rates should be recorded* to indicate if all is well or if there is infection present. Two days following surgery a slightly raised temperature can be expected, but it should begin to return to normal by the fourth day. Increase in pulse rate may be due to fright, disease or haemorrhage.

2. *The environmental temperature should be kept constant* at about 70°F. Barbiturates tend to interfere with the normal functioning of body temperature, and allowances should be made for this.

3. *Haemorrhage* is still a possibility, and the colour of the animal's mucous membranes should be observed. The patient should also be prevented from causing strain to the sutures by struggling.

4. *Fluid intake and output should be noted.* An increase in fluid intake can be expected due to blood loss and a decrease in output can be expected due to loss of fluid by evaporation and bleeding and also because the animal's water intake has been restricted prior to surgery (p. 273).

5. *The wound should be observed for suppuration,* undue inflammation and breaking of the tissues round the sutures. Swelling at the suture line for 48 hours due to fluid is normal and usually subsides. If swelling increases and the area is red, moist and irritable, all is not well. Breaking of the sutures and self-mutilation are also problems to be considered.

6. *Constipation and urine retention should be noted.* Animals often will not soil their kennels and therefore need to be taken out. Bowel activity will be reduced due to fasting before the operation and poor appetite in the 24 hours after. Bowel and bladder activity should be normal by the fourth post-operative day.

The general progress and ability of the patient to recover depend a lot on its health before the operation, duration of the anaesthesia, the nature of the surgery involved and, of course, the post-operative progress and care.

It is quite normal for animals to be depressed during the 24–48 hours following general anaesthesia. Warmth and quiet are necessary and if the cat or dog is immobile it should be turned frequently to prevent muscle stiffness and the risk of hypostatic pneumonia. Patients that are able to move should be encouraged to do so quietly and gently. Violent exercise on a lead is inadvisable due to the possibility of stress on internal sutures, and climbing staircases and jumping into chairs should be severely discouraged. In the case of paraplegic or immobilized animals, care must be taken to prevent bed sores and urine scald. Thin-skinned animals, such as Greyhounds and Dachshunds, are the most susceptible and should be provided with soft bedding. Soiled or wet areas should be washed and dried; talc may be used to avoid chafing.

Veterinary surgeons may order medication to be administered during the post-operative period, and it is the nurse's duty to ensure that these instructions are carried out. These drugs should be recorded on a chart, which is a valuable reference source.

After the post-operative period of 3–5 days, the patient enters a period of convalescence. The appetite increases and the animal becomes brighter and behaves more normally. On discharge of the animal, the veterinary surgeon will probably leave instructions for the owner regarding its diet, exercise and bodily functions.

## Maintenance of Intravenous Drips

During the post-operative period it may be necessary for the patient to have an intravenous drip (in cases of shock, severe blood loss or dehydration). It is normally the duty of the RANA to restrain the patient, ensure the drip remains in place and flows at the required rate.

Unconscious or paraplegic patients do not present any real problem; they will probably lie quietly with the drip in place, secured by a piece of elastoplast. However, there are greater difficulties with the conscious patient.

Sedatives or analgesics may be used to keep the patient quiet, in which case the intravenous needle or catheter secured with tape may be sufficient. Alternatively, the patient may be restrained by hobbling the back legs with bandage or tape. This may be sufficient to stop the patient from moving, but in less-placid patients this may not be so, as they may wriggle and thrash about. Some patients may unwillingly struggle when unconscious due to poisons, anaesthetics which make them react to noise or because they are in shock. In such cases it is advisable for the nurse to sit with and restrain the patient.

When using a giving set or catheter it may be further secured by placing part of the drip tubing parallel to the leg, looping it back and taping or bandaging the loop of the tube in place; this supports the drip and takes some of the strain from the catheter. Plastic venous catheters are becoming increasingly popular in practice due to their advantages over needles (p. 316). They allow some movement of the leg without dislodging the drip, as the cannula moves with the leg and not against it. "Mini-veins" are an alternative but the point of the metal needle may damage the vein but they are not easily dislodged.

Small dogs and cats may be further restrained by placing them in a small cat basket. Space is thus restricted and the patient is less likely to become entangled in the drip set. There is usually sufficient space between the basket and the lid to allow the tubing to be passed through and the bag hung up at the required height. Jugular catheters, inserted in the animal's jugular vein and strapped to the neck, may be used as an alternative to the above methods. It may be necessary to suture a jugular catheter to the skin using a strip of adhesive tape around the catheter as it emerges from the vein, to stitch on to.

The drip sets may be hung on springs, which relieve some of the tension from the tubing if the animal moves. Swivels may also be incorporated in the spring to allow rotation.

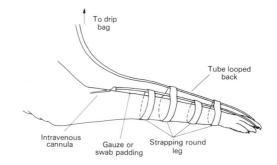

FIG. 10.21.    A method of attaching an intravenous drip to the dog's foreleg.

**Wound Care**

Many sutured wounds are left uncovered and it is the nurse's responsibility to ensure that these are not interfered with and that they remain healthy.

If the patient insists on licking the wound the first resort should be the use of the voice with a stern "No". If this is not successful then other methods have to be used. Plastic skin or an unpleasant tasting application may be enough to deter the patient, but in cases of persistent worrying an Elizabethan collar may be fitted to prevent the patient from reaching the wound (Figs. 10.22 and 10.23). A plastic bucket fitted to the collar is an effective alternative to the Elizabethan collar. Muzzles may be used but must be removed at reasonable intervals to allow eating and drinking. In cases of head and neck wounds, scratching by the patient may also be a problem. Bandaging of the feet often prevents any damage from the claws and distracts the animal's attention from the wound.

Bandaging may be used over the wound itself, often with a Jelonet gauze or powder dressing next to the wound to prevent sticking. Dressings should be changed frequently and kept dry, as wet bandages only act as a wick for infection. Net-type bandages may be used on wounds where ventilation is required, but care should be taken when using these, especially on the head region, as they are made of stretchy material and may become tight and cause respiratory distress.

Tranquillizers may be used post-operatively to prevent wound interference, and analgesics are often an advantage, especially after orthopaedic operations. Orthopaedic patients may require external fixation in the form of a plaster or Hexcelite cast. Care should be taken to ensure that these casts are comfortable and that no irritations or sores occur. Persistent plaster chewers may be restrained as mentioned earlier.

The cleaning of wounds during the post-operative period should be as aseptic as possible. Warm sterile saline should be used to wash away any dirt or debris. The wound should then be dried thoroughly and a wound dressing can be applied if required. Gentleness throughout this task prevents unnecessary damage to tissues and any resentment by the animal. A certain amount of swelling can be expected 48 hours after surgery but this should subside. If the wound appears hot, red, swollen, moist and irritable the veterinary surgeon must be informed and appropriate action taken. Small animals normally tamper with their wounds only if they are uncomfortable. Clean, healthy wounds should cause few problems.

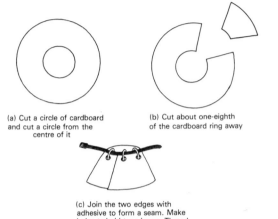

(a) Cut a circle of cardboard and cut a circle from the centre of it

(b) Cut about one-eighth of the cardboard ring away

(c) Join the two edges with adhesive to form a seam. Make holes to hold tape loops. Thread leather collar through tape loops

FIG. 10.22. Prevention of interference with dressings. How to make a cardboard Elizabethan collar.

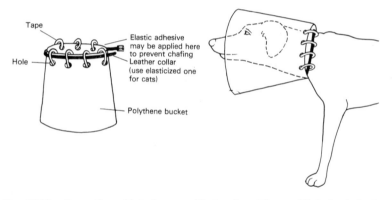

Tape

Hole

Elastic adhesive may be applied here to prevent chafing
Leather collar (use elasticized one for cats)

Polythene bucket

FIG. 10.23. Prevention of interference with dressings. The modified plastic bucket.

## Orthopaedic Nursing

The care of the orthopaedic patient will often consist of a period of hospitalization, followed by a period of convalescence at home, when the patient is considered well enough to benefit from the home environment. The nursing care is then continued by the owner, who must be instructed by the RANA. An assessment of the ability of the owner to care for such a patient is essential. In some cases it may be necessary to keep the patient hospitalized for a longer time if conditions in the home will be unfavourable for the uncomplicated recovery.

Orthopaedic patients usually fall into two categories:

(1) Those who have undergone "elective surgery", such as repair of a ruptured cruciate ligament, or correction of a congenital abnormality, such as patella luxation.

(2) Those who have suffered traumatic injury, such as a road traffic accident.

In the case of the planned orthopaedic

procedure, the owner is prepared in advance for the necessary aftercare of the patient. In the accident case, however, the patient is usually accompanied by a very distressed owner who is totally unprepared, and often unable to cope with an injured animal.

The hospitalization period following any orthopaedic procedure will usually need the confinement of the animal in a restricted area, a supply of adequate and suitable bedding, convalescent feeding and the administration of medication as prescribed by the veterinary surgeon. In some cases, topical applications and dressings may be required as well as external support after surgery.

*Pelvic fractures* often require no more than cage rest. The animal should be restricted in an area or cage to allow the minimum of movement, but enough room to stand and lie comfortably and to accommodate food dishes, and in the case of a cat, a litter tray. The area allowed is gradually increased and the patient given more freedom.

Bedding must be considered carefully. Patients likely to be recumbent for any length of time will need soft and absorbent bedding, so as to avoid the possibility of bed-sores and urine scald. Vetbed is an ideal form of bedding, and foam rubber is a good idea to provide extra padding for fine skinned animals such as greyhounds. Newspaper, if used, should be plentiful and changed frequently, as wet or soiled newspaper is very unpleasant for the patient. Blankets may be used but are less desirable, being harder to replace and keep clean. Heated pads normally have a set temperature, but care must be taken when using hot water bottles, as without the use of sufficient padding they may burn the immobile animal.

It must be remembered that although cats are often content to use a litter tray during their confinement, many dogs refuse to soil their bedding at any cost. Therefore, it may be necessary to take the dog outside, by carrying if required, so that it may relieve itself. In some cases of pelvic injury, there may be a degree of abdominal paralysis. In these cases, regular emptying of the bladder may be necessary, as instructed by the veterinary surgeon. Incontinent patients may tolerate the use of a one-way absorbent nappy to keep them dry and comfortable. A convalescent diet may also be an advantage with the addition of a faecal softener to make defaecation easier.

*Jaw fractures.* A liquid diet such as Complan should be given at first, or in less severe cases, minced or baby food would probably be most palatable. Extremely severe cases may require **pharyngostomy tube feeding**. As when feeding all fracture cases, the veterinary surgeon may also require the addition of bone meal and extra protein to the feed.

*Limb surgery.* Following an internal fixation procedure or elective surgery, the patient will need post-operative observation of the operation site, for swelling and bleeding. If this is apparent, the veterinary surgeon must be informed and subsequent action taken. Analgesics and sedative may be prescribed for the immediate post-operative period.

External fixation of fractured limbs is usually by means of a rigid plaster or Hexcelite cast. The use of a Robert Jones soft padded splint has grown in popularity for fracture support. It must contain a large volume of cotton wool, be tightly overbandaged with a "stove-piped" appearance for both comfort and structural support. However, in some cases the fracture may be further complicated by the presence of an open wound. It is often necessary, in badly mutilated cases, to improvise with a splint and wet saline packs which can be changed frequently and allow access to the wounds for cleaning and any topical applications. These wounds may be repaired at a later date. If only one open wound is concerned, a "window plaster cast" may be used. When nursing a patient with an external support, you must make sure that no sharp edges are exposed on the splint or cast, which will rub the patient. Careful observation is necessary with regard to the circulation of the affected limb: a plaster cast or bandage that is too tight can be disastrous. If the toes are left exposed, check their temperature and watch for any swelling: it may be necessary to loosen or remove the plaster if all is not well. Some patients are persistent plaster chewers, so it may be advisable to cover the plaster with Elastoplast or restrain the patient by means of an Elizabethan collar.

*Home nursing.* When the period of hospitalization is over and the patient is ready to return home to continue its recovery, it is essential that the owner is given explicit instructions with regard to its aftercare. For example, it must be stressed that confinement in the house does not mean free access to the stairs and jumping on to furniture. Likewise, restricted exercise, in the case of the dog, it must be kept on a lead, even when briefly let out in the garden. Gradually increased exercise may be allowed only as the patient progresses: a dog or cat should not be let loose to run around the garden unattended. In the care of the cat, there should be gradual progress from cage to small room and then the ground floor of the house. Access to high obstacles from which they can jump should be prevented, food should not be left out on kitchen tables, whilst partially open windows are another source of temptation for the convalescent cat.

The owner nursing an animal at home, must be instructed to contact the veterinary surgeon if any abnormality in healing is noticed. Regular appointments for re-examination of the orthopaedic case being nursed, should be arranged.

### Further Reading

BEDFORD, P. (1984) *Atlas of Canine Surgical Techniques,* Blackwell, Oxford.

BOSTOCK, D. E. and OWEN, L. N. (1975) *Neoplasia in the dog, cat & horse,* Wolfe Medical Publications, London.

BOJRAB, M. J. (1983) *Current Techniques in Small Animal Surgery,* 2nd Ed, Lea & Fibiger, Philadelphia.

HALL, L and CLARKE, K. (1983) *Veterinary Anaesthesia,* 8th Ed, Bailliere Tindall, London.

HOUGHTON, M. and HUDD, J. (1967) *Theatre Technique,* Bailliere Tindal, London.

HUROV, L. (1978) *Handbook of Veterinary Surgery, Instruments & Glossary of Surgical Terms,* W.B. Saunders, Philadelphia.

KNECH, ALLEN and WILLIAMS (1981) *Fundamental Technique in Veterinary Surgery,* W.B. Saunders Philadelphia.

SETTLER, KNOWLES and WHITTICK (1981) *Veterinary Critical Care,* Lea & Fibiger, Philadelphia.

TRACY, D. L. (1983) *Small Animal Surgical Nursing,* C. V. Mosby, St. Louis.

# CHAPTER 11

# Obstetrical and Paediatric Nursing

G. T. WILKINSON

## Oestrus

### Puberty

In the bitch, puberty, i.e. the ability to reproduce, is normally reached between 7 and 12 months of age, but there is a good deal of variation especially between different breeds. For example, some greyhound bitches may not show signs of oestrus until they are 2 years old.

In the female cat (queen), the age at puberty averages 9–10 months, but again this is dependent upon certain factors, including the time of the year when the kitten was born and its breed. For example, a kitten born in the spring may not come into oestrus until the following spring when she will be 12 months old. This is due to the fact that at the time when she would be attaining puberty, most cats are entering the period of sexual inactivity or anoestrus. On the other hand, it is not unusual for a kitten to have its first oestrous cycle at $3\frac{1}{2}$ months of age. The Colourpoint Long-hair breed ("Himalayan" in the United States) is usually later than other breeds in attaining puberty, averaging about 13 months of age, whereas Burmese kittens tend to reach puberty early when they are about 7 months old.

## The oestrous cycle

The oestrous cycle of the dog and cat depends upon a complex interaction of neural and hormonal factors. In the hypothalamus area of the female brain there is an intrinsic cycling centre which exerts a fundamental control over the reproductive cycle, but which is itself influenced by external stimuli from the environment and by internal stimuli arising from within the animal's body. This hypothalamic control of the reproductive system is mediated through the anterior portion of the pituitary gland, situated at the base of the brain, mainly via the secretion of two hormones, follicle stimulating hormone or FSH, and luteinizing hormone or LH.

FSH stimulates the development of the ovum (egg)-bearing **follicles** in the ovary, which in turn secrete another hormone, oestrogen. Initially the low levels of oestrogen produced stimulate the release of more FSH, resulting in accelerated follicle growth and increasing blood levels of oestrogen. The latter is responsible for the onset and physical signs of oestrus, which make the female attractive to the male and prepare her for mating. High blood levels of oestrogen exert what is termed a "negative feedback" effect on the pituitary gland, shutting off further FSH release and triggering the release of LH. Initially this occurs in the form of a high-level burst or pulse, which causes rupture of the follicles and release of their contained ova (ovulation). The ruptured follicles then become filled with a yellow glandular tissue, the **corpus luteum**, under the influence of continuing low blood levels of LH. The corpus luteum secretes another hormone, progesterone, which prepares the uterus to receive the fertilized ova and plays an important part in maintaining the resulting pregnancy. High blood levels of progesterone exert a negative feedback on the pituitary gland inhibiting the secretion and release of both FSH and LH.

(a) *The bitch* is described as being "monoestrous" in that she only ovulates once during each breeding season. The canine oestrous cycle can be divided into pro-oestrus, oestrus, metoestrus and ano-estrus. Pro-oestrus heralds the start of the cycle and is indicated by swelling of the external genital organs followed in 2–4 days by a blood-stained discharge from the vulva. As the discharge increases, the vulva and neighbouring part of the vagina become more enlarged and turgid, and warm to the touch. This warmth has given rise to the lay term of **heat** to describe oestrus. The bitch becomes restless and excitable, she may wander from the house and does not respond in her usual manner. She drinks more water and urinates more frequently, often passing small quantities of urine. Although the bitch becomes increasingly more attractive to male dogs, she will not accept their advances. Pro-oestrus has an average duration of around 9 days but this varies with different breeds with a range of from 2 to 27 days. Oestrus immediately follows pro-oestrus and is considered to start from the time when the bitch will accept the male. The vulva **remains** swollen but the vaginal discharge

is now clearer and contains less blood. The bitch in oestrus tends to adopt a position with her back arched and with her tail elevated and held horizontally to one side. Oestrus lasts for an average of 9 days with a range of from 3 to 21 days. Dog breeders refer to the combined period of pro-oestrus and oestrus as "heat" or "being in season". Metoestrus* follows oestrus if pregnancy does not ensue. As there are no special physical signs shown by the bitch during this stage, although the vulval swelling and the vaginal discharge diminish considerably, its duration is difficult to determine, but it is thought to average about 30 days although it might extend up to 90 days in some cases. Quite a high proportion of bitches will develop a condition known as "false or phantom pregnancy" or "pseudo-cyesis" during this phase of the cycle.

*False pregnancy* results from the effect of the continued secretion of progesterone by the corpus luteum in the absence of true pregnancy. It occurs with sufficient frequency to be regarded as a normal physiological process under conditions of domestication. The bitch may show all the psychological and physiological signs of pregnancy including abdominal distension, enlargement of the mammary glands with the secretion of milk in some cases, and a maternal instinct manifested by

*There is some controversy regarding the terminology of the oestrus cycle of the bitch partly due to the fact that the bitch is keyed into sexual receptivity by progesterone (after oestrogen priming). This means that the classical division of the cycle into pro-oestrus (period prior to sexual receptivity and associated with follicle growth); oestrus (period of sexual receptivity); metoestrus (period of initial establishment of the corpora lutea) and dioestrus (period of mature luteal activity) does not really fit the pattern shown by the bitch. So the terminology used above, in which metoestrus is used for the whole period of luteal activity, has been evolved. However, it has been suggested that it is simpler to recognize that metoestrus, or early luteal function, occurs during the latter phase of oestrus, and to use dioestrus for the luteal phase of the cycle *beginning* with the *loss of sexual receptivity*.

bedmaking and nursing of soft furry or woolly objects, such as bedroom slippers, children's toys, etc. These signs usually subside spontaneously with time and can be encouraged to do so by simple measures, such as the administration of a mild saline laxative daily coupled with increased exercise. Occasionally the signs persist or the lactation assumes nuisance proportion and treatment with hormonal preparations is required.

Anoestrus is the stage of sexual inactivity and follows metoestrus. During this phase the external genitalia return to normal and the bitch is no longer attractive to male dogs. Duration of anoestrus varies from 2 to 8 months usually averaging about 4 months. The duration of metoestrus plus anoestrus determines the period between "heats" in the bitch.

Although there is no true breeding season in the bitch, there is a tendency for there to be a seasonal incidence of oestrus with a twofold higher incidence in the period from February to May.

(b) *The queen* is said to be "seasonally polyoestrous" in that she undergoes recurrent oestrous cycles at 21-day intervals during the breeding season. The latter usually extends from late January to September in the Northern Hemisphere, with peaks of breeding activity occurring from February to May and from July to August. Many cats, especially of the short-haired breeds and those confined entirely indoors, will continue to cycle throughout the year with no period of sexual rest, but the majority are anoestrus from late September to late January. The anoestrus period is thought to be associated with a decrease in the hours of daylight and it can be shortened, or even eliminated, by the provision of artificial light. This is probably the reason for the absence of an anoestrus period in many cats confined indoors.

The feline oestrus cycle can be divided into pro-oestrus, oestrus and dioestrus. This cycle is repeated until the end of the breeding season when the queen enters anoestrus. In the cat metoestrus coincides with pregnancy and is only occasionally seen in the queen that has not been mated unless ovulation has been induced by some artificial stimulus. Dioestrus is a period of sexual quiescence. Pro-oestrus lasts from 1 to 2 days, oestrus from 1 to 4 days and dioestrus is rather variable in duration, 7 to 12 days being common. In some queens, dioestrus apparently does not occur and oestrous behaviour can continue for 42 days without any obvious interruption.

Unlike the bitch the queen shows little visible signs of oestrus such as swelling of the vulva and vaginal discharge. The behaviour of the cat, however, presents quite striking evidence that she is in oestrus. Usually there is increasing restlessness and the cat may stay out of doors for long periods, sometimes being absent for days at a time. Allied to this restlessness there is an increase in vocal activity, varying from a more frequent "talking" to a raucous shriek or howl, the latter being most marked and distracting in the Siamese breed. This vocal activity gives rise to the lay terms of **calling** or "being on call" to denote oestrus. Some cats will become more affectionate to their owners at this time and a previously unmanageable cat will often allow itself to be groomed, evincing unmistakable signs of pleasure during the procedure. Many cats indulge in frequent rolling and crying, and this may cause inexperienced owners to seek veterinary advice as their cat is "rolling on the floor in agony". Other signs of oestrus are lordosis (concave curvature of the spine), raising of the hindquarters, deflection of the tail horizontally to one side and treading movements with the hindfeet.

## Mating

The optimum time for mating is during the oestrus stage of the reproductive cycle as this is the time in which the female will most readily accept service from the male and also the time when ovulation occurs. Most dog breeders mate their bitches between the 10th and the 14th day from the first signs of vaginal bleeding, i.e. from soon after the start of pro-oestrus, and on average this will coincide with the onset of oestrus. As mentioned earlier, however, there is a wide variation in the duration of pro-oestrus between individual bitches. The most certain method of detecting oestrus is to observe whether the bitch will accept the dog. A common practice is to present the bitch to the dog for mating on alternate days from the 10th day of pro-oestrus and allow two to three matings during the first 4 days from the time when the bitch will accept service. It is advisable to introduce the dog to the bitch whilst both are on leads until one can be satisfied that neither is going to bite the other. Mating should be arranged in an enclosed space where there is adequate room for the participants to move about in the preliminary play and courtship, but where there is a measure of control over the proceedings. The dog will approach the bitch, sniffing and licking at the external genitalia whilst the bitch, if ready, will stand motionless with her tail held horizontally to one side exposing the vulva. Maiden bitches often like to indulge in play, frisking away from the dog and wrestling with him for a little time before accepting service, but the experienced bitch usually mates straight away. An experienced stud dog usually has no difficulty in mounting the bitch by grasping her behind the shoulders with his front legs and inserting the penis into the vagina. He then makes several thrusts with his pelvis and at this time the continuing engorgement and enlargement of the penis coupled with a constriction of the vagina, results in the penis being held securely in the vagina, the so-called **tie**. Ejaculation occurs early in the dog, sometimes before the tie has taken place, so it is possible for conception to occur without a tie. The dog then drops on his forelegs at the side of the bitch, raises the appropriate hindleg over her back and completes a half-circle turn so that the partners now face in opposite directions. They remain in this position locked together by their genitalia for from 5 to 45 minutes until mating is completed. No attempts should be made to separate the two animals or to prevent them from adopting this rather peculiar position as it is thought that it assists in fertilization.

Ovulation occurs spontaneously in the bitch and all the ova are shed simultaneously, or nearly so, within 1–2 days of the onset of oestrus. Fertilization of the ova occurs about 72 hours after mating and implantation of the embryos into the lining of the uterus occurs about 21 days after mating.

The *cat* is a non-spontaneous ovulator, which means that ovulation does not occur automatically when the follicles ripen, as it does in the bitch, but requires some stimulus to trigger it off. It is not known precisely what constitutes this required stimulus, but it has been shown that mechanical stimulation of the cervix will induce ovulation, so it may well be that mating provides the trigger mechanism. This does not account for the fact that whereas the free-roaming queen will almost invariably conceive at every oestrus, the pure-bred cat subjected to controlled mating with one selected male (stud) often fails to conceive although apparently normal mating has occurred. It has been assumed that a single mating will induce ovulation, but it is highly probable that not only are several matings on successive days required, but also that a fairly prolonged period of **courtship** is necessary to ensure maturation of the ovarian follicles to the point when rupture will occur following mating. This courtship period occurs during pro-oestrus and may last for up to 4 days, during which time the female is surrounded by several males and witnesses their frequent battles and confrontations. During the courtship period the queen will reject, often quite aggressively, the advances of any of the males. This is followed by a period when the queen will accept service from a selected suitor and usually she is not promiscuous; although on occasion more than one male will be accepted. Several matings occur daily until oestrus declines. In contrast to this prolonged courtship, queens coming into oestrus within a few days after the birth of a litter, usually disappear briefly and accept service with few preliminaries. Such matings are generally fertile.

During mating the stud mounts the queen, taking a firm hold on the skin of the neck with his teeth and gripping her body between his forelegs, Intromission of the penis is achieved by a rapid thrusting movement and ejaculation occurs almost at once. There is no "tie" as occurs in the dog. The papillae of the glans of the penis would appear to produce a painful stimulus to the queen at the time of mating (p. 82). The queen emits a single, shrill cry and violently disengages herself from the stud, rolling to and fro on her back, with her fore- and hindlegs fully extended and with her front paws turned inwards with splaying of the toes and exposure of the claws. Intermittently she licks frantically at the vulva. Meanwhile the stud has retreated to a safe distance from which he watches the queen cautiously. Any attempt by the stud to reapproach during this "after-reaction" period is met with an aggressive response from the queen. After

an interval of from 15 to 60 minutes, the after-reaction dies down and the queen is ready to mate again. Following the period of acceptance oestrous behaviour usually continues for a further 24 hours, but the male is no longer accepted. Due to the rather peculiar anatomical arrangement of the male external genitalia in the cat, the full co-operation of the female is essential for mating to be possible and forced mating cannot be achieved in the cat as it can in the bitch.

Under controlled breeding, as occurs with pure-bred cats, the queen should always be brought to the male and introduced into his living quarters. Most stud houses incorporate separate accommodation, consisting of sleeping area, sanitary tray, and sufficient space for feeding and stretching, for the visiting queen. Her quarters must be secure and allow easy access for the queen without molestation by the stud. It would appear that the stud must be accustomed to his own quarters and have marked out his territory by spraying the boundaries with urine, before he feels sufficiently assured to mate.

By the end of the breeding season, many free-living males show a marked loss of bodily condition, with a rather staring, hidebound coat, tucked-in abdomen and often the enlarged kidneys, which are characteristic of the breeding male cat, can be seen protruding in the flanks. Owners may think that these prominences are due to tumours in the abdomen.

Ovulation occurs about 24 hours after mating, fertilization taking place 24–48 hours post-mating and implantation of embryos in the uterus occurring about 14 days thereafter.

## Pregnancy

### Normal pregnancy

In the bitch, gestation, i.e. the period between mating and parturition (whelping), averages 63 days with a range of from 59 to 66 days. Bitches of the small breeds tend to whelp slightly earlier than do those of the larger breeds. Puppies born before the 8th week of pregnancy seldom survive.

The bitch pregnant with several foetuses shows progressive signs of abdominal enlargement from the 5th week onwards, but if only one or two foetuses are present then distension of the abdomen may not be noticeable. A bitch pregnant for the first time (primagravida), especially if she is lean, will show more obvious abdominal enlargement than will a fat bitch which has already had several litters (multigravida).

Changes occur in the mammary glands and teats during pregnancy and again these are more noticeable in primagravida. Around the 35th day the teats become enlarged and turgid, protruding from the skin of the lower abdomen and chest. In bitches with unpigmented skin in this area they become bright pink in colour. About the 45th day the teats become still larger but are now softer and more tumefied, and may become pigmented in some bitches. The mammary glands themselves commence to enlarge about the 50th day of pregnancy, the enlargement progressing until by the time the bitch is due to whelp (term), the glands extend from the inguinal to the axillary region as two parallel rows of enlarged, oedematous areas separated by a depression in the midline. Two or 3 days before whelping a water secretion can be expressed from the teats, true milk secretion occurring with parturition. In multigravid bitches mammary enlargement is delayed, occurring from about the 56th day, and milk secretion may commence a few days before whelping.

Pregnancy diagnosis depends upon abdominal palpation, and in a co-operative, lean, small bitch foetal units can be detected as a series of tense, oval swellings in the uterus about 1 cm in diameter at about the 21st day. The best time to diagnose pregnancy, however, is about the 30th day when the foetal units have increased to around 2–3 cm in diameter. After this the uterus between the foetal units dilates and the demarcation between the units is lost. From about the 7th week it should be possible to palpate the actual foetuses, especially the ones nearest the pelvis. Radiography will usually reveal the foetal spines within the last 2 weeks of pregnancy although actual calcification of the skeleton does not occur until the last week. Laboratory pregnancy tests are not applicable to the bitch.

As described in an earlier chapter, the pregnant bitch does not require any increased food intake until about the 4th week, when her requirements will increase by about 20%. This will increase to as much as 66% by the 5th and 6th weeks. During the last 2 weeks food consumption usually decreases, possibly due to pressure of the enlarged uterus on the stomach, and it may be advisable to feed more concentrated, less bulky foods at this time preferably in more frequent, smaller meals. Providing the diet is a balanced one containing optimum amounts of vitamins and minerals, then supplements should not be required.

Normal exercise should be maintained throughout pregnancy but over-boisterous play should be discouraged. The pregnant bitch should be treated for round and hookworm infection twice during pregnancy, the second treatment being administered during the final 2 weeks.

Pregnancy in the cat is usually said to average 63 days, but it seems that this figure is on the low side. A more accurate average would be 65 days with a range of from 61 to 70 days. It is unlikely that kittens born before the 56th day will survive. One survey reported that stillbirth or early postnatal death occurred in all litters of Siamese or Persian kittens born following gestation periods of 60 days or less, whereas kittens born following gestations of 67, 68 or 69 days showed no stillbirths or early mortalities. There may be a genetic factor to length of gestation period as it has been noted that certain males will consistently sire litters of kittens with either shorter or longer gestation periods than average, never a mixture of both. There does not seem to be any correlation between time of year or breed and duration of gestation. Neither does the fact that the queen is pregnant for the first time appear to affect the length of pregnancy. Some pregnant cats will show signs of oestrus about the 21st and 42nd days, which can be confusing as far as pregnancy diagnosis is concerned.

Diagnosis of pregnancy can in the cat be performed by abdominal palpation at 21–35 days, when the foetal units can be appreciated as tense spherical swellings in the uterus, about the size of a pea in the early part of the period increasing to about 2 cm in diameter by the 35th day. After this time the uterus becomes generally enlarged and the constriction between foetal units can no longer be detected. About the 7th week the foetal heads and bodies can be recognized by palpation, and radiography during the final 2 weeks will reveal the skeletons of the kittens. Abdominal distension occurs in queens with several kittens in the litter from between the 5th and 6th weeks. In primagravida the nipples become more prominent and pink after the first 2 weeks. The mammary glands become enlarged mainly during the last week of pregnancy and progressivly assume the appearance as described in the bitch.

The average number of kittens in a litter is 4.5. It is probable that more ova are released and fertilized than kittens are born at full term. This is shown by the greater number of corpora lutea in the ovary than foetuses in the uterus being frequently observed at spaying of pregnant cats. As also occurs in the bitch, it is possible for members of the same litter to have two or more different sires. This is due to a process called "superfecundation", in which two or more ova released at the same ovulation are fertilized during successive matings by different males at the same oestrus.

The cat does not require any special management during a normal pregnancy. She should receive a balanced diet, particular attention being paid to the calcium: phosphorus ratio (Ca:P), which should be as close to 1:1 as possible, and to vitamin A, the requirement here being about 1600–2000 international units per day. It should be remembered that meat is very deficient in calcium and quite high in phosphorus, so that the Ca:P ratio is around 1:10. Milk contains a good supply of calcium and can provide a substantial proportion of the mineral required by the pregnant cat. Cooked fish containing the bones crushed up is another good source of calcium and will also contribute iodine which is almost absent from meat. The vitamin A requirements can be met by feeding a small quantity of liver, preferably raw, two or three times a week. If the cat cannot be persuaded to change from an entirely meat diet, then calcium carbonate should be added to the food at the rate of 0.5 g per 100 g wet weight of food. Usually the actual quantity of food consumed does not increase very much until about the 6th week, from which time it increases until the cat is eating about twice her normal food intake by the 8th to 9th week. It is better to divide the daily ration into two or three smaller meals rather than one big one, to allow for the enlarged uterus occupying most of the abdominal space.

For many years there has been a feeling

that it is detrimental and/or inefficient to mate a queen that is too young (variously interpreted as under 8 months old or during her first oestrus). It is thought that such a queen would produce a smaller litter and would probably care for it less well than a more mature animal. Many veterinarians were of the opinion that queens mated too young were themselves physically stunted by the experience. Recent studies have shown, however, that there is no evidence that queens allowed to mate in their first oestrus will perform poorly. Litter size is related to the number of litters the queen has had rather than her chronological maturity. It has been stated, in fact, that postponing mating a queen, especially of the Siamese or Burmese breeds, until she is more physically mature, might well lead to difficulties in achieving conception later.

Normal exercise, running, jumping and climbing are allowed and, in fact, are beneficial in maintaining the muscle tone of the cat. In the final 2 weeks of pregnancy routine treatment for roundworms should be administered (p. 375).

**Interruptions to pregnancy**

Abortion can be defined as the premature expulsion from the uterus of the products of conception, the embryo, or of a non-viable foetus. It can be expanded legitimately to include those cases in which the product of conception dies and is then resorbed rather than expelled from the uterus.

The causes of abortion in the dog and cat are legion and to a large extent are not yet clearly understood. In the human subject, if 40% of naturally occurring abortion can be explained, this is regarded as highly satisfactory. In the dog and cat the picture appears to be just as complex and abortion in these animals can be divided into two main categories:

(1) *sporadic*—associated with hormonal, nutritional, traumatic and other poorly defined causes;
(2) *infectious*—arising from bacterial, viral or protozoal origins.

*1. Sporadic*

The causes of this type of abortion are not well understood. In the cat **vitamin A deficiency** leads to poor breeding records with failures of implantation and abortions around the 50th day of pregnancy. Such deficiency often occurs following depletion of liver reserves by respiratory virus infections. Vitamin E deficiency may lead to abortion and infertility in rats but has not been implicated in the aetiology of canine of feline abortion. Nevertheless, it is a wise precaution to ensure that all breeding stock should receive sufficient vitamine E as part of a nutritionally adequate diet.

Pregnancy is normally maintained by **progesterone**, which is secreted by the corpora lutea for the first part of pregnancy and by the placenta for the remaining period. Abortions and resorptions before about the 7th week may be associated with defective hormone output of the corpora lutea and may be treated with LH. After this time the placenta may be deficient and pregnancy can often be maintained by the administration of progesterone.

Placental defects of a structural type may cause death of the foetuses due to anoxia. If the tissues between the maternal and foetal blood vessels become thickened for any reason, then proper interchange of oxygen and carbon dioxide is impaired and the foetuses may die from lack of oxygen leading to abortion or resorption.

Probably quite a number of abnormal embryos are conceived, but at a certain stage in their development the abnormality is sufficiently marked as to cause death. This might account for the discrepancies noted earlier between the number of corpora lutea and embryos. A 5% resorption rate of foetuses is considered normal in the bitch.

It is well recognized in human medicine that the age of the mother is an important factor in abortion, viz. with advancing maternal age there is an increasing incidence of abortion, and probably the same holds true for the dog and cat. In fact it has been noted that Beagle bitches over 5 years old have smaller litters than younger animals, probably due to foetal death. In the same way the chances of abortion rise with the number of previous pregnancies.

Severe trauma will almost certainly cause a heavily pregnant animal to abort or commence premature parturition, but this is a relatively infrequent occurrence and the cause is usually obvious in such cases. There is no evidence to suggest that normal running, jumping, and in the case of the cat, climbing trees, etc., increases the risk of abortion.

## 2. Infectious

A severe **viral infection**, such as distemper in the bitch or feline panleucopaenia in the queen, may cause resorption of foetuses or abortion. The feline leukaemia virus is suspected of causing abortion and resorption of foetuses in the cat. Among the bacteria, *Brucella canis* is specifically associated with abortion in the bitch while salmonellae, streptococci and *Escherichia coli* have been incriminated as causing abortion in both dogs and cats. In the cat, the protozoan parasites *Toxoplasma gondii* and *Haemobartonella (Eperythrozoon) felis* have been associated with abortion and stillborn kittens.

## Misalliance (mésalliance, mismating)

Quite frequently, despite all precautions by the owner, a bitch or queen in oestrus will escape surveillance and be mated. In such cases conception can be avoided by the administration of hormones which act by preventing nidation of the fertilized ova in the endometrium of the uterus. In the case of the bitch an injection of the female sex hormone, oestrogen, will prevent conception if given within 48 hours of mating. The effect of the oestrogen is that the oestrus period will be prolonged, and owners should be warned of this as a further mating during this period could prove fertile. In old bitches oestrogen injections have been associated with a high incidence of pyometra, a serious condition of the uterus which necessitates hysterectomy. In the queen oestrogens are rather toxic, and their use is to be avoided if possible. In this species conception can be prevented by the oral administration of a progestogen, megestrol acetate ("Ovarid", Glaxo) either in a single dose within 24 hours of mating or as a smaller dose given daily throughout the oestrus period.

## Abnormalities of pregnancy

The vast majority of pregnancies are completely normal in both the bitch and the queen. Ectopic pregnancies, i.e. where the embryo develop outside the uterus, have occasionally been reported but must be very rare. Rupture of the heavily gravid uterus may occur following crushing road accidents or, in the case of the cat or small bitch, by being grasped across the abdomen between the jaws of a large dog. In such cases the foetuses are liberated into the abdominal cavity and their placentas may adhere to other abdominal organs. As the tear in the uterus usually heals very quickly, if such a situation is revealed on exploratory laparotomy, it might be thought to be a case of ectopic pregnancy. Another accident during pregnancy which is more common in the queen than the bitch, is torsion of the uterus. This probably results from the animal jumping or twisting with the heavy uterus swinging over itself to become twisted. The torsion may involve one horn or the uterine body. The mishap usually occurs about term and parturition commences fairly shortly afterwards. If only one horn is involved then two or three kittens or puppies may be born normally after which labour ceases. Abdominal palpation reveals that there are more foetuses in the uterus which feels tense and painful. Inguinal hernia is not uncommon in the bitch although rare in the cat, and often the hernia contains one or both uterine horns. If the bitch becomes pregnant the hernia will increase rapidly in size and there may be a danger of strangulation of the imprisoned uterus or bowel. These conditions all constitute surgical emergencies and veterinary attention should be sought immediately.

### Parturition

About 10 days prior to the expected date of parturition it is advisable to provide a suitable place for the bitch or queen to give birth. In the bitch a whelping box, usually made of wood, and large enough for the bitch to move around comfortably yet still remain warm should be placed in a quiet room or kennel. The box should be raised off the floor to avoid draughts. The sides of the box should be about 10–15 cm (4–6 in.) high to stop the puppies crawling out of it but should be cut down to about 7.5 cm (3 in.) at one point to form a door for the bitch to enter and leave more easily. Some breeders like to run a wooden or metal rail horizontally around the sides of the box about 2 in. from the sides to allow an escape route for the puppies if the bitch is clumsy and tends to roll or lie on them. Bedding is provided in the form of layers of clean newspaper which can be removed and burned daily and provides good insulation for retention of heat. Provision should be made for heating to ensure an ambient temperature of about 26°C (80°F). Most cats like to find a spot where they are protected on at least three sides and which is in partial darkness. A cardboard box lined with several thicknesses of clean newspaper or wood wool and placed in the bottom of a cupboard makes an ideal nesting place. Long-haired bitches and queens should be clipped around the perineal area a few days before the expected time of parturition.

The approach of parturition is indicated by several signs. Relaxation of the pelvic ligaments cause the hindquarters to assume a rather sunken-in appearance and they feel soft to palpation. The external genitalia becomes swollen and there may be a slight mucous discharge from the vulva. The dam makes frequent visits to her bed and will often tear up the paper in an attempt to form a nest. About 24–48 hours before parturition commences there is a **sudden fall of the body temperature** until it is about 2°F below the normal, but this is often only transitory, so temperatures should be taken twice daily. Most dams will refuse food for 24 hours prior to parturition, while others may eat but often vomit the food soon after.

Parturition can be divided into three stages:

*Stage 1*

In this stage there is relaxation and dilatation of the cervix and the soft tissues of the birth canal. Intermittent uterine contractions occur but there are no observable straining efforts. The contractions must be intermittent at this stage to ensure that the blood supply to the placenta is not interrupted.

The bitch becomes restless, glances frequently at her flanks, shivers and usually pants fairly continually. More vigorous attempts at nest making occur. Some bitches will insist that the owner, or even another bitch, should keep her company, but others prefer solitude and like to seek out shelter under cover and partial darkness. On average the first stage lasts from 6 to 12 hours in the bitch, but it may extend to as much as 36 hours in a nervous animal whelping for the first time. On the other hand, the stage may pass almost unnoticed in a bitch that has borne several litters.

In the cat this stage is marked by the queen becoming restless, occasionally crying and making frequent trips to her box where she may indulge in some bedmaking activity. Usually there is no panting as is so often seen in the bitch, but this may occur during the latter part of the stage. In most cases the first stage in the cat lasts for 12–24 hours.

### Stage 2

In this stage the uterine contractions are intensified and the foetus is propelled through the cervix into the vagina. Its passage through the cervix initiates a neurohormonal reflex response which increases the uterine contractions. The foetus is contained within two fluid-filled sacs, the outer of which is the allantochorion and forms part of the placenta, and the inner the tougher amnion. The uterine contractions squeeze behind these sacs of fluid and exert a hydraulic effect which dilates the cervix and the already relaxed soft tissues of the vagina. This is a most important process, and if fluid is lost from the sacs early in parturition, dilatation of the birth canal does not occur and the birth can be difficult. The foetuses at the start of the second stage are lying in an inverted position with their limbs and head and neck flexed. During their passage out of the uterus they have to rotate and extend their heads and limbs, otherwise obstruction will occur. This rotation and extension is probably initiated by uterine contractions and movement of the fluid in the foetal membranes, but its continuation depends upon movements of the foetus itself to rotate on its long axis and extend its head, neck and limbs. A foetus which has died before passing out of the uterus and is thus incapable of performing these movements, almost invariably remains unrotated and unextended into the correct position for delivery.

By the time the foetus is approaching the pelvic inlet, the sac of the allantochorion is appearing between the lips of the vulva as the "water bag". It either ruptures spontaneously or is torn by the dam, releasing some fluid—the so-called "breaking of the waters". The amniotic sac remains intact and has now passed into the pelvic cavity further dilating the vagina by hydraulic pressure. As the head of the foetus becomes fully into the pelvic inlet, it initiates a reflex which brings into play forceful abdominal straining efforts by the dam to help to propel the foetus through the pelvis. The amnion now bulges through the lips of the vulva, which may present some obstruction to delivery in a primagravid dam, evoking signs of pain and possibly temporary cessation of her straining efforts. Once the head is through the vulva, however, the rest of the foetus slips out easily, lubricated and enclosed by the amniotic fluid. (Quite a high proportion of pups and kittens are born in posterior presentation, i.e. with the hindlegs and tail coming first, and this is of little consequence except that if it occurs with the first foetus of the litter, delivery may be rather protracted due to the absence of the dilating effect of the head on the birth canal. With such presentations death from anoxia is likely to occur especially if delivery is delayed, due to the fact that placental separation or compression of the umbilical cord against the floor of the pelvis cutting off the foetus's oxygen supply may occur before the head gains access to the air.) The dam tears the amniotic sac with her incisor teeth and pushes the membranes back away from the head of the foetus by vigorous licking. The latter action stimulates respiratory movements in the new-born pup or kitten, which is still attached to the placenta within the mother by the umbilical cord at this stage. The dam then bites through the cord with her carnassial teeth.

Most bitches prefer to lie on one side during the second stage, although some will remain standing particularly during straining bouts. Often the bitch will push herself around the periphery of the whelping box during straining, pausing from time to time to lick at the vulva. Straining efforts are characterized by extension of the head, neck, tail and sometimes the limbs, and may be accompanied by a low groan. Nervous or hysterical bitches may emit a shrill cry or even scream during such efforts. Between straining bouts the bitch pants rapidly and fairly continually. Intervals between the births of pups vary and are often dependent upon the number in the litter—if only two or three pups are present the interval tends to be longer than with a larger litter—but usually ranges from 15 to 60 minutes.

The cat behaves very similarly to the bitch in the second stage except that panting is not so marked and an inter-rupted type of labour occurs in the cat in which part of the litter is delivered normally and there is then a period varying from 12 to 24 hours during which the queen behaves as though parturition has been completed. Examination reveals that further kittens are present in the uterus, but the cat is well and the kittens born are apparently normal. Labour is resumed at the end of this period of rest and the remainder of the litter is delivered without difficulty. Uterine rest also occurs in the bitch but it is usually of much shorter duration than in the cat usually extending for only 2 or 3 hours.

The duration of the second stage varies considerably again according to the number in the litter but usually is completed within 4–6 hours in both species.

*Stage 3*

This is the stage of expulsion of the foetal membranes and the placenta. This occurs following involution or contraction of that portion of the uterus from which the foetus has come. The membranes are expelled and are usually eaten by the dam. This is a perfectly natural process although aesthetically unpleasant and should not be interfered with by the attendant. The third stage is short usually lasting from 5 to 15 minutes. Occasionally the next foetus follows on so quickly that the membranes are trapped and may not be delivered until they arrive wrapped around the head of the next but one foetus. More rarely two or three sets of membranes are held up and then expelled together in one mass. In the bitch the vaginal fluids during parturition are dark green in colour due to breakdown of the placental attachment to the lining of the uterus, whereas those in the cat are of a brown colour (p. 100). Appearance of a dark green vaginal discharge in the bitch or a brown one in the queen is evidence that placental separation is occurring and that the foetuses must be delivered fairly rapidly if they are to remain viable.

## Abnormal parturition (dystocia)

In the vast majority of cats, parturition (kittening) is completely normal, but the same cannot be said of the bitch due to the great disparity in size of different breeds and the exaggeration of certain features of conformation which has occurred with selective breeding in pure-bred animals. For instance, the massive head of the bulldog can lead to obstruction to delivery of the pup.

Dystocia can be divided into that of maternal origin and that of foetal origin.

## Maternal dystocia

Maternal dystocia is of two main types:

### 1. Uterine Inertia

This can be defined as the absence or weakness of uterine contractions at or subsequent to parturition. Inertia may be primary, in which case parturition does not commence, or if it does, soon ceases, or secondary, where obstruction to delivery has occurred and exhaustion of the uterine muscle has supervened.

(a) *Primary*—seen mainly in the bitch, the condition being quite rare in the queen. It occurs most frequently in bitches which are over 5 years of age, particularly if they are overweight and also if only two or three pups are present in the litter. Conversely bitches of the small breeds carrying large numbers of pups with consequent gross abdominal and **uterine distension** often show inertia. It is prob-

able that a number of causative factors are involved in the production of inertia including over-stretching of the uterine muscle, age or degenerative changes in the muscle, low blood calcium, hormonal factors and possibly genetic factors.

With complete primary uterine inertia* all the signs of imminent parturition are present but labour does not commence and the expected whelping date comes and goes. Usually a week later a dark-green vaginal discharge appears denoting that placental separation is occurring and that the puppies will soon die unless effective treatment is soon forthcoming. In most cases a Caesarean section is required. It is unwise to breed again from a bitch that has shown uterine inertia as the condition tends to recur at subsequent whelpings. With partial primary inertia, parturition commences but straining efforts are weak and infrequent and little progress is made by the leading foetuses. Providing that the cervix is dilated and there is no obstruction to delivery, such cases often respond to the frequent injection of small doses of oxytocin, a hormone secreted by the pituitary gland which causes uterine contractions. Oxytocin should only be administered at the direction of a veterinary surgeon as it may cause rupture of the uterus if the latter is overdistended, if the cervix is not dilated or if obstruction occurs. Some cases will also respond to the intravenous injection of calcium but again this must only be done under direct veterinary supervision.

(b) *Secondary* uterine inertia is treated by removing the obstruction to delivery, when following a period of uterine rest,

---

*Primary uterine inertia has been successfully treated in the cat by the injection of 0.5–1 mg/kg of prostaglandin $F_{2\alpha}$ repeated if necessary after 24 hours. Side effects consist of some colicky pain, urination and defaecation and the owner should be warned that these will almost certainly occur within a short time after the injection.

parturition will recommence and will usually be completed.

Under the heading **uterine inertia** can be included **nervous inhibition** of labour. In some pure-bred cats, especially the Siamese breed, the first stage of labour can be quite protracted with the queen becoming almost hysterical and following the owner about crying continually. It may be necessary to administer a mild tranquillizer in such cases before parturition can proceed. Both bitches and queens seem to be able to inhibit labour if the environment is not to their liking and, unfortunately, the requirements vary from one individual to another. Some animals like to have the reassuring presence of the owner while others prefer complete solitude and will not commence labour until assured that they are alone. Some will eschew the bed so carefully chosen by the owner and will inhibit parturition until allowed to pick their own site, which is often a most inconvenient one, e.g. the owner's own bed. A bitch or queen with just one or two oversized foetuses may inhibit when such foetuses engage in the pelvic inlet probably in response to pain, and in these cases straining is obviously cut short as pain occurs. Sometimes a primagravida will inhibit straining when the head of the foetus is at the vulva, probably again a pain response due to insufficient vulval dilation. In such cases the head of the foetus is easily palpable in the perineal area and it is essential that delivery should be achieved as quickly as possible if a live foetus is to be born.

In some breeds of dog such as the bulldog where the abdominal floor drops steeply away from the pelvis, the foetus has to be propelled uphill to the pelvis and this can lead to exhaustion of the uterine musculature and a secondary inertia. This can sometimes be prevented by lifting the floor of the abdomen by means of a towel passed around the abdomen or by trying to arrange that the bitch lies with her forequarters higher than the hind during whelping. Poor tone in the abdominal muscles due to lack of exercise during pregnancy or to obesity may result in a lack of effective straining during the second stage.

## 2. Obstructive Dystocia

This is where obstruction to delivery is due to abnormalities of the birth canal either in the soft tissues or in the bony pelvis. Soft tissue abnormality is rare in the cat and uncommon in the bitch, and includes such conditions as tumours within the vagina or encroaching on it from the pelvic soft tissues, a persistent mullerian duct in the form of a band of tissue extending from the roof to the floor of the vagina and occasionally a small or infantile vulva may present an obstacle to delivery. In the cat a deformed bony pelvis often results from calcium deficiency in the diet of the queen when a kitten. This is not uncommon, particularly in the Siamese which often dislikes milk and will only eat meat. In both cat and dog deformity resulting from healed fractures of the pelvis are common. In certain breeds of dog, e.g. the Scottish terrier, the pelvic inlet (p. 39) is flattened from above to below, and this can cause obstruction. Almost all cases of maternal obstructive dystocia require Caesarean section.

## Foetal dystocia

Owing to the fact that the bony maternal pelvis is non-dilatable and that its dimensions are such that the normal full-term foetus can just pass through it, it is essential that (a) the foetus should not be larger than normal, and (b) the foetus must be presented at the pelvic inlet in such a manner as to offer the minimal amount of obstruction. Foetal dystocia can thus be divided into:

(i) *Gross oversize* of the foetus which may be normal or abnormal. Oversize of a normal foetus occurs where there are only one or two foetuses in a litter, in matings between dogs where the sire is much larger than the dam, although pups tend to take after the size of their mother, and in breeds such as the Persian cat and the Pekinese which have a disproportionately large head. Oversize of an abnormal foetus is seen in the case of monsters, in oedematous foetuses and in foetuses which have died and are distended with gas.

(ii) *Abnormal presentation* of the foetus at the pelvic inlet such as deviation of the head to one side, breech presentation where the foetus is coming with the tail first and the two hindlegs extended forwards under the body, or when the foetus remains unrotated.

Dystocia can usually be recognized as delay in the process of parturition, and observation of the type of delay can indicate the type of dystocia. For example, delay in onset of parturition suggests primary uterine inertia, delay in delivery associated with weak or sporadic straining indicates partial primary, or possibly secondary uterine inertia if some foetuses have already been born, and, finally, delay in delivery despite forceful straining efforts is indicative of obstructive dystocia.

The RANA can be of great assistance to the veterinary surgeon in cases suspected of dystocia by **obtaining as much information as possible** to enable him or her to assess the situation and determine the best course of action. First it is essential to obtain as complete a history of the animal as possible, particularly in regard to previous breeding performance both of the dam and related animals, temperament, previous illnesses and behaviour during pregnancy and during the first stage if started. The time of onset of the three stages should be noted. The dam should be observed closely to determine whether straining is occurring and the character of any straining efforts, i.e. whether they are forceful and regular, weak and sporadic, or appear to be interrupted in mid-strain. The state of the vulva and perineum should be assessed and the presence and character of any vaginal discharge or fluid noted. The abdomen should be palpated gently to try to determine how near the leading foetus is to the pelvic inlet, to detect foetal movement and possibly uterine contractions, and to discover whether there are only one or two or many foetuses present in the uterus. The perineal area is palpated to determine whether any parts of the foetus have passed through the pelvis. Finally, if the results of such observations indicate a need, a digital exploration of the vagina should be performed. This procedure should only be performed by the RANA in the bitch, as the conscious cat strongly resents and resists such investigation.

*Vaginal exploration* requires care and attention to surgical cleanliness. The bitch is placed on a suitable table in a good light and the perineal area is cleaned with an antiseptic wash such as "Phisohex". The nurse's hands are scrubbed thoroughly in an antiseptic solution and any long fingernails are trimmed back so as to avoid trauma to the vagina. A lubricant, such as "KY Jelly" or an obstetrical cream, may be applied to the exploring finger if required. The forefinger is inserted into the vagina; most right-handed people find the left forefinger to be more sensitive than the right but this is a matter of personal choice, and the degree of dilation of the vagina is assessed and the presence of any soft tissue obstructions or bony deformities of the pelvis is determined. Foetal membranes may be palpable imparting a feeling of floating tendrils of tissue followed by a thin-walled, fluid filled bag. It may be difficult to distinguish the membranes from the walls of the vagina, but the latter are much thicker and firmer. The forefinger can be insinuated between the membranes and the vaginal walls, allowing a comparison to be made between the two structures. If the finger is raised so as to press on the roof of the vagina a straining reflex will be stimulated and this will often bring a portion of the foetus within reach, as well as indicating the strength of the straining effort. Sometimes raising of the abdominal floor with the other hand, or getting an assistant to raise the bitch's forequarters, will also bring the foetus within reach.

An attempt should be made to try to determine which portion of the foetus is presenting. If the presentation is correct, the blunt nose should be palpable through the membranes. The latter should be ruptured with the fingertip and the finger inserted in the mouth of the foetus. If it is alive it will usually make sucking movements and by feeling the ridges of the hard palate dorsally and the tongue and the lower jaw ventrally, one can determine that the foetus is in the normal rotated position; these structures are reversed in position in the unrotated foetus. If the head has not extended then the top of the head and the ears are presented. Deviation of the head and neck to one side often occurs in foetuses occupying the extremities of the uterine horns, possibly due to the lack of room for extension to take place, and also in short-faced breeds, where the absence of a long nose leads to failure of the head to engage correctly into the pelvic inlet. The deviation is often accompanied by extension of the foreleg opposite to the side to which the head is turned, so often one can palpate one foreleg and a rather shapeless mass just in front of the pelvic brim. With posterior presentation the tail and the two hindfeet can be palpated whilst in a breech presentation only the tail is palpable. Partial breech presentation is indicated by the presence of the tail and one hindfoot. Very rarely the foetus is transversely presented in which case one may be able to feel a rather shapeless mass just anterior to the pelvic brim in which it might be possible to detect the outline of the spine and the ribs.

Correction of any of these **foetal malpresentations** is outside the competence of the RANA, but she should be able to present a valuable report to the attending veterinary surgeon on her findings. Any digital vaginal examination should be performed as gently as possible and in as short a time as practicable, otherwise swelling of the vaginal lining and consequent further obstruction to delivery may be provoked.

Where a foetus is palpable in the perineal area or a part is visible at the vulva, the RANA must assist delivery if delay has occurred as the veterinary surgeon will be unable to arrive in time to save that particular foetus. If the nose is present at the vulva, the amnion is ruptured so that the foetus can have access to air when the maternal blood supply is cut off by compression of the umbilical cord in the pelvis. The head is fixed by holding it between thumb and forefinger through the perineal tissues and an attempt is made to gently push the lips of the vulva back over the head. This can be difficult in a primagravida but can be assisted by rubbing a little lubricating jelly around between the vulval lips and the head. Once the head is free it should be grasped in the right hand with the thumb under the lower jaw and two fingers hooked behind the ears. Gentle easing of the foetus is then applied in a downwards direction, i.e. towards the dam's hocks, and slightly towards the dam's right side so as to allow the shoulders to pass through one at a time. Pulling must only be applied during straining efforts and should be of a smooth, gentle, non-jerky nature. As the foetus begins to emerge, the left foreleg can be hooked forward with the left forefinger and the lateral traction is then exerted towards the dam's left side so as to free the right foreleg. Once the shoulders are free the remainder of the foetus slips out easily. In a posterior presentation, the tail and two hindfeet appear at the vulva. The feet are grasped with a dry cloth to avoid slipping and the vulva lips are pushed back over the foetus's hindquarters. When the hocks come into view the grip is shifted to them and foetus eased, again in a downwards and lateral direction, this time to ensure that the hips pass through alternately. With posterior presentation the head may become obstructed at the vulva, in which case the vulva lips are again pushed back over the head as already described.

## Post-parturient care

Once parturition has been completed, it is advisable to palpate the abdomen to ensure that all the foetuses have been delivered. Whilst this is comparatively easy in the cat and the small breeds of dog, larger bitches, especially if obese, present considerable problems in detection of a single foetus. If any doubt exists then veterinary advice should be sought.

The perineal area of the dam should be washed and dried and clean paper laid in the bed. The litter should be placed in contact with the mammary area and a watch kept to ensure that none are rejected. If a pup or kitten is persistently rejected then hand-rearing will probably

be required after a careful examination has revealed no obvious defects. The dam will usually accept a drink of water or milk but will seldom eat at this time. She may vomit some of the ingested foetal membranes, which should then be disposed of before she can re-ingest them. Most dams are reluctant to leave the litter for the first few hours so a sanitary tray should be provided near to the bed in the case of the cat, and the bitch coaxed outside on a lead to urinate and possibly defaecate. The dam's stools are often rather loose and blackish in colour for a few days post-partum.

Rectal temperature should be taken twice daily for 1 week following parturition. A rise to over 39.5°C (103°F) indicates the need for veterinary advice.

A reddish vaginal discharge is normal for up to 3 weeks after parturition but if it persists after that time, or if it appears to be composed of frank blood, then advice should be sought. Persistence of a dark green or brown vaginal discharge in the bitch or a brown one in the queen suggests retention of a foetus or foetal membranes in the uterus.

**Retention of foetal membranes** occassionally occurs but may remain unsuspected unless the attendant has observed each birth and counted the placentas. Suspicion should be aroused if the dam is restless, shows signs of abdominal discomfort, neglects her litter, has a slight temperature rise or shows a green or brown vaginal discharge.

Puerperal **metritis** is not common and is due to infection gaining access to the uterus whilst its powers of resistance are lowered by fatigue. This may occur following a protracted labour, uterine inertia, or where there have been manipulations per vagina or forceps delivery. The condition usually occurs within 3 days of parturition. There is a high temperature, loss of appetite, although the animal is often very thirsty, neglect of the litter and an offensive reddish-brown vaginal discharge which soils the perineum, hocks and tail. Nursing measures should include regular cleaning away of discharges to keep the patient as comfortable and clean as possible, tempting the appetite and possibly hand-rearing the litter.

**Mastitis** (inflammation of the mammary gland) may occur, often only one gland being affected, and may cause rejection of the litter. The affected gland is swollen, hard, reddened, hot and tender, and a brownish or blood-stained watery fluid can be expressed through the nipple. More rarely a definite abscess forms which will "point" and rupture with the discharge of creamy, offensive pus. On very rare occasions an acute necrotic mastitis may affect all the glands with the consequence that the dam becomes extremely ill from absorption of toxins. In such cases the glands turn black and eventually slough away leaving large areas of raw tissue. Treatment of the usual form of mastitis consists of hot fomentations of the affected gland to ease the pain and to bring blood to the area, gentle expression of the infected fluid through the teat and the administration of antibiotics. The litter should be removed and either hand-reared or weaned as soon as possible.

Lactation or puerperal tetany (**eclampsia**) occurs occasionally in the bitch but is rare in the cat. It usually occurs within 3 weeks of parturition but it has been recorded during the latter stages of pregnancy. The condition is due to a low calcium concentration in the extracellular fluid leading to muscle twitching and spasms. Affected bitches are restless and nervous, evidenced by whining, panting and pacing about. They become ataxic showing a stiff-legged, apparently painful gait and progress quite rapidly into a state of lateral recumbency with the limbs extended and the head, neck and tail arched upwards. Due to the muscle spasms the temperature may be very high, 41–42°C (106–108°F). Sometimes the central nervous system becomes involved and there are epileptiform convulsions although the bitch appears to retain consciousness. Loud noises or touching the animal will often stimulate tetanic or epileptiform attacks. In the cat signs vary from case to case but are again essentially nervous in character, and take the form of ataxia, muscular twitching and tonic spasms. There may be vomiting, rapid shallow breathing and very high temperatures. There may be unusual dryness of the sclerotic of the eye and the mouth. In both species treatment consists of the intravenous injection of a 10% solution of calcium borogluconate, up to 5 ml in the cat and up to 10 ml in the bitch. The injection must be made slowly, otherwise vomiting will occur and there may be serious effects on the heart. It is advisable to monitor the heart whilst making the injection, and the latter should be stopped if there are any signs of slowing of the heart rate or any arrhythmic heart sounds. Cats will respond to the subcutaneous injection of calcium borogluconate. The litter should be removed for 24 hours and the dam placed in a quiet, darkened room. If the temperature remains high then the patient should be cooled by the application of ice bags, especially to the head region. If the litter is old enough weaning should be achieved as quickly as possible, but younger pups and kittens can be hand-fed and suckled alternately for a day or two before returning them to the care of the dam.

### Lactation

It is important to realize that the nutritional demands on the dam are much greater during lactation than they are during pregnancy. In the bitch, depending on the number of pups in the litter, the nutritional requirements in the first week of lactation are **double the normal** maintenance requirements and these are trebled between the 4th to 7th weeks. In the cat in full lactation the nutritional requirements exceed the capacity of the cat to consume and digest food, so she has to mobilize her fat reserves and break down body protein to make up the deficit. Consequently there is loss of body weight but this is soon made up after the kittens are weaned.

Another phenomenon which is often seen during lactation is an excessive shedding of hair—a pronounced moult. This is due to the hormonal changes which occur at parturition and lactation and is a normal physiological process. The dam will regrow her coat quite rapidly after weaning has occurred.

## Management of the Newly Born

### Care of the newly born (neonate)

Normally the dam will free the neonate from the foetal membranes which may envelop it at birth. If she does not do this fairly promptly then the RANA must, as delay may result in asphyxiation. One should not be in too much of a hurry to sever the umbilical cord as there is evidence that a valuable amount of blood is expressed from the placenta and augments the neonate's blood supply in the first few minutes after birth. If necessary the cord should be torn between thumb and forefinger of both hands about 1 cm from the neonate's abdomen. Rarely the dam fails to sever the cord of three or four neonates, and the cords may become twisted around each other resulting in the neonates being drawn together as they crawl around. They are thus unable to get to the dam to suckle and will starve unless released by cutting the tangled cords.

Occasionally apparently lifeless young are born, but the vigorous licking action of the mother's tongue will usually revive them. If no sign of life appears within a short time the RANA must intervene. First ascertain whether there is a heartbeat by holding the chest lightly between the thumb and forefinger. If no beat is discernible the neonate should be put to one side. It is advisable to check whether there are any obvious abnormalities, such as cleft palate, before proceeding with **resuscitation**. Clear the airway by swabbing out the mouth and pharynx with cotton wool or by sucking out the back of the pharynx with a drinking straw with the neonate held head down and then compressing the chest gently a few times. Another useful method is to hold the neonate in the hand with the head between the finger tips and swing it head down in an arc three or four times. The "kiss of life" may be attempted, but it is important to allow the angles of neonate's mouth to remain open and to give very short, light puffs of breath, otherwise there is a danger of causing over-expansion and possibly rupture of the lung alveoli. The neonate should be rubbed briskly with a warm, dry towel, especially in the umbilical area, and this will often provoke indignant cries. Other useful measures to induce that important first gasp are to pinch the loose skin at the back of the neck fairly hard, to compress the chest gently in the region of the heart, or to dip the neonate in hot and cold water alternately. Once revived, the young one should be placed in a box on a **well-padded hot-water bottle** until sufficiently strong to be returned to the mother.

If the dam is very restive between births, it is advisable to remove any young already born to a warm box or an incubator (Fig. 11.1) until parturition is completed. Providing the mother is calm then the neonates should be allowed to remain

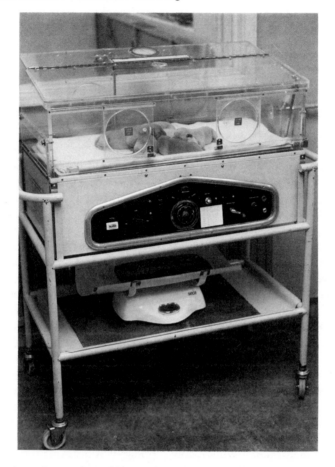

FIG. 11.1.   An incubator for puppies or kittens. (Courtesy of the Guide Dogs for the Blind Association.)

and encouraged to suckle as this tends to stimulate uterine contractions.

Newly born pups and kittens commence suckling immediately after they have been licked clean by the dam. In the 1st week of life suckling occurs about every 2 hours, after which the frequency falls off to around every 4 hours. If the mother's milk supply is inadequate, the litter appears hungry, nosing around the mother and crying continually. A check can be made on the adequacy of the milk supply by daily weighing of the young. They should gain weight every day and should have doubled their birth weight by about the 8th day. Weighing is best performed by suspending the young in a net suspended from a spring balance calibrated from 0 to 500 g, as the usual household scales are not sufficiently sensitive for kittens and pups of small breeds of dogs.

Healthy neonates spend a lot of the time sleeping. They tend to lie on their sides with limbs extended and relaxed showing occasional involuntary muscle spasms. They do not cry and crying should always be regarded as a warning sign that something is amiss. The mucous membrane of the mouth is bright pink in colour, the coat looks sleek and the body feels warm and firm to the touch. If roused they become quite vigorous and may indulge in high pitched squealing but soon settle down and relax when placed in contact with the mother.

For the first 3 days of life it is critical that the pup or kitten obtains access to a source of heat as at this age they are unable to raise their body temperature by shivering. The best source of heat is the mammary area of the mother, but some dams deny this to their offspring by restlessness, lying on their abdomen or pushing the young away. If this occurs, the pup or kitten soon shows signs that something is wrong. There is increase in activity and a high-pitched crying which occurs with every expiration. The respiratory rate increases and the neonate feels cool to the touch. In these cases it is essential that heat should be provided probably most conveniently in the form of a hot-water bottle. If the mother persists in denying access to the mammary area then it is advisable to keep the litter in a warmed bed returning them to the dam every 2 hours for suckling.

Both pups and kittens are born with their eyelids fused together, but these gradually part until the eyes are fully open, usually by about the 10th to the 14th day although it may occur as early as the 7th day in some litters. Certain breeds of dog are required by the show standards to have their tails amputated to a prescribed length. There is a good deal of controversy at present as to the ethics of performing this mutilating operation. However, if it has to be performed the optimum age for the operation is 4 days old. Dewclaws may be removed at the same time if necessary. Kittens and pups, especially the latter, should be treated for roundworms at 3 weeks of age, the treatment then being repeated every fortnight from 4 to 12 weeks of age. This régime will minimize the dangers of infection of human contacts, especially children, with the larvae of *Toxocara* spp.

## Care of the orphaned animal

Orphaned animals can be successfully reared by hand, but it is obviously much easier if a suitable foster-mother can be found. This can sometimes be achieved by advertising in a local paper or there are some kennels and catteries which supply foster-mothers for a fee. A pseudo-pregnant bitch may be used as a foster-mother. A foster-mother should always be examined for any sign of infectious disease and for the presence of ectoparasites, e.g. fleas, ear mites, etc., before putting the litter in contact with them.

The main aim of hand-rearing is to provide an acceptable substitute for the milk of the bitch or the queen and also to supply, as far as possible, those attentions normally given by the dam.

Table 11.1 shows the comparison between the milk of the cow, the bitch and the cat.

As can be seen from Table 11.1 the chief differences between the milk of the different species are that canine and feline milk are much more concentrated than bovine milk, containing more than **twice as much protein** and, in the case of the bitch, more than twice as much fat. In addition, the milk of the bitch and the queen contains more than twice the calcium and phosphorus content of cow's milk. Powdered evaporated cow's milk intended for human babies ("Ostermilk No. 2", Glaxo) reconstituted at twice the concentration recommended for babies and supplemented with 8 g of calcium phosphate per litre, constitutes a good substitute for bitch's or queen's milk. The powder may be difficult to dissolve at this strength and it is easier to dissolve skim

Table 11.1

|          | Cow's milk % | Bitch's milk % | Cat's milk % |
|----------|:---:|:---:|:---:|
| Protein  | 3.2 | 7.5 | 9.5 |
| Fat      | 3.9 | 8.3 | 4.8 |
| Lactose  | 4.9 | 3.7 | 4.9 |

milk powder at double strength. Then add 10 ml of vegetable oil, which may be olive or corn oil, to 90 ml of the mixture at blood-heat. The oil should contain 80 μg of vitamin A per ml for the first 2 days followed by 50 μg/ml. The vitamin can be supplied in the form of "Abidec" (Parke, Davis) or "Adexalin" (Glaxo) drops. Another satisfactory substitute for bitch's milk can be made up by adding 200 ml of single cream and one egg yolk to 800 ml of whole cow's milk and carefully stirring into the mixture 6 g of sterilized bone flour and 4 g of citric acid in that order. The mixture will keep for a few days in the refrigerator. Commercial canine and feline milk substitutes are also now available, e.g. "Cimicat" (Hoechst) (see also p. 203).

The milk substitute should be heated slowly to about blood-heat (37°C), and can then be fed to the orphaned animals through a foster feeding bottle ("Catac" Foster Feeding Bottle, Cats Accessories Ltd, 1 Newnham Street, Bedford, England), which is available with different sizes of teats for dogs and cats, or through a doll's plastic feeding bottle. A more rapid method of feeding, which can easily be mastered with a little practice, is to pass a length of soft rubber or polythene tubing, about 2 mm in diameter, down the oesophagus into the stomach and then inject the milk mixture through a syringe. Mark the tube with marking ink at a point three-quarters of the distance from the pup's or kitten's nose to its last rib. Attach the **feeding tube** to the syringe and draw up the appropriate amount of mixture. Hold the orphan's head with the index finger and thumb of the left hand just wedging the mouth open and pass the tube gently over the tongue into the back of the throat, where it will be instinctively swallowed and can be passed down until the mark on the tube is at the nose. The tube should slide in easily and if it sticks after only an inch or two have been passed, **do not force it** as it may have entered the trachea, although this is unlikely in the kitten, withdraw it and try again. Once the tube is in position the syringe is then emptied gently. The amount of mixture to be given is calculated on the calorific requirement of the orphan and this is different in the pup and the kitten. Whereas the pup requires around 60 kcal per 500 g body weight daily the kitten needs much more at 200 kcal per 500 g body weight daily. The milk mixture recommended contains about 1 kcal/ml. Kittens weigh around 100 g at birth and require feeding every 2 hours for the 1st week during the day and every 4 hours at night, say ten feeds per day. From this we can estimate that the total daily calorific intake is 40 kcal = 40 ml of mixture divided by ten feeds = 4 ml per feed. Pups vary in birth weight according to breed, but the same principles can be used to determine the amount to be given per feed. These quantities will have to be increased as the orphan animal gains weight. After the 1st week the frequency of feeding can be reduced to every 4 hours during the day and every 6 hours at night. By the 4th week feeds should be at 8-hour intervals day and night. If diarrhoea develops dilute the mixture to half strength then gradually increase it up to the recommended concentration. Defaecation and urination must be stimulated after each meal by gently stroking the perineal area with a paper tissue. The

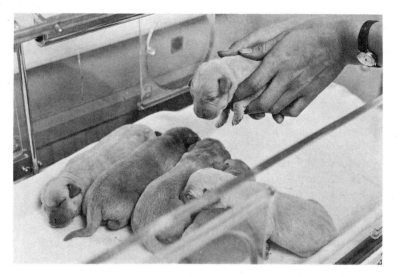

Fig. 11.2. Handling new-born puppies. (Courtesy of the Guide Dogs for the Blind Association.)

latter is preferable to cotton wool which may give rise to a type of "nappy rash".

Orphaned litters require an ambient temperature of about 30°C (86°F) and this can best be monitored by placing a thermometer in the bed. Heat can be supplied by means of an infra-red lamp, hot-water bottle, reading light, etc. Probably the best bed is a large cardboard box lined with cotton wool. In such draught-free surroundings the orphans should be able to keep themselves warm by 3–4 weeks of age.

## Weaning

Weaning is the transition from a very low fibre milk diet to a more solid, adult diet, which is considerably higher in fibre content. This transition must be made gradually to avoid gastrointestinal disturbances. The foods used for weaning should be high in protein and calories as the energy and protein requirements of the young growing animal are about twice the adult animal's needs.

The weaning period should start when the litter is 3 weeks old but it can be commenced earlier in certain circumstances, e.g. orphaned animals, lactation tetany in the dam, etc. It is first necessary to teach the pup or kitten to lap milk from a saucer. This can be done by allowing the young to suck on one's finger which is then brought into contact with the surface of the milk. Once lapping has been achieved then a weaner powder, such as "Farex" (Glaxo), and some dissolved meat jelly, derived from any proprietary tinned cat or dog food, can be added to the milk to make it more solid. Later some scraped cooked beef can be added to the mixture and gradually the diet is made more solid in consistency. Good quality canned dog or cat food can be made into a gruel or porridge-like consistency by the addition of reconstituted dried milk, meat broth or soup. Strained baby foods can be very useful at this stage. During the period of weaning the litter is allowed access to the mother and continues to suckle although at lengthening intervals as the young's hunger is satisfied increasingly with the more solid food. Except for immediately before and after feeding, clean water should be available to the litter at all times.

The frequency of feeding during weaning depends upon the dam's milk supply and the ambient temperature. If these are satisfactory then the litter will need about 3 meals daily, but if the milk supply is poor and the temperature low, then 5 meals a day may be required. As the demands on the dam decrease, the milk supply begins to wane and the dam herself tends to lose interest in the litter, leaving the young to their own devices for increasing periods of time. Eventually, usually by about the 6th week, the dam will reject the young which should by this time be weaned on to a solid diet, although still drinking cow's milk as a nutritional supplement. When weaning kittens it is important to accustom them to as wide a variety of foods as possible, as once food fads have developed it is very difficult to make changes in the diet which may be necessary for medical reasons. Weaned pups and kittens require about five meals daily of a sufficient quantity which can be eaten within 5 minutes. The frequency of feeds should be gradually reduced so that by the time the young animals attain maturity they should be receiving 2 meals daily. Young growing animals require a diet with a high content of protein of good biological quality, a high calorific value and with a calcium:phosphorus ratio as near to 1:1 as possible.

### Common congenital abnormalities and deformities

Congenital abnormalities, i.e. abnormalities that are present at birth, are more common in dogs than in cats, probably due to the fact that until recently there has been less human intervention in feline breeding (p. 211). Cleft palate, which is due to a failure of the two halves of the hard palate to fuse together, is seen quite frequently in the brachycephalic breeds such as the Pekingese, Pug, etc. Pups of these breeds should always be examined for this defect as soon as possible after birth. It is kinder to destroy affected animals as they are unable to suckle due to their inability to form a vacuum within the mouth and will die slowly of starvation. The condition occurs in the cat especially in the Long-hair (Persian) breed and in kittens where the dam has been treated with certain drugs during pregnancy. Failure of the bones of the cranium to fuse may cause a defect in the skull through which a portion of the brain bulges (encephalocoele). Similarly, failure of the vertebral arches of the spine to join together leads to a condition called spina bifida, which is commonly seen in the Manx cat.

Infection of the queen with the virus of feline panleucopaenia may result in the birth of kittens in which that part of the brain concerned with balance, the cerebellum, is poorly developed. This defect results in disturbances of balance, ataxia and fine tremors of the head and neck, which are especially noticeable when the kitten attempts to feed.

Hydrocephalus, or the accumulation of fluid in the ventricles of the brain, occurs in both species and may be hereditary in nature in the cat. The condition is more common in certain canine breeds such as the Chihuahua. The cranium is enlarged and dome-shaped and the whole head may be enlarged and oedematous.

Microphthalmos, a condition in which the eyes are very small and may be cystic, is a relatively common abnormality occurring most often in the Pekingese but also an hereditary type occurs in the Great Dane, Shetland Sheepdog and the Collie. Anophthalmos, or complete absence of the eyes, is rare.

Congenital malformations of the heart occur occasionally and are usually manifested by stunting of growth, respiratory distress, a very rapid heart beat, sometimes clearly audible abnormal heart sounds and the accumulation of fluid in the abdomen or thorax.

In the kitten especially, some congenital abnormalities are associated with deficient feeding of the mother during pregnancy. In vitamin-A deficiency, kittens may be born with chests flattened dorso-ventrally, hydrocephalus, deafness, ataxia, intention tremors and spasticity of the tail and hindlegs. Where there is calcium deficiency there is malformation of the scapula, the chest and the pelvis, and growth ceases. In iodine deficiency kittens may be born almost hairless and with open eyes and cleft palates.

Obvious monsters are occasionally seen and are usually stillborn. They include such malformations as "Siamese twins", in which two foetuses are joined together by some parts of their anatomy; schistosoma reflexus, in which the spine is angulated so that the head and tail are brought close together dorsally and there is incomplete closure of the thorax and abdomen ventrally with exposure of the viscera; and one-eyed or "cyclops" monsters.

Finally, an important inherited defect which may not be noticed for several days or more is atresia anus, in which the anus is absent. This means that faeces cannot be passed so that there is a build-up of waste material in the rectum and colon leading to abdominal distension and failure to thrive.

## Further Reading

ARTHUR, *et al.* (1982) *Veterinary Reproduction and Obstetrics,* 5th edn., Baillière Tindall, London.

FREAK, M. J. (1975) Practitioners'–breeders' approach to canine parturition, *Veterinary Record* **96**, 303–8.

JONES, D. E. and JOSHUA, J. O. (1982) *Reproductive and Clinical Problems in the Dog,* Wright, Bristol.

UNIVERSITIES FEDERATION FOR ANIMAL WELFARE. (1972) *The UFAW Handbook on the Care and Management of Laboratory Animals,* 4th edn., Churchill Livingstone, Edinburgh.

# Glossary

**abdomen**  The cavity of the body that lies between diaphragm and the pelvis.

**albuminuria**  albumin (a protein) in the urine.

**alopecia**  Loss of hair.

**anaesthesia**  Temporary loss of conscious sensations, especially touch and pain.

**analgesia**  Absence of pain.

**anorexia**  Loss of appetite for food.

**anoxia**  Lack of oxygen.

**anthelminthic**  A drug which kills parasitic worms.

**antibiotic**  A drug produced by a micro-organism which is antagonistic to the growth or life of other micro-organisms. Some are now produced synthetically.

**antibody**  A protein fraction formed by plasma cells, which specifically combines with an antigen, in order to eliminate it from the body.

**anticoagulant**  A drug that prevents the clotting of blood.

**antidote**  An agent that counteracts the effects of a poison.

**antigen**  Any substance (e.g. in bacteria) that stimulates the production of an antibody.

**antiseptic**  A substance, usually a chemical solution, which will destroy micro-organisms, but not necessarily bacterial spores, on living tissue without damaging that tissue.

**antiserum**  A drug, derived from the blood of an immune animal which contains a high concentration of antibodies against a disease producing agent, usually a micro-organism or its toxin.

**antitoxin**  A drug containing a high concentration of antibodies against a specific toxin.

**apnoea**  The cessation of breathing—often temporary, during anaesthesia due to reduced carbon dioxide in the blood.

**arthritis**  Inflammation of a joint.

**ascites**  The presence of oedema fluid (transudate) in the abdominal cavity, producing a swollen abdomen.

**asepsis**  Absence of "sepsis" or of pathogenic micro-organisms.

**auto-immune disease**  A disorder produced by anti-bodies (or sensitized lymphocytes) that are produced by an animal against its own cells or tissues.

**bile duct**  The tube that conveys bile from the liver and gall bladder to the duodenum (first part of small intestine).

**blood platelets**  (thrombocytes)  Small particles of cytoplasm present in the blood that are concerned in the arrest of haemorrhage including blood clotting.

**bronchi**  The two tubes into which the trachea divides. They lead into the bronchioles within the lungs.

**cachexia**  Extreme debility and emaciation.

**calculus**  A concretion of mineral salts, or "stone", formed within an organ—principally the urinary bladder.

**callus**  The tissue which forms around the fractured ends of a bone and ultimately develops into hard bone to repair the fracture.

**carcinogenic**  Cancer-producing. A number of agents (e.g. feline leukaemia virus, radiation, tar compounds) are known to cause or predispose to the development of cancer.

**cardiac**  Relating to the heart.

**carnassial teeth**  The largest in the jaw; in the dog they are the 4th premolar teeth in the upper jaw and the 1st molar teeth in the lower jaw.

**caudal**  Relating to the tail or directed towards the tail end of the body.

**cautery**  The application of a caustic substance or a heated instrument to destroy tissue.

**cephalic**  Relating to the head, or directed to the head end of the body. One of the foreleg veins, used for injections, is called the cephalic vein.

**Cheyne-Stokes respiration**  A rhythmic waxing and waning of the depth of respiration. Short periods when the depth of respiration gradually increases and then decreases again are separated by short periods when breathing ceases.

**chorea**  Involuntary twitching of muscle, often seen in dogs after distemper infection.

**cirrhosis**  Chronic inflammatory disease of the liver that causes destruction of liver cells and scarring (fibrosis).

**cloaca**  An opening, e.g. in birds, which is common for both the alimentary canal and the urinogenital system.

**commensalism**  A state in which a parasitic organism does no damage to its host but is no advantage to it either.

**condyle**  A rounded articular surface on a bone which forms part of a synovial joint.

**constipation**  Infrequent or incomplete passage of faeces.

**cortex**  The outer zone of an organ as distinguished from the inner part or medulla.

**cranial**  Relating to the skull or directed to the head end of the body.

**crepitus**  The grating noise produced by the rubbing together of the parts of a fractured bone.

**cryosurgery**  (or cryotherapy)  A technique in which intense cold is applied in a controlled manner to kill diseased cells while producing the minimum of damage to healthy tissue.

**cyanosis**  A bluish-purple colour of mucous membranes or skin due to an inadequate oxygen supply to the tissues.

**cyst**  A closed cavity filled with fluid.

**dermatomycosis**  An infection of the skin with ringworm fungus.

**diaphysis**  The shaft of a long bone.

**diastole**  Those stages of the heart cycle when the heart muscle relaxes so allowing the atria or ventricles to fill with blood again.

**diathermy**  The generation of heat in a tissue using a high frequency electric current, e.g. to destroy tissue or stop bleeding.

**diphasic**  Occurring in two stages or phases e.g. the dog's temperature rise in canine distemper.

**diuretic**  A drug which increases the volume of urine produced.

**dysphagia**  Difficulty in eating, particularly in swallowing.

**dyspnoea**  Difficulty in breathing.

**dystocia**  Difficult or abnormally slow parturition.

**dystrophy**  Wasting of muscles or other organs, often due to defective nutrition of the organ.

**eclampsia**  A twitching condition in the lactating female that will progress to convulsions; it is due to a fall in blood calcium (from a Greek word meaning "sudden development").

**ectropion**  Eversion or outward turning of the eyelids.

**eczema**  A general term for forms of non-contagious skin inflammation, characterized by irritation, discharge and/or the development of crusts and pustules.

**embolus**  An amount of material (blood clot, fat, air, etc) which, after circulating in the bloodstream, blocks a small blood vessel.

**empyema**  An accumulation of pus in a body cavity, usually the thoracic cavity.

**epididymis**  A convoluted tubule outside the testicle in which the sperm mature.

**epiphora**  Persistent overflow of tears (lacrimal fluid). The cause of a brown streak down the face of many white dogs.

**epiphysis**  An end of a long bone, initially separated from the shaft.

**epistaxis**  Bleeding from the nose (nasal chamber).

**erythema**  Superficial reddening of the skin.

**ESR**  An abbreviation used for the rate at which red blood cells sink or sediment through plasma, (=erythrocyte sedimentation rate).

**fertilization**  The fusion of the sperm and egg.

**fever**  A complex disorder of the body's metabolism. It is usually characterized by a high temperature (called pyrexia) and other changes including increased pulse and respiratory rates and loss of appetite.

**fistula**  An abnormal passage connecting the cavities of two internal organs or connecting the cavity of an internal organ to the surface.

**foetus**  An unborn animal after the main anatomical regions can be distinguished. In the dog and cat the embryo is known as a foetus after about 3 weeks of pregnancy.

**foramen**  A hole, as in a bone (foramen magnum) or other tissue, e.g. the foramen ovale of the heart.

**furunculosis**  Rupture of hair follicles; usually the result of bacterial infection producing multiple openings through which pus drains (e.g. anal furunculosis).

**gamete**  Either of the two mature sex cells (egg or sperm) each of which carries half the normal number of chromosomes.

**gangrene**  Death of tissue accompanied by bacterial decomposition (putrefaction).

**general anaesthesia**  A temporary loss of sensation accompanied by unconsciousness, produced by a reversible and controlled depression of the central nervous system.

**granulation**  The growth of vascular connective tissue as seen in the healing of open wounds by second intention.

**haematocrit**  A test to separate the blood into its various parts, used mainly for the measurement of the packed cell volume (PCV).

**haematoma**  A swelling containing blood; *plural*: haematomata.

**haematuria**  Red blood cells in the urine.

**haemoglobin**  The oxygen carrying red pigment of the red blood cells.

**haemolysis**  The breakdown or lysis of red blood cells.

**haemopoiesis**  The formation of blood cells both red and white.

**hepatitis**  Inflammation of the liver.

**hibernation** A dormant state in which the metabolism is slowed down. Used by some animals during a winter period when food supplies are short.

**hypotension** Abnormally low blood pressure.

**hypothermia** Abnormally low body temperature.

**icterus** Yellow coloration of the skin and mucous membranes due to an excess of bile pigments. Also known as jaundice.

**immunity** Some form of body resistance to infection.

**implantation** The time early in pregnancy when the fertilized egg (zygote) becomes attached to the wall of the uterus.

**inspiration** The flow of air (or gases) into the lungs during breathing.

**intussusception** The passage of a length of intestine into the length lying just beyond it.

**ischaemia** A localized deficiency in the blood flow to an organ.

**ischium** The most posterior of the three bones which are joined to form the pelvic bone.

**keratitis** Inflammation of the cornea of the eye.

**lacrimal ducts** Two small tubes in each eye which connect the lacrimal puncta in the corner of the eye to the nasolacrimal duct. This drains the tears to the nasal chamber.

**lesion** Any injury, wound or other damage to a tissue or organ.

**leukaemia** The presence in the circulating blood of white blood cells showing characteristic cancerous changes.

**local analgesic** A type of temporary loss of sensation, usually known as local anaesthesia. A drug is used to prevent the conduction of nerve impulses; both sensory and motor fibres may be affected.

**lymphocytes** A type of white blood cell produced by lymphoid tissue and concerned with the development of immunity.

**malignant** A virulent disease or condition which gets worse and is usually fatal. Usually applied to tumours or to severe infections.

**median** In the middle or midline, e.g. a median section of the brain.

**mediastinum** The midline space of the thorax between the two pleural sacs.

**melanoma** A tumour of melanin pigmented cells.

**meningitis** Inflammation of the membranes around the brain and spinal cord.

**metastasis** Transfer of disease from one part of the body to another—usually applied to the spread of tumour cells.

**metritis** Inflammation of the uterus.

**mycosis** A fungal disease.

**myocardium** The heart muscle which makes up most of the heart's total volume.

**narcotic** A drug which produces heavy sedation resulting in stupor and insensibility to pain.

**neoplasm** A new and abnormal growth of cells in the body.

**nictating membrane** The third eyelid. Consists of a fold of conjunctiva over a plate of cartilage in the medial angle of the eye.

**nystagmus** Rapid involuntary movement of the eyeball.

**oliguria** Decreased urine production.

**opisthotonus** A generalized muscular spasm causing both head and tail to be raised and drawn towards each other.

**ornithosis** A disease of birds, particularly the parrot family. It is also known as psittacosis.

**ossification** The formation of bone.

**osteophytes** Small outgrowths of bone, often seen on radiographs.

**otitis externa** Inflammation of the external part of the ear canal, i.e. above the ear drum.

**paediatrics** The branch of medicine concerned with young animals (more strictly with young children).

**panleukopenia** A decrease in the total number of all types of white blood cells (leukocytes). This is seen during the disease of feline infectious enteritis which is then also known as feline panleukopenia.

**pannus** An infiltration of the cornea of the eye with blood vessels.

**paraplegia** Paralysis, with loss of sensation, of the posterior or caudal part of the body.

**parasitism** An association between two different living organisms in which the smaller (the parasite) lives upon or within the larger (or host) and receives food and/or shelter.

**parturition** The act of giving birth.

**pathogen** A disease-producing micro-organism.

**pericardium** The double membrane that surrounds and encloses the heart.

**peristalsis** A wave of muscle contraction as occurs in the intestine, oesophagus and ureters.

**peritonitis** Inflammation of the peritoneum, the serous membrane that lines the abdominal cavity and covers the abdominal organs.

**petachiae** Small pinpoint haemorrhages; a feature of certain infectious diseases.

**pleurisy** Inflammation of the pleura, the serous membrane that lines the thoracic cavity and covers the lung surface.

**portal vein** A large vein which carries blood from the intestines, stomach, spleen and pancreas to the liver.

**prodromal** Preceding, premonitory. As in the prodomal stage of rabies,—a stage between the appearance of abnormal behaviour and the onset of diagnostic signs.

**prognosis** A forecast of the outcome of a disease or condition.

**prophylaxis** (adjective prophylactic) Measures taken to prevent a disease.

**puberty** The age at which the reproductive organs

become functional and mating can be followed by the development of the young.

**pyaemia**   The generalized circulation of pus-producing bacteria in the circulating blood which will result in multiple abscesses forming.

**pyelonephritis**   An inflammation of the kidney tissue where the renal pelvis is most affected by bacteria.

**pyometra**   A pus producing inflammation of the uterus.

**pyrexia**   The elevation of body temperature associated with fever conditions (though often used to indicate any abnormal increase in body temperature).

**quadriplegia**   Paralysis of all four limbs.

**ranula**   A cyst, usually occurring beneath the tongue, due to distension of a salivary duct.

**retina**   The innermost coat of the eyeball containing the light-sensitive nerve-endings.

**rhinitis**   An inflammation of the mucous membrane lining the nasal cavities.

**ringworm**   A contagious skin disease due to a parasitic fungus.

**roundworms**   Worms that are found in the intestine of animals; this word usually refers to the ascarid worms of dogs and other domestic pets.

**sarcoma**   A malignant tumour of connective tissue.

**scabies**   A skin disease of man caused by the human sarcoptic mange mite.

**sclera**   Known as the "white" of the eye. It is the outermost tough fibrous coat of the eyeball often only seen clearly in dogs when the eyelids are pulled open wide.

**sclerosis**   Hardening due to increased production of fibrous tissue, usually following chronic inflammation.

**septicaemia**   A condition arising as the result of the continuous invasion of the bloodstream by pathogenic organisms and their toxins.

**serum**   The liquid that separates from a blood clot as it contracts.

**sinusitis**   The inflammation of a sinus. The sinuses are air cavities in the skull.

**spondylitis**   Inflammation of a vertebra.

**sprain**   Tearing or over-stretching of the ligaments surrounding a joint.

**stenosis**   Narrowing or contraction of a channel or opening.

**stercoraceous vomiting**   Vomiting of material which is, or resembles, faeces.

**strain**   The tearing or overstretching of a muscle.

**superficial**   Means on or near the surface, usually a tissue or organ surface.

**suppuration**   The production of pus as seen in an infected wound.

**symbiosis**   An association between parasite and host, whether harmful or beneficial; where both derive some advantage from the association, it is known as "mutualism".

**symphysis**   The line of fusion between two bones which were at one time separated.

**syndrome**   A set of clinical signs which occurs often to suggest one particular disorder.

**systole**   The time when the heart muscle contracts.

**tenesmus**   Straining, particularly if painful and ineffective.

**tetanus**   An infectious disease with muscle spasm caused by the toxin of a bacterium *Clostridium tetani*.

**tetany**   A state of the body where violent repeated muscle spasms occur (twitching), usually due to a low calcium level in the blood.

**thrombus**   A blood clot occurring in a blood vessel or one of the chambers of the heart.

**toxaemia**   A condition in which the blood is "poisoned" by the absorption of bacterial toxins.

**trachea**   The tube connecting the larynx to the bronchii that is commonly known as the "windpipe".

**transudate**   A fluid which passes through a membrane.

**trauma**   Wounding or injury.

**ulcer**   Erosion of a surface e.g. of the tongue or stomach lining.

**ulceration**   A condition where there is a break in the surface of the skin or mucous membrane. Often seen in the mouth or ear.

**umbilicus**   The point of connection on the abdominal wall of the umbilical cord.

**uraemia**   An abnormally high level of urea in the blood. The term includes the syndrome of vomiting, listlessness and loss of appetite that arises from the high level of urea and other protein breakdown products in the blood.

**urethritis**   Inflammation of the urethra.

**urolithiasis**   The formation of urinary calculi.

**urticaria**   A skin condition characterized by weals and severe itching.

**vasoconstrictor**   A drug which produces constriction of blood vessels.

**vesicle**   A blister or a small sac containing fluid.

**villus**   A minute finger-shaped projection on the surface of the intestine; it forms the specialized absorption areas of the alimentary canal.

**virulence**   The capacity of a micro-organism to produce disease, this reflects its ability to invade and become established within the host and its ability to produce toxins.

**viscera**   The organs of the three body cavities; usually used when referring to the contents of the abdomen.

**vitamin**   An organic compound essential to normal tissue metabolism; required in very small quantities.

**zoonosis** A disease that can be transmitted from animal to man.

**zygote** A single cell that results from the fusion of male and female gametes (sperm and egg).

**Other Descriptive Terms**
See list p. 682.

**Common Prefixes, Suffixes**
See list p. 681.

This list of words commonly used in veterinary work is provided to help the reader understand the text but it does not comprise all the technical terms used in the fourth edition. It may also prove of value as revision notes for the trainee nurse and the list and that on p. 412–417 can be used for self-testing by candidates for the RANA examinations. The list can be added to by the reader as the various chapters of the book are read according to individual needs.

# Common Prefixes and Suffixes and Other Descriptive Terms

Certain syllables are commonly used as the beginning or ending of medical terms, in many cases being added to a word stem which denotes a particular organ or part of the body. The meaning of some of the most frequently encountered prefixes and suffixes are given in this section.

### Prefixes

*a-* or *an-*  lack of (e.g. anorexia, loss of appetite; analgesia, absence of pain; ataxia, lack of muscular co-ordination; avitaminosis, vitamin deficiency).

*chole-*  bile (e.g. cholestasis, stoppage of bile flow).

*dys-*  difficult or defective (e.g. dystocia, difficulty in giving birth; dysphagia, difficulty in swallowing).

*endo-*  within (e.g. endometrium, the mucous membrane lining of the uterus; endoscope, an instrument for examining the interior of a hollow organ or cavity; endocrine, secreting internally—relating to hormones).

*ex-*  out, away from (e.g. excision, cutting out; exostosis, a bony outgrowth).

*haema-* or *haemo-*  blood (e.g. haemolysis, the breakdown of red blood cells; haematemesis, the vomiting of blood).

*hydro-*  water (e.g. hydrothorax, fluid in the thoracic cavity; hydrocephalus, an accumulation of fluid in the brain).

*peri-*  around (e.g. pericardium, the sac surrounding the heart; periosteum, the specialized connective tissue covering bones).

*poly-*  many or much e.g. polydipsia, increased thirst; polyarthritis, inflammation in several joints (5 or more).

*pyo-*  pus (e.g. pyometra, pus in the uterus; pyotho-rax, pus in the thoracic cavity; pyuria, pus—or white blood cells—in the urine).

*steat-*  fat (e.g. steatorrhoea, excessive loss of undigested fat in the faeces; steatitis, inflammation of adipose tissue).

*sub-*  beneath (e.g. sublingual, beneath the tongue; subcutaneous, beneath the skin) *OR* partial or moderate (e.g. subluxation, a partial dislocation; subacute, moderately acute).

*uro-*  urine or urination (e.g. urolith, urinary calculus or stone; urochrome, the yellow pigment in urine).

### Prefixes which are sometimes confused are:

*hyper-*  above or excessive (e.g. hyperactive, excessively active; hypercalcaemia, an abnormally high level of calcium in the blood).

*hypo-*  beneath or deficient (e.g. hypodermic, beneath the skin; hypothyroidism, decreased activity of the thyroid gland).

*inter-*  between (e.g. intercostal, between the ribs; interdigital, between the digits (toes)).

*intra-*  within (e.g. intravenous, inside a vein; intra-abdominal, within the abdomen).

*super-*  usually meaning excessive though occasionally meaning above (e.g. supernumerary digits, more than the normal number of toes).

*supra-*  above (e.g. supraorbital, above the orbit).

### Suffixes

*-aemia*  blood (e.g. anaemia, lack of blood; septicaemia, bacteria and their toxins in the blood;

uraemia, accumulation of urea in the blood and also the clinical signs that develop as a result). Used with hypo- and hyper- to indicate the abnormal levels of various blood constituents (e.g. hypoproteinaemia, abnormally low level of protein in the blood; hyperglycaemia, abnormally high level of glucose in the blood).

*-ectomy*   surgical removal (excision) of part of the body (e.g. tonsillectomy, cutting out one or both tonsils; gastrectomy, excising, all or part of, the stomach).

*-graphy*   writing or recording. Often refers to radiography of a part of the body (e.g. urography, radiography of the urinary tract). But preceded by electro- indicates the recording of electrical signals from part of the body (e.g. electrocardiography (ECG), from the heart; electroencephalography (EEG), from the brain).

*-itis*   inflammation, of a part of the body denoted by the word stem (e.g. gastritis, inflammation of the stomach; dermatitis, of the skin; nephritis, of the kidney; arthritis of a joint).
**But note** pruritus (meaning itching) ends in -itus not -itis.

*-logy*   science or study of (e.g. pathology, the study of disease—especially changes in structure and function; dermatology, the study of skin diseases).

*-oma*   a swelling—in almost all cases a tumour (neoplasm) of a type of tissue, or a part of the body, denoted by the word stem (e.g. adenoma, a benign tumour of epithelial tissue; carcinoma, a malignant tumour of epithelial tissue; lipoma, a benign tumour of fat; lymphosarcoma, a malignant tumour of lymphoid tissue).
**But note** haematoma, a swelling containing blood, and hygroma, a fluid-filled swelling.

*-osis*   denotes a particular specific disease process (e.g. nephrosis, degeneration of the renal tubules). It may be associated with some abnormal increase (e.g. fibrosis, increased formation of fibrous tissue; acidosis, an accumulation of acid in the body).

*-pathy*   general term for *any* disease condition of a part of the body denoted by the word stem (e.g. enteropathy, an intestinal disease; myopathy, a muscular disease).

*-phagia*   eating (e.g. coprophagia, eating faeces; polyphagia, increased appetite).

*-plasia*   development (e.g. aplasia, failure to develop; dysplasia, abnormal development; hypoplasia, underdevelopment; hyperplasia, overdevelopment).

*-pnoea*   breathing (e.g. dyspnoea, difficulty in breathing; hyperpnoea, abnormally deep and rapid breathing).

*-rrhoea*   increased flow or discharge (e.g. seborrhoea, excessive secretion of sebum; diarrhoea, frequent discharge (and/or increased liquidity) of the faeces).

*-rrhage* or *-rrhagia*   excessive flow (e.g. haemorrhage, bleeding; rhinorrhagia, nose-bleed).

*-scopy*   examination of a part of the body, usually inspection of the interior of a hollow organ or cavity with an endoscope (e.g. bronchoscopy, examination of the bronchi; proctoscopy, of the rectum).

*-tomy*   cutting (incising) part of the body (e.g. laparotomy, cutting through the abdominal wall—usually to explore the abdominal cavity; cystotomy, incision of the bladder).

*-uria*   urine or urination (e.g. haematuria, red blood cells in the urine; bilirubinuria, bilirubin in the urine; polyuria, increased production of urine; stranguria, slow and painful urination).
**But note:** urea (the substance found in blood and urine) ends in -ea not -ia.

## Other Descriptive Terms

### Disease conditions may be referred to as:

*acute*   a condition of relatively sudden onset and lasting a short time, in which the signs are severe.

*chronic*   a condition present for a long time. Usually of slower onset with less pronounced signs.

Less commonly used are the descriptive terms:

*peracute*   a condition that is extremely acute, with very sudden onset and signs of great severity.

*subacute*   a condition that is moderately acute, i.e. intermediate between acute and chronic.

*congenital*   one that is present at birth. It may be inherited or the result of some influence during pregnancy or injury in the birth process.

*inherited*   or genetic or hereditary; one that arises from, or is predisposed to by, the genetic constitution of that individual

*acquired*   one that develops due to external factors such as infection or trauma (i.e. is not inherited). Usually it arises after birth.

*primary*   a condition which precedes another *or* which arises from changes occurring solely within the part of the body affected, rather than resulting from changes elsewhere (e.g. primary hypothyroidism which is due to changes occurring in the thyroid gland itself).

*secondary*   a condition that occurs as the result of another (e.g. a secondary bacterial pneumonia following infection with canine distemper virus, *or* renal secondary hyperparathyroidism in which changes in the parathyroid glands result from changes in the kidneys).

*Note* (1) Some signs may also be termed primary or secondary when the appearance of the first is linked to the appearance of the second (e.g. primary polyuria and secondary polydipsia).

(2) Tumours (neoplasms) may also be termed primary (the initial tumour growth) and secondary (arising from a group of cells that have become detached from the primary tumour and carried in the blood or lymph streams to another site. A secondary tumour is also known as a metastasis).

# Author Index

* Denotes joint authorship.

# Subject Index

References in **bold** type are to complete sections of more important references.